PUBLIC HEALTH AND THE LAW

Issues and Trends

Edited by
L. Lynn Hogue, Ph.D., J.D.
Assistant Professor of Law
School of Law
University of Arkansas at Little Rock
Little Rock, Arkansas

AN ASPEN PUBLICATION®
Aspen Systems Corporation
Rockville, Maryland
London
1980

Library of Congress Cataloging in Publication Data
Main entry under title:

Public health and the law.

Includes bibliographical references and index.

1. Public health laws—United States—Addresses,
essays, lectures. 2. Medical care—Law and legislation—
United States—Addresses, essays, lectures. I. Hogue,
L. Lynn.
KF3775.A75P8   344.73'04   80-15041
ISBN:0-89443-289-3

Copyright © 1980 by Aspen Systems Corporation

Library of Congress Catalog Card Number: 80-15041
ISBN: 0-89443-289-3

Printed in the United States of America

1 2 3 4 5

To my parents,
Benton and Maxine Otey Hogue,
and my wife,
Dr. Carol Rowland Hogue,
whose dedication to epidemiology and public health
inspired me to investigate the
legal dimensions of this important field.

CONTENTS

CONTRIBUTORS X

ANNETTE K. ALTSCHULER, M.S.W.
Consultant
Philadelphia, Pennsylvania

DAN E. BEAUCHAMP, PH.D.
Department of Health Administration
School of Public Health
University of North Carolina at Chapel Hill
Chapel Hill, North Carolina

JAMES F. BLUMSTEIN, LL.B.
School of Law
Vanderbilt University
Nashville, Tennessee

IRENE BUTTER, PH.D.
Department of Hospital Administration
School of Public Health
University of Michigan at Ann Arbor
Ann Arbor, Michigan

ROBERT S. CATZ, J.D., LL.M.
Cleveland-Marshall College of Law
Cleveland State University
Cleveland, Ohio

SUSAN M. CHALKER, J.D.
Civil Division
U.S. Department of Justice
Washington, D.C.

HARRIS S. COHEN, PH.D.
U.S. Department of Health, Education and
Welfare
Rockville, Maryland

WILLIAM J. CURRAN, J.D., LL.M., S.M.
HYGIENE
Harvard Medical School and School of Public
Health
Cambridge, Massachusetts

WINSTON J. DEAN, J.D., M.P.H.
U.S. Department of Health, Education and
Welfare
Rockville, Maryland

ROBERT C. DERBYSHIRE, M.D.
Santa Fe, New Mexico

DAVID D. DONIGER, J.D., M.C.P.
Staff Attorney
Natural Resources Defense Council
Washington, D.C.

JONATHAN E. FIELDING, M.D., M.P.H.
Los Angeles, California

WARREN GREENBERG, PH.D.
Center for Metropolitan Planning and
Research
The John Hopkins University
Baltimore, Maryland

LAWRENCE G. GOLDBERG, PH.D.
Department of Economics
New York University
New York, New York

CLARK C. HAVIGHURST, J.D.
School of Law
Duke University
Durham, North Carolina

L. LYNN HOGUE, J.D., PH.D.
School of Law
University of Arkansas at Little Rock
Little Rock, Arkansas

RONALD P. KAPLAN, J.D.
Attorney
Sheppard, Mullin, Richter, & Hampton
Los Angeles, California

STEPHEN J. MORSE, J.D., PH.D.
University of Southern California Law Center
Los Angeles, California

GEORGE B. MOSELEY, III, J.D., M.B.A.
Attorney and Lecturer
Harvard Law School
Cambridge, Massachusetts

RICHARD A. MUELLER, J.D.
Attorney
Shepherd, Sandberg and Phoenix
St. Louis, Missouri

G. KEITH PHOENIX, J.D.
Attorney
Shepherd, Sandberg & Phoenix
St. Louis, Missouri

MARILYN G. ROSE, LL.B.
Staff Attorney
Center for Law and Social Policy
Washington, D.C.

JEFFREY B. SCHWARTZ, J.D., M.B.A.
Attorney
Berriman & Schwartz
King of Prussia, Pennsylvania

SIDNEY A. SHAPIRO, J.D.
School of Law
University of Kansas
Lawrence, Kansas

FRANK A. SLOAN, PH.D.
Department of Economics
Vanderbilt University
Nashville, Tennessee

REBECCA G. SWEET
Ann Arbor, Michigan

LAURENCE R. TANCREDI, J.D., M.D.
Department of Psychiatry
Yale University
New Haven, Connecticut

CYRIL H. WECHT, J.D., M.D.
Allegheny County Commissioner
Pittsburgh, Pennsylvania

STEPHEN M. WEINER, LL.B.
School of Law
Boston University
Boston, Massachusetts

PREFACE

This anthology of articles and cases on public health and the law was developed to meet the need for a useful collection of materials for courses on the legal aspects of health care administration, hospitals, and public health. The book covers six significant areas of interaction between law and the health care delivery system: economic and regulatory concerns; law and the administration of health care; the role of law in protecting the public's health; health and the role of law and ethics in channeling behavior; the interaction of ethics and law as related to health; and the regulation of public health research. It is intended to serve the needs of a broad readership, including students in health care and health sciences administration programs, law schools, and medical schools. It is hoped that the collection will also meet the needs of professionals and other individuals interested in the area who will turn to it for a survey of major topics in the law of public health. A special section on "Issues for Consideration and Suggestions for Further Reading" is included at the end of each chapter to foster student discussion and inquiry and serve, together with the authorities cited in the articles, as a beginning point for the development of papers for courses in which this is appropriate. I anticipate that these suggestions will be liberally augmented with ones developed from the interests of individual instructors.

A NOTE ON LOCATING AND UTILIZING LEGAL SOURCE MATERIALS

The sources cited in this collection will be available in most law libraries. They are of five principal types: cases, statutes, administrative regulations, books or treatises, and periodicals.

Legal citation generally follows a simple format: volume number, name or title of the work, page number on which the particular item begins, and date in parenthesis. Cases are generally cited by the name of the litigant parties, or in some instances the subject matter of the dispute, followed by the name of the reporter (volume or set of volumes in which the case is printed or reported) or reporters (if reproduced in more than one place) in which the case is found, the name of the court and jurisdiction deciding the case in the form it is reported, and the date of decision. Statutes are usually cited by section (§) in the appropriate code or codification (a collection of laws—whether state or federal—arranged by subject), and the date of publication of the volume. Federal administrative regulations are principally found in the *Federal Register* (Fed. Reg.) or its codification the *Code of Federal Regulations* (C.F.R.). Books are generally cited by author's first initial and last name, together with the book's title, date of publication, and the page referred to. Periodicals, particularly law journals and law reviews, are cited by the author's last name only, title, the periodical's name, page (the first page of the article only if the reference is to the entire article), and date. Generally the volume number precedes the name of the reporter, book, or periodical, and the page, section, or paragraph (¶) number follows.

The subject of legal citation is, of course, far more complex and refined than this cursory survey suggests. The reference librarian at the law library will be invaluable in assisting with specific inquiries. Citations herein generally conform to the accepted standard for legal writing, although some liberty has been taken when necessary to assure clarity as many readers will not be familiar with legal citation. Abbreviations are minimal. No effort has been made to alter or renumber citations in articles included in this book that follow different citation or footnoting formats.

Special acknowledgments go to the journals listed below for permission to reprint articles:

American Journal of Law and Medicine; Clearinghouse Review; Duke Law Journal; Ecology Law Quarterly; Inquiry; Journal of Health Politics, Policy and Law; Law & Liberty; MMFQ/Health & Society; Northwestern University Law Review; St. Louis University Law Journal; Southern California Law Review; UALR Law Journal; Utah Law Review.

L. Lynn Hogue
Little Rock, Arkansas
July 1980

CHAPTER 1

THE REGULATION OF HEALTH CARE DELIVERY: ECONOMIC ISSUES

OVERVIEW

The economic regulation of the health care industry uniquely fuses law and policy issues. Increased public awareness of the rising proportion that medical and health-related expenditures represent in the Gross National Product has stimulated interest in a variety of measures designed to reduce health costs. Some efforts have been voluntary, but most at some level have involved the coercive power of the law to assist in the attainment of their objectives.

Health care in America has long been subject to the economic forces of market conditions. Writers generally concede that the ability of health providers to respond to market demands has been largely preempted by the combined roles of reduced market entry by new providers (restricted medical school enrollment,[1] licensure and specialty certification rules, and controls on new professionals). Likewise, traditional consumer checks on prices in the health marketplace are absent because of the importance of third party payment through, for example, medical insurance that pays for services, drugs, and equipment not purchased *by* the consumer but *for* him by the provider who is thought largely immune from traditional market constraints since health insurance or transfer payments to the needy simply disseminate the costs broadly on all insureds or taxpayers and fail to produce a pressure sufficient to check rising prices.

The articles presented in this chapter explore the economic issues of health care from a variety of perspectives. Beauchamp's thesis is that the egalitarian ethic of social justice, not market justice—entitlement based on "individual efforts, actions or abilities"—should govern the provision of public health.[2] This ethical viewpoint toward health and the right of each person to enjoy it contrasts with the approaches of the remaining authors, who deal in varying ways with the market aspects of the health care system and consider techniques for rectifying its malfunction.

Blumstein and Sloan suggest that replacing market forces with regulation will correct the imbalance between consumer and provider. This is the theory of certificate-of-need requirements, for example, that restrict the number of hospital beds or technological innovations permitted in a given area or for a given population base. Another approach represented here in the writings of Havighurst would seek to foster the responsiveness of the health care industry to market forces and attenuate the role of regulation.

Two of the articles explore the effects of cost-control innovations from a historical perspective. Goldberg and Greenberg report on the success of a cost-control program attempted by Oregon health insurers in the 1930s and 1940s. The final article in this chapter, by Curran and Moseley, examines the malpractice experience of one of the major proposals for reintroducing market forces into the health care system—the health maintenance organization or HMO. HMOs are health care providers that contract with patients to provide health care for a fixed price.[3] HMOs differ from insurance schemes in that, rather than paying physicians or hospitals to provide services to those covered by the plan, the HMO provides them directly. Cost effectiveness results because the HMO's prices are fixed and therefore the HMO has an incentive to detect illness as early as possible and to treat it in the least costly manner consistent with good medical practice. The savings from keeping patients healthy at a lower cost represent the HMO's profit, which it retains. HMOs compete, of course, with private physicians and hospitals for patients and also among themselves. Poor patients may be enrolled into some plans under federally mandated open enrollment periods.[4]

NOTES

1. Kessel, "The A.M.A. and the Supply of Physicians," 35 *Law & Contemporary Problems* 267 (1970).

2. A fundamental characteristic differentiating "public health" from other health and medical disciplines is its corporate focus or emphasis on the group rather than the individual.

In scientific public health, we no longer treat the individual—the segment of the community—but the total body politic—mental, physical, social, and economic. We no longer treat individuals with communicable diseases, but we prevent, control, or eradicate the disease in the body politic. The total patient is our responsibility [i.e. the community], and not the individuals who are a part of it. McGavran, "What Is Public Health?" 44 *Canadian J. Pub. Health,* 441, 444 (1953).

3. [T]he HMO itself and/or participating physicians accept contracted responsibility to assure the delivery of a stated range of health services, including at least ambulatory and in-hospital care to a voluntarily enrolled population in exchange for an advance capitation payment (and assumes at least part of the financial risk and/or shares in the surplus for the delivery of ambulatory and hospital services).
R. Wetherille & J. Nordby, *A Census of HMOs: October 1974,* 1–2 (1974) (Interstudy).

4. See 42 U.S.C.A. §300e (c)(3)(A) and (B), but note a waiver of the requirement is available where compliance would endanger the HMO's economic viability, 42 U.S.C.A. §300e(d)(1)(A) and (B). A thorough treatment of the prospects of the needy for benefiting from HMOs is presented in Schneider and Stern, "Health Maintenance Organizations and the Poor: Problems and Prospects," 70 *Nw. U.L. Rev.* 90 (1975).

1.1 Public Health as Social Justice*

DAN E. BEAUCHAMP

Reprinted with permission of the Blue Cross Association, from *Inquiry*, Vol. XIII, No. 1 (March 1976), pp. 3–14. Copyright © 1976 by the Blue Cross Association. All rights reserved.

Anthony Downs[1] has observed that our most intractable public problems have two significant characteristics. First, they occur to a relative minority of our population (even though that minority may number millions of people). Second, they result in significant part from arrangements that are providing substantial benefits or advantages to a majority or to a powerful minority of citizens. Thus solving or minimizing these problems requires painful losses, the restructuring of society and the acceptance of new burdens by the most powerful and the most numerous on behalf of the least powerful or the least numerous. As Downs notes, this bleak reality has resulted in recent years in cycles of public attention to such problems as poverty, racial discrimination, poor housing, unemployment or the abandonment of the aged; however, this attention and interest rapidly wane when it becomes clear that solving these problems requires painful costs that the dominant interests in society are unwilling to pay. Our public ethics do not seem to fit our public problems.

It is not sufficiently appreciated that these same bleak realities plague attempts to protect the public's health. Automobile-related injury and death; tobacco, alcohol and other drug damage; the perils of the workplace; environmental

*This paper is a slightly revised version of a paper presented at the annual meeting of the American Public Health Association in Chicago, November 18, 1975, entitled, "Health Policy and the Politics of Prevention: Breaking the Ethical and Political Barriers to Public Health."

pollution; the inequitable and ineffective distribution of medical care services; the hazards of biomedicine—all of these threats inflict death and disability on a minority of our society at any given time. Further, minimizing or even significantly reducing the death and disability from these perils entails that the majority or powerful minorities accept new burdens or relinquish existing privileges that they presently enjoy. Typically, these new burdens or restrictions involve more stringent controls over these and other hazards of the world.

This somber reality suggests that our fundamental attention in public health policy and prevention should not be directed toward a search for new technology, but rather toward breaking existing ethical and political barriers to minimizing death and disability. This is not to say that technology will never again help avoid painful social and political adjustments.[2] Nonetheless, only the technological Pollyannas will ignore the mounting evidence that the critical barriers to protecting the public against death and disability are not the barriers to technological progress— indeed the evidence is that it is often technology itself that is our own worst enemy. The critical barrier to dramatic reductions in death and disability is a social ethic that unfairly protects the most numerous or the most powerful from the burdens of prevention.

This is the issue of justice. In the broadest sense, justice means that each person in society ought to receive his due and that the burdens and benefits of society should be fairly and equitably distributed.[3] But what criteria should be followed in allocating burdens and benefits: Merit, equality or need?[4] What end or goal in life should receive our highest priority: Life, liberty or the pursuit of happiness? The answer to these questions can be found in our prevailing theories or models of justice. These models of justice, roughly speaking, form the foundation of our politics and public policy in general, and our health policy (including our prevention policy) specifically. Here I am speaking of politics not as partisan politics but rather the more ancient and venerable meaning of the political as the search for the common good and the just society.

These methods of justice furnish a symbolic framework or blueprint with which to think about and react to the problems of the public, providing the basic rules to classify and categorize problems of society as to whether they necessitate public and collective protection, or whether individual responsibility should prevail. These models function as a sort of map or guide to the common world of members of society, making visible some conditions in society as public issues and concerns, and hiding, obscuring or concealing other conditions that might otherwise emerge as public issues or problems were a different map or model of justice in hand.

In the case of health, these models of justice form the basis for thinking about and reacting to the problems of disability and premature death in society. Thus, if public health policy requires that the majority or a powerful minority accept their fair share of the burdens of protecting a relative minority threatened with death or disability, we need to ask if our prevailing model of justice contemplates and legitimates such sacrifices.

MARKET-JUSTICE

The dominant model of justice in the American experience has been market-justice.[5] Under the norms of market-justice people are entitled only to those valued ends such as status, income, happiness, etc., that they have acquired by fair rules of entitlement, e.g., by their own individual efforts, actions or abilities. Market-justice emphasizes individual responsibility, minimal collective action and freedom from collective obligations except to respect other persons' fundamental rights.

While we have as a society compromised pure market-justice in many ways to protect the public's health, we are far from recognizing the principle that death and disability are collective problems and that all persons are entitled to health protection. Society does not recognize a general obligation to protect the individual against disease and injury. While society does prohibit individuals from causing direct harm to others, and has in many instances regulated clear public health hazards, the norm of market-justice is still dominant and the primary duty to avert disease and injury still rests with the individual. The individual is ultimately alone in his or her struggle against death.

Barriers to Protection

This individual isolation creates a powerful barrier to the goal of protecting all human life by magnifying the power of death, granting to death an almost supernatural reality.[6] Death has throughout history presented a basic problem to humankind,[7] but even in an advanced society with enormous biomedical technology, the individualism of market-justice tends to retain and exaggerate pessimistic and fatalistic attitudes toward death and injury. This fatalism leads to a sense of powerlessness, to the acceptance of risk as an essential element of life, to resignation in the face of calamity, and to a weakening of collective impulses to confront the problems of premature death and disability.

Perhaps the most direct way in which market-justice undermines our resolve to preserve and protect human life lies in the primary freedom this ethic extends to all individuals and groups to act with minimal obligations to protect the common good.[8] Despite the fact that this rule of self-interest predictably fails to protect adequately the safety of our workplaces, our modes of transportation, the physical environment, the commodities we consume, or the equitable and effective distribution of medical care, these failures have resulted so far in only half-hearted attempts at regulation and control. This response is explained in large part by the powerful sway market-justice holds over our imagination, granting fundamental freedom to all individuals to be left alone—even if the "individuals" in question are giant producer groups with enormous capacities to create great public harm through sheer inadvertence. Efforts for truly effective controls over these perils must constantly struggle against a prevailing ethical paradigm that defines as threats to fundamental freedoms attempts to assure that all groups—even powerful producer groups—accept their fair share of the burdens of prevention.

Market-justice is also the source of another major barrier to public health measures to minimize death and disability—the category of voluntary behavior. Market-justice forces a basic distinction between the harm caused by a factory polluting the atmosphere and the harm caused by the cigarette or alcohol industries, because in the latter case those that are harmed are perceived as engaged in "voluntary" behavior.[9] It is the radical individualism inherent in the market model that encourages attention to the individual's behavior and inattention to the social preconditions of that behavior. In the case of smoking, these preconditions include a powerful cigarette industry and accompanying social and cultural forces encouraging the practice of smoking. These social forces include norms sanctioning smoking as well as all forms of media, advertising, literature, movies, folklore, etc. Since the smoker is free in some ultimate sense to not smoke, the norms of market-justice force the conclusion that the individual voluntarily "chooses" to smoke; and we are prevented from taking strong collective action against the powerful structures encouraging this so-called voluntary behavior.

Yet another way in which the market ethic obstructs the possibilities for minimizing death and disability, and alibis the need for structural change, is through explanations for death and disability that "blame the victim."[10] Victim-blaming misdefines structural and collective problems of the entire society as individual problems, seeing these problems as caused by the behavioral failures or deficiencies of the victims. These behavioral explanations for public problems tend to protect the larger society and powerful interests from the burdens of collective action, and instead encourage attempts to change the "faulty" behavior of victims.

Market-justice is perhaps the major cause for our over-investment and over-confidence in curative medical services. It is not obvious that the rise of medical science and the physician, taken alone, should become fundamental obsta-cles to collective action to prevent death and injury. But the prejudice found in market-justice against collective action perverts these scientific advances into an unrealistic hope for "technological shortcuts"[11] to painful social change. Moreover, the great emphasis placed on individual achievement in market-justice has further diverted attention and interest away from primary prevention and collective action by dramatizing the role of the solitary physician-scientist, picturing him as our primary weapon and first line of defense against the threat of death and injury.

The prestige of medical care encouraged by market-justice prevents large-scale research to determine whether, in fact, our medical care technology actually brings about the result desired—a significant reduction in the damage and losses suffered from disease and injury. The model conceals questions about our pervasive use of drugs, our intense specialization, and our seemingly boundless commitment to biomedical technology. Instead, the market model of justice encourages us to see problems as due primarily to the failure of individual doctors and the quality of their care, rather than to recognize the possibility of failure from the structure of medical care itself.[12] Consequently, we seek to remedy problems by trying to change individual doctors through appeals to their ethical sensibilities, or by reshaping their education, or by creating new financial incentives.

Government Health Policy

The vast expansion of government in health policy over the past decades might seem to signal the demise of the market ethic for health. But it is important to remember that the preponderance of our public policy for health continues to define health care as a consumption good to be allocated primarily by private decisions and markets, and only interferes with this market with public policy to subsidize, supplement or extend the market system when private decisions result in sufficient imperfections or inequities to be of public concern. Medicare and Medicaid are examples. Other examples include subsidizing or stimulating the private sector through public support for research, education of professionals, limited areawide planning, and the construction of facilities. Even national health insurance is largely a public financing mechanism to subsidize private markets in the hope that curative health services will be more equitably distributed. None of these policies is likely to bring dramatic reductions in rates of death and disability.

Our current efforts to reform the so-called health system are little more than the use of public authority to perpetuate essentially private mechanisms for allocating curative health services. These reforms are paraded as evidence that the system is capable of functioning equitably. But, as Barthes[13] points out (in a different context), reform measures may merely serve to "inoculate" the larger society against the suspicion that it is the model itself (in our case, market-justice) that is at fault. In fact, the constant reform efforts designed to "save the system" may better be viewed as an attempt to expand the hegemony of the key actors in the present system—especially the medical care complex. As McKnight says, the medical care complex may need the hot air of reform if its ballooning empire is to continue to inflate.[14]

Public Health Measures

I have saved for last an important class of health policies—public health measures to protect the environment, the workplace, or the commodities we purchase and consume. Are these not signs that the American society is willing to accept collective action in the face of clear public health hazards?

I do not wish to minimize the importance of these advances to protect the public in many domains. But these separate reforms, taken alone, should be cautiously received. This is because each reform effort is perceived as an isolated exception to the norm of market-justice; the norm itself still stands. Consequently, the predictable career of such measures is to see enthusiasm for enforcement peak and wane. These public health measures are clear signs of hope. But as long as these actions are seen as merely minor exceptions to the rule of individual responsibility, the goals of public health will remain beyond our reach. What is required is for the public to see that protecting the public's health takes us beyond the norms of market-justice categorically, and necessitates a completely new health ethic.

I return to my original point: Market-justice is the primary roadblock to dramatic reductions in preventable injury and death. More than this, market-justice is a pervasive ideology protecting the most powerful or the most numerous from the burdens of collective action. If this be true, the central goal of public health should be ethical in nature: The challenging of market-justice as fatally deficient in protecting the health of the public. Further, public health should advocate a "counter-ethic" for protecting the public's health, one articulated in a different tradition of justice and one designed to give the highest priority in minimizing death and disability and to the protection of all human life against the hazards of this world.

SOCIAL JUSTICE

The fundamental critique of market-justice found in the Western liberal tradition is social justice. Under social justice all persons are entitled equally to key ends such as health protection or minimum standards of income. Further, unless collective burdens are accepted, powerful forces of environment, heredity or social structure will preclude a fair distribution of these ends.[15–17] While many forces influenced the development of public health, the historic dream of public health that preventable death and disability ought to be minimized is a dream of social justice.[18] Yet these egalitarian and social justice implications of the public health vision are either still not widely recognized or are conveniently ignored.

Seeing the public health vision as ultimately rooted in an egalitarian tradition that conflicts directly with the norms of market-justice is often glossed over and obscured by referring to public health as a general strategy to control the "environment." For example, Canada's "New Perspectives on the Health of Canadians,"[19] correctly notes that major reductions in death and disability cannot be expected from curative health services. Future progress will have to result from alterations in the "environment" and "lifestyle." But if we substitute the words "market-justice" for environment or lifestyle, "New Perspectives" becomes a very radical document indeed. Ideally, then, the public health ethic[20] is not simply an alternative to the market ethic for health—it is a fundamental critique of that ethic as it unjustly protects powerful interests from the burdens of prevention and as that ethic serves to legitimate a mindless and extravagant faith in the efficacy of medical care. In other words, the public health ethic is a *counter-ethic* to market-justice and the ethics of individualism as these are applied to the health problems of the public.

This view of public health is admittedly not widely accepted. Indeed, in recent times the mission of public health has been viewed by many as limited to that minority of health problems that cannot be solved by the market provision of medical care services and that necessitate organized community action.[21] It is interesting to speculate why many in the public health profession have come to accept this narrow view of public health—a view that is obviously influenced and shaped by the market model as it attempts to limit the burdens placed on powerful groups.[22]

Nonetheless, the broader view of public health set out here is logically and ethically justified if one accepts the vision of public health as being the protection of all human life. The central task of public health, then, is to complete its unfinished revolution: The elaboration of a health ethic adequate to protect and preserve all human life. This new ethic has several key implications which are referred to here as "principles"[23]: 1) Controlling the hazards of this world, 2) to prevent death and disability, 3) through organized collective action, 4) shared equally by all except where unequal burdens result in increased protection of everyone's health and especially potential victims of death and disability.

These ethical principles are not new to public health. To the contrary, making the ethical foundations of public health visible only serves to highlight the social justice influences at work behind pre-existing principles.

Controlling the Hazards

A key principle of the public health ethic is the focus on the identification and control of the hazards of this world rather than a focus on the behavioral defects of those individuals damaged by these hazards. Against this principle it is often argued that today the causes of death and disability are multiple and frequently behavioral in origin.[24] Further, since it is usually only a minority of the public that fails to protect itself against most known hazards, additional controls over these perilous sources would not seem to

be effective or just. We should look instead for the behavioral origins of most public health problems,[25] asking why some people expose themselves to known hazards or perils, or act in an unsafe or careless manner.

Public health should—at least ideally—be suspicious of behavioral paradigms for viewing public health problems since they tend to "blame the victim" and unfairly protect majorities and powerful interests from the burdens of prevention.[26] It is clear that behavioral models of public health problems are rooted in the tradition of market-justice, where the emphasis is upon individual ability and capacity, and individual success and failure.

Public health, ideally, should not be concerned with explaining the successes and failures of differing individuals (dispositional explanations)[27] in controlling the hazards of this world. Rather these failures should be seen as signs of still weak and ineffective controls or limits over those conditions, commodities, services, products or practices that are either hazardous for the health and safety of members of the public, or that are vital to protect the public's health.

Prevention

Like the other principles of public health, prevention is a logical consequence of the ethical goal of minimizing the numbers of persons suffering death and disability. The only known way to minimize these adverse events is to prevent the occurrence of damaging exchanges or exposures in the first place, or to seek to minimize damage when exposures cannot be controlled.

Prevention, then, is that set of priority rules for restructuring existing market rules in order to maximally protect the public. These rules seek to create policies and obligations to replace the norm of market-justice, where the latter permits specific conditions, commodities, services, products, activities or practices to pose a direct threat or hazard to the health and safety of members of the public, or where the market norm fails to allocate effectively and equitably those services (such as medical care) that are necessary to attend to disease at hand.

Thus, the familiar public health options:[28]

1. Creating rules to minimize exposure of the public to hazards (kinetic, chemical, ioniz-

ing, biological, etc.) so as to reduce the rates of hazardous exchanges.

2. Creating rules to strengthen the public against damage in the event damaging exchanges occur anyway, where such techniques (fluoridation, seat-belts, immunization) are feasible.

3. Creating rules to organize treatment resources in the community so as to minimize damage that does occur since we can rarely prevent all damage.

Collective Action

Another principle of the public health ethic is that the control of hazards cannot be achieved through voluntary mechanisms but must be undertaken by governmental or non-governmental agencies through planned, organized and collective action that is obligatory or nonvoluntary in nature. This is for two reasons.

The first is because market or voluntary action is typically inadequate for providing what are called public goods.[29] Public goods are those public policies (national defense, police and fire protection, or the protection of all persons against preventable death and disability) that are universal in their impacts and effects, affecting everyone equally. These kinds of goods cannot easily be withheld from those individuals in the community who choose not to support these services (this is typically called the "free rider" problem). Also, individual holdouts might plausibly reason that their small contribution might not prevent the public good from being offered.

The second reason why self-regarding individuals might refuse to voluntarily pay the costs of such public goods as public health policies is because these policies frequently require burdens that self-interest or self-protection might see as too stringent. For example, the minimization of rates of alcoholism in a community clearly seems to require norms or controls over the substance of alcohol that limit the use of this substance to levels that are far below what would be safe for individual drinkers.[30]

With these temptations for individual noncompliance, justice demands assurance that all persons share equally the costs of collective action through obligatory and sanctioned social and public policy.

Fair-Sharing of the Burdens

A final principle of the public health ethic is that all persons are equally responsible for sharing the burdens—as well as the benefits—of protection against death and disability, except where unequal burdens result in greater protection for every person and especially potential victims of death and disability.[31] In practice this means that policies to control the hazards of a given substance, service or commodity fall unequally (but still fairly) on those involved in the production, provision or consumption of the service, commodity or substance. The clear implication of this principle is that the automotive industry, the tobacco industry, the coal industry and the medical care industry—to mention only a few key groups—have an unequal responsibility to bear the costs of reducing death and disability since their actions have far greater impact than those of individual citizens.

DOING JUSTICE: BUILDING A NEW PUBLIC HEALTH

I have attempted to show the broad implications of a public health commitment to protect and preserve human life, setting out tentatively the logical consequences of that commitment in the form of some general principles. We need, however, to go beyond these broad principles and ask more specifically: What implications does this model have for doing public health and the public health profession?

The central implication of the view set out here is that doing public health should not be narrowly conceived as an instrumental or technical activity. Public health should be a way of doing justice, a way of asserting the value and priority of all human life. The primary aim of all public health activity should be the elaboration and adoption of a new ethical model or paradigm for protecting the public's health. This new ethical paradigm will necessitate a heightened consciousness of the manifold forces threatening human life, and will require thinking about and reacting to the problems of disability and premature death as primarily collective problems of the entire society.

Right-to-Health

What concrete steps can public health take to accomplish this dramatic shift? Perhaps the most important step that public health might take to overturn the application of market-justice to the category of health protection would be to centrally challenge the absence of a right to health. Historically, the way in which inequality in American society has been confronted is by asserting the need for additional rights beyond basic political freedoms. (By a right to health, I do not mean anything so limited as the current assertion of a right to payment for medical care services.) Public health should immediately lay plans for a national campaign for a new public entitlement—the right to full and equal protection for all persons against preventable disease and disability.

This new public commitment needs more than merely organizational and symbolic expression; ultimately, it needs fundamental statutory and perhaps even constitutional protection. I can think of nothing more helpful to the goal of challenging the application of market-justice to the domain of health than to see public health enter into a protracted and lengthy struggle to secure a Right-to-Health Amendment.[32] This campaign would in and of itself signal the failure of market-justice to protect the health of all the public. Once secured, this legislation could serve as the basic counterpoise to our numerous and countless policies sanctioning unreflecting growth, uncontrolled technology or unrelenting individualism. Such an amendment could enable public health in all of its activity to constantly, relentlessly, stubbornly, militantly confront and resist all efforts to dishonor the integrity of human life in the name of progress, convenience, security and prosperity, as well as assist public health in challenging the dubious stretching of the principle of personal freedom to protect every corner of social life.[33]

A second step on the path to a fundamental paradigm change is the work of constructing collective definitions of public health problems.[34] Creating and disseminating collective definitions of the problems of death and disability would clearly communicate that the origins of these fates plainly lie beyond merely individual factors (but, as always, some individual factors cannot be totally ignored), and are to be found in structural features of the society such as the rules that govern exposure to the hazards of this world. These new collective descriptions, as they create more accurate explanations of public health problems, would in and of themselves expose the weakness of the norm of individual responsibility and point to the need for collective solutions.

These new definitions of public health problems are especially needed to challenge the ultimately arbitrary distinction between voluntary and involuntary hazards, especially since the former category (recently termed "lifestyle") looms so large in terms of death and disease.[35] Under the current definition of the situation, more stringent controls over involuntary risks are acceptable (if still strenuously resisted by producer groups), while controls over voluntary risks (smoking, alcohol, recreational risks) are viewed as infringements of basic personal rights and freedoms.

These new definitions would reveal the collective and structural aspects of what are termed voluntary risks, challenging attempts to narrowly and persuasively limit public attention to the behavior of the smoker or the drinker, and exposing pervasive myths that "blame the victim."[36] These collective definitions and descriptions would focus attention on the industry behind these activities, asking whether powerful producer groups and supporting cultural and social norms are not primary factors encouraging individuals to accept unreasonable risks to life and limb, and whether these groups or norms constitute aggressive collective structures threatening human life.

A case in point: Under the present definition of the situation, alcoholism is mostly defined in individual terms, mainly in terms of the attributes of those persons who are "unable" to control their drinking. But I have shown elsewhere that this argument is both conceptually and empirically erroneous. Alcohol problems are collective problems that require more adequate controls over this important hazard.[37]

This is not to say that there are no important issues of liberty and freedom in these areas. It is rather to say that viewing the use of, for example, alcohol or cigarettes by millions of American adults as "voluntary" behavior, and somehow fundamentally different from other public health hazards, impoverishes the public health approach, tending (as Terris has suggested)[38] to divorce the behavior of the individual from its social base.

In building these collective redefinitions of health problems, however, public health must take care to do more than merely shed light on specific public health problems. The central problems remain the injustice of a market ethic that unfairly protects majorities and powerful interests from their fair share of the burdens of prevention, and of convincing the public that the task of protecting the public's health lies categorically beyond the norms of market-justice. This means that the function of each different redefinition of a specific problem must be to raise the common and recurrent issue of justice by exposing the aggressive and powerful structures implicated in all instances of preventable death and disability, and further to point to the necessity for collective measures to confront and resist these structures.

Political Struggle

Doing public health involves more than merely elaborating a new social ethic; doing public health involves the political process and the challenging of some very important and powerful interests in society. The public health model involves at its very center the commitment to a very controversial ethic—the radical commitment to protect and preserve human life. To realize and make visible this commitment means challenging the embedded and structured values—as well as sheer political power—of dominant interests. These interests will not yield their influence without struggle.

This political struggle for a *truly* public health policy crucially involves bringing the medical care complex under the control of a new public health ethic. The medical care industry, like other powerful groups, must bear its fair share of the burdens of minimizing death and disability. Of all the perils presently confronting the public health community, there is none greater than that of gradually limiting and diminishing its mission to that of public medical care. I am deeply concerned that national health insurance—and here I have the Kennedy plan in mind—will become a vehicle to be used by what Alford has labelled the "corporate rationalizers"[39] to further finance, extend, solidify and entrench the power of the medical care complex. The nation's leading medical care issue is not to expand the

medical care service market; the central issue is to control a powerful and expansionist medical care industry. Challenging medical dominance could go a long way toward reclaiming health as a public concern and an issue of social justice.

Challenging these centers of power in order to incarnate the priority of human life requires not only a new ethic but a supporting base of power. I believe that while professional prestige is an important attribute in the modern day public policy process, public health is ultimately better understood as a broad social movement. There is simply no way that we can hope to capture public health under a defining set of competences, skills and professional backgrounds. The political potential of public health goes beyond professionalism; at its very heart is advocacy of an explosive and radical ethic. Doing public health should be a ubiquitous, pervasive, common and routine activity accomplished in every public and private agency, at every level of government, among all peoples, and at every moment of our common history. Health policy is most decidedly not the sole preserve of physicians, schools of public health, health educators, consumer groups or any other special interest group; rather it is a fundamental concern of all human activity and a distinguishing sign of a just community. By stressing the pervasive character of public health and the problems of death and disability, the foundation for a broad social movement can be established.

At the same time, public health should always hold in mind that this power struggle is meant to be not only instrumental but also dialectical, informative and symbolic. The point of the struggle is not merely to assure that producer interests accept their fair share of the costs of minimizing death and disability, but also—and once again—to reveal through the process of confrontation and challenge the structured and collective nature of the problems of death and disability and the urgency for more adequate structures to protect all human life.

I also believe that the realism inherent in the public health ethic dictates that the foundation of all public health policy should be primarily (but not exclusively) national in locus. I simply disagree with the current tendency, rooted in misguided pluralism and market metaphors, to build from the bottom up. This current drift will, in my opinion, simply provide the medical care industry and its acolytes (to cite only one powerful group) with the tools necessary to further elaborate and extend its hegemony. Confronting organizations, interests, ideologies and alliances that are national and even international in scope with such limited resources seems hopelessly sentimental. We must always remember that the forces opposed to full protection of the public's health are fundamental and powerful, deeply rooted in our national character. We are unlikely to successfully oppose these forces with appeals or strategies more appropriate for an earlier and more provincial time.

Finally, the public health movement must cease being defensive about the wisdom or the necessity of collective action. One of the most interesting aspects of market-justice—and particularly its ideological thrusts—is that it makes collective or governmental activity seem unwise if not dangerous. Such rhetoric predictably ignores the influence of private power over the health and safety of every individual. Public health need not be oblivious to the very real concerns about a proliferating bureaucracy in the emergent welfare state. In point of fact, however, the preventive thrust of public health transcends the notion of the welfare or service state and its most recent variant, the human services society. Much as the ideals of service and welfare are improvements over the simple working of market-justice, the service society frequently functions to spread the costs of public problems among the entire public while permitting the interests, industries, or professions who might remedy or prevent many of these problems to operate with expanding power and autonomy.

CONCLUSION

The central thesis of this article is that public health is ultimately and essentially an ethical enterprise committed to the notion that all persons are entitled to protection against the hazards of this world and to the minimization of death and disability in society. I have tried to make the implications of this ethical vision manifest, especially as the public health ethic challenges and confronts the norms of market-justice.

I do not see these goals of public health as hopelessly unrealistic nor destructive of fundamental liberties. Public health may be an "alien ethic in a strange land."[40] Yet, if anything, the public health ethic is more faithful to the traditions of Judeao-Christian ethics than is market-justice.

The image of public health that I have drawn here does raise legitimate questions about what it is to be a professional, and legitimate questions about reasonable limits to restrictions on human liberty. These questions must be addressed more thoroughly than I have done here. Nonetheless, we must never pass over the chaos of preventable disease and disability in our society by simply celebrating the benefits of our prosperity and abundance, or our technological advances. What are these benefits worth if they have been purchased at the price of human lives?

Nothing written here should be construed as a per se attack on the market system. I have, rather, surfaced the moral and ethical norms of that system and argued that, whatever other benefits might accrue from those norms, they are woefully inadequate to assure full and equal protection of all human life.

The adoption of a new public health ethic and a new public health policy must and should occur within the context of a democratic polity. I agree with Terris[41] that the central task of the public health movement is to persuade society to accept these measures.

Finally, it is a peculiarity of the word freedom that its meaning has become so distorted and stretched as to lend itself as a defense against nearly every attempt to extend equal health protection to all persons. This is the ultimate irony. The idea of liberty should mean, above all else, the liberation of society from the injustice of preventable disability and early death. Instead, the concept of freedom has become a defense and protection of powerful vested interests, and the central issue is viewed as a choice between freedom on the one hand, and health and safety on the other. I am confident that ultimately the public will come to see that extending life and health to all persons will require some diminution of personal choices, but that such restrictions are not only fair and do not constitute abridgement of fundamental liberties, they are a basic sign and imprint of a just society and a guarantee of that most basic of all freedom—protection against man's most ancient foe.

REFERENCES AND NOTES

1. Downs, A. "The Issue-Attention Cycle and the Political Economy of Improving Our Environment,"

revised version of the Royer Lectures presented at the University of California at Berkeley, April 13–14, 1970.

2. Etzioni, A. and Remp, R. "Technological 'Shortcuts' to Social Change," *Science* 175:31–38 (1972).

3. Jonsen, A.R. and Hellegers, A.E. "Conceptual Foundations for an Ethics of Medical Care," in: Tancredi, L.R. (ed.) *Ethics of Health Care* (Washington, D.C.: National Academy of Sciences, 1974).

4. Outka, E. "Social Justice and Equal Access to Health Care," *The Journal of Religious Ethics* 2: 11–32 (1974).

5. Some might object strenuously to the marriage of the two terms "market" and "justice." One theory of the market holds that it is a blind hand that rewards without regard to merit or individual effort. For this point of view, see: Friedman, M. *Capitalism and Freedom* (Chicago: University of Chicago Press, 1962); and Hayek, F. *The Constitution of Liberty* (Chicago: University of Chicago Press, 1960). But Irving Kristol, in his "When Virtue Loses All Her Loveliness," [*The Public Interest* 21:3–15 (1970)], argues that this is a minority view; most accept the marriage of the market ideal and the merits of individual effort and performance. I agree with this point of view—which is to say I see the dominant model of justice in America as a merger of the notions of meritarian and market norms.

6. Marcuse, H. "The Ideology of Death," in: Feifel, H. *The Meaning of Death* (New York: McGraw-Hill, 1959).

7. Illich, I. "The Political Uses of Natural Death," *Hastings Center Studies* 2:3–20 (1974).

8. For excellent discussions of the notion of market "externalities," see: Hardin, G. *Exploring New Ethics for Survival* (Baltimore, Md.: Penguin Books, 1972); Mishan, E. *The Costs of Economic Growth* (New York: Praeger, 1967); and Kapp, W. *Social Costs of Business Enterprise,* 2d ed. (New York: Asia Publishing House, 1964).

9. Brotman, R. and Suffet, F. "The Concept of Prevention and Its Limitations," *The Annals of the American Academy of Political and Social Science* 417:53–65 (1975).

10. Ryan, W. *Blaming the Victim* (New York: Vintage Books, 1971). See Barry, P. "Individual Versus Community Orientation in the Prevention of Injuries," *Preventive Medicine* 4:45–56 (1975), for an excellent discussion of "victim-blaming" in the field of injury-control. Also, see Beauchamp, D. "Alcoholism As Blaming the Alcoholic," *The International Journal of Addictions* 11 (1) (1976); and "The Alcohol Alibi: Blaming Alcoholics," *Society* 12:12–17 (1975), for discussion of the process of victim-blaming in the area of alcoholism policy.

11. Etzioni and Remp, *op. cit.*

12. Freidson, E. *Professional Dominance* (Chicago: Aldine, 1971).

13. Barthes, R. *Mythologies* (New York: Hill and Wang, 1972).

14. McKnight, J. "The Medicalization of Politics," *Christian Century* 92:785–787 (1975).

15. Tawney, R. *Equality* (London: G. Allen and Unwin, 1964).

16. Hobhouse, L.T. *Liberalism* (New York: Oxford University Press, 1964).

17. Rawls, J. *A Theory of Justice* (Cambridge: Harvard University Press, 1971).

18. I am aware that I am passing too quickly over a very complex subject: The formative influences for public health. I am simply asserting that the dream of eliminating or minimizing preventable death and disability involves a radical commitment to the protection and preservation of human life and that this vision ultimately belongs to the tradition of social justice. Further, one can clearly find social justice influences in the classics of the public health literature. For example, see: Smith, S. *The City That Was* (Metuchen, N.J.: Scarecrow Reprint Corporation, 1973); and Winslow, C.-E.A. *The Life of Hermann Biggs, Physician and Statesman of the Public Health* (Philadelphia: Lea and Febiger, 1929).

There are several reasons why public health has seldom been treated as standing in the tradition of social justice. Public health usually entails public or collective goods (such as clean air and water supplies) where the question of distributive shares seems not important. However, for collective goods and in the case of death and disability, the key distributive questions are the *numbers* or *rates* of persons who suffer these fates, that no group or individual be unfairly or arbitrarily excluded from protection, and that the *burdens* of collective policies be fairly distributed. Writers in the tradition of social justice (such as Rawls) do not pay sufficient attention to the social justice implications of public or collective goods. This helps explain in part why many in the public health movement seldom saw themselves as involved in a drive for social justice—their work was defined as protection for the entire community (and often the entire community, rather than a minority, seem threatened in the age of acute infectious epidemics or in the drive for sanitary reform). Further, while there was opposition to even these reforms, the question of distributing the burdens of collective action did not arise so acutely as it does in the present period.

19. Government of Canada. *A New Perspective on the Health of Canadians* (Ottawa, Ontario, Canada: Ministry of National Health and Welfare, 1974).

20. By the "public health ethic" I mean several things: The assignment of the highest priority to the preservation of human life, the assurance that this protection is extended maximally (consistent with main-

taining basic political liberties: See Rawls, *op. cit., and* note 33), that no person or group should be arbitrarily excluded, and finally that all persons ought accept these burdens of preserving life as just.

21. Two examples of this point: A standard text in health administration, John Hanlon's *Public Health Administration and Practice* (St. Louis, Missouri: C.V. Mosby, 1974), does reference very broad definitions of public health but quickly settles down to discussing public health in terms of those various programs designed to deal with market failures or inadequacies. Nowhere does Hanlon seem to view the concept of public health as an ethical concept standing as a fundamental critique of the existing measures to protect human life. Second, a recent proposed policy statement on prevention for adoption by the American Public Health Association (*The Nation's Health*, October 1975), does give a very high priority to prevention but contains within it a major concession to the norm of market-justice—the category of voluntary or self-imposed risks and the treatment of this category as distinctively different from other public health hazards.

22. Beauchamp, D. "Public Health: Alien Ethic in a Strange Land?" *American Journal of Public Health* 65:1338–1339 (December 1975).

23. I hasten to add that I am not arguing that there are exactly four principles of the public health ethic. Actually, the four offered here can be easily collapsed to two—controls over the hazards of this world and the fair sharing of the burdens of these controls. However, the reason for expanding these two key principles is to draw out the character of the public health ethic as a counter-ethic or counter-paradigm to the market model, and to demonstrate that the public health ethic focuses on different aspects of the world, asserts different priorities and imposes different obligations than the market ethic.

24. Brotman and Suffet, *op. cit.*

25. Sade, R. "Medical Care As A Right: A Refutation," *The New England Journal of Medicine* 285:1288–1292 (1971).

26. Ryan, *op. cit.* See also: Terris, M. "A Social Policy for Health," *American Journal of Public Health* 58: 5–12 (1968).

27. See Brown, R. *Explanation in Social Science* (Chicago: Aldine, 1963) for an excellent discussion of the limitations of dispositional explanations in social science. Also, see Beauchamp, D. "Alcoholism as Blaming the Alcoholic," *op. cit.*, for a further discussion of the pitfalls of dispositional explanations in the specific area of alcohol policy.

28. For excellent discussions of the strategies of public health, see: Haddon, W., Jr. "Energy Damage and the Ten Countermeasure Strategies," *The Journal of Trauma* 13:321–331 (1973); Haddon, W., Jr. "The

Changing Approach to the Epidemiology, Prevention, and Amelioration of Trauma," *American Journal of Public Health* 58:1431–1438 (1968); and Terris, M. "Breaking the Barriers to Prevention," paper presented to the Annual Health Conference, New York Academy of Medicine, April 26, 1974.

29. Olson, M. *The Logic of Collective Action* (Cambridge: Harvard University Press, 1965).

30. Beauchamp, D. "Federal Alcohol Policy: Captive to an Industry and a Myth," *Christian Century* 92:788–791 (1975).

31. This principle is similar to Rawls' "difference principle." See Rawls, *op. cit.*

32. I must confess a certain ambivalence about the term "right to health." This expression is not only confused with a right to payment for medical care services, it suffers the further limitation of not conveying the full intent of the public health ethic which, at least as I see it, is to give the highest priority to life and to assure collective rules and arrangements that embody and incarnate that priority. The term "right to health" could easily be construed as something far less ambitious than these goals.

33. I am not unaware that I have not begun to clarify the issue of just how far a society can go in protecting life and limb without jeopardizing political liberty. I agree with Rawls, *op. cit.*, as to the priority of liberty. However, I tend to think of liberty in terms of specific constitutional guarantees (freedom of speech, religion, due process, etc.) rather than in the more extensive sense of a positive freedom to act as one chooses except where one's actions bring harm to others. Also, shedding light on this issue of the conflict between liberty and the protection of the public's health would help shed light on just what "minimizing" death and disability specifically entails. I am satisfied at this point however that the public health ethic would move us much further toward protecting all of the public's health, without relinquishing those basic liberties and freedoms that are the attributes of a just political community and without which the very notion of social justice itself would be in jeopardy.

34. Friedmann, J. *Retracking America: A Theory of Transactive Planning* (Garden City, New York: Doubleday Anchor Books, 1973).

35. See: *A New Perspective on the Health of Canadians, op. cit.*

36. Destroying these "myths" could be a major task of public health activity. See Ryan, *op. cit.*, for the best discussion of "victim-blaming" myths. See Beauchamp, "The Alcohol Alibi," *op. cit.*, for a foray against the "myth" of alcoholism. I am using myth here in the specific sense: The confusion and false definitions that arise when we discuss a *public* problem in an individual idiom. For a good discussion of the con-

cept of myths in general, see Ryle, G. *The Concept of Mind* (New York: Barnes and Noble, 1949).

37. Beauchamp, "The Alcohol Alibi," *op. cit.*

38. Terris, "A Social Policy For Health," *op. cit.*

39. Alford, R. "The Political Economy of Health Care: Dynamics Without Change," *Politics and Society* 2: 127–164 (1972).

40. Beauchamp, "Public Health: Alien Ethic in a Strange Land?" *op. cit.*

41. Terris, "A Social Policy For Health," *op. cit.*

1.2 Health Planning and Regulation through Certificate of Need: An Overview*

JAMES F. BLUMSTEIN and FRANK A. SLOAN

Reprinted with permission from 1978 *Utah Law Review* 3–23, 30–33. Copyright © 1978 by the *Utah Law Review*. All rights reserved.

Certificate-of-need laws have now been enacted in over two-thirds of the states.[1] An integral part of the local, state, and national health planning scheme, certificate-of-need statutes are intended to establish a review process by which the proliferation of health care facilities may be controlled. As an introduction to health planning and regulation through certificate-of-need laws, this Article will discuss the rationale for government health planning; the intent and effect of the National Health Planning and Resources Development Act of 1974; the 1974 Act in light of policy perspectives; the evaluation of certificate-of-need initiatives by the states; the effect of these initiatives; and the newly proposed Hospital Cost Containment Act.

I. WHY PLANNING?

In a nation whose institutions have relied on market mechanisms for making basic economic choices, governmental imposition of planning bears a burden of persuasion.[2] Justification for planning in the health sector is typically founded on two rationales. First, government intervention traditionally follows as a remedy for some market failure. The medical marketplace deviates in some significant ways from classical market assumptions,[3] and planning is often promoted as a replacement for the dysfunctional market. A second rationale is found in the economist's view of a "merit good."[4] This is basically an equity argument, that planning can help to achieve important health policy goals established by government.

Proponents of planning who stress efficiency objectives focus primarily on deviations from competitive market conditions as a rationale for government intervention.[5] One fundamental assumption in the competitive market model is that consumers are sufficiently knowledgeable and competent to make rational and informed choices about what, when, where, and why to buy.[6] Advocates of planning argue that in the medical sector, however, consumers lack the expertise necessary to make informed judgments.[7] As a result, they contend, patients must delegate much decision-making authority to physicians, who thereby become the primary determiners of patient demand. If one accepts this premise, it follows that the number of visits to the physician, the kinds of laboratory tests ordered, the decision to hospitalize and for how long, and even the use of surgical procedures are based largely on the judgment of physician-suppliers, not "sovereign" consumers.[8]

Another deviation from the competitive model results from the important role played by non-profit institutions in the medical care sector.[9] The profit motive encourages technical efficiency and low-cost production. The marketplace disciplines firms that become overly in-

*Work on this article was supported in part by the Vanderbilt Institute for Public Policy Studies and by Grant No. 7-R01-HS 02590 from the National Center for Health Services Research, United States Department of Health, Education, and Welfare.

efficient. Nonprofit producers, however, do not have the same pressures for efficient production nor the same incentives to adjust output in order to achieve higher profit.[10] This problem is exacerbated by the form of nearly complete[11] third-party payment that characterizes existing health insurance plans. Such a system of reimbursement provides few incentives for either the hospital or the physician to achieve greater efficiency, and inexorably leads to higher overall consumer costs.[12]

Indeed, the peculiar characteristics of the traditional physician-hospital and physician-patient relationships result in increased costs. Physicians generally cannot admit or treat patients at hospitals where they do not have staff privileges. By the same token, a major source of patients for hospitals is the roster of physicians who have staff privileges.[13] Consequently, hospitals have a strong incentive to compete for physicians' goodwill by accommodating their requests for new or improved facilities or equipment. The combination of nonprofit institutions and third-party payment seems to countenance a form of "quality imperative"[14] that leads to excessive expansion of facilities and to the purchase of specialized, expensive equipment, even if these are not fully justified by utilization projections.[15]

Although these defects[16] are widely recognized, not all agree that the solution is to impose rationality on the health "nonsystem" through a centralized bureaucratic system of controls. Some would suggest that attention be directed initially at remedying the imperfections in the market, rather than substituting a regulatory system for the market.[17] These marketeers call for the use of health education programs to improve patient knowledge; the erosion of entry barriers and restrictions on the substitution of inputs by modifying excessively rigid licensure rules; and the promotion of competition through advertising and the fostering of a pluralistic delivery system[18] comprised of alternative modes of health care delivery such as health maintenance organizations.[19]

Planning proponents reason that the defects, in a fundamental sense, are incurable through market-perfecting techniques and that if left on its own, the medical marketplace would perpetuate inefficiency, fail to curtail unnecessary duplication, and permit excessive cost escalation.[20] The National Health Planning and Resources Development Act of 1974,[21] signed into law on January 4, 1975, adopted the planners' strategy for remedying market failure. The Planning Act abandons the market and superimposes on the medical marketplace a "command-and-control"[22] bureaucratic regulatory apparatus.[23]

In addition to arguments based on efficiency in resource allocation, proponents justify planning as a tool for improving the distribution of services to so-called underserved areas, defined by location and income status.[24] The major goals of the Planning Act include achieving "equal access to quality health care at a reasonable cost"[25] and remedying the "maldistribution of health care facilities and manpower."[26] Indeed, the first priority listed in the Act is the "provision of primary care services for medically underserved populations."[27] . . . These are not efficiency (or allocative) targets; rather, they reflect politically determined substantive health policy objectives which conform to equitable principles of distributive justice.

The goal of achieving greater equity in access to medical care is perhaps the major energizing force underlying the health planning movement.[28] Distribution of income and other life chances is not equal. A significant segment of the population has been designated indigent and an even larger number medically indigent. Since the enactment of the Medicaid and Medicare legislation, the federal government has been committed to providing financial support for groups of eligible and needy recipients. The Planning Act similarly makes a commitment to provide care to those in underserved areas, especially in rural or economically depressed regions. Viewed abstractly, the market system takes the pattern of income distribution as given. To the extent that society determines that current resource distribution patterns are inequitable and that the resulting distribution of services is unfair, some mode of government intervention becomes necessary. Thus, a commitment to alter the distribution of medical care so as to include those currently receiving inadequate access to medical services necessitates some mode of government involvement. The financing mechanisms of Medicaid and Medicare have had a major effect on improving and equalizing access for underserved populations;[29] but because of what are perceived as structural problems in the market, proponents of planning conclude that the financing and taxation approaches of the

Medicaid and Medicare legislation are insufficient and that more direct techniques of resource redistribution are needed.[30]

Thus, health planning has two different though usually complementary purposes: improving the allocative efficiency of resources in the market and achieving specific outcome objectives in terms of delivery of health care to previously underserved populations. We now turn our attention to an analysis of the National Health Planning and Resources Development Act of 1974, focusing initially on its responses to criticisms of earlier health planning legislation, then describing its mechanisms and considering the extent to which it has sufficient tools to achieve its general goals.

II. ANALYSIS OF THE NATIONAL HEALTH PLANNING AND RESOURCES DEVELOPMENT ACT OF 1974

Critics have noted a number of deficiencies in earlier health planning laws[31] which Congress sought to remedy by enacting the National Health Planning and Resources Development Act of 1974.[32] In summary form, these criticisms included:

1. The absence of a definition of health planning.[33]
2. The absence of processes or procedures for planning.[34]
3. The absence of goals or criteria for success.[35]
4. The lack of sufficient powers of the planning agencies.[36]
5. The lack of adequate professional staff.[37]
6. Excessive dependence on local sources of funding.[38]

The Planning Act specifically focuses on the identified deficiencies of the earlier Comprehensive Health Planning and Public Health Services Amendments of 1966[39] (CHP legislation). While from the planners' perspective, some definite improvements have been made, many of the planners' hopes remain unrealized.

A. Definition of Health Planning

The statute requires that the Secretary of the Department of Health, Education, and Welfare (HEW) issue guidelines concerning national health planning policy. Section 1501(b)[40] of the Act explicitly requires that these guidelines include "[s]tandards respecting the appropriate supply, distribution, and organization of health resources,"[41] and a statement of national health planning goals which, to the maximum extent practicable, should be expressed in quantitative terms.[42] Moreover, section 1513(b)[43] establishes specific functions that will be performed by health systems agencies (HSAs), the new areawide planning bodies.[44]

B. Processes and Procedures for Planning

The 1974 Act establishes detailed processes and procedures for planning. The HSA . . . must develop a health systems plan (HSP). It is to include "a detailed statement of goals . . . describing a healthful environment and health systems in the area which, when developed, will assure that quality health services will be available and accessible in a manner which assures continuity of care, at reasonable costs, for all residents of the area."[45] These goals must be responsive to the area's unique needs and resources and must take into account and be consistent with the national guidelines for health planning policy, when issued by the Secretary of HEW, respecting the supply, distribution, and organization of health resources and services.[46] The Act requires a public hearing, with adequate notice,[47] to secure public comment on a proposed HSP.

In addition to the HSP, the HSA must establish and review annual implementation plans (AIPs), which describe objectives to achieve the goals of the HSP and identify priorities among the objectives. The Act specifies that priority must be given to those objectives that will "maximally improve the health of the residents of the area, as determined on the basis of the relation of the cost of attaining such objectives to their benefits."[48]

At the state level, the law requires the establishment of a health planning and development agency (SHPDA) . . . , which must prepare a *preliminary* state health plan, made up primarily from HSPs of the health systems agencies within the state.[49] It must also review on a periodic basis all the institutional health services being offered in the state, considering recommendations submitted by the HSAs.[50] The state agency must make public its findings[51] and must submit to the appropriate HSA a detailed statement of the reasons for any inconsistency between its action and the goals of the applicable HSP or the priorities of the applicable AIP.[52]

The Act also provides for the establishment of an advisory Statewide Health Coordinating Council (SHCC) . . . , which comments on the HSPs and AIPs of each HSA within the state and reports to the Secretary, with comments, for his review purposes.[53] Also, the SHCC prepares, reviews, and revises a state health plan which is to be made up of the HSPs of the HSAs within the state.[54] The Act provides for a public hearing on the proposal with notice and opportunity for interested persons to submit their views orally and in writing.[55] The Act's processes and procedures for planning establish a broad framework within which planning can proceed at the state and regional levels.

C. Specific Goals and Success Criteria

In contrast to the CHP legislation, the Planning Act establishes specific goals and success criteria. In the Act, Congress made explicit legislative findings of (1) a lack of uniformly effective methods of delivering health care,[56] (2) a maldistribution of health care facilities and manpower,[57] and (3) an increasing cost of health care,[58] none of which were being addressed in a comprehensive or rational manner. In addition to these findings, there is an explicit statement of national health priorities, emphasizing "[t]he provision of primary care services for medically underserved populations, especially those which are located in rural or economically depressed areas."[59] Encouraging the development of medical group practices and health maintenance organizations,[60] and "the training and increased utilization of physician assistants, especially nurse clinicians,"[61] are among other priorities established under section 1502[62] of the Act.

Each HSP must conform to the priorities established by the Act and to the health planning guidelines as they are promulgated by the Secretary.[63] In addition, the Secretary must establish performance standards that cover the structure, operation, and performance of the functions of each designated HSA and SHPDA.[64] These review criteria are spelled out in detail in section 1535(c); they include such factors as the adequacy of the HSP;[65] the structure, operation, and performance of the functions of the

agency;[66] the representativeness of the agency's governing body;[67] the appropriateness of the data assembled and the quality of the analysis of such data;[68] the professional credentials and competence of the staff of the agency;[69] the extent to which technical and financial assistance have been utilized effectively;[70] and the extent to which it can be shown that the health of the residents in the agency's area has been improved,[71] and that health care has been made more accessible and acceptable, with greater continuity and improved quality[72] without excessive increases in costs.[73] Thus, the Act purports to provide specific goals, priorities, and criteria for planning[74] (for example, cost-benefit analysis)[75] as well as specific performance standards by which the agencies created by the Act will be evaluated.

D. Increased Regulatory Authority

Unlike the CHP agencies, the state and areawide planning agencies under the 1974 Act have some regulatory as well as planning functions and powers. Specifically, an HSA has the power to review and approve or disapprove a proposed use of specified federal funds within its health service area.[76] The HSA also reviews and makes recommendations concerning the need for new institutional health services which a certificate-of-need applicant proposes to offer and develop within the HSA's health services area.[77] If the recommendations of an HSA regarding a certificate of need are not accepted, the statute and the regulations permit an HSA to press an administrative appeal.[78] In addition, an HSA is expected to review periodically all existing institutional health services offered in its area and to make recommendations to the SHPDA concerning the appropriateness of such services.[79] The HSA can recommend projects for the modernization, construction, and conversion of medical facilities that will achieve the planning and implementation objectives of the HSA. The HSA also designates priorities among such projects.[80] The HSA, however, has no authority under federal law to close existing hospitals or services.

At the state level, the SHCC must review and approve or disapprove any state plan and any state application for the receipt of funds under allotments made to the states under specified federal programs.[81] The SHPDA is charged with the extremely important regulatory function of administering a mandatory state certificate-of-need program.[82] Moreover, the SHPDA reviews all institutional health services being offered in the state and is expected to publish its findings concerning their appropriateness.[83] Thus, the health planning agencies under the new statute have considerably more regulatory authority than did the agencies under the CHP legislation.

E. HSA Staff

No HSA can have a professional staff of fewer than five persons.[84] The Act specifies that the staff must have expertise in at least four areas: (1) administration;[85] (2) the gathering and analysis of data;[86] (3) health planning;[87] and (4) development and use of health resources.[88] The law also requires that the functions of planning and development of health resources be conducted by staffs with skills appropriate to each function.[89] Moreover, the HSAs have express statutory authority to employ consultants and contract with individuals and entities for the provision of services.[90] These provisions for staff size and expertise, the authority to contract for consultant services, and the backup support provided by the Regional Health Planning Centers[91] and the National Health Planning Information Center[92] should allow the HSAs to improve the quality of health planning, at least to the extent that the state of the art and the existence of adequate data permit.

F. HSA Financing

Finally, the financing mechanisms under the Act provide HSAs with significantly more autonomy than earlier planning agencies had. HSAs are authorized funds for contracting with outside consultants to the extent that such expertise is necessary[93] and are empowered to provide technical assistance to other elements in the community.[94] These provisions are designed to allow an HSA to assume a more autonomous and professional stature and allow its influence as a source of technical assistance to be felt more pervasively in the medical community.

III. POLICY PERSPECTIVES ON THE ACT

The processes and procedures established in the Act provide a broad framework for state and regional planning. As HEW proceeds with promulgation of National Guidelines for health planning, the substantive criteria by which state and regional plans are developed will likely become further clarified.[95] Despite the greater specificity in planning processes and procedures, the planning agencies will undoubtedly be frustrated in seeking to fulfill their statutory mandate.[96]

First, as a mechanical matter, the government has been slow in promulgating regulations. The initial proposed health planning guidelines were not published until more than two and one-half years had elapsed, and were not finalized until more than three years after the Planning Act became law. Moreover, these guidelines are themselves modest initial steps in the development of comprehensive regulations in fulfillment of the statutory mandate.[97] They reflect HEW's perception that the designated issues of utilization of hospital resources "present important short-term opportunities for the containment of costs and the enhancement of the quality of care."[98] HEW's objective is to develop a "comprehensive statement of national health planning goals and resource standards" which "will provide health policy direction and guidance."[99] There is, however, a very real problem of securing consensus on such broad objectives, at least in a sufficiently specific manner so as to serve a useful planning function—a point recognized by HEW: "[T]he development of such a comprehensive statement will be a long-term, progressive process. In many cases, there is currently incomplete agreement respecting health goals and resource standards. Thus, as local and State health plans are extended and refined over many years, so will the National Guidelines."[100]

A second concern, acknowledged forthrightly by Dr. Julius B. Richmond, HEW Assistant Secretary for Health, under whose jurisdiction the planning guidelines are formulated, is that the state of the art of planning is rudimentary. In promulgating the initial proposed resource standards for nine categories of services and facilities, Dr. Richmond admitted "[t]he state of the art of establishing specific quantitative resource standards is still in its infancy."[101] Despite negative comments received during the period for commenting on the initial set of proposed planning guidelines, Dr. Richmond concluded there was sufficient justification to issue the proposed standards.[102] The concession that there is a large amount of guesswork and considerable room for arbitrariness—even on the initial, relatively straight-forward issues of institutional resources—suggests that local HSAs will be operating with considerable autonomy and flexibility, which the proposed regulations certainly guarantee.

In addition to the state of the art problems, there is a lack of an adequate data base on which to premise planning. An important function of HSAs will be the assembly of data to improve the foundation of knowledge about various health care regions.[103] In this regard, however, there is a lurking jurisdictional issue between HSAs and the federal planning apparatus on the one hand and Professional Standards Review Organizations (PSROs), the Medicare and Medicaid peer review agencies, on the other.[104] PSROs are charged with gathering data as part of their mission to establish appropriate ranges of treatment for specific episodes of illness. The composition and constituencies of HSAs and PSROs are very different, however, and the control of data seems to be viewed as a potential source of institutional self-aggrandizement.[105] The Planning Act contemplates cooperation between PSROs and HSAs,[106] but there is a serious question whether this type of mutual cooperation will be forthcoming.[107]

Apart from concerns with the logistics of the planning process, the analyst must wonder whether the tools of implementation, even including the much-heralded certificate-of-need authority, are adequate to achieve the Act's lofty objective—"equal access to quality health care at a reasonable cost." The national health priorities set forth in the Act are an interesting melange of goals and means. . . . But one can hardly help pondering these priorities and asking whether an HSA or a SHPDA can realistically be expected to accomplish what it is mandated to achieve. The planning bodies, to be sure, have some negative authority through the certificate-of-need program and the power to approve or disapprove the proposed use of federal funds in specified programs. However, while the HSAs and the SHPDAs are empowered to make findings as to the appropriateness of institutional health services, and the HSAs are expected to make recommendations to the SHPDAs with respect to priorities for facility construction in their area, neither the HSAs nor the SHPDAs

have authority under federal law to decertify or to engage in outright entrepreneurial activity. In short, these planning agencies have veto power but do not have the ability to initiate or to act affirmatively.[108] HEW has recognized that "HSAs do not have all the means that may be necessary to achieve such targets."[109] Rather, the HSPs are seen as political, catalytic documents which "can and should be important occasions and vehicles for advancing public understanding of these issues."[110] This is action by coaxing and cajolery, not by the "teeth" planners typically seek.[111]

Perhaps an equally serious problem is the limited jurisdiction of the planning agencies. Under federal law, they have no direct control over pricing decisions of providers;[112] they have no regulatory authority over private third-party insurance companies, which control might help curtail excessive health spending;[113] they do not have any direct input on utilization or quality decisions for federal third-party payment programs (Medicare and Medicaid);[114] and they have little influence on the type of research that is funded, which ultimately produces a new piece of high-cost, high-style technology equipment for which a hospital seeks approval. Furthermore, the regionalized structure and the deference that HEW necessarily grants to HSAs encourages the same type of "more and better" attitude that PSROs are likely to have.[115] As the law is currently written and implemented, there is realistically no incentive for an HSA to make hard decisions that would deprive its constituents of a benefit when another region will capture the reward.[116] Furthermore, there is no incentive for an HSA to be "hard nosed" in its certificate-of-need decision making or its review of existing facilities when there is a real and often political cost in saying "no," and very little real harm will result from saying "yes." As in the case of PSROs, HSAs cannot capture and reallocate savings that stem from choosing to forgo increments of quality or access for their region.[117] Any diminution in quality or access, when costs are borne by the federal government, for example, results in net harm to the area and can only be justified by the most romantic resort to idealistic goals of general public responsibility.[118] In the crunch, however, when identifiable regional interests are being threatened, consideration for the overall general welfare is not likely to be much of a restraint.

Thus, the 1974 Act provides more implementation tools than planning agencies previously had. Yet, there remain significant limitations on the ability of planning agencies to pursue the statutory mandate of providing expanded access and of controlling increases in overall outlays, many of which stem from rapidly rising prices.[119] These limitations derive from technical insufficiencies in the current state of the art of planning and from political and structural characteristics built into the scope of the planning process and the geographical and substantive jurisdictions of planning agencies.

From this general discussion of planning and the current structure imposed by the federal planning legislation, we now turn to consideration of the certificate-of-need program mandated by the Act as a tool for implementing statutorily-established policy objectives.

IV. EVOLUTION OF CERTIFICATE-OF-NEED INITIATIVES BY THE STATES

Largely in response to dissatisfaction with rapidly rising hospital costs and excessive facility duplication, campaigns for certificate-of-need laws began to gain momentum at the state level in the mid-1960s and early 1970s.[120] Although the certificate-of-need laws that have emerged are heterogeneous in several ways to be described, as a group they constitute, to date, the strictest form of health care capital expenditures regulation implemented on a widespread basis.

Generally stated, certificate-of-need laws involve the regulation by state-designated agencies of the building, expansion, and modernization of health care facilities and capital equipment on the part of institutional health care providers—principally hospitals and nursing homes.[121] On the whole, these programs have emphasized bed-size changes.[122] The certification process relies primarily on the institution's initiative in proposing a change in beds, facilities, and/or services. In this sense, certificate-of-need programs are reactive.[123] Actions by certificate-of-need agencies to initiate capital projects in "underserved" areas are essentially unknown phenomena. State sanctions under certificate-of-need programs involve a mixture of legal prohibitions of unnecessary capital investment, often linked to licensure and financial controls, whereby the eligibility of health care institutions for funds relating to a specific investment hinges on approval of the investment.[124]

As of January 31, 1978, thirty-six states had enacted certificate-of-need laws.[125] Before that date the Supreme Court of North Carolina had ruled that its certificate-of-need law was unconstitutional.[126] There is substantial interstate variation in terms of comprehensiveness, thresholds for review, and review and appeals procedures. However, most certificate-of-need laws provide a specific expenditure threshold above which the review program applies. Also, many state laws provide detailed surveillance of health services, even where substantial capital expenditures are not involved. In these cases, the appropriate agency must approve any significant change in special services offered by the covered institution.[127]

There are formal links between certificate-of-need programs and the state health planning process. A three-tier application and review process is common (though not always in the sequence mentioned): review by an areawide or regional planning agency with frequent provision for public hearings; approval by the state comprehensive health planning board; and issuance of the certificate of need by the authority of the appropriate state department.[128] Certificate-of-need statutes also allow appeals from adverse decisions.[129]

Certificate-of-need programs are by no means the only regulatory programs operated by the states. In fact, the simultaneous operation of several regulatory programs makes it all the more difficult to isolate the effects directly attributable to certificate-of-need laws. Certainly the effectiveness of a certificate-of-need statute in meeting its objectives may well vary with the presence (or absence) of other regulatory devices. Important among these are the 1122 Review Programs which are subject to adoption on a voluntary basis by the states,[130] but which exist in most states that have adopted a certificate-of-need law.[131] These programs require that a state-designated agency approve: (1) capital expenditures in excess of $100,000, (2) changes in bed complement, or (3) addition of services. Without such approval, expenses related to the investment such as depreciation and interest, and the return on equity capital are not eligible for reimbursement under Social Security

Act programs (principally Medicare and Medicaid).[132] Blue Cross can deny reimbursement for capital costs attributable to unapproved hospital investments and can deny participatory status to non-conforming hospitals.[133] Usually, approval is linked to areawide health planning agencies, and/or certificate-of-need and 1122 programs.[134] Prospective budgeting systems, that establish payment formulas or designate actual payment amounts in advance on a hospital-by-hospital basis, now exist in a few states.[135] Annual budget reviews, conducted under prospective budgeting, can potentially assist certificate-of-need programs in assuring industry compliance. Conversely, a stringent rate review program may render certificate-of-need review unnecessary.

The federal planning law builds on certificate-of-need initiatives in many states, by requiring that all states adopt a certificate-of-need program. The statute and regulations require that the certificate-of-need law apply to "[t]he construction, development, or other establishment of a new health care facility or health maintenance organization."[136] The regulations do not require, however, that a certificate of need be granted for expenditures below $150,000, although states may be more restrictive.[137] As originally promulgated in the waning days of the Ford Administration,[138] the regulations would have permitted a health care facility to change its bed capacity or redistribute or relocate beds without obtaining a certificate, provided that the number involved was fewer than forty beds or less than twenty-five percent of capacity.[139] This reflected a change from the initial proposal which apparently would have required certificate-of-need review for even a single bed.[140] Under Secretary Califano's modifications, certificate-of-need review is triggered by changes involving ten beds or ten percent of capacity.[141] Secretary Califano reasoned that although bed conversions may not necessitate sufficient capital expenditures to trigger review under the $150,000 standard, they nevertheless could impose significantly increased operating costs. Thus, "a change in the use of acute care beds . . . from one service to another, can have significant impact on operational costs."[142]

The federal regulations also establish criteria for certificate-of-need review by HSAs[143] and by SHPDAs.[144] These reviewing agencies must determine whether there is need for the new facil-

ity or equipment and whether the proposal conforms to the applicable plans developed for the region. Importantly, the reviewing agencies are directed to consider not only the merits of a particular application but also alternatives that could be adopted. For example, one consideration is "[t]he availability of less costly or more effective alternative methods of providing such services."[145] Another is "[t]he availability of resources . . . for the provision of the services proposed to be provided and the availability of alternative uses of such resources for the provision of other health services."[146] These provisions requiring the consideration of alternatives, which are drawn directly from the language of the federal planning act, apparently drew criticism when issued as proposals. It was argued "that the possibility that a less costly alternative service could be developed is too theoretical a ground for determining that a proposed service is not needed."[147] The Secretary responded by indicating that consideration was only to be given to "existing alternative services or those alternatives which have a reasonable opportunity of being developed, not services which theoretically might be developed in the community."[148] HEW has also emphasized that the consideration of alternative uses for proposed expenditures "is only one of twelve" factors in evaluating a proposal.[149] Since there are no limitations on the proposed expenditures that HSAs and SHPDAs can recommend and approve, the concept of opportunity cost, incorporated in the regulations, may be difficult to implement in practice.[150]

The federal regulations, in general, seek to "delineate a minimum set of considerations to be included in the review criteria."[151] HEW is encouraging HSAs and SHPDAs to develop and apply their own more elaborate and particularized standards in the review process, utilizing technical assistance from the various support centers that have been established for this purpose.[152]

* * *

VI. THE HOSPITAL COST CONTAINMENT ACT

The Carter Administration proposed the Hospital Cost Containment Act in April, 1977.[174] The original bill has undergone revisions since then and is unlikely to pass in the form in which it was initially introduced. Yet, since the Act includes provisions on capital expenditures regulation which go far beyond past legislation at both federal and state levels, it clearly merits brief comment here.

The proposed Act requires the Secretary of HEW to promulgate an annual nationwide hospital capital expenditure limit, not to exceed $2.5 billion.[175] As originally proposed, the Secretary would be required to apportion this capital expenditure limit among the states on the basis of state population;[176] this provision was modified in an amended version to account for widespread crossing of state lines to receive hospital services.[177] Starting eighteen months after enactment, the Secretary would be directed to take account of interstate variations in construction costs, population patterns, need for modernization, and "other factors important to equitable apportionment of such sum."[178] Furthermore, the Secretary would determine a national ceiling on the number of hospital beds and a standard for hospital occupancy. In no case would the bed ceiling exceed four hospital beds per 1,000 population and occupancy would not be less than 80 percent, except in exceptional circumstances determined by the Secretary. These standards conform to those in the health planning guidelines. In areas where the bed-population ratio is exceeded, a certificate of need could be issued for new beds if, for every new bed authorized, at least two beds were decertified. The proposed Act defines capital expenditures as those (a) which are not for operation and maintenance and which exceed $100,000; (b) which change bed capacity; or (c) which substantially alter the services of the hospital.[179]

If state certificate-of-need programs represent "planning with teeth,"[180] the Hospital Cost Containment Act represents "planning with incisors." Certainly, the Act contains more definite limits and in this way would substantially reduce discretion at the local level. In developing planning guidelines, HEW has been very wary of imposing rigid, cost-conscious standards on local planning agencies. The proposed Act, however, would require that planners-regulators at the local level pay a price for certifying a project. Under the current system, a certificate-of-need agency suffers no penalty for approving a project and is essentially at liberty to disregard national guidelines when faced with an application for an expensive new project. Disapprovals often involve lengthy justification, loss of political capital, and in some cases litigation, which burden agencies that may have meager budgets. The ceiling provisions in the proposed Act mean that an agency would be required to judge which projects it must deny or which beds must be decertified when it approves a project. By giving a state a limited approval budget for hospital capital expenditures, the proposed Act would provide greater incentive for agencies to take seriously their charge in the statute and regulations to consider opportunity costs—that is, available alternatives.

Tough restraints on beds and large investments in equipment and services may have unintended side effects, however. Non-institutional settings, especially physicians' offices, would remain unregulated. Thus, physicians may form groups for purposes of purchasing expensive capital items and continue to pass through the operating costs to third party payers. In addition, the proposed Act may promote compensatory responses on the part of hospitals. For example, some funds displaced from the capital expenditures column may well find their way into improved staffing. It is virtually impossible to avoid such unintended side effects without promulgating lengthy lists of regulations; yet this too has its costs.

The proposed Act, in sum, would add an important dimension to certificate-of-need programs—an expenditure cap. This would encourage agencies to think in terms of trade-offs,[181] but it would leave open many opportunities for by-pass.

VII. CONCLUSION

The 1974 Planning Act is a noble attempt at augmenting the authority of planners-regulators to implement their plans. However, there is no denying that the largely reactive authority granted planning agencies leaves conscientious planners in a dilemma as to how to achieve the lofty goals of the Act, which would necessitate aggressive, affirmative steps. Moreover, the one strong regulatory authority mandated by the 1974 Act—certificate of need—may not turn out to achieve the cost-containment objectives its proponents had anticipated. Even the proposed Hospital Cost Containment Act, with its emphasis on fixed expenditure and revenue ceilings, has sufficiently broad loopholes so that its effectiveness would be a question. This assessment leads us to question the political likelihood of enacting a successful cost-containment regulatory program,[182] and in turn suggests that perhaps the inexorable pull toward regulation in the health sector should be re-evaluated.[183]

NOTES

1. As of January 31, 1978, thirty-six states had enacted certificate-of-need laws. DIVISION OF REGULATORY ACTIVITIES, BUREAU OF HEALTH PLANNING AND RESOURCES DEVELOPMENT, DEP'T OF HEALTH, EDUCATION AND WELFARE, STATUS OF CERTIFICATE OF NEED AND SECTION 1122 PROGRAMS IN THE STATES (1978).

2. See generally Blumstein & Zubkoff, Public Choice in Health: Problems, Politics and Perspectives on Formulating National Health Policy, INT'L J. HEALTH SERVICES (1978) (forthcoming); Blumstein & Zubkoff, Perspectives on Government Policy in the Health Sector, 51 MILBANK MEM. FUND Q.: HEALTH & SOC'Y 395 (1973).

3. Blumstein & Zubkoff, Perspectives, supra note 2, at 405-07.

4. Id. at 407-12.

5. See, e.g., Grosse, The Need for Health Planning, in REGULATING HEALTH FACILITIES CONSTRUCTION 27 (C. Havighurst ed. 1974).

6. See Pauly, The Behavior of Nonprofit Hospital Monopolies: Alternative Models of the Hospital, in REGULATING HEALTH FACILITIES CONSTRUCTION 143, 145-46 (C. Havighurst ed. 1974).

7. See Grosse, supra note 5, at 27.

8. There is a lively empirical debate on the importance of physician-induced demand. Compare Sloan & Feldman, Competition Among Physicians, in FEDERAL TRADE COMM'N, BUREAU OF ECONOMICS, COMPETITION IN THE HEALTH CARE SECTOR: PAST, PRESENT AND FUTURE 57-131 (W. Greenberg ed. 1978) [hereinafter cited as HEALTH CARE COMPETITION] with Reinhardt, Comment on Competition Among Physicians in HEALTH CARE COMPETITION, supra, at 156-90 and Green, Physician-Induced Demand for Medical Care, J. HUMAN RESOURCES (1978) (forthcoming).

9. See Arrow, Uncertainty and the Welfare Economics of Medical Care, 53 AM. ECON. REV. 941, 950 & n.20 (1963).

10. Pauly, Efficiency, Incentives and Reimbursement for Health Care, 7 INQUIRY 114 (1970).

11. See Gibson & Mueller, National Health Expenditures, Fiscal Year 1976, 40 SOC. SEC. BULL. 3, 9-10 (Apr. 1977).

12. See Feldstein, Hospital Cost Inflation: A Study of Nonprofit Price Dynamics, 61 AM. ECON. REV. 853, 870 (1971).

13. See generally Ludlam, Physician-Hospital Relations: The Role of Staff Privileges, 35 L. & CONTEMP. PROB. 879 (1970).

14. This term is used by Havighurst & Blumstein, Coping with Quality/Cost Trade-Offs in Medical Care; The Role of PSROs, 70 NW. U.L. REV. 6, 20-30 (1975). Victor Fuchs has used a similar term, the "technological imperative." V. FUCHS, WHO SHALL LIVE? 60 (1974); Fuchs, The Growing Demand for Medical Care, in ESSAYS IN THE ECONOMICS OF HEALTH AND MEDICAL CARE 61, 66 (V. Fuchs ed. 1972).

15. See Salkever, Competition Among Hospitals, in HEALTH CARE COMPETITION, supra note 8, at 191-206.

16. Monopoly elements also exist in the physician market through restriction on entry. For example, restrictive licensure laws often make substitution of less expensive for more costly factors of production impossible. These can serve as a barrier to the use of more efficient production technologies and may inhibit full utilization, for example, of nurse clinicians practicing in an expanded role. See generally Sloan & Feldman, supra note 8; Lipscomb, Legal Restrictions on Input Substitution in Production: The Case of General Dentistry (Mar. 1977) (Working Paper No. 3371; Duke Institute of Policy Sciences and Public Affairs).

17. See Blumstein & Zubkoff, Public Choice, supra note 2; Ellwood, Alternatives to Regulation: Improving the Market, in INSTITUTE OF MEDICINE, NAT'L ACADEMY OF SCIENCES, CONTROLS ON HEALTH CARE 49 (1975); Havighurst, The Role of Competition in Containing Health Care Costs, in HEALTH CARE COMPETITION, supra note 8.

18. See generally Havighurst, Blumstein & Bovbjerg, Strategies in Underwriting the Costs of Catastrophic Disease, 40 L. & CONTEMP. PROB. 122, 188-95 (1976).

19. See generally INSTITUTE OF MEDICINE, NAT'L ACADEMY OF SCIENCES, HMOs: TOWARD A FAIR MARKET TEST (policy statement 1974).

20. For a discussion of the varying strategies for health care reform, see R. ALFORD, HEALTH CARE POLITICS: IDEOLOGICAL AND INTEREST GROUP BARRIERS TO REFORM (1975).

21. Pub. L. No. 93-641, 88 Stat. 2225 (codified at 42 U.S.C. §§300k to 300t (Supp. V 1975)).

22. See C. SCHULTZE, THE PUBLIC USE OF PRIVATE INTEREST (1977).

23. For a discussion of the problems of regulation, see Havighurst, Federal Regulation of the Health Care Delivery System: A Foreword in the Nature of a "Package Insert," 6 U. TOLEDO L. REV. 578 (1975).

Cf. Altman & Weiner, *Constraining the Medical Care System: Regulation as a Second Best Strategy,* in HEALTH CARE COMPETITION, *supra* note 8, at _____ ; Ball, *Background of Regulation in Health Care,* in INSTITUTE OF MEDICINE, NAT'L ACADEMY OF SCIENCE, CONTROLS ON HEALTH CARE 3 (1975).

24. *See, e.g.,* Navarro, *National Health Insurance and the Strategy for Change,* 51 MILBANK MEM. FUND Q: HEALTH & SOC'Y 223, 230–37 (1973).

25. 42 U.S.C. §300k(a)(1) (Supp. V 1975).

26. *Id.* §300k(a)(3)(B).

27. *Id.* §300k-2(1).

28. COMMITTEE FOR ECONOMIC DEVELOPMENT, BUILDING A NATIONAL HEALTH CARE SYSTEM 16–19 (Apr. 1973).

29. *See, e.g.,* R. ANDERSEN, J. LION, & O. ANDERSON, TWO DECADES OF HEALTH SERVICES: SOCIAL SURVEY TRENDS IN USE AND EXPENDITURE 30, 190 (1976); THE ROBERT WOOD JOHNSON FOUNDATION, A NEW SURVEY ON ACCESS TO MEDICAL CARE 4 (Special Report No. 1, 1978); Benham & Benham, *Utilization of Physician Services Across Income Groups,* 1963–1970, in EQUITY IN HEALTH SERVICES 97 (R. Andersen, J. Kravits, & O. Anderson eds. 1975); Davis, *The Impact of Inflation and Unemployment on Health Care of Low-Income Families,* in HEALTH: A VICTIM OR CAUSE OF INFLATION? 55 (M. Zubkoff ed. 1976); Rogers & Blendon, *The Changing American Health Scene: Sometimes Things Gets Better,* 237 J.A.M.A. 1710, 1714 (1977); Sloan & Bentkover, Access to Ambulatory Care and the U.S. Economy (1977) (Final Report on Contract HRA 230-75-0125 to National Center for Health Services Research, Dep't of Health, Education, & Welfare).

30. *See, e.g.,* Navarro, *Social Class, Political Power, and the State: Their Implications in Medicine* (pts. 1–3), 1 J. HEALTH POL., POL'Y & L. 256, 267, 499 (1976–1977).

31. *See generally* Atkisson & Grimes, *Health Planning in the United States: An Old Idea with New Significance,* 1 J. HEALTH POL., POL'Y & L. 295 (1976); May, *The Planning and Licensing Agencies,* in REGULATING HEALTH FACILITIES CONSTRUCTION 47 (C. Havighurst ed. 1974); O'Connor, *Comprehensive Health Planning: Dreams and Realities,* 52 MILBANK MEM. FUND Q.: HEALTH & SOC'Y 391 (1974); West & Stevens, *Comparative Analysis of Community Health Planning Transition from CHPs to HSAs,* 1 J. HEALTH POL., POL'Y & L. 173 (1976).

32. 42 U.S.C. §§300k to 300t (Supp. V 1975).

33. O'Connor, *supra* note 31, at 401.

34. *Id.*

35. *Id.*

36. The planning agencies created under prior laws acted in a hostile political atmosphere. The Comprehensive Health Planning and Public Health Services Amendments of 1966 (CHP), Pub. L. No. 89–749, 80 Stat. 1180 (1966) (codified in scattered sections of 42 U.S.C.), for example, explicitly stated that there was to be no interference "with existing patterns of private professional practice of medicine." 80 Stat. 1180 (1966). Thus, the only power granted to the CHP agencies was that of commenting on and recommending uses for federal funds such as those available through the Hill-Burton program. The statute provided no authority and established no mechanisms for implementation by the planning agency. In short, the CHP law relied on a "political" model of regulation with its attendant weaknesses, aggravated by the absence of any significant regulatory controls or any financial inducements to secure community support. *See* O'Connor, *supra* note 31, at 401–02.

37. Many of the areawide planning agencies, the so called "b" agencies, had a staff of two or fewer persons. Such small agency staffs could not adequately cope with the task of carrying out health planning. *See generally* O'Connor, *supra* note 31, at 402–03; P. O'DONOGHUE, EVIDENCE ABOUT THE EFFECTS OF HEALTH CARE REGULATION 65 (1974).

38. The Comprehensive Health Planning and Public Health Services Amendments of 1966, see note 36 *supra,* required that the regional planning agencies rely on local matching funds, typically provided by health care institutions. This raised several problems for the "b" agencies. First, since funding was uncertain and job positions insecure, fund raising was a major work activity of a "b" agency staff. This extremely time-consuming enterprise diverted time resources from the task of health planning. Second, the need to raise funds locally tended to detract from the independence of areawide agencies from their funding sources. This was a particular problem when the agency was placed in the position of having to recommend policies which were not in the interests of the funding institutions. Third, the funding uncertainty left staff personnel in a great state of personal anxiety. As a result they often spent a good deal of time considering their own future, instead of their task of planning. *See* O'Connor, *supra* note 31, at 402–03; P. O'DONOGHUE, *supra* note 37, at 65.

39. See note 36 *supra.*

40. 42 U.S.C. §300k-1(b) (Supp. V 1975).

41. *Id.* §300k-1(b)(1).

42. *Id.* §300k-1(b)(2).

43. *Id.* §300*l*-2(b).

44. The HSAs have four types of authority: (1) the power of persuasion; (2) the power to approve or disapprove certain federal spending in the region; (3) the power to make recommendations about the necessity for new institutional services and facilities and to comment on the appropriateness of existing facilities and services; and (4) the responsibility for developing

health plans and implementation plans. *See* West & Stevens, *supra* note 31, at 184.

45. 42 U.S.C. §300*l*-2(b)(2) (Supp. V 1975).

46. *Id.* §§300*l*-2(b)(2)(B),(C). On September 23, 1977, HEW issued proposed National Guidelines for Health Planning, and, on January 20, 1978, the Department issued revised proposals. 42 Fed. Reg. 48,502 (1977); 43 Fed. Reg. 3056 (1978). On March 15, 1978, these proposals were issued in final form. 43 Fed. Reg. 13,040, 13,044 (1978).

The initial set of standards is intended to be part of a "rational, comprehensive set of health planning goals and standards." 43 Fed. Reg. 3056 (1978). The Department apparently expects to formulate National Guidelines that will include "such issues as cost containment, access to care, availability and distribution of health care resources, quality of care and health status." *Id.* However, the initial set of guidelines is much more modest in scope, limited to "certain institutional resources, the excess supplies of which need to be contained if the rapid escalation of health care costs is to be moderated." 42 Fed. Reg. 48,502 (1977).

47. There must be publication in at least two newspapers of general circulation throughout the HSA's area. 42 U.S.C. §300*l*-2(b)(2) (Supp. V 1975).

48. *Id.* §300*l*-2(b)(3).

49. *Id.* §300m-2(a)(2).

50. *Id.* §300m-2(a)(6).

51. *Id.*

52. *Id.* §300m-2(c).

53. *Id.* §300m-3(c)(1).

54. *Id.* §300m-3(c)(2)(A).

55. This hearing must be announced at least 30 days in advance, and the announcement must be published in at least two newspapers of general circulation in the state, giving the time and place of the hearings. *Id.* §300m-3(c)(2)(B).

56. *Id.* §300k(a)(3)(A).

57. *Id.* §300k(a)(3)(B).

58. *Id.* §300k(a)(3)(C).

59. *Id.* §300k-2(1).

60. *Id.* §300k-2(3).

61. *Id.* §300k-2(4).

62. *Id.* §300k-2.

63. *Id.* §300*l*-2(b)(2)(C).

64. *Id.* §300n-4(b).

65. *Id.* §300n-4(c)(1).

66. *Id.* §300n-4(c)(2).

67. *Id.* §300n-4(c)(3).

68. *Id.* §300n-4(c)(5).

69. *Id.* §300n-4(c)(4).

70. *Id.* §300n-4(c)(6).

71. *Id.* §300n-4(c)(7)(A).

72. *Id.* §300n-4(c)(7)(B).

73. *Id.* §300n-4(c)(7)(C).

74. *Id.* §300n-1(c).

75. *Id.* §300*l*-2(b)(3).

76. *Id.* §300*l*-2(e)(1)(A). These include funds appropriated out of the Public Health Service Act, the Community Mental Health Centers Act, or the Comprehensive Alcohol Abuse and Alcoholism Prevention, Treatment, and Rehabilitation Act of 1970 for grants, contracts, loans, or loan guarantees for the development, expansion or support of health resources. They also include federal funds made available by the state under state allotments from these same federal programs.

77. *Id.* §300*l*-2(f).

78. *Id.* §300m-1(b)(13). *See also* 42 Fed. Reg. 4031 (1977) (to be codified in 42 C.F.R. §123.407(9)).

79. 42 U.S.C. §300*l*-2(g) (Supp. V 1975).

80. *Id.* §300*l*-2(h).

81. These are the Public Health Service Act, the Community Mental Health Centers Act, or the Comprehensive Alcohol Abuse and Alcoholism Prevention, Treatment, and Rehabilitation Act of 1970. *Id.* §300m-3(c)(6).

82. *Id.* §300m-2(a)(4)(B).

83. *Id.* §300m-2(a)(6).

84. *Id.* §300*l*-1(b)(2)(B).

85. *Id.* §300*l*-1(b)(2)(A)(i).

86. *Id.* §300*l*-1(b)(2)(A)(ii).

87. *Id.* §300*l*-1(b)(2)(A)(iii).

88. *Id.* §300*l*-1(b)(2)(A)(iv).

89. *Id.* §300*l*-1(b)(2)(A).

90. *Id.* §300*l*-1(b)(2)(B).

91. *Id.* §300n-3.

92. *Id.* §300n-2(c).

93. *Id.* §300*l*-5(a). The Act specifically restricts the type of private contributions an HSA can accept. *Id.* §300*l*-1(b)(5).

94. *Id.* §300*l*-2(c)(2).

95. See note 46 *supra*.

96. *See* West & Stevens, *supra* note 31, at 193–94. *See also* Glantz, *Legal Aspects of Health Facilities Regulation,* in HEALTH REGULATION: CERTIFICATE OF NEED AND 1122 75, 96–99 (H. Hyman ed. 1977).

97. See note 46 *supra*.

98. 43 Fed. Reg. 3056 (1978). HEW has been quite candid in indicating that these initial proposed guidelines "do not constitute a full array of National Guidelines for Health Planning." *Id.* at 3058.

99. *Id.*

100. *Id.*

101. 42 Fed. Reg. 48,502, 48,503 (1977).

102. "While it is recognized that the process of developing quantitative standards is still in its early stages, the Department believes that sufficient progress has been made to support the standards as issued." 43 Fed. Reg. 3056, 3058 (1978).

103. 42 U.S.C. §300*l*-2(b)(1) (Supp. V 1975).

104. *See* Blumstein, *The Role of PSROs in Hospital Cost Containment,* in HOSPITAL COST CONTAINMENT: SELECTED NOTES FOR FUTURE POLICY 461, 479–81 (M. Zubkoff, I. Raskin, R. Hanft eds. 1978).

105. For example, the following resolution was adopted on April 16, 1977 by the Tennessee Medical Association House of Delegates:

WHEREAS, the State Center for Health Statistics (SCHS), Tennessee Department of Public Health, in accordance with P.L. 93-353, is being supported by the National Center for Health Statistics (NCHS) as part of the Cooperative Health Statistics System (CHSS) activity in Tennessee; and

WHEREAS, P.L. 93-641 and its legislative history relate that a Health System [sic] Agency (HSA) should not engage in data collection activities, but should, to the maximum extent feasible, obtain information from existing data systems, such as PSRO and CHSS; and

WHEREAS, The American Medical Association policy is:

1. A primary responsibility of the physician controlled local PSRO is the ownership, maintenance, and the prudent dissemination of data generated by medical providers within the PSRO.
2. The pathway of data flow for PSRO decisions and documentation thereof shall be delineated and controlled by PSRO.
3. Routine reports of data that are required by statute should be furnished in accordance with the law, but these reports shall not identify the specific patient, physician or hospital.
4. It must be the prerogative of the PSRO to choose its data processor.

WHEREAS, all providers and users of data desire to avoid any unnecessary and duplicative efforts devoted by each agency in data collection, processing and dissemination; and

WHEREAS, The Tennessee Foundation for Medical Care, Inc. has been collecting PSRO information for all Title XVIII (Medicaid) and Title XIX (Medicare) patients and provides a data abstracting service to hospitals in Tennessee for all patients. Now, therefore be it

RESOLVED, that the Tennessee Medical Association supports the concept of "Single Statewide Health Statistics System" so long as the Tennessee Foundation for Medical Care, Inc., is responsible for and controls the collection, and

performs the processing and provides the statistics on patterns of utilization and quality of care including those required and requested by the Bureau of Health Planning and Resources Development (BHPRD), HEW Recommended Data Sets; and be it further

RESOLVED, That the sharing of data and information such as statistics on patterns of utilization and quality of care will be subject to approval by the Board of Directors of the Tennessee Foundation for Medical Care, Inc., for PSRO Area II and the Board of Directors of Shelby County Foundation for Medical Care, Inc., for PSRO Area I.

Tennessee Medical Association Res. 9–77.

106. 42 U.S.C. §300*l*-2(d)(1). *Cf. id.* §300*l*-2(b)(1) (charging HSAs to assemble and analyze data).

107. HEALTH POLICY PROGRAM, SCHOOL OF MEDICINE, UNIVERSITY OF CALIFORNIA-SAN FRANCISCO, COOPERATION BETWEEN HEALTH SYSTEMS AGENCIES AND PROFESSIONAL STANDARDS REVIEW ORGANIZATIONS (Jan. 1977) (HEW Contract No. HRA-230-75-0071). *See also* M. Goran & H. Cain, Health Systems Agencies/Professional Standards Review Organizations Relationships (Dec. 6, 1976) (draft joint memorandum).

108. Dr. Richmond has recognized this limitation, conceding that "[w]ith respect to the roles of Health Systems Agencies in achieving their established target levels, it is clear that their current authority is limited." 43 Fed. Reg. 3056, 3058 (1978).

109. *Id.* at 3059.

110. *Id.* at 3058.

111. There is a so-called "forum" function for health planning, that is, "a common meeting ground where individuals and institutions with their own vested interests can be exposed to the proposals and rationales of other groups within the community." O'Connor, *supra* note 31, at 407. "Closely related to the forum function of health planning is its educational function. This function must be performed in such a way that all segments of the community are informed of both the issues and the alternatives involved in particular decision-making situations." *Id.* at 408. It was the forum and educational functions of health planning that the 1974 Act was meant to strengthen by adding "teeth;" it is ironic to see the proposed planning guidelines justified in no small measure by resort to these forum and educational functions.

112. For general discussions of state-administered rate-review programs, see S. LAUDICINA, PROSPECTIVE REIMBURSEMENT FOR HOSPITALS: A GUIDE FOR POLICYMAKERS (Department of Public Affairs, Community Service Society of N.Y., 1976); P. O'DONOGHUE, *supra* note 37, at 47–57.

113. Dowling, *Prospective Reimbursement of Hospitals,* 11 INQUIRY 163 (1974). *See generally* Goldberg &

Greenberg, *The Effect of Physician-Controlled Health Insurance; U.S. v. Oregon State Medical Society*, 2 J. HEALTH POL., POL'Y & L. 48 (1977); Havighurst, *Controlling Health Care Costs: Strengthening the Private Sector's Hand*, 1 J. HEALTH POL., POL'Y & L. 471 (1977).

114. This function is performed by PSROs. *See generally* Havighurst & Blumstein, *supra* note 14, at 38–51.

115. *Id.* at 60–68.

116. *Cf.* Blumstein, *Inflation and Quality: The Case of PSROs*, in HEALTH: A VICTIM OR CAUSE OF INFLATION? 245, 284 (M. Zubkoff ed. 1976) (discussing the same problem in the context of PSROs).

117. *Id.* at 283–84.

118. *Id.* at 271.

119. During the 1960's, about half the increase in expenditures resulted from increases in utilization and the other half from increases in price. *See* Stuart & Stockton, *Control Over the Utilization of Medical Services*, 51 MILBANK MEM. FUND Q: HEALTH & SOC'Y 341 (1973). On trends in health care costs, see COUNCIL ON WAGE AND PRICE STABILITY, THE PROBLEM OF RISING HEALTH CARE COSTS (1976).

120. Curran, *A National Survey and Analysis of State Certificate-of-Need Laws for Health Facilities*, in REGULATING HEALTH FACILITIES CONSTRUCTION 85 (C. Havighurst, ed. 1974); Curran, Steele & Ober, *Government Intervention on Increase*, 49 HOSPITALS 57 (May 16, 1975); Elsasser & Galinski, *Status of State Legislation*, 45 HOSPITALS 54 (Dec. 16, 1971).

121. *See generally* P. O'DONOGHUE, *supra* note 37, at 59.

122. *See* LEWIN AND ASSOCIATES, INC., AN ANALYSIS OF STATE AND REGIONAL HEALTH REGULATION, pt. 1, 4–28 (Nat'l Technical Information Service PB-240 966, 1974); Bicknell & Walsh, *Certification-of-Need: The Massachusetts Experience*, 292 NEW ENGLAND J. MED. 1054 (1975); Salkever & Bice, *The Impact of Certificate-of-Need Controls on Hospital Investment*, 54 MILBANK MEM. FUND Q.: HEALTH & SOC'Y 185, 190 (1976).

123. *See* Elsasser & Galinski, *supra* note 120, at 55.

124. *See* Curran, *A National Survey and Analysis*, *supra* note 120.

125. See note 1 *supra*.

126. *In re* Certificate of Need for Aston Park Hosp., Inc., 282 N.C. 542, 193 S.E.2d 729 (1973).

127. *See generally* LEWIN AND ASSOCIATES INC., *supra* note 122, pt. 3, vols. 1–2.

128. *See* Elsasser & Galinski, *supra* note 120, at 56.

129. *See* Curran, *A National Survey and Analysis*, *supra* note 120, at 98–103; Havighurst, *Regulation of Health Facilities and Services by "Certificate of Need,"* 59 VA. L. REV. 1143, 1173–76 (1973).

130. Social Security Amendments of 1972, 42 U.S.C. §1320a-1 (Supp. V 1975).

131. *See* Curran, Steele, & Ober, *supra* note 120, at 58.

132. *See generally* P. O'DONOGHUE, *supra* note 37, at 59.

133. F. SLOAN & B. STEINWALD, HOSPITAL DEMAND FOR LABOR AND NON-LABOR INPUTS: A TIME SERIES CROSS-SECTION ANALYSIS (in process of preparation).

134. *See* Curran, *A National Survey and Analysis*, *supra* note 120, at 1175–76.

135. *See* authorities cited at note 112 *supra*.

136. 42 Fed. Reg. 4002, 4025, 4029 (1977).

137. *Id.*

138. The final regulations were approved on January 11, 1977 but were not published until January 21, 1977, after President Ford left office.

139. 42 Fed. Reg. 4002, 4025, 4029 (1977).

140. 42 Fed. Reg. 18,606 (1977).

141. 42 Fed. Reg. 18,605, 18,606, 18,607 (1977) (to be codified in 42 C.F.R. §§122.304(a)(3), .404(a)(3)).

142. 42 Fed. Reg. 18,606 (1977).

143. 42 Fed. Reg. 4002, 4027 (1977) (to be codified in 42 C.F.R. §122.308).

144. 42 Fed. Reg. 4002, 4031 (1977) (to be codified in 42 C.F.R. §123.409).

145. 42 Fed. Reg. 4002, 4027, 4031 (1977) (to be codified in 42 C.F.R. §§122.308(a)(4), .409(a)(4)). *See* 42 U.S.C. §300n-1(c)(4) (Supp. V 1975).

146. 42 Fed. Reg. 4002, 4027, 4031 (1977) (to be codified in 42 C.F.R. §§122.308(a)(7), .409(a)(7)). *See* 42 U.S.C. §300n-1(c)(4) (Supp. V 1975).

147. 42 Fed. Reg. 4002, 4019 (1977).

148. *Id.*

149. *Id.* at 4020.

150. *See* notes 174–81 *infra* and accompanying text.

151. 42 Fed. Reg. 4002, 4017 (1977).

152. These centers are funded under the federal planning act. 42 U.S.C. §300n-3 (Supp. V 1975). Additional technical assistance is available from the National Health Planning Information Center, provided for under 42 U.S.C. §300n-2(c) (Supp. V 1975).

* * *

174. H.R. 6575, S. 1391, 95th Cong., 1st Sess. (1977).

175. H.R. 6575, 95th Cong., 1st Sess. (1977). §1504(a)(1) (1977).

176. *Id.* §1504(a)(2).

177. H.R. 9717, 95th Cong., 2d Sess. §1504(a)(3) (1977).

178. H.R. 6575, 95th Cong., 1st Sess. §1504(a)(2) (1977).

179. *Id.* §1527(c)(7).

180. *See, e.g.*, Havighurst, *supra* note 129, at 1153.

181. Title I of the proposed Act would seek to curtail increases in hospital revenues directly. A tough revenue policy could be a very effective cost-containment technique.

182. *See* Marmor, Wittman, & Heagy, *Politics, Public Policy, and Medical Inflation*, in HEALTH: A VICTIM OR CAUSE OF INFLATION? 299, 305–13 (M. Zubkoff ed. 1976).

183. *See* authorities cited at notes 2, 17–20, 22–23, 113 *supra*.

1.3 Health Care Cost-Containment Regulation: Prospects and an Alternative*

CLARK C. HAVIGHURST, J.D.

Reprinted with permission from 3 *American Journal of Law & Medicine* 309–322 (1977). Copyright © 1977 by the *American Journal of Law & Medicine* and Clark C. Havighurst. All rights reserved.

ABSTRACT

Regulation of the health care system to achieve appropriate containment of overall costs is characterized by Professor Havighurst as requiring public officials to engage, directly or indirectly, in the rationing of medical services. This rationing function is seen by the author as peculiarly difficult for political institutions to perform, given the public's expectations and the symbolic importance of health care. An effort on the part of regulators to shift the rationing burden to providers is detected, as is a trend toward increasingly arbitrary regulation, designed to minimize regulators' confrontations with sensitive issues. Irrationality and ignorance are found to plague regulatory decision making on health-related issues, even though it is the consumer who is usually thought to suffer most from these disabilities. The author argues that consumer choice under some cost constraints is a preferable mechanism for allocating resources because it better reflects individuals' subjective preferences, has a greater capacity for facing trade-offs realistically, and can better contend with professional dominance of the resource allocation process.

In view of the unlikelihood of regulation that is both sensitive and effective in containing costs, the author proposes that we rely primarily on consumer incentives to reform the system. A simple change in the tax treatment of health insurance or other health plan premiums, to strengthen consumers' interest in cost containment while also subsidizing needy consumers, is advocated. Steps to improve opportunities for innovation in cost containment by health insurers, HMOs, and other actors are outlined briefly.

*This Comment copyright © 1977 by the *American Journal of Law & Medicine* and Clark C. Havighurst. The paper was adapted from a study prepared for the Federal Trade Commission with support from Grant HS01539 from the National Center for Health Services Research, HEW.

I. INTRODUCTION

Regulation to contain the costs of medical care is appropriately viewed as a response to a perceived failure of the "market" to allocate resources to, and within, the health care sector of the economy in accordance with the public's true wishes. The problem is not so much the absolute level of health care spending—although that is disturbingly high—as our increasing lack of confidence in the mechanisms by which the private sector decides what services should and should not be purchased.[1] Even casual observation reveals, on the one hand, large expenditures on care whose value is very much in doubt and, on the other hand, clear needs that are being neglected.[2] The desire to meet unmet needs is being frustrated by our recognition that giving the system more resources will simply encourage more waste as undue availability of resources induces the system to increase further both the quantity and the quality of its output without regard to the relation between marginal costs and marginal benefits. Cost-containment regulation, in seeking to prevent the misallocation of resources within the health care industry, ostensibly sets out to solve an important public problem.

This Comment seeks to provide an overview of the cost-containment effort in the health care industry in order that its substantial limitations and its more troublesome implications can be appreciated. My purpose is to dispel the optimism of those observers of regulation who tend to view its disappointing performance to date simply as a challenge to try harder and to invest more money in the effort. Moreover, because these observers persist in the belief that regulation is inevitable and that there is no choice but to redouble our efforts, I have also felt it necessary to argue that a better approach is in fact available. My view is that we would be well advised to regard the regulatory effort only as a stop-gap and to turn our major attention toward changing the incentives of consumers and providers and toward improving their opportunities to express their preferences in a competitive marketplace.

My objective in proposing an alternative that is preferable to regulation is to counteract, if possible, our political institutions' perhaps insuperable bias toward solving problems by direct regulation even when better solutions are readily available. In his recent Godkin Lectures at Harvard, Charles L. Schultze, the chairman of the President's Council of Economic Advisers, noted and deplored government's undue propensity to adopt a "black box" approach to social intervention, "grafting a specific command-and-control module onto the private enterprise incentive-oriented system"[3] instead of intervening to preserve and improve, and even affirmatively employ, market forces as instruments of social control. Health policy issues, so far treated as resolvable only by regulatory means, provide a dramatic illustration of Schultze's thesis and a test of his hope that a "steady maturing of both the electorate and political leaders"[4] is improving our ability to make sensible choices between public regulation and private incentives.

II. ASSESSING REGULATION'S PROSPECTS

Early doubts about the probable efficacy of regulation in the health care industry were somewhat unfocused because they were necessarily based on extrapolation from experience in dissimilar industries, such as those regulated as public utilities and common carriers.[5] Those early doubts were not wide of the mark, however, and accumulating evidence about health sector regulation has done nothing to dispel them. Indeed, whereas the early critics anticipated some beneficial impact from regulation and argued only that it would be woefully inadequate to the need, the most careful studies that have been done so far have shown practically no measurable effects.[6] But such early returns have not much dampened enthusiasm for regulation, because it is possible to argue that it is too soon to tell. But, of course, if we must wait for a conclusive demonstration of regulation's inadequacies, it will then be too late to do anything about it—just as it is now virtually impossible to make major deregulation moves in those industries that came under regulation in the New Deal.

Because the impending choices in health policy could commit us irrevocably to a regulatory course, a new evaluation of regulation, moving beyond analogies to regulation in other industries, now seems in order. Although data are still inconclusive and experiments are still incomplete, we are nevertheless in a better position than ever before to evaluate health sector regulation on its own merits, with improved understanding of what it must seek to achieve and what specific obstacles it must confront. While the earlier analogies were useful in framing the pertinent questions, it is clear that health sector regulation is in many respects *sui generis*. Among other things, it employs some unusual and perhaps promising regulatory mechanisms—particularly the health systems agencies, or HSAs—which were designed in large measure specifically to avoid some of the problems which regulation has encountered in other settings and about which the early critics of regulation warned.[7] But, while such institutional factors may suggest that regulation in the health sector could outperform regulation in other industries, the cost-containment job that regulators have been asked to do with respect to health care is far from easy compared to other regulatory assignments.

some cutbacks are certainly essential if costs are to be appropriately controlled.

III. COST CONTAINMENT AS RATIONING

Although the regulators' task in the health care industry is variously stated, the job to be done involves nothing less than rationing health care—preventing patients from receiving and providers from providing care that they believe would be beneficial. This is not a regulatory function that will be popular with or easily understood by a public which has been told that there is a right to health care and which has come to expect a high standard of care and easy access to it.[8] In effect, the regulators have been charged with reducing, one way or another, what has come to be seen as the most tangible indicium of "quality" in medical care—namely the quantity of services rendered both in the individual case and in the aggregate. They have been asked to say "no" to more and better health services under circumstances where everyone immediately concerned in a specific treatment decision is inclined—because they do not face the costs—to say "yes." Although some means of limiting the consumption of health services is clearly required, public regulation may be incapable of achieving this specific goal.

The rationing objective is usually obscured in the rhetoric describing the function of various regulatory programs in the health sector. Thus, Professional Standards Review Organizations (PSROs) are said to be primarily concerned with the quality of care, not cost containment; under the banner of quality assurance some "unnecessary" care and "overutilization" can perhaps be eliminated, but the medical profession's *de facto* control of PSROs assures that cost considerations and the rationing objective will be kept distinctly secondary.[9] Certificate-of-need agencies are usually charged with preventing "duplication" and forestalling the construction of "unneeded" facilities but are seldom, if ever, publicly instructed to create artificial shortages; yet meaningful cost containment requires that supply be curtailed not to meet, but to contain, demand.[10] Similarly, the ostensible purpose of most hospital rate-setting agencies is to squeeze "inefficiency" out of the system, not to force hospitals to cut back services; nevertheless,

IV. RATIONING AS A POLITICAL "HOT POTATO"

The semantic obscurity under which regulation is practiced reveals the political and social touchiness of the subject being regulated. A powerful taboo surrounds public discussion of trade-offs between citizens' lives and health on the one hand and the public's financial resources on the other. This taboo causes regulators to be reluctant to fight many battles in the "quality/cost no man's land"—that area where, although additional medical inputs are undeniably beneficial, there is real doubt that the benefits are worth the cost.[11] Even though effective cost-containment regulation seems to call for the sophisticated techniques of benefit/cost analysis, regulators will naturally shy away from such tools, because their use would require placing explicit values on individuals' lives and health.[12] Given their political vulnerability, the lack of public understanding, and their own moral trepidation in the face of providers' claims, regulators are unlikely to be able to consistently and forthrightly address the trade-offs involved in rationing health care and to have due regard for other uses of resources.

One consequence of regulators' difficulties in challenging directly what passes for "quality" in medical care is that, to be effective, regulation must somehow avoid addressing the medical merits of specific cases and concentrate on grosser forms of control. One reason why almost no one expects PSROs to make more than a marginal contribution to cost containment is that they purport to assess the medical merits of individual utilization decisions, which can usually be questioned only if one is willing to compare the benefits and costs of treating an individual patient. Much greater hope is currently reposed in limiting the availability of health facilities (through certificate-of-need programs) and the amount of hospital budgets (through rate setting), two approaches that impose resource constraints on providers and thereby shift to them the difficult task of rationing care among those who seek it. Indeed, regulation in the health sector has shied away from asking public authorities to make the hard case-by-case decisions and has moved in subtle ways towards making providers do the rationing. Precisely because the regulators, like Ado Annie in *Oklahoma,* "cain't say 'no,'" they have sought to shift the burden of doing so to the providers. The PSRO program does this explicitly, but certification of need and hospital rate setting programs do it as well.

The policy of forcing providers to do the rationing job is based on an unarticulated assumption that limiting the resources available to providers can induce them to allocate those resources to their best uses, providing those services that are most valuable to patients and omitting those services that are least valuable. But hardly any thought has been given to whether providers can realistically be expected to serve primarily public needs rather than their own preferences and values in performing this allocative function. Despite the lack of assurance on this score, regulation is being implemented in a way that perpetuates the very provider dominance which has produced excessive emphasis on high-technology acute care rendered in institutional settings while neglecting more routine needs of large populations and which has therefore been an important source of the health sector's problems in the first place. It is far from clear that the limited consumer participation provided for in health planning and resource development can overcome provider influence on any issue where the claims of "quality" are plausible.

Providers' economic interests and their traditional "cost-is-no-object" orientation make it doubtful that they can be counted on to cooperate fully in helping the regulators achieve their rationing objective. Indeed, far from sparing the regulators embarrassment in their efforts to limit the health sector's spending proclivities, providers can be expected to expose the regulators' veiled attempts to erode what providers will characterize as the quality of care. In exercising their substantial discretion in the allocation of regulation-limited resources, providers may find it convenient to threaten cutbacks in just those highly visible areas where the regulators are most vulnerable and under the most pressure to keep the resources flowing. Thus, the politics of such regulation could easily produce a "hot potato" game in which providers are better insulated against political pressures and can force public decision makers to take the heat. Under these circumstances, socially appropriate stringency will not often be achieved.

V. JUDGING REGULATION'S EFFECTIVENESS

Even the most pessimistic observer cannot be sure that regulation will be totally ineffective in the health care industry or that no change in the direction or pace of cost escalation will occur as controls take hold. Some regulators may prove adept in managing the political environment and in developing a constituency for cost-containment efforts, and some providers may adopt relatively responsible attitudes toward regulation and change their behavior in material respects. For these reasons, regulation sometimes will seem to have had a beneficial effect when compared with past experience in a particular area or with contemporaneous experience in places where regulation has been less skillful or providers more recalcitrant. But such apparent successes are likely to be marginal in magnitude and difficult to replicate universally. Proponents of regulation will nevertheless single out the more successful programs to prove the efficacy of their chosen methods and will view unimpressive average performance only as evidence of the need to try harder and to invest more money in the regulatory effort. They may also yield to the temptation to equate vigorous regulatory activity, such as frequent denial of certificate-of-need applications, with regulatory success, when in fact regulation may have had only minimal impact on its most important targets—that is, on cost and capital investment.[13]

Regulation will frequently seem advantageous because it is measured only against the alternative of doing nothing, not against other promising policies that might have been, but were not, tried. Indeed, when adopted at the national level, regulation forecloses experimentation, not only making success or failure hard to recognize but also making the optimum strategy undiscoverable. While it is quite possible that some kind of equilibrium eventually will be reached where pressures to control costs and pressures to increase them will be in rough balance, there is no reason whatsoever to think that the political processes yielding that result will have come anywhere near finding the socially optimal level of spending on health care. Instead, excessive spending on health care, buying too much of a good thing, is likely to continue as a direct consequence of the strategic advantage that providers enjoy as a result of their control of the high ground overlooking the quality/cost no-man's-land.

VI. ESCALATING ARBITRARINESS IN REGULATION

Because it is unlikely that the present regulatory facade will be finally accepted as legitimizing the costs now being incurred, government, in seeking more effective control, can be expected to turn increasingly to its only available counterstrategy against providers' refusal to accept the rationing burden. That strategy is to move toward more arbitrary forms of regulation, thereby reducing the potential for confrontations with providers over specific quality/cost trade-offs and increasing the necessity for providers to accept without recourse the unwanted burden of rationing services. This expectation of escalating arbitrariness is confirmed by the Carter Administration's recent proposals to put a 9 percent "cap" on annual hospital cost increases and another "cap" on aggregate capital investments by hospitals.[14]

Arbitrariness of the sort reflected in the Carter proposals can be publicly justified only by charging providers with gross irresponsibility, and Secretary Califano's assertions about the "fat" and inefficiency in hospitals,[15] although a distortion, can be seen both as an attempt to justify extreme measures and as an expression of frustration about regulatory achievements to date. Indeed, the Carter proposals are themselves a confession of the failure of the regulatory approaches originally conceived for the health sector. Although regulation was intended to embody a toughminded, planning-oriented approach to medical care, this has not materialized and, for the reasons stated above, seems not to be in the political cards. Judging from Secretary Califano's remarks, it may be that, rather than face the hard trade-offs openly on their merits, government regulators will find it politically preferable to appear overtly antiprovider, even dictatorial, and to have their adverse impacts on "quality" chalked up to general obtuseness rather than to callous cost-consciousness in resolving health care spending issues on a case-by-case basis. Even though such arbitrariness

may in fact be the most responsible regulatory policy because it is the most likely to be effective, the courts may be hard to convince that they should tolerate regulation that misrepresents the facts and avoids the hard decisions. But too much "due process," openness, and explicitness will preclude stringency, which, although socially appropriate, is politically unpalatable.[16]

The scenario of escalating arbitrariness as a strategic response to providers' ability to force the implications of health care spending issues into the open leads ultimately to an approach similar to that offered in Senator Kennedy's proposed Health Security Act: a fixed budget for the health care system as a whole. While achieving absolute control over total health care costs, that proposed solution would leave internal allocation of the system's resources largely to political processes that are extremely difficult to assess. Many of the same intractable decision-making difficulties that currently exist would remain, and it seems likely that, despite all efforts to introduce citizen participation, providers would continue to exercise disproportionate influence over the uses to which resources are put, if not over absolute levels of spending. Thus, despite long experience with a fixed budget and central planning, the British National Health Service remains more heavily committed to high-technology acute care than seems appropriate given that system's limited resources and unmet needs in such areas as long-term care for the elderly, the chronically and mentally ill, and the handicapped.[17] Even if professional influence could be overcome in the world of Health Security, it is unrealistic to think that a public consensus exists about the standard and style of medicine to be provided. Treating the allocation of health care resources as a subject for political compromise means depriving some of what they would willingly purchase and giving others what they would not, even if their resources were adequate. Moreover, the equality among income classes striven for in such a system could easily prove more symbolic than real, as qualitative differences prove resistant to change.

VII. REGULATION VERSUS PRIVATE CHOICE

Health care varies greatly in value, some of it being of priceless benefit and other care not being, in any defensible sense, worth its cost. Although versions of this long-neglected insight have been increasingly embraced in health policy discussions in the 1970s, its full implications have yet to sink in. For example, many observers who give lip service to the insight that only limited benefits are yielded by much health care remain fervently attached to the symbolic goal of comprehensive benefits and equality of access to high-quality services. Yet the emerging sophistication about health care's value should suggest placing less emphasis on providing the poor with an ideal standard of health care and more emphasis on providing them with other things, many of which, such as better housing and nutrition, might be more productive of improved health.

The new awareness about medicine's uncertain benefits also has yet to overcome the tendency of policy makers and other observers to disparage private choices between health care and other things. Yet increasing skepticism among commonly recognized authorities about the value of health care at the margin suggests (1) that the range and subjectivity of consumers' preferences with respect to medical care does not necessarily signify consumer ignorance or irrationality and (2) that different people can come rationally to different conclusions about what quantity and quality of services to buy. Although individual consumers' decisions can always be questioned, most consumer choices are made with the benefit of professional advice, or by employment (or other) groups whose sophistication cannot be doubted. Moreover, private choices are made with information concerning personal preferences that obviously is not available to anyone except the individuals involved. In a democratic society, private decisions might be viewed as having comparative or even absolute legitimacy on this account alone.

As a substitute for private decisions, regulation leaves much to be desired. Not only does it suffer from almost totally irremediable ignorance about individual cases—both the precise medical circumstances and the subjective preferences of the parties affected—but it also lacks data on societal preferences concerning the value of health care in comparison with other possible uses of society's limited productive capacity. Although it is common to attribute irrationality only to consumers, it is clear that irrationality systematically afflicts health system regulators because politicized regulation allows symbolism to overwhelm forthright benefit/cost comparisons. Moreover, the interest-group bargaining implicit in the American concept of regulation perpetuates a high degree of provider influence, leaves out many other pertinent values and interests, and assigns weights on the basis of "clout," not merit. It is doubtful that health sector regulators can earn higher marks for knowledge, rationality, general soundness, or democratic validity than consumers making decisions with professional and other available advice and under appropriate incentives to conserve resources.

Regulation is failing to solve the resource allocation problem in the health sector because it proceeds on wrong premises concerning the capabilities of public decision makers. But, even if it should succeed in imposing effective controls, it would do so at the expense of important values. While holding out the promise of a "right to health care," it would simultaneously define that right narrowly and arbitrarily and would almost certainly deny or indirectly curtail the consumer's right to purchase care that he might wish to have but which the regulators chose not to make available. Regulation's chief tendency is thus toward narrowing consumers' range of choice, enforcing a false consensus, and obscuring the wide variations that exist in both consumer preferences and medical practice. Contrary to what both the political debate and professional ideology imply, there is no "one right way" to deal with most health problems. Rather than relying on government alone to chart our course, it may seem more appropriate in a pluralistic society to widen opportunities for consumer choice under meaningful cost constraints.

VIII. OUTLINE OF A MARKET ALTERNATIVE

As some of the foregoing truths begin to dawn, the logic of turning resource allocation decisions in the health sector over to public decision makers may no longer seem as unassailable as it once did. At the very least, we should be led to look with renewed interest at the possibility that workable alternatives to regulation may exist. If they exist anywhere, they most likely lie in the direction of strengthening market incentives and assuring competition at critical points in the market for health services and health services financing. Although this Comment is not the place to make the complete case for a new departure in health policy,[18] it should at least be observed that a case can be made for seeking to improve the private market's resource-allocation capability through a program based on the following elements:

(1) Change in the tax law to eliminate the current incentive to overinsure against health care needs. Although seldom recognized as the distorting force it is, the tax law is a major contributor to unwarranted cost escalation in the health sector. By making health insurance a tax-free fringe benefit for both income tax and Social Security tax purposes, the tax law has long stimulated the purchase of more insurance—that is, more comprehensive coverage—than people would otherwise purchase. This excessively comprehensive insurance has in turn increasingly allowed providers to prescribe and render more services of a more expensive variety than people would be willing to pay for out of pocket, thus misallocating resources. Even more importantly, the tax law penalizes health insurers' cost-containment efforts by taxing as wages any saving in health insurance premiums that an employer might pass on to his employees. For these reasons, the prevailing belief that regulation is required to solve the cost problem, because the private sector cannot do the job, is in large measure traceable to the tax law's excessive subsidization of health insurance.

To correct the problem, it is not necessary to eliminate the tax subsidy altogether, but a limit on the amount of the subsidy is essential to deter excessive coverage—by making it purchasable only with after-tax dollars. A shift to a system of limited tax credits could achieve the desired effect without increasing the tax bill of the average taxpayer. Moreover, the subsidy thus provided would be uniform for all taxpayers, instead of larger for those in higher brackets, and would cause underinsured persons to increase their coverage. By allowing lower-income people larger credits and refunding the credit in cash if the tax due did not absorb it, a kind of "national health insurance" could be achieved. Most important, use of tax policy as a vehicle for national health insurance would strengthen, rather than destroy, private incentives for cost containment and reduce, rather than increase, the need for regulation.

(2) Encouragement of active competition between and among health insurers, HMOs, and new models of health care financing and delivery, such as Dr. Paul Ellwood's "health care alliances."[19] It is in choosing a prepaid health plan or health insurance coverage that consumers are in the best position to give effect to their preferences and to face, at least indirectly, the trade-offs among the quantity, quality, efficacy, style, and cost of services. It is important to realize that, partly because of the tax-induced distortions of demand described above, competition among health plans has in the past been weak in stimulating innovations to contain costs, and many promising approaches have heretofore never been tried. Private cost-containment efforts, while a kind of rationing, are preferable to public controls because they are essentially consensual, not coercive, and permit the benefits of economizing to accrue to the affected group. The sensitive politics of cost containment, though still a factor in the administration of private controls, are less likely to prevent appropriate levels of stringency from being approached.

(3) Removal of legal and other restraints on innovation in cost containment by employers, unions, health insurers, and others. Aside from the tax laws, the greatest obstacles to private cost-containment initiatives are the restraints long practiced by members of the medical profession against unwanted limitations on their freedom to ignore costs. The antitrust laws are conveniently available to overcome such restraints and clear the way for competitive innovation by insurers and others.[20] With the antitrust laws and competition at work, provider dominance could be undercut to a degree not possible in a regulated system. Indeed, it is an important insight that, in a system dominated by government, concerted political action by providers is constitutionally protected and bound to have a powerful effect, whereas in a market-oriented system providers are prohibited from taking collective action to prevent change in the consumer's interest.

(4) Change in the means of subsidizing the purchasing power of Medicare and Medicaid eligible

persons so as to allow their cost consciousness to play some part in the containment of health care costs. A voucher system (or a system of refundable tax credits) could be designed to permit Medicare and Medicaid beneficiaries to exercise, within limits, a choice between additional health benefits and cash. Although it seems sensible to encourage the private sector to offer a range of options to voucher-carrying beneficiaries of public programs, the existing Medicare and Medicaid programs would also be improved by revitalizing the remainder of the market, because that step would make such concepts as "usual and customary fees" and "customary practice" meaningful once again and therefore valuable as yardsticks for public programs.

Although interest in strengthening competition in the health sector has recently picked up a bit, no one in Congress or in the Carter administration is currently working on the design of a legislative program based on the foregoing principles.[21] Our vast policymaking apparatus appears instead to be pursuing the impossible dream of effective regulation and, trapped by self-fulfilling prophecies about regulation's inevitability, is letting slip past the last clear chance to organize a health care system in which consumers with professional help, rather than regulators or organized providers, would dictate the appropriate level and type of health care spending and the appropriate degree and methods of cost containment. Perhaps the scenario presented here of increasingly limited freedom of choice, increasingly arbitrary regulation, and an increasing squeeze on providers, designed to force them to accept the burden of rationing care, may yet scare some influential and far-sighted providers, employers, and consumer groups into seeking a responsible and workable alternative that would keep more of the crucial decisions in the hands of the individuals directly concerned.

NOTES

1. Economist Uwe E. Reinhardt describes the issue in this way, capturing the essential point that it is market failure, not cost alone, that matters. Address by Uwe E. Reinhardt, National Health Leadership Conference on Controlling Health Care Costs, Washington, D.C. (June 26, 1977).

2. The classic demonstration of these problems, which reviews the technical literature, is A.L. COCHRANE, EFFECTIVENESS AND EFFICIENCY: RANDOM REFLECTIONS ON HEALTH SERVICES (1972).

3. Schultze, *The Public Use of Private Interest*, HARPER'S, May 1977, at 43, 44.

4. *Id.* at 62.

5. *See, e.g.*, Havighurst, *Regulation of Health Facilities and Services by "Certificate of Need,"* 59 VA. L. REV. 1143 (1973); Noll, *The Consequences of Public Utility Regulation of Hospitals*, in INSTITUTE OF MEDICINE, CONTROLS ON HEALTH CARE (1975).

6. *E.g.*, Salkever and Bice, *The Impact of Certificate-of-Need Controls on Hospital Investment*, 54 MILBANK MEMORIAL FUND Q.: HEALTH AND SOCIETY 185 (1976); Hellinger, *The Effect of Certificate-of-Need Legislation on Hospital Investment*, 13 INQUIRY 187 (1976): Special Section, *Prospective Reimbursement*, 13 INQUIRY 274 (1976) (results here are mixed but hardly reassuring). Unpublished studies of the PSRO program, conducted under the auspices of the Health Services Administration of HEW, show negligible impact on utilization and costs.

This is not the place to examine these and other studies, which give rise to substantial disputes over methodology and other factors. The text statement is perhaps debatable, but the lack of demonstrable success is striking.

7. The HSAs, as local planning agencies, could make an interesting difference if they were dedicated to "hard" planning, but there are many signs that planning methodologies are weak and that politics plays a predominant role. On the general problem, see Havighurst, *supra* note 5, at 1194–1204.

8. Usually rationing involves simply giving equal portions to each within broad functional categories defined by objective circumstances. Rationing health care requires parcelling out medical services in accordance with relative need, which entails comparing incommensurables and making myriad social valuations, all in a context fraught with potential personal tragedy.

9. *See* Havighurst and Blumstein, *Coping with Quality/Cost Trade-Offs in Medicare Care: The Role of PSROs*, 70 Nw. U.L. REV. 6 (1975); Havighurst, Blumstein and Bovbjerg, *Strategies in Underwriting the Costs of Catastrophic Disease*, 40 LAW AND CONTEMPORARY PROB. 122, 150–53 (1976). These sources argue, among other things, that PSROs could "ration" better if they were seen not as regulatory agencies but as agencies to define and appropriately limit the coverage of federal health programs.

10. Responses to a questionnaire recently circulated by the author indicated that 40 of 44 HSA administrators feel that "to eliminate duplication of services and save the costs of underutilized capital assets" is a better statement of the purpose of certificate-of-need

laws than "to limit the availability of facilities as a means of forcing providers to make hard choices about their use." *See also* Havighurst and Blumstein, *The Role of PSROs, supra* note 9, at 33–35; Havighurst, Blumstein, and Bovbjerg, *Catastrophic Disease, supra* note 9, at 145–50.

11. *See* Havighurst and Blumstein, *The Role of PSROs, supra* note 9, at 17.

12. *See generally* Havighurst, Blumstein, and Bovbjerg, *Catastrophic Disease, supra* note 9, at 138–53.

13. George Stigler and Claire Friedland have observed that "innumerable regulatory actions are conclusive proof, not of effective regulation, but of the desire to regulate." Stigler and Friedland, *What Can Regulators Regulate? The Case of Electricity,* 5 J. Law & Econ. 1 (1962). Counting applications and denials may be meaningless since multiple applications to build a certain facility or to invest the same funds are possible. Also, applications granted are not always acted on, suggesting that not all are equally serious. Furthermore, planners take credit for modifying proposals— *e.g.*, cutting a 10-story hospital down to 5—yet applicants may have inflated their requests. Empirical studies are necessary to document real changes. *Compare* Salkever and Bice, *Impact of Certificate-of-Need, supra* note 6, with Bicknell and Walsh, *Certification-of-Need: The Massachusetts Experience,* 292 New Eng. J. Med. 1054 (1975).

14. "The Hospital Cost-Containment Act of 1977," H.R. 6575, 95th Cong., 1st Sess. (1977). Another current example of emerging arbitrariness in regulation is National Guidelines for Health Planning, 42 Fed. Reg. 48,501 (1977). *See "Numbers Game" by HEW Concerns Critics of Draft Guidelines for Health Planning,* Health Planning and Manpower Reports, November 28, 1977, at 2.

15. *E.g.,* Interview with Joseph A. Califano, Jr., Secretary of HEW, on NBC's "Today" Show (October 11, 1977).

16. *See* Havighurst, Blumstein, and Bovbjerg, *Catastrophic Disease, supra* note 9, at 155–57; Blumstein, *Constitutional Perspectives on Government Decisions Affecting Human Life and Health,* 40 Law and Contemp. Prob. 237 (1976).

17. *See* R. Crossman, A Politician's View of Health Service Planning 26 (1972); Bosanquet, *Inequities in the Health Service,* 17 New Society 809, 912 (1974). Moreover, even though Britain has achieved a commendable emphasis on primary care and family practice, this allocational success resulted more from the preexisting and largely fortuitous subdivision of the medical profession into consultants and general practitioners than from any special success in combatting professional solidarity or in changing professional values.

18. For a fuller discussion of this issue, *see* Havighurst, *Controlling Health Care Costs: Strengthening the Private Sector's Hand,* 1 J. Health Politics, Policy & Law 471 (1977); Havighurst, The Role of Competition in Containing Health Care Costs, Address to the Federal Trade Commission Conference on Competition in the Health Care Sector, Washington, D.C. (June 1–2, 1977).

19. *See A New Scheme to Force You to Compete for Patients,* Medical Economics, March 21, 1977, at 23.

20. *See* Havighurst, The Role of Competition, *supra* note 18.

21. However, Professor Alain Enthoven, working as a part time consultant for HEW, has developed a substantial proposal for a "Consumer Choice Health Plan" that is currently being circulated in the bureaucracy. While this proposal contemplates somewhat less competition and somewhat more regulatory dictation than the proposal sketched here, it is unique among national health insurance proposals in the extent to which it would permit resources to be allocated by relying on the decisions of cost-conscious consumers.

1.4 Governmental Regulation of Health Care: A Response to Some Criticisms Voiced by Proponents of a "Free Market"

STEPHEN M. WEINER, LL.B.

Reprinted with permission of the American Society of Law & Medicine, Inc. and the Massachusetts Institute of Technology, from 4 *American Journal of Law & Medicine* 15–33 (1978). Copyright © 1978 by the American Society of Law & Medicine, Inc. and the Massachusetts Institute of Technology. All rights reserved.

ABSTRACT

In this Comment, the Massachusetts Rate Setting Commissioner takes issue with the criticism of health care cost-containment regulation that was expressed by Professor Clark C. Havighurst in a recent edition of the *Journal,* and argues that instead of abandoning regulation in favor of various "free market" alternatives recommended by Professor Havighurst, the nation should find ways to make regulation work more effectively in the public interest. The author challenges Professor Havighurst on the ground that he fails to recognize (1) that the free market model is inadequate for evaluating regulatory activity and (2) that regulation is essentially a political process, and therefore regulatory objectives cannot and should not be defined in economic terms alone. What is needed, suggests Mr. Weiner, is acceptance of the need for, and validity of, regulation, and an examination of how regulation can best achieve its economic and political objectives. The key challenge for policy makers in the health care regulatory field, he asserts, is the clarification and implementation of appropriate relationships (1) between health care regulation and health care rationing; (2) between health care regulation and health care planning; and (3) between health care regulation and health care competition.

I. INTRODUCTION

In a recent *American Journal of Law & Medicine* Comment entitled *Health Care Cost-Containment Regulation: Prospects and an Alternative,*[1] Professor Clark C. Havighurst, one of the nation's best known proponents of a "free market" approach to the delivery of health services, once again sounds his two basic themes: (1) governmental regulation of the health care delivery system inevitably will fail in its cost-containment objectives; and (2) free market alternatives should actively be developed to supplant current regulatory initiatives. To these points he now adds a third: cost control through governmental regulation has a chance of being effective only if it is accompanied by an explicit political decision in favor of true rationing of health care resources. Professor Havighurst suggests that such a decision is not likely to occur; therefore, inferentially, the frail reed upon which potentially successful regulation could lean will break.

Unfortunately, Professor Havighurst's analyses do not provide any practical solutions to current health policy problems, nor do they even adequately frame the kinds of questions one must ask in order to produce such solutions. The purpose of this Comment is to identify the critical questions related to sound policy development in areas affecting health care delivery, and to offer alternative solutions to the public regulatory issues they raise.

This Comment focuses on four matters of immediate concern to health care policy makers: the likelihood that health care policies relying upon governmental regulation will succeed (Part II); the relationship between health care rationing and health care regulation (Part III); the relationship between health care planning and health care regulation (Part IV); and the viability of the market approaches espoused by Professor Havighurst as alternatives to regulation (Part V). At times in the discussion, Professor Havighurst's positions will be analyzed critically; at other times they will be utilized as a starting point for the exploration of pertinent topics. This Comment concludes with a summary of key questions confronting policy making in the health care regulatory field.

II. ASSESSING REGULATION'S PROSPECTS: THE IMPORTANCE OF USING CORRECT CRITERIA

Professor Havighurst rightly asserts that many of the recent regulatory initiatives affecting the health care delivery system are aimed at cost containment.[2] But the correctness of his analysis ends there. Deriving his analytic framework from theories developed in studies of regulation in other sectors of the economy, he wrongly assumes that the conclusion reached in each of those studies—that regulation has "failed"— must apply to regulation in the health care system as well.[3]

Professor Havighurst's assumptions are incorrect, in part, because they are developed from a narrow base. The analyses upon which he relies were undertaken by a group of economists who pursue the ideal of the "free market." They tend to analyze regulation by postulating what economic results would have occurred in a free market and contrasting those results with the outputs of governmental regulation. There are two major difficulties with their analyses that Professor Havighurst fails to avoid: they make use of a market model that is not well suited to an evaluation of regulatory activity; and they assume that regulatory objectives can and should be defined in economic terms alone.

A. The Free Market Bias

Professor Havighurst fails to note that alternative economic models of equal or superior intellectual validity are available that do not produce the same pessimistic outlook on regulation as does his free market model. Professor Victor Goldberg, for example, observes that the "tradi-

tional" economic criticism of regulation uses as its model the notion of a "discrete transaction" between a buyer and a seller who conduct their transactions in the market place at a fixed point in time.[4] Criticizing this approach, he suggests that the "discrete transaction" model inadequately characterizes the complex interrelationships that exist between buyers and sellers in many modern marketplaces.[5] Increasingly more common is an economic relationship defined by an "administered contract." The "administered contract" exhibits either or both of two elements. First, it involves a contractual relationship between principals that continues for an extended period of time, rather than occurring only at a fixed point in time, and that establishes a framework for redefining contractual terms and conditions as circumstances change over time. Second, this relationship involves a reliance upon agents for the fulfillment of such functions as gathering and analyzing essential information, making binding decisions, and adjusting the terms of the ongoing contractual relationships between the principals.[6]

Professor Goldberg notes that regulation "can be viewed as an [implied] administered contract in which both elements [described above] are significant."[7] He states:[8]

By attempting to analyze regulation within a discrete transaction framework, economists have suppressed the most significant aspects of the regulatory arrangement and this has led to an overstatement of the case against regulation. First, that framework generates the wrong criteria against which regulation is to be evaluated. Second, when viewed in an administered contracts perspective, regulatory policies that would appear indefensible in a discrete transactions world can be seen to have a (loose) efficiency rationale. And finally, a failure to appreciate the complexity of contractual arrangements in the private sector is apt to leave the analyst unduly sanguine as to the efficacy of private market solutions to problems in the regulatory sector.

The analysis offered by Professor Goldberg, while not providing a rationale for extending regulation further into all segments of the economy,[9] does persuasively argue that regulation is not by its nature an economically, or for that matter, socially, irrational activity. In addition, Professor Goldberg's analysis underscores the importance of making explicit, and evaluating the validity of, the economic models used to analyze and to critique regulation.

No model can lay sole claim to legitimacy. Professor Havighurst fails to recognize this. What's worse, he fails to assess the significant deficiencies of his own model, which appears to be based on the "discrete transaction" approach. Therefore, he develops what are at best partial perceptions of the economic implications of regulation in health care and, at worst, distortions of the proper role and function of health care regulation.

B. Beyond Economics

More broadly, it is not clear that regulation should or can be evaluated in strictly economic terms. Although analysis of regulation seems to have moved in recent years from the political scientists to the economists,[10] regulation is fundamentally a political process, and the decision to regulate is a political decision.[11]

The rhetoric supporting the decision to regulate may rely primarily or even exclusively upon economic terminology, but the process producing a regulatory program involves conflict, cooperation, and compromise among diverse interests, each concerned with its own set of issues relating to status, power, and economics. Only economic determinists could conclude that the decision is solely economic in nature. Because of the political nature of the decision, it may be possible to identify the motivation for a regulatory program, but it is likely to be very difficult to identify its objectives with great precision. The definition of objectives varies with the interest groups involved in the process, and the ambiguity of enabling act language resulting from political compromise increases the difficulty of developing an objective statement of goals.[12]

Indeed, in many situations, the only discernible objective of legislation establishing a regulatory program is to delegate to administrative agencies the responsibility and authority to deal with the problems and issues that created the need for legislation in the first place. In functioning on the basis of that delegation, the agency develops policy, and thereby defines the regulatory program's objectives. The reasons for such delegation vary. For example, the legislative forum may be poorly suited to resolving the competing interests affected by the program, so that broad or vague language serves to remove the resolution to the administrative level; or the nature of the problem or of the affected interests may preclude the fixing of specific and long-term solutions in legislative form.

Whatever the cause, delegation of regulatory authority to an administrative agency involves the transfer of a political (and therefore a bargaining) process from a legislative arena to an administrative one. The process of administrative decision making, the process by which the agency exercises the discretion vested in it by the legislature, encompasses outcomes, generally viewed as economic in nature because they impact on the distribution of economic resources, that result from the relative political or power relationships among the parties who are benefited, protected, or harmed by the process. There is no preordained outcome, in the sense that there is no inevitability that one party to the process will always be predominant. Social policy and values become articulated and implemented through the shifting power relationships among the parties interested in and affected by the regulatory process, including the administrative agency itself. It is through this activity that policy objectives are determined and refined.

The process of regulation, then, requires the development of a long-term set of relationships among public and private parties. How the regulatory agency balances those varying interests at any one point in time with respect to any one decision is the proper subject of legal, political, and economic analyses of the regulatory process. For purposes of this Comment, though, it is important to perceive that the political nature of that process precludes the facile positing of a static "optimal result" of the regulatory process.[13] The individual outcomes of regulatory activities, and therefore the de facto definition of regulatory objectives, are a function of the current status of the various fluid relationships within the process at the time the decision is made.[14] In such a situation, it is inappropriate to evaluate regulation against any abstracted standards or norms, including the use of a preconceived economic model as the referent, without acknowledging that any such effort reflects the value structure of the commentator, and not necessarily the value structure of the agency.

Because of the described political nature of the regulatory process, the defining of regulatory *objectives* is far more complex than many economic analysts suggest.[15] Analyses of the administration of regulatory programs should focus on understanding the tools available to the parties for defining and effecting those objectives and the factors that make a difference in using those tools.

Professor Havighurst's analysis lacks concern for these types of issues. His ideological preference is antiregulation. But that orientation does not relieve him of some responsibility for (1) examining the processes by which the objectives of regulatory agencies are specified, (2) identifying those objectives most likely to emerge in the health care regulatory setting, and (3) proposing constructive changes in the process to achieve whatever different objectives he may feel are more appropriate for the agencies under review. This is particularly so, given the current realities of active health care regulation and of the likelihood that such active regulation will continue into the future.

III. RATIONING AND REGULATION: PROVIDERS' ROLE IN AN EXPLICIT RELATIONSHIP

In his Comment, Professor Havighurst recognizes and examines the link between rationing and cost-containment regulation in the health care delivery system. Unfortunately, he does not explore the full subtleties of that relationship. According to Professor Havighurst, cost-containment regulation of health care is a rationing process, but, because of the political sensitivity associated with rationing of health care, regulators do not want the general public to understand that.[16] As a result, says Professor Havighurst, regulators attempt to shift responsibility for rationing onto the providers, thereby guaranteeing a perpetuation of "the very provider dominance which has . . . been an important source of the health sector's problems in the first place."[17]

Several responses to Professor Havighurst's points about rationing are appropriate. As to the first part of his argument (that cost-containment regulation is really rationing), it is naive to state

that public agencies try to obscure the fact that rationing may result from cost-containment regulation. That cost containment entails rationing is tautological, and regulatory agencies have not avoided recognizing and acknowledging the rationing implications of their actions.

"Cost containment" implies the need to conserve a resource—namely, the services of facilities and personnel that otherwise would be expended by the health care sector of our economy, and that, due to their conservation, may be utilized elsewhere. Its implementation requires the presence of strategies for determining who is entitled to use available resources and when they may use them, that is, strategies for rationing.

For example, the primary thrust of current cost-containment regulation is directed toward the hospital sector. Hospital cost-containment regulation has attempted to place very clearly articulated constraints on economic resources available to hospitals, in terms both of capital and of operating revenue.[18] Such regulatory programs as hospital rate-setting programs and state certificate-of-need programs are evolving increasingly sophisticated techniques for measuring the legitimacy of hospitals' demands for economic resurces.[19] One of the stated objectives of hospital-cost regulation is to restrain further increases in that most expensive and most rapidly escalating segment of the health system, and thereby achieve savings which could be reallocated to less costly, but equally appropriate, modalities of providing service.[20] There is an explicit link between hospital regulation and the need to allocate, reallocate, and limit health care resources, that is, to ration.[21]

In the second part of his argument, Professor Havighurst states that regulators seek to avoid facing up to the present realities and to the future implications of rationing by shifting responsibility for it onto the providers of care. He sees such a strategy as permitting the regulatory agency to avoid making the hard decisions,[22] and suggests that this is an inappropriate course to follow. But in fact it is an appropriate strategy, for three principal reasons.

First, as a political process, health care regulation—like regulation in other spheres—functions best when it establishes parameters within which the parties to the process are to operate. Those parameters represent politically agreed-upon limitations on the delivery system.

The development of such limitations is fundamentally a governmental process because it is unlikely that private groups, absent the potentiality of coercive governmental action, could produce such consensus. Individual case judgments within those parameters, however, need not necessarily be made by governmental action. If the parameters represent a public decision concerning resource allocation generally, the specific allocation of those resources need not be a public concern, so long as the parameters are not violated.[23] Further, government is better suited to deal with aggregated abstracts. Where decisions affect identifiable individuals, the political process invariably produces a skewing of resources in support of the individual, regardless of the social and economic cost.[24] Focused judgments affecting individuals or specific cases should be left to private providers who understand both the subtleties of the immediate case and the general parameters developed within the socially and politically agreed-upon process. The potential for an individual provider to undermine the parameters by exploitation of the individual case—a matter of some apparent concern to Professor Havighurst[25]—is itself a factor in the political calculus producing the rules.

Second, Professor Havighurst expresses concern that a regulatory strategy shifting rationing responsibilities to providers will reinforce their proclivity for costly approaches to health care. This argument, though, does not recognize the importance of the fact that the primary focus of cost-containment regulation is on hospitals. Existing reimbursement systems have tended to provide a substantial incentive for high-cost activities among physicians in a hospital setting. Cost-containment regulation, by attempting to limit the otherwise unlimited resources available to hospitals, should revise that trend and create competition among physicians for access to those available resources. Under such circumstances, high-cost behavior would not be rewarded. Indeed, one would expect a number of phenomena to occur over a period of time, specifically (1) high-cost physicians would be viewed increasingly by their peers as disproportionate users of resources and therefore as threats to the ability of their peers to obtain desired resources, and (2) some internal mechanism, either through the medical staff, the administrator, or the trustees, would have to be found for establishing an effective intrahospital

allocation system that considers the physician, patient, and other interests that are at play. The result of such a process might be a very balanced private decision-making process for determining the usage of each institution's available resources according to need, a result not likely to be achieved in systems in which supply is not constrained.

Third, Professor Havighurst would prefer to use consumer choice, not government constraint of supply, as the allocating mechanism.[26] This goal is laudable except for one problem with his analysis: he says that consumer choice is to be exercised with the benefit of "professional advice." In that context, the "professional" being referred to must be the health care provider, especially the physician. Yet is it likely, given their natural economic instincts, that providers' advice to individual patients will produce "socially optimal" results? If informed consumer choice in the health field is largely a function of receiving good "professional advice," why won't the very education, training, and orientation of providers toward high-cost, relatively inefficient forms of treatment, which necessitated the recent growth in regulation, also structure the advice they give patients in the absence of regulatory programs constraining supply?

In summary, Professor Havighurst is correct in seeing rationing as an objective of *hospital* cost-containment regulation, although he overstates the extent to which the nature of that objective has been obscured by policy makers and implementers. He is wrong, however, in his apparent assumption that the "success or failure" of regulation in the hospital sector is predetermined. It is not. Its success or failure is dependent upon the agency's capacity, through the regulatory process, (1) to identify objectives that may, from the point of view of political analysis, be considered as conducive to the "public interest,"[27] (2) to secure political acceptance of the objectives by taking measures to insure that they are perceived as in the "public interest," and (3) to fulfill the objectives.

This "political" process of regulation means that there can be no *a priori* decision with respect to regulation's success or failure. It also means, though, that the process functions most expeditiously when the major interest groups affected by the regulatory decision are relatively few in number. Some of Professor Havighurst's pessimism may be warranted, however, if one recognizes that the *likelihood* of successful regulation *diminishes* (although, as will be seen, neither total, nor even partial failure becomes inevitable) as cost-containment forms of regulation, entailing rationing concepts, extend beyond the hospital sector of the health care system. Hospital regulation, while complex technically, involves the traditional discretely defined triad of interest groups present in most regulatory processes: one class of providers,[28] affected consumers,[29] and the agency.[30] The preceding sentence may contain something of an oversimplification. But it does present a relatively simple structure in contrast to the complexity of interests that would be involved in and affected by regulation of the *health system* generally.

The traditional procedural mechanisms available to a regulatory agency could very well become overloaded if they were to serve as the sole channel for allocating limited dollars among the vast array of competing demands in the health system. Once beyond the hospital sector, the trade-offs involved in health regulation, and the ethical dilemmas that rationing and resource allocation genuinely raise, may become too complex to be handled by a governmental process most capable of dealing with relatively discretely defined interests.

This observation, though, does not suggest that the failure of system-wide cost-containment regulation is a foregone conclusion. The point is simply that in classing all cost-containment regulation together, Professor Havighurst fails to discern that the tasks required for successful hospital regulation may be different from the tasks required for successful health care regulation more generally. This distinction suggests that, as the political decision is made to extend cost-containment regulation beyond hospitals, it is necessary to examine traditional regulatory organization and process to determine what types of changes may be appropriate to adapt them to the particular features of the health delivery system. What is needed, at least in part, is the development of some structure better suited than the traditional regulatory agency to handle the complexity of interests normally involved in decision making. The necessity of this analysis is one of the more exciting intellectual challenges facing students of regulation generally and of health regulation specifically. It raises foursquare the importance of linking two of the most significant structures to emerge in health

policy: regulation and planning. Yet Professor Havighurst, because of his preconceived notion of regulation, fails to identify and to address the importance of this linkage. The next Part of this Comment focuses on the relationship between regulation and planning in the context specifically of the foregoing analysis of regulation.

IV. HEALTH REGULATION AND HEALTH PLANNING: FORGING A NEW LINK

Congress recognizes that the health care delivery segment of the economy raises unique questions for public policy. By passing P.L. 93-641 (the National Health Planning and Resources Development Act of 1974),[31] it created a nationwide network of (1) regional (within states) health planning agencies called health systems agencies (HSAs), which are required by law to be governed by boards widely representative of the diverse interests involved in health care delivery,[32] (2) state health planning and development agencies (SHPDAs),[33] and (3) statewide health coordinating councils (SHCCs).[34] The HSAs are responsible for developing regional health plans;[35] the SHCC, in conjunction with the SHPDA, for developing a state health plan.[36] The plans are expected to contain objectives, agreed upon by the members of the respective responsible bodies, for allocating health care resources, that is, for the rationing of health dollars among the various sectors of the system, based on standards and criteria or predetermined priorities developed by the organizations after consideration of national health planning guidelines and priorities.[37]

The planning system created by P.L. 93-641 is a somewhat unusual phenomenon. Resource allocation decisions in the United States traditionally have occurred either through direct government regulation or through voluntary decisions by private individuals or organizations (the market). Under P.L. 93-641, government requires that the resource allocation decisions be made; yet the agencies primarily responsible for making those decisions are themselves private (although some might say that they are "quasi-private" or even "quasi-public") organizations[38] or have a majority of members designated by private organizations,[39] and have no regulatory authority to enforce their decisions.[40]

This new health planning structure does, though, present challenges and opportunities for health care regulation. As was suggested above, regulation, as a political process, is expected to evaluate diverse and often conflicting views, to weight them, and to produce a result that represents some balance among them. Traditional regulatory structure may not be sufficiently flexible to deal directly with the multiplicity of interests involved in health care delivery. The planning structure, particularly the organizational composition of the HSAs, may provide an appropriate alternative forum for working out many of the differing or conflicting views. If the system "worked well,"[41] it would likely be possible to view the state and regional plans as expressions of public policy that provide generally acceptable guidelines for regulatory decision making. The resource allocation (*i.e.,* rationing) decisions contained in such plans, representing the end product of a consensual process, would bear a certain political legitimacy, and therefore political acceptability, that strictly governmental decisions might lack.

Such a relationship between planning and regulation raises a constellation of problems requiring immediate study.[42] One set of problems concerns how to cope in the *private* HSA arena with the kinds of problems also faced by *public* regulatory bodies, such as (1) assuring adequate access for all affected interests,[43] (2) avoiding provider dominance (for example, by offering incentives for nonprovider participation), and (3) assuring adequate competency of staff. As to the first concern, the extent to which the privately organized planning agencies, as they become increasingly involved in regulatory activities, will become subject to due process or access requirements similar to those imposed on public agencies remains to be worked out. As to the second and third concerns, it is possible that the opportunity of enforcing planning decisions through regulatory decisions may provide sufficient incentive to attract broad public (especially nonprovider) participation in, and competent staff for, the planning agencies. Reinforcement of this incentive, and mechanisms for addressing all three of the enumerated concerns, must be carefully developed.

Another set of problems arising from linking planning with regulation relates to the legal competence of regulatory agencies to rely on the health systems plans developed by HSAs, and state plans adopted by SHCCs on the basis of HSA plans, as policy guidelines for decision making. Such reliance on the HSA and SHCC plans may raise a question as to whether the regulatory agency has in fact unlawfully delegated its responsibility for policy development to private organizations. This question, in turn, requires that consideration be given to the process for incorporating HSA and SHCC policies into regulatory decisions without undermining or avoiding the usual administrative law requirements. Such a process should include specification as to the type of review the regulatory agency will undertake of planning agency determinations and the extent to which parties dissatisfied with planning agency recommendations or findings may use regulatory agency procedures as an appeal mechanism. In short, any formal interlinking of the regulatory and planning processes poses unusual questions for traditional administrative law.

Related to these problems is the broader question of the extent to which planning agencies and regulatory agencies in fact share common objectives. Briefly put, the question is: How likely are planning agencies to share the orientation of cost-containment regulation? In relying on planning processes, would cost-containment regulatory agencies be taking a risk that planning outcomes may produce cost pressures that are undesirable from the point of view of these agencies?[44]

In spite of the problems, however, there is some basis for expecting a sharing of objectives between the two systems. Rapid increases in the cost of health care, and government's increasing unwillingness (political) or inability (economic) to pay more for it, have created a very real need to limit further increases and to reallocate existing levels of spending to more cost-effective modalities of care. Cost containment is explicitly viewed as an alternative to reductions in health benefit entitlements or as a prerequisite for further extensions in such entitlements.[45] Planning agencies, because they are concerned with benefits and entitlements, should become increasingly sensitized to the need to pursue cost-containment objectives in order to redirect current levels of spending toward needed new services. Also, and somewhat more cynically, in the final analysis the willingness of regulatory agencies to rely on planning agency work product is a function of the extent to which planning agencies develop objectives that are acceptable to the regulatory agencies. Any significant and continuing divergencies could eventually overcome the political desire of the regulatory agency to use the "political" structure of the planning agencies, and thereby deprive the planning agencies of their ability to use the regulatory process for implementation of their goals.

While complex, the problems discussed above should not be permitted to overly discourage us from striving to link cost-containment regulation and planning. From the planning standpoint, the linkage presents the possibility of planning outputs and priorities being directly translated into action that structures and shapes the health care delivery system. From the regulation standpoint, the linkage establishes a capacity to handle politically the multiplicity of interests in the health field and to produce intelligent, legitimate, and accepted policies.

Furthermore, such a link could help health care regulatory agencies to take more risks and to function more flexibly than regulatory agencies operating in other economic sectors. The fact that the health system has a far greater diversity of actors than other sectors of the economy, and that there is a planning structure available that provides for representation of these diverse actors, suggests that the public need not rely exclusively on regulation to achieve policy objectives. Regulation could in fact interact with nonregulatory mechanisms to coordinate the attainment of policy objectives. The existence of such possibilities makes the prospect of future studies of health care regulation especially exciting. Yet the position taken by Professor Havighurst virtually excludes exploring these possibilities, and therefore will tend to be increasingly irrelevant as evolving concepts of sound public policy continue to support the use of regulation.

Professor Havighurst's emphasis on competitive mechanisms as alternatives to regulation, then, avoids his addressing the relevant questions facing regulation. But even given this, it is necessary to consider whether his proposals contain real alternatives to regulation and, if so, what the relationship should be between them and regulation.

V. REGULATION AND COMPETITION

Professor Havighurst proposes that we replace regulation with competitive mechanisms.

But in some cases his proposed mechanisms are qualitatively no different from direct regulation. For example, he proposes a restructuring of what he perceives in the Internal Revenue Code to be unhealthy incentives for excess purchase of health insurance. He cites no empirical evidence in his Comment to demonstrate the effect of these incentives. His tax proposal is weak on two grounds. First, he overstates the extent to which the tax laws produce such a result. Health insurance is technically a tax-free benefit when purchased by employers, because the premium expense may be claimed as a business deduction. But the premiums are still an expense which employers, interested in maximizing profit, presumably will try to avoid,[46] and this expense has in fact become a major concern of employers.[47] Health insurance coverage has emerged as a significant issue in collective bargaining.[48] Even without changes in the tax laws, the high cost of health care, and particularly hospital care, is already forcing employers to reevaluate the scope of coverage they are willing to provide to their employees.

Further, existing tax laws are not structured to encourage excessive purchases of health insurance by individuals, as even a cursory reading of Form 1040 indicates. For individual taxpayers, health insurance expense is not treated as a business deduction but as a medical deduction subject to specific limitations. Only one-half of health insurance premiums up to $150 is deductible. The balance is deductible only if medical expenses exceed 3 percent of adjusted gross income, and even these benefits are available only to taxpayers who itemize deductions. Thus, individuals do bear a real economic burden in purchasing health insurance.

Second, Professor Havighurst's tax proposal is puzzling even in terms of his own biases. Manipulation of spending habits by use of the tax system is no less economically coercive than direct governmental regulation,[49] and is no more immune to unpredictable effects. What appears to be a simple approach masks the very complex necessity of *someone* (1) determining for purposes of a credit structure what is an adequate or appropriate level of coverage, so that the tax structure does not encourage underinsurance, (2) structuring a precisely defined system of tax credits to produce the desired result, and (3) doing all of this without increasing the tax bill of the "average taxpayer."[50]

The decision as to the amount of the credit, which in effect is a decision as to who will be able to afford significant coverage, is made either legislatively or by regulation. It is not a matter for private choice, although private choice concerning insurance purchases will be based on it. As such, the credit system moves very close to direct regulation of the availability and price of insurance policies, but is different from current cost-containment approaches in a significant way not mentioned by Professor Havighurst: it moves critical health policy decisions away from the agencies directly concerned with the health care delivery system to a terrain (*i.e.,* tax law) unfamiliar to most health experts and health consumers. The tax manipulation approach could thereby unproductively or unnecessarily distort market decision making as well as reduce public scrutiny of governmental decisions.

Some of Professor Havighurst's proposals do, of course, have merit. For example, he notes the important cost-containment pressures inherent in prepaid group medical practices, generally known as health maintenance organizations (HMOs).[51] But without belaboring the advantages or disadvantages of his various proposals, it is sufficient to note that all of his proposals contain a common defect: his analysis concentrates to the exclusion of other essential considerations, on his preference to pursue market alternatives to regulation and, therefore, he chooses to ignore the policy problems raised by the existence and the realities of regulation. As a result, he makes no effort either to explore in what ways regulation and market alternatives can be integrated within a consistent framework, or to view regulation as a device with the potential for establishing, reinforcing, or protecting, market approaches.[52] The very heterogeneity of the health care system suggests that, like planning and regulation, both the market and regulation may have roles to play, roles that could be mutually reinforcing.

Much analytic effort is required to define the respective roles of regulation and competition, including ways in which regulation can foster more competitive incentives. True, such health interactions have not characterized other regulated sectors of the economy. But the health care delivery system has some special characteristics, for example, heterogeneity, diversity of products, difficulty of defining product, and dif-

ferentiation between need and demand. These characteristics suggest the possibility of a mutually reinforcing and successful interaction between regulation and competition, so that efforts to establish such an interaction could be quite productive.

VI. CONCLUSION

Professor Havighurst's approach to health care policy focuses too narrowly on the necessity of developing "free choice" market mechanisms as alternatives to cost-containment regulation. In effect, he acknowledges that cost-containment regulation is an increasingly dominant force in the health care delivery system, but he fails to raise and to address the questions that should flow from that acknowledgment. Certainly the development of effective competitive mechanisms is important to achieve cost-containment objectives of public policy. But equally important is a more careful analysis to determine the appropriate role for regulation and the implications of that role for the health care system generally. Because health care regulation, and especially cost-containment regulation, is still in a relatively early stage of development, it is almost irresponsible to classify it as a "stopgap" without dealing with how it might be restructured or better managed so as to produce more desirable results. In this context, this Comment has attempted to identify a number of policy questions relating to cost-containment regulation that require more sustained attention and analysis. These questions are the following:

1. What are the appropriate criteria for evaluating the "success" of regulation in the health care delivery sector of our economy? Are any of the economic models relied upon by economists to analyze other sectors appropriate?
2. What modifications, if any, in the "traditional" structure and process of regulation are appropriate and desirable as a function of the peculiar characteristics of the health care delivery system?
3. How can a workable political process be structured around cost-containment regulation of the entire health care system, as opposed to merely the hospital sector? What mechanisms are available for assur-

ing that such regulation can, and indeed, will, function in the "public interest"?

4. What are the appropriate linkages between regulation and planning? To what extent can and should regulation rely on the output of the health planning process for policy guidance or direction?

5. What is the appropriate relationship between regulation and competition in achieving cost-containment objectives? To what extent can they coexist, and in what ways can they be mutually reinforcing in attaining their common objectives?

To give regulation of the health care delivery system a reasonable chance of being intelligent, sensitive, rational, and ultimately "successful," it is necessary to find answers to these questions. It is hoped that this Comment will stimulate and facilitate the search for such answers.

NOTES

1. Havighurst, *Health Care Cost-Containment Regulation: Prospects and an Alternative,* 3 AM. J.L. & MED. 309 (1977).

2. *Id.* at 309–10.

3. While Professor Havighurst does not specifically reference his intellectual antecedents in his Comment, except for a quotation from Charles Schultze, it is clear that they may be found in Chicago and at The Brookings Institute. *See, e.g.,* NOLL, REFORMING REGULATION (1971); Schultze, *The Public Use of the Private Interest,* HARPER'S, May 1977, at 43; Stigler, *The Theory of Economic Regulation,* 2 THE BELL JOURNAL OF ECONOMICS 3 (1971).

4. Goldberg, *Regulation and Administered Contracts,* 7 THE BELL JOURNAL OF ECONOMICS 426, 426 (1976).

5. *Id.* at 426–28.

6. *Id.* at 426–27.

7. *Id.* at 427.

8. *Id.*

9. Goldberg specifically warns that his argument "should not be construed as a brief for wall-to-wall regulation." *Id.*

10. Much of the recent literature on regulation appears either in economics-oriented journals, such as *The Bell Journal of Economics* or *The Journal of Law and Economics,* or in law reviews (*see, e.g., Symposium— Federal Regulatory Agencies: A Response to the Ash Report,* 57 VA. L. REV. 923 (1971) and the discussions of regulation and competition appearing at 82 YALE L.J. 871 (1973)). One of the most respected political science analysts of regulation complains about the paucity of good empirical research about regulatory process. Bernstein, *Independent Regulatory Agencies: A Perspective on Their Reform,* THE ANNALS OF THE AMERICAN ACADEMY OF POLITICAL AND SOCIAL SCIENCE, March 1972, at 14, 21.

11. An argument can even be made that there is no economic reason to regulate at all, that even the paradigmatic "natural monopoly" does not impel a public policy supporting governmental regulation. *See* Demsetz, *Why Regulate Utilities?* 11 J.L. & ECON. 55 (1968).

12. More often than not, enabling acts contain no specific economic criteria for regulatory decision making. For example, the Massachusetts Rate Setting Commission has the authority to establish "fair, reasonable and adequate" rates. MASS. GEN. LAWS ANN. ch. 6A, §32 (West Supp. 1977–1978). Is that an economic, political, social, or ethical criterion? Contrast this language with the very specific language governing the Massachusetts determination-of-need program for health care facilities:

> The [Massachusetts Department of Public Health], in making any [determination of need], shall encourage appropriate allocation of private and public health care resources and the development of alternative or substitute methods of delivering health care services so that adequate health care services will be made reasonably available to every person in the Commonwealth at the lowest reasonable aggregate cost.

MASS. GEN. LAWS ANN. ch. 111, §25C, para. 2 (West Supp. 1977–1978).

13. Professor Havighurst, for example, refers to the "socially optimal level of spending on health care." Havighurst, *supra* note 1, at 316.

14. For this reason, legal analysis tends to focus upon issues of access to and openness of the regulatory process and upon the avoidance of arbitrary action on the part of agencies. DAVIS, ADMINISTRATIVE LAW OF THE SEVENTIES 167–76 (1976); Davis, *A New Approach to Delegation,* 36 U. CHI. L. REV. 713 (1969); Lazarus & Onek, *The Regulators and the People,* 57 VA. L. REV. 1069, 1092–108 (1971).

15. In this context, one of the more pertinent aspects of Goldberg's argument is his use of an economic model that can be analyzed in political terms. Goldberg, *supra* note 4, at 445.

16. Havighurst, *supra* note 1, at 312–13.

17. *Id.* at 314.

18. *See, e.g.,* MASS. GEN. LAWS ANN. ch. 6A, §37 (West Supp. 1977–1978), which authorizes the Massachusetts Rate Setting Commission to approve hospital charge increases which are justified by (1) cost increases that are a function of inflation in the economy generally, (2) net volume increases, and (3) cost increases that are beyond the reasonable control of the individual hospital; and Massachusetts Rate Setting

Commission Regulation 14 CHSR 11 (1977), which sets out in detail the specific criteria which may permit a hospital's charges to increase. *See also* the proposed Hospital Cost Containment Act of 1977, H.R. 6575, 95th Cong., 1st Sess., introduced by the Carter Administration in April, 1977. Title I of the proposal would, over time, have the effect of limiting hospital revenue increases to changes in the Gross National Product deflator (*id.* §§111, 112), with certain specified exceptions, *see, e.g., id.* §124; Title II would establish an annual ceiling, proposed to be $2.5 billion, on capital investment in hospitals.

19. *See generally* Weiner, *"Reasonable Cost" Reimbursement Under Medicare and Medicaid: The Emergence of Public Control,* 3 AM. J.L. & MED. 1, 37–42 (1977).

20. COMMONWEALTH OF MASSACHUSETTS, HEALTH CARE EXPENDITURES IN MASSACHUSETTS: A WHITE PAPER DEVELOPED BY THE HEALTH PLANNING AND POLICY COMMITTEE 8 (1976).

21. The issue of whether cost-containment regulation does or does not entail rationing may be clouded by the existence of two different approaches to rationing. One approach involves establishing a flat dollar amount for resources flowing into the particular system, whether it be health care generally or the hospital sector specifically. Title II of the Administration's cost containment bill, *see* note 18, *supra,* is one of the rare examples of a proposal to cap the system with a flat dollar amount, although rhetoric expressing concern about the proportion of the Gross National Product going to health care does imply a proposal to limit health care resources to a specific dollar amount based on the GNP. This first approach requires political decisions as to the dollar amount and a process for allocating the specified resources.

A second approach involves identifying those factors that are considered to justify an increased investment of resources. The system in Massachusetts is of this type. *See* note 18, *supra.* Once the factors are identified, whatever dollar amounts they produce are held to be acceptable. (The GNP-based approach could fall into this model if it were viewed as saying that increased investment in health care resources is acceptable so long as it is directly related to increases in the GNP). In this approach, the actual dollars are not fixed for extended periods of time (usually no more than a year), and negotiation over the factors to be recognized can occur continuously.

22. Havighurst, *supra* note 1, at 314.

23. An analogy is the Massachusetts charge and budget review program administered by the Massachusetts Rate Setting Commission, referred to in note 18, *supra.* This program is organized to determine an acceptable level of total patient care charges, *see* 1976 Mass. Acts ch. 409, §5, on the basis of which unit charges are developed. The acceptable figure is an aggregated "bottom-line" figure representing total allowable revenue resources available to a hospital. The Massachusetts Rate Setting Commission does not require the hospital to expend the revenue in specific areas or for specific purposes. Those decisions, within the parameters of the allowable revenue figures, are to be made by each hospital's administration.

24. *See* Weiner, *State Regulation and Health Technology,* in TECHNOLOGY AND THE QUALITY OF HEALTH CARE 407, 421–23 (Egdahl & Gertman eds. to be published).

25. Havighurst, *supra* note 1, at 314–15.

26. *Id.* at 319.

27. There are at least two approaches to defining "the public interest." It may be equated with the interests of only one group in the regulatory process (consider, *e.g.,* recent tendencies to equate consumer interests with the "public interest," or, in a somewhat different context, the famous equation of the interests of General Motors with the interests of the United States). Or it may be determined by the regulatory agency weighing and melding the various conflicting interests surrounding it (including its own predilections as a bureaucratic interest). The two approaches become one if, in the first approach, the agency is viewed as placing full weight on the interests of one group and none on the others' interests. It is important, in analyzing an agency's process of defining objectives, to identify its approach to weighing and balancing interests.

28. The providers are, of course, never a monolith. Sensitive regulatory agencies—and analysts of same—need to be aware of discrete differences of interest among members of the supplier class. *See, e.g.,* Geller, *A Modest Proposal for Modest Reform of the Federal Communications Commission,* 63 GEO. L.J. 705 (1975), noting different interests among members of the communications industry and suggesting a certain level of competition among those interests for the favor of the Federal Communications Commission.

29. The consumers tend ordinarily to be represented, if at all, by third party payers, particularly the governmental health care programs, such as Medicare and Medicaid.

30. A peculiar feature of hospital regulation is that there are actually two classes of affected providers: hospitals and physicians. One could view the regulatory strategy of forcing "providers"—both classes—to make the discrete rationing decisions as in part aimed at minimizing the number of actors directly involved with the agency: as a result of the strategy, the hospital tends to represent both itself and the physicians before the agency and to take on the responsibility of dealing directly with the physicians.

31. Title XV of the Public Health Service Act, added by P.L. 93-641, §3, 88 Stat. 2227 (codified at 42 U.S.C. §§300k-300t (Supp. V 1975)). Title XVI of the Public

Health Service Act, inserted by P.L. 93-641, §4, is not germane to the discussion in the text.

32. HSAs may be private nonprofit organizations, public regional planning bodies, or single units of general local government. Public Health Service Act, Title XV, §1512(b)(c), 88 Stat. 2232 (codified at 42 U.S.C. §300*l*-1(b)(c)). Of the 205 HSAs that to date have received conditional or full designation from HEW, 180 are private nonprofit organizations, 4 are units of local government, and 21 are regional planning agencies. (Personal communications from the Boston University Center for Health Planning based upon information obtained from HEW's Bureau of Health Planning and Resource Development.) Regardless of form, HSAs must have a governing body that meets explicit requirements. A majority (but not more than 60 percent) of its members are to be (1) residents of the area served by the HSA, (2) consumers of health care, and (3) "broadly representative of the social, economic, linguistic and racial populations, geographic areas of the health service area, and major purchasers of health care." The remainder are to be residents of the area and "providers of health care who represent (I) physicians (particularly practicing physicians), dentists, nurses, and other health professionals, (II) health care institutions (particularly hospitals, long-term care facilities, and health maintenance organizations), (III) health care insurers, (IV) health professional schools; and (V) the allied health professions." Government representation and a balance between metropolitan and nonmetropolitan areas also are required. *Id.* Title XV, §1512(b)(3)(c), 88 Stat. 2233 (codified at 42 U.S.C. §300*l*(b)(3)(c) (Supp. V 1975)).

33. *Id.* §1521, 88 Stat. 2242 (codified at 42 U.S.C. §300m (Supp. V 1975)).

34. *Id.* §1524, 88 Stat. 2247 (codified at 42 U.S.C. §300m-3 (Supp. V 1975)).

35. *Id.* §1513(b)(2), 88 Stat. 2236 (codified at 42 U.S.C. §300*l*-2(b)(2) (Supp. V 1975)).

36. *Id.* §1524(c)(2), 88 Stat. 2248 (codified at 42 U.S.C. §300m-3(c)(2) (Supp. V 1975)).

37. *Id.* §1513(b)(2), 88 Stat. 2236 (codified at 42 U.S.C. §300*l*-2(b)(2) (Supp. V 1975)).

38. Despite the option of an HSA being a public regional planning body or a general unit of local government, most are private nonprofit organizations. *See* note 32 *supra.*

39. At least 60 percent of the members of the SHCC are appointed by the state governor from lists submitted by HSAs whose areas are wholly or partially within the state. Public Health Service Act, Title XV, §1524(b)(1), 88 Stat. 2247 (codified at 42 U.S.C. §300m-3(b)(1) (Supp. V 1975)).

40. Title XV of the Public Health Service Act establishes two types of authority that could be considered regulatory in nature. One, certificate of need, is exercised by the SHPDA, *id.* §1523(a)(4)(B), 88 Stat. 2246 (codified at 42 U.S.C. §300m-2(a)(4)(B) (Supp. V 1975)), which is the only agency in the planning structure not responsible for adopting a plan. The other is the right of the HSAs to disapprove of applications, emanating from the area, for certain federal program funds, although any HSA disapproval is subject to review and reversal by the Secretary of HEW. *Id.* §1513(e), 88 Stat. 2238 (codified at 42 U.S.C. 300*l*-2(c) (Supp. V 1975)).

41. The concept of the planning process "working well" is as yet undefined. *See* the remainder of this part for additional comments relevant to this concept.

42. For an excellent discussion of a number of issues involved in linking planning and regulation, *see* BAUER, THE ARRANGED MARRIAGE OF HEALTH PLANNING AND REGULATION FOR COST CONTAINMENT UNDER P.L. 93-641—SOME ISSUES TO BE FACED (1977).

43. The principal "due process"-type statutory requirements applicable to HSAs appear in the requirements (1) that governing body meetings be conducted in public, with adequate notice to the public, and that the governing body make its records and data available, upon request, to the public, Public Health Service Act, §1512(b)(3)(viii), 88 Stat. 2234 (codified at 42 U.S.C. §300*l*-1(b)(3)(B)(viii) (Supp. V 1975)); and (2) that public notice be given and public hearings be conducted with respect to proposed health systems plans before adoption of a final document, *id.* §1513(b)(2), 88 Stat. 2236 (codified at 42 U.S.C. §300*l*-2(b)(2) (Supp. V 1975)).

44. See in this context the Opinion of the Attorney General of Maryland providing an answer to an inquiry about the relationship of the Maryland Health Services Cost Review Commission to the Comprehensive Health Planning Agency, [1976] 2 Medicare and Medicaid Guide (CCH) ¶ 14,725.69.

45. *See, e.g.,* testimony of Governor Michael S. Dukakis of Massachusetts before the Health Subcommittee of the Senate Human Resources Committee, May 24, 1977. *HEW Seeks Agency with Power to Limit Cost of Health Care,* New York Times, Feb. 16, 1977, at Al, col. 3.

46. Havighurst does not present any evidence that savings in health insurance premiums through bargaining for reductions in coverage are provided, dollar for dollar, to employees in wages or other fringe benefits. To the extent such savings are not passed on dollar for dollar, even without changes in the tax laws, the employer has an incentive for reducing premium expense.

47. Much publicity was generated by General Motors' announcement in March 1976 that it was paying more to Blue Cross for employee health insurance coverage than it was spending on steel purchases from United States Steel. Statement of Victor Zink, Director of Employee Benefits and Services, before U.S. Senate Committee on Labor and Public Welfare, Sub-

committee on Health, April 19, 1976. Private communications between this author and local General Motors representatives in Massachusetts revealed that the company took the position that its local representatives should become more actively involved in initiatives focusing on changes that would constrain health insurance premium increases.

48. *See, e.g.,* references to negotiations between the United Auto Workers and General Motors, Health Lawyers News Report, September 1976, at 4; HEALTH CARE EXPENDITURES IN MASSACHUSETTS, *supra* note 20, at 1.

49. *See, e.g.,* Posner, *Theories of Economic Regula-* *tion,* 5 BELL JOURNAL OF ECONOMICS AND MANAGEMENT 335 (1974).

50. Havighurst, *supra* note 1, at 320.

51. *Id.* It is interesting that Professor Havighurst recognizes HMO-type approaches to be a "kind of rationing," although he prefers that to governmental rationing because it is "consensual" in nature. If consensual rationing can be as stringent as government rationing, it is undoubtedly to be preferred.

52. For an introductory exploration of these kinds of questions, see Kingsdale, Marrying Regulatory and Competitive Approaches to Health Care Cost Containment (to be published in the *Journal of Health Politics, Policy and Law*).

1.5 More on Regulation: A Reply to Stephen Weiner

CLARK C. HAVIGHURST, J.D.

Reprinted with permission of the American Society of Law & Medicine, Inc. and the Massachusetts Institute of Technology, from 4 *American Journal of Law & Medicine* 243–253 (1978) (Editor's Note omitted). Copyright © 1978 by the American Society of Law & Medicine, Inc. and the Massachusetts Institute of Technology. All rights reserved.

I was not flattered by the attention Stephen Weiner, writing in this journal,[1] paid to my work, mostly because he paid so little. While purporting to discuss a brief editorial Comment[2] that I wrote for an earlier edition, his attack clearly was aimed at a larger target. Had that target been the totality of my writing on health care regulation, I could not have complained, but he makes no reference to any of my lengthier papers, which were cited in my Comment and which provide a foundation for most of the conclusions it reached. Moreover, Mr. Weiner's specific complaints about gaps in my argument, and his apparent misunderstanding of my positions and of my mode of analysis, indicate, at best, a poorly recollected reading of my more deliberate work. It appears that Weiner became absorbed in attacking a different target, namely his own stereotype of a "free market" advocate. That he had a stereotype in mind appears in his tracing of my "intellectual antecedents" to "Chicago and The Brookings Institute [sic]." Such an indiscriminate lumping of the University of Chicago school of economics and The Brookings Institution, which are usually thought to be ideologically opposed, indicates either a weak knowledge of the ideological landscape[3] or an attempt to isolate a substantial number of respected scholars.

I felt called upon to reply to Mr. Weiner's paper because it has a patina of scholarship that will make it popular among those who need the comfort of his conclusions. Perhaps it will be possible, in addition to setting the record straight on some specific points, to reveal the substance of his dispute with me so that the true issues will appear and some false ones can be put aside.

Before getting to the finer points, I must challenge some direct misstatements. Weiner accuses me of "assuming" that, because other kinds of regulation have failed, health sector regulation also must fail.[4] What I said, at the outset of my analysis, was that, "[w]hile the earlier analogies [to older regulatory efforts] were useful in framing the pertinent questions, it is clear that health sector regulation is in many respects *sui generis*,"[5] and my argument proceeded exclusively on that basis. Weiner criticizes me at length for ignoring the possibility that combining planning and regulation may pay great dividends,[6] but I said, "The HSAs, as local planning agencies, could make an interesting difference if they were dedicated to 'hard' planning. . . ."[7] I also concluded that "a toughminded, planning-oriented approach . . . seems not to be in the political cards."[8] I have more fully explored this matter, which I find to be of great interest, in other writing.[9]

Weiner seems to argue that, working from an economic model, I fail to appreciate the importance of politics and political bargaining in determining the outcome of regulatory processes. But, by my count, I have published roughly 160 pages in numerous journals specifically considering health sector regulation as a political process.[10] This figure excludes the Comment that Weiner purports to be criticizing, which analyzed regulation *exclusively* in political terms.

My goal throughout has been to do precisely what Weiner says that I have a "responsibility"[11] to do. Given the amount of ink I have used in trying to assess the politics of regulation in the health sector, I am surprised by Weiner's reference to my conclusions as "assumptions"[12] and his attribution to me of a belief that government regulation is always economically and socially irrational[13] and of an *"a priori"* belief that regulation is doomed to fail.[14] Contrary to Weiner's repeated assertions, I believe the record will show that my criticisms of regulation have been constructive and that the design of regulation today reflects many steps taken in an attempt to avert hazards that I helped to point out.

My assessment of health sector cost-containment regulation was gloomy precisely because I regard rationing health care, reducing what passes for "the quality of care," to be a particularly difficult *political* assignment, as compared, say, with limiting the profits of a public utility. I tried to prove that obvious point by analyzing the highly instructive rhetoric surrounding cost-containment regulation, which is usually described as having as its noncontroversial goals the *improvement* of the quality of care and the elimination of "inefficiency," "fat," "unnecessary care," and "duplication." Weiner contradicts, without evidence,[15] my documented observation that politically exposed regulators are reticent about acknowledging their rationing function.[16] The point is not crucial, but it still seems to me to be correct. (Indeed, the subject's political touchiness was confirmed again recently when Senator Kennedy, on the Public Broadcasting System's *MacNeil/Lehrer Report*, dodged a direct question by the AMA's executive vice president about his views on rationing.) I cannot tell whether, in disputing my argument that politics makes it hard for regulators to be candid and therefore, presumably, to be effective rationers of care, Weiner intends to deny my larger point that the cost-containment job is difficult. Probably he would take the position that most regulators take—namely that the job is difficult but not impossible. Such a stance conveniently explains past deficiencies while also justifying a larger regulatory budget for the future.

Weiner attributes to me the view that it is inappropriate for regulators to seek to shift the rationing burden to providers.[17] While I did question some of the assumptions behind that strategy and doubted its success (because of the politics of what I called a "'hot potato' game"), I denied neither the need to push ahead with this approach nor the conscientiousness of the regulators who have adopted it. Indeed, I characterized regulatory "arbitrariness," designed to clamp a lid on the resources available to providers and thus force rationing, as probably *"the most responsible regulatory policy because it is the most likely to be effective."*[18] The probable defeat, as of this writing, of the Carter Administration's hospital cost-containment bill, which would have overcome some of the political difficulties in rationing care (though it had other defects), vindicates my political assessment that providers, by talking about the quality of care, usually can avoid having the rationing burden imposed on them. I do not disagree with Weiner's reasons for supporting provider rationing, mostly because they are close to ideas that were alluded to in my Comment and that James Blumstein and I elaborated fully some time ago.[19]

My further points should help to isolate Weiner's real basis for resisting the logic of my arguments. Weiner's reference[20] to Victor Goldberg's article,[21] which analogizes regulation to an "administered contract," was interesting to me, though not because it proves any of Weiner's points. Weiner's description of relations under private "administered contracts"[22] is very close to what I believe relations should be between consumers and providers, on the one hand, and competing health plans, on the other—whether they are of the insurance, the service-plan, the HMO, or some new hybrid variety. Adequate attention to my work would have led Weiner to perceive that, far from wishing to return exclusively to "discrete transactions"[23]—whatever that term means in this context[24]—I regard "administered contracts" as the best available mechanism for resolving most of the problems of the health care industry. Indeed, it is the proponents of regulation who need a lesson in "administered contracts," for they regularly cite consumer ignorance, third-party payment, and physician control of demand as making regulation inevitable, and they refuse to see the myriad possibilities for overcoming these problems that are inherent in the institution of private contract. I differ with such persons not over the consumer's need to escape the "discrete transactions" marketplace and to have the aid of an expert intermediary in dealing with providers, but over whether that intermediary must be a public rather than a private entity.

The advantages of private administered contracts over public regulation are too numerous to go into here. In any event, Weiner, surprisingly, appears to agree with me, for in his footnote 51, crediting me with "recognizing" that HMOs are a private, consensual vehicle for rationing care—that is, an administered contract—, he says, "If consensual rationing can be as stringent as government rationing, it is undoubtedly to be preferred."[25] But my argument was that, if only government did not distort private incentives through its tax rules governing employer-paid insurance premiums, private rationing could be not merely as stringent as government rationing but more so (because it would be less political and therefore less concerned with symbolism)[26] Weiner cannot accept my argument because he cannot conceive of this possibility as a general proposition, though he must concede it with respect to HMOs because they have economized circles around the regulated system. The main apparent reason for his underestimating the power of private incentives as embodied in administered contracts is that he seems not to understand the mechanism—let alone appreciate the impact—of the tax law.

My paper sketched the market-oriented alternative only briefly, but apparently I should have explained more fully how it is that the tax law encourages over-insurance (including excessive liberality in claims payment) and thus why changing that law probably would make a greater difference than regulation can make. Weiner devotes two paragraphs[27] to disputing that the employer's business deduction and the employee's limited personal deduction of their respective health insurance premiums create any significant problem. But it is not these deductions so much as the total and unlimited *exclusion* of the employer's contributions from the employee's taxable wages (for both income and payroll tax purposes) that induces the purchase of excessive insurance. By this mechanism, the tax law makes it highly advantageous for as much health care as possible to be paid for through employer-purchased insurance. A further result is that private incentives to reduce premiums through cost-containment efforts are impaired, leaving us no apparent alternative but to turn to government for help. My argument is

that, with the right incentives and more room for competition, the private sector could discharge the responsibility for cost-containment better than government—though it may not, for complex reasons, be anxious to do so.[28]

There is plenty to argue about in this conclusion, but, if one uses Weiner's own test from his footnote 51, the issues are strictly empirical, not theoretical: Would private-sector cost containment in fact be as stringent, or more so, than government regulation? Is competitive innovation in cost containment feasible? Could provider cartels be prevented from continuing to call the tune?

Weiner never joins the issue on these interesting empirical questions because he persists in thinking that I, true to his stereotype, perceive the issue only in theoretical, even ideological, terms. Yet it would appear from Weiner's footnote 51 that he and I share a philosophical preference for private over governmental solutions to problems of public policy. Perhaps the only problem is that Weiner has yet to appreciate the practical value of removing distortions of private incentives so that market forces can stimulate the complex world to conform more nearly to people's desires.

There appears, however, to be a more fundamental blind spot in Weiner's thinking, one so pervasive that it causes him to deny the very legitimacy of thinking about nonregulatory alternatives. He seems to believe that a political choice of regulation (a) has been made and (b) must be respected, and that therefore my broad skepticism, whether right or wrong, is not only irrelevant but a bit subversive. This view may be challenged on two levels.

First, it is far from clear that a definitive and final decision to rely solely on regulation has in fact been made. Indeed, many cumulatively crucial choices—for more or less regulation, for broader or narrower regulatory coverage (of HMOs, home health services, doctors' offices, and so forth), for liberality or strictness in particular regulatory decisions, for tolerating, encouraging, or suppressing various forms of competition, for one or another model of national health insurance, and so on—remain to be faced. Weiner admits that some of this agenda is open when he asks me to consider how competition and regulation can be blended usefully.[29] But surely my Comment, showing why regulation of the supply side of the market in order to control demand is an imperfect tool, is an essential preamble to any such effort to reconcile seemingly conflicting approaches. Weiner's criticism that I have neglected this dimension in analyzing regulation is easily refuted by reference to my other writings, which have highlighted the ways in which regulation may, but need not, suppress such useful forms of competition as HMOs.[30] Moreover, although Weiner had no way of knowing it, the paper he was criticizing is to be a chapter in my forthcoming book tentatively entitled *Competition in a Regulated Health Care System.*

Much more serious are the implications of Mr. Weiner's refusal to concede that I have a clear right, as a scholar, to question government's choice of regulation once that choice has been made. The source of this vague but distinctly repressive impulse lies in Weiner's apparent reverence for the political process, as revealed in his lengthy recitation of the theory of interest-group liberalism—the idea that competing interests will all balance out in the political process and approximate the "public interest."[31] This discussion reveals no awareness of the large volume of scholarship by political scientists and economists that casts grave doubts on the theoretical as well as the empirical reliability of that model as a vehicle for advancing the public welfare. Consider, for example, the phenomenon of "pork barrel" legislation and the difficulty of aggregating interests and registering the respective strengths of competing preferences. Weiner and other critics who rightly regard the "free market" model as too simplistic to substitute for policy should be wary of accepting uncritically a textbook model of the political process.

Weiner's acceptance of the output of political institutions, particularly regulatory institutions, is not shaken by the poor performance of regulation in other industries, by health sector regulation's unimpressive performance to date, or by my showing of the substantial political difficulties of doing the cost-containment job. The reason for his—and perhaps for many other people's—unshakeable acceptance of regulation is that in their view regulation, by definition, cannot fail: As a political enterprise, its results are automatically legitimized and can be challenged only in the particular, not in the aggregate. Consider, for example, this explicit attempt by Weiner to limit the scholar's agenda:

"How the regulatory agency balances . . . varying interests at any one point in time with respect to any one decision is *the proper subject* of legal, political, and economic analyses of the regulatory process."[32] A careful reading of Weiner indicates that he is saying much more than that I should accept regulation as a *fait accompli* and get on to more practical matters.

Weiner also takes the view that a scholar who disputes the need for a regulatory scheme that is already in place is expressing a counter-revolutionary political preference only, and is sailing under false colors if he cloaks his argument as academic analysis. Thus, he says that, given the political context, "*it is inappropriate* to evaluate regulation against any abstracted standards or norms . . . without acknowledging that any such effort reflects the value structure of the commentator, and not necessarily the value structure of the [regulating] agency."[33] Specifically, Weiner is objecting to my statement that "there is no reason whatsoever to think that the political processes yielding [through regulation some ultimately stable share of GNP devoted to health] . . . will have come anywhere near finding *the socially optimal level of spending on health care.*"[34] The objection to my passing reference to a social optimum is fully answered in an earlier article in which James Blumstein and I carefully discussed the use of such a purely hypothetical benchmark in thinking about public policy towards health care.[35]

I would readily admit that measuring regulation by the yardstick of theoretical optimality—a highly and perhaps perfectly democratic yardstick, it should be noted—would not justify overturning a regulatory scheme unless (1) that scheme could not be improved and (2) there was a better way to approach the posited objective. But I have argued, first, that health care regulation *cannot* be sufficiently strengthened without greatly increased arbitrariness and the sacrifice of values that most people would regard as important and, second, that a system affording consumers a wide range of choice under appropriate cost constraints would outperform any acceptable form of regulation.

Once my own positions are correctly stated, it turns out that Weiner agrees with me on several points. Thus, despite his sweeping attempt to discredit my analysis, he ends up by accepting my gloomy assessment of regulation for all aspects of the health care enterprise except hospitals.[36] This indicates that the real differences between us may be less fundamental than his tone would suggest. That he agrees with me on the potential utility of HMOs has already been noted. Finally, if Weiner could get over his romantic or merely ill-considered acceptance of the processes of interest-group liberalism and accept the need to demand that government do as well (by *some* standard, which the political process may help to define) as some realistic alternative, there seems some chance that he would accept at least the theoretical framework of my analysis and my definition of the empirical issues.

Despite our areas of agreement, however, Weiner and I might still differ over the allocation of decision-making responsibility on some significant matters. It is regrettable that he did not respond to my discussion[37] of the desirability of leaving room for individuals to express (with costs in view) their widely varying preferences about the highly personal matter of health care. Since it was my stated position that there is no "one right way" to deal with health problems and that the system can safely be arranged to permit a considerable range of individual choice, we need to know why Weiner might think that collective decisions, restricting choice, would be preferable. What worries me is that, in passing over my arguments for facilitating individual choice, Weiner may have signified a disinterest in people's preferences comparable to that which characterizes that shadowy cultural elite increasingly being referred to as "the new class."[38] This "new class" was recently described by Paul H. Weaver, in an illuminating article on the social issues involved in government regulation, as "that rapidly growing and increasingly influential part of the upper-middle class that feels itself to be in a more or less adversary posture vis-à-vis American society and that tends to make its vocation in the public and not-for-profit sectors."[39] Weaver sees "the real animus of the new class . . . [as being] against the liberal values served by corporate capitalism and the benefits these institutions provide to the broad mass of the American people: economic growth, widespread prosperity, material satisfactions, a sense of nationhood, a belief in an open and self-determined future, and the many options and freedoms that these make possible for ordinary citizens."[40]

There is, unfortunately, some slight evidence—again in the unconsciously revealing footnote 51—that Weiner shares this "new class's" antagonism toward what Weaver calls "acts of consumption by consenting adults."[41] In conditioning his acceptance of "consensual rationing" on whether it "can be as stringent as government rationing," Weiner is, like the new class, "working against the widespread enjoyment of consumer goods and services that liberal capitalism makes possible."[42] My own view is that the ultimate goal is not stringency for its own sake but an allocation of resources in accordance with people's revealed preferences and that political processes are incapable of determining, measuring, and giving appropriate effect to those preferences. Indeed, as political processes fall more and more under the control and influence of "the new class," they seem less and less likely to serve pluralistic values that I regard as important, more stifling indeed than mere "bureaucracy" ever was. There is no doubt that "the new class" is highly active in health sector regulation and that important values are at stake. Perhaps it is as well to draw these lines explicitly and to let the overriding issue concerning the future scope of health care regulation be seen as, quite simply, whether this is any longer a liberal democracy in which there is a presumption in favor of the individual's right to choose for himself and to have his preferences catered to in the economic marketplace.

To conclude, Weiner's Comment reflects fairly accurately the conventional wisdom favoring regulation in the health care industry, and is also a typical expression of the prevailing bias in favor of "black box" solutions to policy problems, using "command-and-control modules," that is deplored by Charles L. Schultze in *The Public Use of Private Interest*. If Weiner's definition of the issues and his strictures on scholarship were to be accepted, it would seriously narrow the range of the health policy debate, which I firmly believe should be expanded both into the value questions alluded to above and into the practical problems of restoring competition and fostering privately initiated change. Thus, while Weiner has asked me to join the throng of people already engaged in trying to make regulation work within the context of the conventional wisdom, I would suggest that he join the small cadre that is working on neglected alternatives. I still do not know for certain whether there is some basic value preference, or only a debatable (though potentially self-fulfilling) prophecy of future political choices, that keeps him from joining in this effort.

NOTES

1. Weiner, *Governmental Regulation of Health Care: A Response to Some Criticisms Voiced by Proponents of a "Free Market,"* 4 AM. J.L. & MED. 15 (1978).

2. Havighurst, *Health Care Cost-Containment Regulation: Prospects and an Alternative,* 3 AM. J.L. & MED. 309 (1977).

3. At one point, Weiner tries to score a debating point by claiming that my proposal to use limited tax credits to subsidize health insurance purchases is inconsistent with my "biases." Weiner, *supra* note 1, at 31. In order to lecture me on the implications of my own supposed philosophy, Weiner must be wedded very firmly to his stereotype, since one would expect my philosophy to be revealed in its application. In any event, my proposal was to remove an existing distortion of private incentives (see text accompanying notes 27–28 *infra*), not to manipulate them, as Weiner suggests. Further, there is an important distinction between the conservative *laissez faire* tradition, with which Mr. Weiner seems to think he is contending, and the approach of a pragmatic liberal such as Charles L. Schultze (formerly of Brookings) in his 1977 book *The Public Use of Private Interest.* Indeed, this title, suggesting that private interest is not sacrosanct but is there to be *used* by the public, probably would offend a true conservative. I am myself quite comfortable with a pragmatic approach that would provide for direct government intervention only where indirect approaches—ordering incentives and strengthening competitive forces—are demonstrably inadequate. Later discussion in the present Comment suggests the possibility that Weiner himself could be philosophically content with this approach.

4. Weiner, *supra* note 1, at 16.

5. Havighurst, *supra* note 2, at 312.

6. Weiner, *supra* note 1, at 26–30.

7. Havighurst, *supra* note 2, at 312 n.7.

8. *Id.* at 316.

9. Havighurst, *Regulation of Health Facilities and Services by "Certificate of Need,"* 59 VA L. REV. 1143, 1194–1204 (1973).

10. Havighurst, Blumstein, & Bovbjerg, *Strategies in Underwriting the Costs of Catastrophic Disease,* L. & CONTEMP. PROB., Autumn 1976, at 122, 138–65 (1976); Havighurst & Blumstein, *Coping with Quality/Cost Trade-Offs in Medical Care: The Role of PSROs,* 70 NW. U.L. REV. 6, 20–68 (1975); Havighurst, *Federal Regulation of the Health Care*

Delivery System: A Foreword in the Nature of a "Package Insert," 6 U. TOL. L. REV. 577 (1975); Havighurst & Bovbjerg, *Professional Standards Review Organizations and Health Maintenance Organizations: Are They Compatible?* 1975 UTAH L. REV. 381, 401–21 (1975); Havighurst, *Health Maintenance Organizations and the Health Planners,* 1978 UTAH L. REV. 123, 140–54 (1978); Havighurst, *supra* note 9, at 1178–1218.

11. Weiner, *supra* note 1, at 20.

12. *Id.* at 16.

13. *Id.* at 18.

14. *Id.* at 24.

15. *Id.* at 21.

16. Havighurst, *supra* note 2, at 313.

17. Weiner, *supra* note 1, at 22.

18. Havighurst, *supra* note 2, at 317 (emphasis added).

19. Havighurst & Blumstein, *Coping with Quality/Cost Trade-Offs in Medical Care: The Role of PSROs,* 70 NW. U.L. REV. 6 (1975).

20. Weiner, *supra* note 1, at 17–18.

21. Goldberg, *Regulation and Administered Contracts,* 7 THE BELL JOURNAL OF ECONOMICS 426 (1976).

22.   The "administered contract" exhibits either or both of two elements. First, it involves a contractual relationship between principals that continues for an extended period of time, rather than occurring only at a fixed point in time, and that establishes a framework for redefining contractual terms and conditions as circumstances change over time. Second, this relationship involves a reliance upon agents for the fulfillment of such functions as gathering and analyzing essential information, making binding decisions, and adjusting the terms of the ongoing contractual relationships between the principals.

Weiner, *supra* note 1, at 17 (footnote omitted).

23. *Id.*

24. Presumably it would refer to doctor-patient transactions conducted on a fee-for-service basis without third-party financing.

25. Weiner, *supra* note 1, at 32 n.51.

26. It should be recognized that unions and employers have a "political" relationship with the workers and necessarily are concerned with symbolism in providing health benefits. The tax law exacerbates this problem by transferring some of the cost of eschewing stringency from the parties to the federal government. If the tax law were changed and if the union leadership still preferred lavish health care at the expense of increased take-home pay, the high cost would be borne solely by the rank and file, who would have an incentive to demand a different plan. If they failed to do so,

that presumably would reflect their choice, and, even if we did not agree with it, it would be hard to find any reason to intervene.

27. Weiner, *supra* note 1, at 30–31.

28. Insurance companies, in particular, would rather not have this ticklish responsibility. Competition should force them to accept it, however. *See* Havighurst, *Professional Restraints on Innovation in Health Care Financing,* 1978 Duke L.J. 321 (1978).

29. Weiner, *supra* note 1, at 32.

30. Havighurst & Bovbjerg, *Professional Standards Review Organizations and Health Maintenance Organizations: Are They Compatible?* 1975 Utah L. Rev. 381 (1975); Havighurst, *Health Maintenance Organizations and the Health Planners,* 1978 Utah L. Rev. 123 (1978); Havighurst, *supra* note 9, at 1204–15.

31. Weiner, *supra* note 1, at 18–20.

32. *Id.* at 20 (emphasis added).

33. *Id.* (emphasis added).

34. Havighurst, *supra* note 2, at 315–16 (emphasis added).

35. Havighurst & Blumstein, *supra* note 19, at 15–20.

36. Weiner, *supra* note 1, at 25.

37. Havighurst, *supra* note 2, at 317–19.

38. *See, e.g.,* I. Kristol, Two Cheers for Capitalism 27–31 (1978).

39. Weaver, *Regulation, Social Policy, and Class Conflict,* Pub. Interest, Winter 1978, at 45, 59.

40. *Id.* at 60.

41. *Id.* at 61.

42. *Id.* at 60–61.

1.6 The Effect of Physician-Controlled Health Insurance: *U.S. v. Oregon State Medical Society**

LAWRENCE G. GOLDBERG and
WARREN GREENBERG

Reprinted with permission of the Department of Health Administration, Duke University, from 2 *Journal of Health Politics, Policy and Law* 48–52, 54–69, 73–78 (1977). Copyright © 1977 by the Department of Health Administration, Duke University. All rights reserved.

ABSTRACT

The trial record in an antitrust case against the Oregon State Medical Society, finally decided in 1952, was examined to reconstruct the behavior of a competitive market for health insurance coverage. Health insurers, called "hospital associations," were found to have engaged individually in cost-control efforts similar to, but possibly more aggressive than, today's utilization review under professional sponsorship. The subsequent disappearance of these insurer-initiated cost controls in Oregon is traced to the medical society's organization of a competing Blue Shield plan as a model of insurer conduct and to a simultaneous boycott by physicians of the hospital associations as long as they persisted in questioning doctors' practices. Some modern parallels are noted, and the advantages of fostering privately sponsored cost-control efforts are suggested.

Health care costs in the United States have risen considerably faster than the cost of living

*The views expressed herein are those of the authors and are not necessarily those of the Bureau of Economics or the Federal Trade Commission. The authors wish to thank Professor Clark C. Havighurst for suggesting this case as an area for research and for extensive comments on an earlier draft. The authors also are indebted to M. Glassman, L. Oliver, L. Silversin, P. Buck, C. McCormick, J. Seigfreid and colleagues at the Federal Trade Commission for helpful advice.

in recent years,[1] and much of the increased spending is believed by many experts to be socially inappropriate, in the sense that the health benefits obtained have not been equal to the costs incurred.[2] The conclusion that resources have been increasingly misallocated is based on recognition of the substantial expansion of health insurance coverage over this period[3] and on the perception that consumers and providers of health care increasingly have been freed by such insurance from cost constraints on their consumption decisions. Economist Martin Feldstein has demonstrated convincingly that private health insurance has resulted in the provision of more services of a more expensive variety than consumers would have elected to purchase in a market based on out-of-pocket payment.[4]

Economic theory suggests and experience confirms that the injection of insurance into a marketplace need not result in uncontrolled cost escalation. Automobile insurers, for example, control the cost of collision-damage claims by requiring multiple estimates or by directly inspecting damage prior to repair.[5] Workmen's compensation insurers conduct safety inspections and use experience-rated premiums to stimulate accident prevention.[6] Manufacturers offering warranties covering repairs by independent dealers have developed a variety of techniques to prevent abuse.[7] In each case, competitive pressure to provide essential protection at the lowest possible price induces cost-cutting actions which are both acceptable to insureds and effective enough to warrant incurring the administrative costs involved. Although "moral hazard"—the economist's term for the propensity of insurance beneficiaries to exploit the insurance fund[8]—does add to the cost of insurance, it also poses a challenge which insurers must meet as part of their service to the public. The specific techniques they might adopt are practically numberless and dependent on a wide variety of circumstances that include: the technology and cost of monitoring expenditures, consumer and service providers' preferences regarding claims handling, and the legal environment in which insurers find themselves.

Because a competitive insurance industry should feature cost-control measures to offset the temptation to incur unjustified expenses, it is significant that health care insurers have not exerted much pressure to control health care costs.[9] This paper is an investigation of some reasons why this departure from rational competitive behavior has occurred. One reason seems to be that there are legal restrictions on what insurers can do, but these seem not to be so totally disabling in every state as to explain the almost total abdication of cost-control responsibility.[10] Another reason why insurers may not have been aggressive in cost control is the relatively weak incentives of their customers, primarily employers and employees, to seek lower-cost insurance coverage. Favorable tax treatment of health insurance premiums, particularly when paid by employers, has diluted pressure to control costs, since the federal government would share in any savings achieved.[11] Benefit packages have been designed to permit even routine expenditures to be paid with untaxed insurance dollars rather than out-of-pocket funds previously depleted by income and FICA taxes.

This article, in presenting historical experience from the State of Oregon in the 1930s and 1940s, reveals another aspect of the problem of encouraging insurer-initiated cost controls. It shows that, in at least one time and place, the insurance market was competitive and free enough to generate the spontaneous cost-control efforts which theory and experience in other insurance markets lead one to expect. The reasons why those efforts came to an end in Oregon have important implications for health policy today. Among other things, they suggest an important role for the antitrust laws in improving the cli-

mate for private sector initiatives to solve a problem which, despite a variety of costly and ambitious regulatory programs, still seems to confound government.[12] The history recounted is taken in large measure from the record of an antitrust case, *United States v. Oregon State Medical Society*,[13] which resulted in a decision adverse to the government in 1952.

"CONTRACT MEDICINE" AND THE "HOSPITAL ASSOCIATIONS"

In the early part of the twentieth century, a system of contract medicine developed in both Oregon and Washington State in response to hazardous working conditions in the lumber, railroad, and mining industries. Employers in these industries contracted with so-called "hospital associations" for comprehensive medical and hospital care to be provided by the association for a fixed fee paid jointly by employer and employee.[14] Most of these associations were begun by physicians but later were managed by lay personnel. While some of them were financially strong enough to operate their own hospitals, others used the facilities of community hospitals. Originally designed to provide health care for employees injured on the job, the hospital associations gradually undertook to insure all the health care needs of employees and their dependents.

The hospital associations bore some similarities to the health maintenance organizations (HMOs) of the present.[15] Like an HMO, the hospital association guaranteed a stated range of medical services and assumed the financial risk in health care delivery. Because of competitive pressures and the associations' for-profit nature, there were incentives to control the cost of medical care. Physicians worked either full- or part-time for the hospital associations as they do now for HMOs. Although, like HMOs, the plans began with closed panels of physicians, the associations gradually allowed freer choice of physicians and switched to paying on a fee-for-service basis while maintaining only a few physicians on their own staff. This was in part a response to consumers' preferences but also reflected a concession to the preferences of organized medicine.

National Hospital Association, the largest hospital association, was formed in 1906, while the physician-controlled Prudential Association was organized in 1913. The for-profit hospital association movement gained momentum in 1917 with the passage of the so-called Hospital Association Act which expressly permitted corporations to contract to provide medical and allied services without a medical license (the "corporate practice of medicine").[16] In 1923, the Industrial Hospital Association, also physician-controlled, was begun. Two smaller hospital associations, Weston and Pumphrey, entered in 1904 and 1926 respectively but ceased operations in 1939 and 1940.[17] By 1935, these for-profit hospital associations had disbursements of $843,727 or sixty percent of total health insurer disbursements in Oregon.[18] The balance of the health insurance business belonged to plans operated by local medical societies, the so-called service bureaus.

The aggressive approach to cost control taken by the hospital associations is revealed in the following letter which the Industrial Hospital Association sent to physicians in November 1935:

We solicit your cooperation in adhering to the following regulations:

1. All cases requiring major surgery, except in actual emergency, must be reported to the Association for authority before operation is performed.
2. It will be the policy of the Association to require consultation before authorizing major surgery.
3. No operation for hernia will be authorized until the same has been approved by the State Industrial Accident Commission or the Association has had opportunity to make satisfactory investigation.
4. Hospital ticket or treatment order must be obtained in advance of giving treatments, except in cases of actual emergencies. No bills will be paid without tickets being attached.[19]

Thus, the hospital associations threatened to limit the doctor's clinical freedom, which was then and is now considered by the profession a vital feature of medical practice. Doctors were not accustomed to, and did not like, having others, especially third parties, question their medical procedures. They apparently preferred to deal directly with patients whose medical ignorance frequently allowed doctors to make decisions without having to justify them fully.[20] Technically, of course, the doctor was not bound to obey the association's rules if the patient agreed to pay himself, but physicians did not regard this as a sufficient answer to what they saw as an infringement on their professional role.

Physicians' fees were also affected by the associations. Typically, when dealing with patients on a fee-for-service basis, physicians were accustomed to exercising some monopoly power through the practice of price discrimination—that is, charging non-uniform fees scaled according to the patient's ability to pay.[21] Patients were generally reluctant to shop for the lowest-priced physician, since they had neither sufficient knowledge nor information available to be sure that they were not unduly sacrificing quality. Patients' ignorance in this regard was, and is, fostered by the profession's prohibitions against advertising[22] and ethics forestalling criticism of fellow professionals. The monopoly power thus possessed by physicians could not be exercised as readily in the presence of the hospital associations. Not only did the associations closely scrutinize particular fees, but contract practice itself impaired the physician's ability to discriminate in the prices charged to different patients and therefore his opportunity to maximize income. Because physicians either were paid a fixed salary or billed the plan and not the patient, they could not charge different fees based on the patient's income for the same services. In general, the introduction of the for-profit hospital associations as interested and informed third parties acting on the premium payer's behalf seems to have resulted in a substantial infringement on the physician's market power.

The letters set forth below, which are typical of those in the record in the Justice Department's case against the Oregon State Medical Society,[23] illustrate how the hospital associations were able to restrain the exercise of physicians' market power as well as the overutilization of health facilities. One letter, written by the Industrial Hospital Association (IHA) to a physician, indicates that certain procedures would not be authorized without further investigation:

In regard to the case of Ira Smith . . . we are assuming no responsibility for a hernia operation for any employee of a company outside of your district without having an opportunity to investigate the case before authorizing operation.[24]

* * *

In an exchange of letters between the IHA and a doctor, the doctor did agree to lower his fees. IHA to the doctor:

A fee of $150.00 which you have charged for the Winn case is undoubtedly in line with your private fees, but it is higher than any Hospital Association can expect to pay under their medical contracts.[32]

Reply by the doctor:

In reply to your letter regarding the fees in the above account, I wish to let you know that I will accept the mastoid fee of $75.00 for the operation and an additional fee of $6.00 for the x-rays taken.[33]

Two final letters illustrate how deeply involved hospital associations became in the practice of medicine. In the beginning of the first letter, the NHA stated that the organization would pay for shots of cold serum for the treatment of a cold but would not pay for preventive shots since this was not in the contract:

Concerning the advisability of cold shots, we recently noticed an article in *The Journal of the American Medical Association* dated September 24 which would indicate that cold shots, either orally or by injection, are of little or no value. Have you read this article and, if so, what is your opinion?[34]

The associations' letter writers were not physicians but had access to medical advice, as shown in this letter, again relating to shots:

. . . [W]e have investigated the matter of these shots for the treatment of the condition, and the advice we have from medical men here is that while the shots are many times effective as a prevention of hay fever the proper time to use them is before the hay fever season . . . . Under the circumstances the Association would not feel justified in paying for this service.[35]

It should be apparent from these letters that hospital associations were behaving as informed consumers might behave. Their activities, while perhaps unsophisticated when viewed now,[36] were similar in nature to the reviews conducted currently by hospital utilization review committees[37] and Professional Standards Review Organizations (PSROs).[38] But, unlike such committees and PSROs, the hospital associations, in acting as proxies for consumers, had to compete on the basis of quality as well as price, and therefore had to follow consumer desires or lose their insureds to competitors.[39]

The question arises as to why doctors continued to cooperate with the hospital associations even though the association policies interfered with the doctor-patient relationship. The answer seems to be that doctors found it necessary to accommodate their patients enrolled with the associations and were tempted by the prospect of attracting additional paying patients. Indeed, the hospital associations were serving a useful economic purpose for doctors as well as for patients in guaranteeing payment for services by patients struck with a need for medical treatment which they might not otherwise have been able to afford. This was especially true during the Great Depression, when doctors found it more difficult than usual to collect their bills. In order to be able to ignore the hospital associations, the doctors needed an alternative form of payment guarantee to which patients could be steered. They began to develop this in the 1930s and finally made it effective in the 1940s.[40]

ORGANIZED MEDICINE'S RESPONSE

As contract medicine began to evolve in Oregon, it developed, according to the Oregon State Medical Society, "commercial features which are in distinct contravention of established professional standards."[41] These objectionable features, as listed in the minority report filed with the famous 1932 report of the Committee on the Costs of Medical Care, were as follows: (1) "solicitation of patients, either directly or indirectly;" (2) "competition and underbidding;" (3) "compensation . . . inadequate to secure good medical service;" (4) "interference with reasonable competition in a community;" and (5) impairment of "free choice of physicians"[42] Though termed unethical by the American Medical Association (AMA),[43] items (1) and (2) are simply elements typical of a healthy competitive market. Items (3) and (4) substitute organized medicine's judgment of adequacy and reasonableness for impersonal market forces. Item (5) reflects the profession's preference that consumers not be offered the option of giving up freedom to choose a physician in return for other benefits.

The reaction of organized medicine in Oregon to the practices of the for-profit hospital associations can be divided into two periods. In the first period (prior to 1941), the strategy consisted of: (1) policy statements issued by the medical societies to warn physicians that contract medicine was unethical; (2) expulsion of "unethical" physicians—i.e., those engaging in contract practice—from the county medical societies; and (3) formation of alternative prepaid plans sponsored by the county medical bureaus. In the second period, organized medicine began its own statewide insurance company in order to eliminate the controls which the hospital associations imposed on health care costs and their unwanted interference with medical decisions.

Prior to 1941

In February 1936, the Council of the Oregon State Medical Society, cognizant of the growth of the hospital associations, adopted a *Statement Concerning the Enforcement of the Principles of Medical Ethics*. Essentially, the *Statement* condemned commercial hospital associations for engaging in unethical practices such as the "employment of paid lay solicitors, advertising in newspapers and periodicals, and pamphlets distributed to employers and employees."[44] In addition, the Council found it unprofessional for a physician to be employed by an association "which permit[s] a direct profit from the fees . . . to accrue to . . . [the] individual employing him."[45] Finally, the Council recommended "that the members of component societies engaged in unethical contract practice through association with . . . [a] proprietary hospital association . . . cease such activities"[46] and that a "copy of *The Principles of Medical Ethics* be supplied to every member of the component societies."[47]

Apparently prepaid hospital and medical care was ethical only in the hands of physicians.[48] For example, as early as 1931, a medical service bureau organized by physicians "to provide

prepaid medical, surgical and hospital care to low-wage industrial and commercial groups" in Salem was readily approved by the Oregon State Medical Society.[49] In August 1938, the Oregon State Medical Society adopted a formal policy and program which encouraged local or component prepaid medical care plans.[50] In June 1939, the Oregon State Medical Society attempted to encourage the Industrial Hospital Association, one of its chief competitors, to become an approved agency "consistent with the policy and program of the Oregon State Medical Society and the *Principles of Medical Ethics*."[51]

The policies of the Oregon State Medical Society coincided with the stance taken by the AMA, which first opposed all contract medicine and then reluctantly accepted voluntary insurance, but only under the control of the local medical societies. In 1932, the AMA based its opposition to voluntary health insurance on past experience with contract practice: "wherever they are established there is solicitation of patients, destructive competition among professional groups, inferior medical service, loss of personal relationship of patient and physician, and demoralization of the profession."[52] Faced with the threat of nationwide compulsory health insurance in the depression-ridden 1930s, the AMA finally endorsed the voluntary health insurance concept so long as it was under the control of the medical profession.[53] In 1937, the AMA, in view of increasing physician support of voluntary insurance, accepted group hospitalization insurance under the control of hospital and physician personnel.[54]

The actions of Oregon's medical societies were similar. In a direct step to limit physician participation in contract medicine, the Multnomah County Medical Society, the largest county medical society in Oregon with more than fifty percent of state society physicians, first attempted to expel physicians because of a "violation of the *Principles of Medical Ethics* in connection with contract practice."[55] Initially, the Multnomah Medical Society established the Multnomah Industrial Health Association in 1932 to eliminate the lay-owned commercial hospital associations as well as to provide a prepaid medical care plan for those with incomes below $1500 a year (in order to insure payments to physicians without disrupting opportunities for price discrimination).[56] After only three years of operation, however, a county medical society report stated that the Plan "resulted in a decreased income for that part of the profession within the Multnomah Industrial Health Association from patients who are able to pay customary fees and in the loss of some of these patients by doctors outside the Association."[57] Furthermore, the Plan had "no appreciable effect" on commercial hospital associations.[58] In view of these "failures," the Society began to censure and expel physicians connected with commercial hospital associations for violation of medical ethics.[59] In addition, the Society required members of its own Multnomah Industrial Health Association to appear before the Board of Censors for unethical tactics.[60] Moreover, for some physicians, the mere threat of expulsion or censure was great enough to prompt resignation from the associations, although the absence of an insurance-guaranteed payment undoubtedly hurt physicians.[61] By late 1939, the Oregon State Medical Society was urging all local societies to take "disciplinary action" against their members for unethical practice.[62]

The results of the attack of the Oregon State Medical Society on contract medicine in the 1930s were mixed. Though some physicians were willing to resign from the hospital associations, the associations still grew. In 1935, the five for-profit hospital associations had disbursed a total of $843,727 or sixty percent of all insurance company disbursements. For 1940, the three remaining for-profit hospital associations disbursed $1,045,914 or fifty-one percent of all insurance company disbursements.[63] Apparently the hospital associations were still able to grow and to retain a significant market share, suggesting that they were able to satisfy their customers. One advantage they had was their ability to provide broader and more complete coverage throughout the state than the local county medical organizations, which were confined to single geographic areas.[64]

The 1941 Change of Policy

In 1940, boycott and expulsion tactics of the kind being practiced by the Multnomah County Medical Society were held to be in violation of the Sherman Act by the United States Circuit Court of Appeals for the District of Columbia.[65] In that case, a criminal antitrust proceeding, the AMA was convicted of restraining trade by preventing practicing physicians from accepting employment with Group Health Association, Inc., a non-profit corporation organized to provide prepaid medical and hospital services. The Supreme Court later affirmed, ruling that the defendants' status as physicians and medical organizations did not exempt them from the law "if the purpose and effect of their conspiracy was such obstruction and restraint of Group Health."[66] As a result of this ruling, it appeared that, if the growth of hospital associations was to be curtailed in Oregon, a new strategy would have to be developed by the doctors' organizations.

That new strategy, initiated in 1941, included the introduction by the state medical society of a statewide prepaid medical service plan, the Oregon Physicians Service (OPS), accompanied by a widespread refusal by physicians to deal directly with hospital associations, effectively destroying the ability of the private plans to control costs. Since subscribers could use the services of OPS throughout the state, hospitalization in a county other than that of residence would not preclude collection of benefits. Moreover, doctors could now identify a single plan as the preferred prepayment vehicle and could promote it as such.[67] In order to make the plan more attractive to doctors, stock in OPS would be controlled by physicians, who would thus be able to control any attempts to interfere in the doctor-patient relationship. The prospect of wide enrollment, of assured payment for services, of noninterference in clinical decisions, and of increased professional solidarity made the plan sufficiently attractive that only the most renegade physicians would not value membership. For those who could not or would not understand the value of OPS and the importance to the profession of making it the model of insurer behavior, the threatened denial of OPS membership could be a severe discipline,[68] forcing them to choose between OPS, with its wide coverage and professional approval, and the "unethical" plans. As more patients were enrolled in the physician-controlled plan the less costly it became for individual physicians to reject the hospital associations and their cost-cutting efforts. OPS's growth at the expense of the hospital associations was thus assured.

OPS began in December 1941 as a prepaid medical, surgical, and hospital plan. In addition, special services such as x-rays, physical therapy, and ambulance services were included.[69]

By the mid-1940s, OPS operated in thirty-two of Oregon's thirty-six counties, while cooperating fully with the county medical society plans of Clackamas, Coos, Lane, and Klamath counties.[70] Each local society controlled the day-to-day activities of OPS in its district, although the state medical society seemed to control overall policy in matters such as territorial allocations, fees, and coverage.[71] Like most present Blue Shield arrangements, OPS reimbursed cooperating physicians and hospitals on a service basis (claims paid directly to providers) rather than an indemnity basis (claims paid directly to patients). A flat fee schedule was used to determine payment for each medical or surgical procedure. Physicians who were not "cooperating" had to incur the additional expense of billing patients directly. Membership and eligibility for stockholder status were open only to physicians who were members in good standing of the local medical society,[72] a circumstance strengthening the profession's hold over individual practitioners who might continue to cooperate with the hospital associations.

OPS grew dramatically between its formation in 1941 and the filing of the Justice Department complaint in 1948. In early 1943, OPS had fewer than 5,000 subscribers, but by July 1943 had 70,000 and by July 1948 this figure had risen to nearly 100,000.[73] In 1948, its disbursements were nearly one-third of total health insurance disbursements in the state.[74] This growth was undoubtedly the result of the medical profession's preference for OPS over other insurers. The physicians finally had a statewide insurance plan which usually would cover their charges and would not question their procedures. For example, a witness for the defense testified that OPS never questioned the number of gastrointestinal tests performed on a patient in a single year.

> A. Well, we have never had to write in for authority on that. We go ahead and do the work and give them our reasons for doing it and it's always been satisfactory.[75]

This lack of third-party control was verified by the general manager of OPS:

> Q. Well, does OPS ever try to regulate doctors in the manner in which they treat patients who are subscribers to OPS?
> A. No, we don't.[76]

Although it did not interfere with physicians' procedures, OPS did not always pay whatever the physician billed. A few physicians were disappointed by its failure to pay the full amount of their charges. A letter from a physician illustrates this point, and reveals some reasons for the founding of OPS:

> I have refused to be on the panel of the [OPS] because fees allowed for Internists have been ridiculously small. The fee schedule makes it impossible for me to participate in your activities.
> Just why we should have cut-rate fees in order to fight hospital associations (it was the original purpose in organizing the OPS), I cannot see, but I do wish you to bring this letter before the attention of your board and see if some just method of compensation can be arrived at for Internists.[77]

By and large, however, the great majority of the active membership of the Oregon State Medical Society became members of the OPS. By the middle of the first year in operation, ninety-five percent of the membership of the Society and eighty-five percent of all licensed practitioners in Oregon belonged to OPS.[78]

THE CONSEQUENCES OF OPS'S APPEARANCE

As OPS became established, the importance of the hospital associations began to diminish. By June 1944, the general manager of OPS was able to boast that his plan was already larger than all of the commercial organizations combined.[79] In 1948, the three remaining for-profit hospital associations made approximately twenty-four percent of total health insurance disbursements, down from fifty-one percent of all disbursements at the end of 1940.[80] Moreover, during this period the level of health insurance disbursements increased nearly five-fold in Oregon.

The reasons for the relative decline in hospital association disbursements can be readily understood. One had to be a member in "good standing" of the county medical societies in order to be eligible for OPS membership. Although there were no outright expulsions from any society for cooperating with the hospital associations, it seems that noncooperation with associations was, at least, an implicit requirement for membership and for a "good standing" rating.[81] In addition, county medical societies inhibited the growth of the associations by their encouragement of physician refusal to accept "tickets" for medical work performed. Tickets were provided to patients by the associations to be shown as evidence to the physician that the patient belonged to such an association. A cooperating physician would take the ticket and bill the association directly. If the physician refused to accept the ticket the patient would be liable for payment to the physician. An association which would subsequently reimburse the patient for less than the physician's charge (after a determination that a physician's procedures were unwarranted or too costly) would find itself in disfavor with the patient.

A letter from a physician to the National Hospital Association is illustrative of a physician's refusal to accept tickets:

In answer to your letter of December 27, I wish to state that it is through no fault of the Association that I am not taking any more slips [tickets] by them, but I promised the Oregon Physicians' Service that when all the other doctors quit the National I would also. I am the last doctor to do so.[82]

Another letter from a physician to a patient demonstrates the importance to the physician of the OPS membership:

Enclosed is the check which came in this morning to pay your bill. As I am on the list of the Oregon Physicians' Service, I am not allowed to sign a check of any other health association operating in the same district.[83]

Further evidence that physicians were willing to go along with the county medical societies even in the absence of any viable threat of expulsion is provided in the following letters to a patient and a lumber company:

1. This letter will serve as a means of establishing a diagnosis in your case with the National Hospital Association. Due to the fact that this hospital association is operated for a profit, members of the Medical Society are not allowed to make direct reports to them or to receive remuneration from them directly.[84]

2. It is a rule of the Douglas County Medical Society that its practicing physicians do not do any business with the National Hospital Association.

However, the patient, who is responsible to us for his own bill, is entitled to an itemized statement for his treatment. Such a statement is enclosed.[85]

Another reason for the relative decline in hospital association disbursements was the Oregon State Medical Society's support of its first statewide medical plan. OPS was given special permission to advertise in order to inform prospective patients about the "doctors'" plan.[86] Before OPS, only a threatened expulsion from a medical society could influence a physician to renounce the benefits of insurance of the associations; after its formation, the inducements to leave the private groups were far greater.

Faced with a rapidly declining market share, the for-profit hospital associations in Oregon could either persist in their traditional cost-cutting procedures or abandon their aggressive tactics in anticipation of future doctor cooperation. Dr. Pitman, a witness on behalf of the defendants and former president of the Washington County Medical Society, indicated that the associations chose the latter approach:

I started taking tickets again about March of 1948. By that time the hospital associations themselves had assumed the role of insurance companies. They no longer interfered with the relationship of the physician with the patient. They allowed the patient to choose any doctor in the community. . . . They did not attempt to dictate to the physician what he should do for the patient. Their fee schedule had been adjusted upward so that it was comparable to the schedule of OPS, which is our own organization. It ran a little less, but they usually pay 100 per cent, so it balanced out about the same.[87]

In reply to a question about whether his experience with the hospital associations in 1948 was different from that in previous years, he stated:

It is very much different, yes. I think it was only the opposition of the doctors and the organization of competing hospital associations that has brought about that difference in the relationship.[88]

Thus, the refusal of physicians to "take tickets" forced the hospital associations to reimburse the patient directly rather than to reimburse the physician. This put the onus of controlling physician charges and practices upon the patient and largely eliminated the ability of the hospital associations to control costs.

Though their market shares decreased, the three remaining for-profit hospital associations were able to continue in the market by changing their methods of operation.[89] The elimination of severe competitive pressures enabled the hospital associations to lead the "quiet life" under an OPS umbrella. In addition, in the early 1950s the commercial insurance companies entered the prepaid health insurance market in Oregon and were able to secure more than half of the total membership in health plans by 1957.[90]

In 1946, OPS became a charter member of the National Association of Blue Shield Plans, which coordinates the activities of local plans throughout the United States.[91] In some states, Blue Shield covers only physician services and Blue Cross covers hospitalization, while in others, such as Oregon, Blue Shield may cover both physician services and hospitalization.[92] There is little evidence of active oversight of medical decision making by Blue Shield or the commercial insurers,[93] in Oregon or elsewhere. The Oregon situation thus came to resemble the universal pattern of health insurer behavior.

A MODERN PARALLEL

Recent history has revealed increased private interest in controlling health care costs. Insurance companies offering dental insurance plans, for example, actively monitor dental treatment plans before authorizing payment for treatments expected to cost $100 or more. Under Aetna Life and Casualty's United Automobile Workers' benefits plan, several techniques are available for the investigation of questionable claims. Among them are "(a) discussion with the attending dentist; (b) examination of dental x-rays, study models, etc.; (c) case review by the Aetna's dental consultant when professional judgment is required."[94] In addition, Connecticut General Life Insurance Company has a well-advertised pre-treatment review program in which dentists send to Connecticut General a description of work to be done prior to treatment.[95]

One incident in particular, involving physicians, serves to illustrate the relevance of the Oregon experience to the current problem of health care costs. In that instance, as in Oregon in the 1940s, a private insurer which indicated some willingness to monitor costs was forced by the reaction of doctors and organized medicine to curtail its effort substantially and submit to professional control. Other private-sector cost-control efforts are reported to have encountered similar difficulties with professional groups.[96]

In the early 1970s, Aetna Life and Casualty Company, one of the largest private insurers, with nearly 12 million insureds, attempted to inject itself into disputes between doctors and patients. At that time, Aetna "had agreements with its usual and customary policyholders stating that where (1) Aetna disallowed a portion of the fee for exceeding prevailing limits, (2) attempts to resolve the difference with the doctor failed, (3) the patient refused to pay the balance himself, and (4) the doctor then sued him for it, Aetna would pay to defend the suit."[97] Since all these circumstances occurred infrequently, little attention was focused initially upon this Aetna policy. Aetna also sent form letters to insureds whose claims were not fully paid by Aetna, notifying the patients that the doctors were charging more than the prevailing rates in the area and thus encouraging nonpayment of bills.

As doctors became aware of the Aetna policy, individual physicians and medical societies made public protests. The AMA convention in June 1972 adopted a resolution that:

> took the position that *all* health insurers should consult with organized medicine in developing their fee profiles. It further declared that "the medical profession will not condone or tolerate action on the part of any third party that would encourage or promulgate [sic] litigation" in fee disputes and called for meetings between A.M.A. and Aetna representatives "to satisfactorily resolve the current problem."[98]

The following week in Florida a urologist sued the father of a five-year-old patient in small claims court for paying the physician only Aetna's prevailing rate rather than the full charge. Consistent with its policy, Aetna paid the policyholder's legal expenses. Two practicing specialists in the area testified that the fee was not unreasonable, and this influenced the judge to rule in favor of the plaintiff, forcing Aetna to pay attorney's fees, court costs, and the balance of the disputed bill.

The reaction of doctors to the publication of an article in *Medical Economics* describing the Florida case can be found in the letters-to-the-editor section of a later issue of the magazine. These letters show that the action taken by organized medicine in Oregon could be repeated against a cost-cutting insurer today:

> One obvious method of fighting Aetna's hard-line fee policy would be for doctors to refuse to perform life insurance physicals for Aetna, refuse to send any medical reports on a patient's health history to Aetna, and advise all patients who are Aetna policyholders to change carriers. I have adopted this policy in my office.[99]

In addition, Aetna, according to the letters of enraged doctors, was trying to cut costs in ways reminiscent of the Oregon experience:

> 1. Here's the latest from the Aetna audacity department! Now they are not only challenging fees, but in a recent experience of mine they challenged a diagnosis as well. They refused to pay my patient's claim because a lab report didn't support *their* ideas of what the diagnosis might be.
>
>   Now's the time to ostracize Aetna and consider them non-existent. If doctors and hospitals simply ignored them and refused any communication with them, we might then retain control of our rights and privileges in the practice of medicine.[100]
>
> 2. It seems that Aetna Life and Casualty is attempting to set itself up as a rate-setting commission, but until I read your special report, I thought this policy was limited to the Commonwealth of Massachusetts. Now I find it's nationwide.
>
>   . . . Our patients are admitted with validation forms approved by Aetna, but lately the majority of these claims have

been rejected for the most arbitrary reasons.

> Frankly, I can't tell whether Aetna is trying to set nationwide rate schedules or merely avoid payment responsibilities. If it's the latter, I'd like to know about it because then we could set our own new policy of not accepting patients who have coverage with Aetna.[101]

Under pressure from organized medicine, Aetna completely retreated from its original position. Apparently the threats of boycott did not appear to be empty threats to Aetna, since Blue Shield plans controlled by doctors were in existence throughout the country as a safe alternative to Aetna or any other carrier which dared get tough with physicians. In a meeting between representatives of Aetna and the AMA on August 3, 1972, Aetna affirmed the following:

> 1. Aetna has discontinued a standard practice of sending letters to patients offering to pay legal expenses should legal action be brought against one of its insureds. . . . It never has been and is not now Aetna's policy to encourage or to aid its insureds to bring legal action against physicians.
>
> 2. In the event a physician's charge exceeds in a significant amount Aetna's calculation of the upper limit of the range of prevailing fees for the procedure performed, Aetna will contact the physician prior to communicating its benefit determination to the claimant; however, contact will not necessarily be made when an individual physician's usual charge has been documented through past experience as routinely above the prevailing range as calculated by Aetna. . . .
>
> 3. When, following discussion with the physician, Aetna is unable to accept the full amount of a charge as within the range of prevailing fees, it will ordinarily seek the advice of a peer review committee or other review mechanism of the appropriate medical society before finally determining its benefit payment. . . .
>
> 4. In any instance involving a question of types of treatments, alternative types of

services, or volume of services ordered or provided, it is the policy of Aetna to make inquiry of the physician first and, if necessary, to seek supplemental advice through peer review. . . .[102]

As a result of the reaction to their more aggressive policy, Aetna today apparently does little (compared to the Oregon Hospital Association of the 1930s) to reduce physician charges and to limit unnecessary procedures.[103] For example, the company has reported that "in 5 percent of all claims Aetna processes for physicians' charges, Aetna's prevailing fee is less than the actual physician charge. Peer review is infrequently used in reconciling these two figures (peer review is used in less than 2/10 of one percent of all claims processed for surgical charges)."[104]

THE COURT DECISIONS IN THE OREGON CASE

In our description of the Oregon case, we have focused on the cost-reducing activities of the hospital associations as an important competitive development. Since the creation of OPS brought an end to this type of competition among hospital associations, we believe the mere existence of OPS as an instrument of organized medicine and a response to competitive developments that were not to doctors' liking should have been the crucial issue in the antitrust case. It was not.

The Justice Department complaint charged the defendant state and local medical societies with the monopolization of prepaid medical care (the more important part of the charge) and agreements not to compete among themselves for the prepaid medical care business.[105] The Department further alleged that "prepaid medical care organizations other than those sponsored by the defendants have been prevented and hindered in entering into or expanding their business in Oregon."[106] The relief sought by the government was consistent with its view of the case. There was no proposal to eliminate the physician control of the OPS. Rather, the defendants were to be "perpetually enjoined from further engaging in or carrying out said restraints and conspiracy, from doing any act in furtherance thereof, and from engaging in any similar conspiracy or course of conduct."[107]

The district judge ruled against the Justice Department in a misguided, sometimes irrelevant, opinion.[108] Unconcerned that cost cutting by the hospital associations had ended, the court was more disturbed by the "trend and drift towards Socialized Medicine."[109] Apparently the court was convinced that "the purpose of the doctors in OPS was to save themselves and their profession from threatened socialization."[110]

In the main body of its opinion, the court contrasted the events in Oregon prior to and subsequent to the formation of OPS in December 1941. The court acknowledged that prior to OPS some physicians would not cooperate with the associations out of fear of professional sanctions but noted that subsequent to the formation of OPS expulsions from medical societies ceased. Moreover, the court thought that the formation of OPS simply placed a new competitor into competition with the privately owned insurance firms.[111] In any event, according to the court, OPS could not be a monopoly "since only 120,000 of 1,510,000 people" in Oregon belonged to the organization.[112]

The trial court also ruled against the government's allegation that the state and local medical societies had agreed not to compete among themselves in any specific territory in Oregon. The court concluded that "if the needs of the public are adequately taken care of in a particular county through the activities of local physicians, the profession's duty as to prepaid medical care in that particular county is fully discharged."[113] This view of the matter ignores any benefits from competition among physicians or among insurers.

In April 1952, the Supreme Court, in a seven to one decision, upheld the district court.[114] The Court seemed to be persuaded by the argument that, since any anticompetitive behavior by the Oregon State Medical Society and its members was abandoned with the establishment of OPS, relief that might be ordered would be unnecessary. It held that the trial court's refusal to find an organized boycott against the hospital associations was not "clearly erroneous" despite evidence of the kind presented earlier. In a widely quoted dictum reflecting the government's failure to pierce the profession's "ethical" defenses, the Court said,

We might observe in passing, however, that there are ethical considerations where the historic direct relationship between patient and physician is involved which are quite different than the usual considerations prevailing in ordinary commercial matters. This Court has recognized that forms of competition usual in the business world may be demoralizing to the ethical standards of a profession.[115]

If the suit had been brought in today's climate of intense concern over rising health care costs, perhaps the government would have had more success in persuading the courts that insurer-sponsored cost controls are not an undesirable development.

SUMMARY ANALYSIS AND CONCLUSIONS

The record in this antitrust case, in contrast to the opinions and conclusions of the courts, reveals a great deal about the workings of the market for health services and health insurance and the incentives which face the major participants. A full understanding of the Oregon experience could lead to the development of an effective remedy for some of the current cost-escalation problems of the health care sector.

Before the development of OPS, the policy of the private hospital associations to control and reduce their payments to physicians was consistent with individual firms' efforts in any competitive industry to reduce input costs in order to remain competitive. This active competition appeared to benefit consumers by reducing the number of unnecessary (or cost-ineffective) procedures done by doctors and ultimately by reducing insurance premiums. By restraining demand for medical services, by substituting informed for ignorant buyers, and by curtailing opportunities for price discrimination, the hospital associations were able to reduce the prices which could be charged by physicians.

It is not difficult to understand why doctors were so vehemently opposed to the practices of the hospital associations. For one thing, physicians are taught to think that their profession is essentially different from any other profession or business because medicine deals directly with human life; the sentiment expressed by physicians and the medical societies that no one should make a profit from health care appears throughout the record of the case. However, it is essential to recognize the economic motives of

physicians themselves.[116] Evidence of physician concern for their economic well-being is revealed in the letters and other materials presented in this paper. In fact, the physicians appeared to behave in the manner which one would predict for any group which felt threatened economically—and which also considered itself exempt from antitrust prosecution.

As shown, the reaction of health care providers to the practices of the hospital associations in Oregon may be split into two periods. In the 1930s, the main weapon used was expulsion or threat of expulsion from county medical societies of doctors who worked for hospital associations or cooperated with them. The loss of medical society membership could have serious consequences for a doctor. He could lose his hospital privileges, his prestige in the eyes of his patients, and his access to the physician-controlled county medical service bureaus. After the *AMA* decision of 1940, however, the Oregon medical establishment had to end these practices and find an alternative way to combat the hospital associations. Moreover, the methods used prior to 1940 had not been very successful in encouraging doctors to stop cooperating with the hospital associations, for, without an alternative system of health insurance, the typical physician found it too costly to discontinue his relationship with the associations even though he despised their interference in his practice.

OPS finally provided the needed alternative to the hospital associations. Although several county medical bureaus were already in existence, the formation of a statewide company greatly strengthened the attractiveness of the doctor-run plans since patients could be treated throughout the state. Now organized medicine in Oregon could effectively encourage the boycotting of hospital associations by doctors and could successfully urge patients to join OPS. As OPS grew, physicians found that their need for hospital associations to guarantee payment became less urgent, and they could increasingly afford to refuse to deal with them directly.

It is important to recognize that the refusal of doctors to deal directly with the hospital associations was the factor which finally made it impossible for the associations to continue to serve as a cost-cutting instrument. The hospital associations could still indemnify the patient for expenditures incurred, but if an association felt that a patient had been overcharged or treated unnecessarily, it could do little about it. As previously described, Aetna's undertaking to assist its insureds in resisting doctor's legal actions reveals the limits on insurers' power where doctors' cooperation cannot be enlisted in advance. Moreover, insurers may find it impossible to obtain from noncooperating doctors the records needed to restrict unnecessary procedures. Faced with such difficulties, today's health insurers cannot be blamed for not attempting much in the area of cost control.

A question which arises from the Oregon experience is whether physician control of the dominant insurer is an essential condition for preventing cost-cutting initiatives by the other insurers. Without a physician-controlled insurance company, one might expect the market to produce an array of private insurers which would offer a variety of price/quality packages to consumers. Those firms which offered a high-premium/mild-surveillance package would be preferred by physicians; yet, without an insurer controlled by physicians, the possibility remains that any individual insurer might attempt to monitor physician decision making if competitive pressures or temptations became too intense. It seems possible, for example, that the absence of a professionally controlled insurer may explain, at least in part, the comparatively greater surveillance exercised by insurers over dentists. If it were clearly recognized that the medical profession is prohibited under antitrust principles from organizing or even encouraging provider resistance against unorthodox plans, perhaps the expected variety of insurance packages would begin to appear.

The *Oregon State Medical Society* case illustrates that competitive cost cutting by private insurers can indeed occur under certain circumstances. Doctors would be unhappy about such a development, but this is not surprising. All suppliers of services would prefer to deal with acquiescent consumers from whom monopoly rents can be extracted rather than with knowledgable buyers who have incentives to question the value and price of what is being sold. In showing that a strong doctor-controlled insurance company can compel private insurers to curtail their cost-cutting procedures, the experience in Oregon suggests that competition among health insurers is apt to be more effective in the absence of physician control of any carrier.

Rather than adding to health costs, the existence of a competitive insurance market might well prove to be an effective force in containing them.

NOTES

1. In 1975, spending on health care rose to an annual rate of 12.6 percent compared to a 7.3 percent rise in the consumer price index. Council on Wage & Price Stability, *The Problem of Rising Health Care Costs* (Washington: Executive Office of the President, April 1976); Council of Economic Advisers, *Economic Report of the President* (Washington: U.S. Government Printing Office, 1976), p. 124, Tables 27 and 71. Table 12 (hereinafter cited as *1976 Economic Report of the President*). Whereas in 1965 health care expenditures were 5.9 percent of gross national product, in 1975 they were 8.3 percent or more than $118 billion. Ibid., p. 118, Table 35.

2. Most of the increase in health care costs apparently has not contributed to a commensurate increase in the public's health. See V. Fuchs, *Who Shall Live?* (New York: Basic Books, 1974), especially pp. 30–55. In the past few years there has been little increase in life expectancy. Mortality rates in countries which spend far less than the United States on health care are lower. In addition, critics of the health delivery system remain dissatisfied with the level of medical care available to various segments of the population.

3. Between 1960 and 1975, third-party payments (both public and private) grew from 44.6 percent to 67.4 percent of personal health expenditures, and from 81.4 percent to 92.0 percent of hospital expenditures. *1976 Economic Report of the President,* p. 118, Table 35.

4. M. Feldstein, *The Rising Cost of Hospital Care* (Washington: Information Resources Press, 1971), pp. 27–28. Medicare and Medicaid—public programs modeled after private health insurance—also have contributed to the problem.

5. Apparently auto insurers also attempt to minimize automobile accident costs. Allstate, the largest stock company auto insurer, has led a nationwide campaign to require air bags in automobiles.

6. See National Commission on State Workmen's Compensation Laws, *Report 87-98* (Washington: U.S. Government Printing Office, 1972).

7. For example, automobile manufacturers deter dealer abuses by such techniques as auditing those dealers whose average-warranty-work-per-car is high, or requiring "prior approval" by a local representative of all repair work likely to cost above a certain amount. See D. Randall and A. Glickman, *The Great American Auto Repair Robbery* (New York: Charterhouse, 1972), pp. 44–46.

8. See M. Pauly, "The Economics of Moral Hazard: Comment," *American Economic Review* 58 (June 1968): 531–537.

9. Data from Blue Shield reveal that only 0.04 percent of benefit claims paid to physicians are disallowed because of questionable patterns of practice. Though it is difficult to suggest a hypothetical standard to which these savings may be compared, they appear negligible relative to the cost-cutting procedures of the hospital associations in the 1930s in Oregon. See Ohio Medical Indemnity, Inc. (Blue Shield), *Cost Containment Reports-Second Quarter 1975,* submitted in *Ohio v. Ohio Medical Indemnity, Inc.,* No. C2-75-473 (S.D. Ohio, filed July 9, 1975). See also "Blue Cross Called Lax on Curbing Health Costs," *The New York Times,* August 4, 1975, p. 40, and "Deneberg Uses Travelers–Blue Cross Decision to Blast Private Insurers," *The National Underwriter,* January 22, 1972, p. 1. For an instance in which a private insurer attempted to restrain costs, see text accompanying notes infra.

10. While many states have restrictions upon the employment of physicians by a corporation, many cost-saving possibilities are still available through other means. A compendium of the alternatives open to insurers can be found in Council on Wage and Price Stability, *Labor-Management Innovations in Controlling Cost of Employee Health Care Benefits,* 41 *Fed. Reg.* 40298 (September 17, 1976). Importantly, none of these types of procedures is expressly forbidden by state insurance laws.

11. Council on Wage and Price Stability, *The Problem of Rising Health Care Costs,* pp. 16 ff.

12. See D. Salkever and T. Bice, "The Impact of Certificate-of-Need Controls on Hospital Investment," *Milbank Memorial Fund Quarterly* 54 (Spring, 1975): 185; and C. Havighurst and J. Blumstein, "Coping with Quality/Cost Trade-Offs in Medical Care: The Role of PSROs," *Northwestern University Law Review* 70 (March-April 1975): 6.

13. 343 U.S. 326 (1952), affirming 95 F. Supp. 103 (D. Or. 1950).

14. See L. Reed, *Blue Cross and Medical Service Plans* (Washington: U.S. Public Health Service, 1947); pp. 136–37; and G. Shipman, R. Lampman, and S. Miyamato, *Medical Service Corporation in the State of Washington* (Cambridge: Harvard University Press, 1962), pp. 7–9, for an early history of the hospital associations.

15. For a description of the health maintenance organizations concept, see C. Havighurst, "Health Maintenance Organizations and the Market for Health Services," *Law and Contemporary Problems* 35 (Autumn, 1970): 716.

16. Ch. 173 (1917) *Ore. Gen. Laws* 218; 2158, *United States v. Oregon State Medical Society,* 343 U.S. 326 (1952). For convenience, the *Record* will be cited, without further item and footnote citations to the mi-

crocard upon which it appears rather than to the original printed record.

17. See T. Hammond, "Corporate and Organizational History of OPS and Other Hospital Associations in Oregon," Speech before OPS Annual Statewide Staff Meeting (February 27, 1958), pp. 1,2. In addition to the for-profit hospital associations, two physician-sponsored contract practice associations, Eugene Hospital and Clinic and Hillside Hospital Corp., also were in the market. Finally, three medical service bureaus, approved by the Oregon State Medical Society, in which physicians practiced solely on a fee-for-service basis, sold prepaid insurance. These medical service bureaus were merged into OPS in the early 1940s. Ibid., pp. 2, 3.

18. R. 4810. Market shares are calculated here on a disbursement rather than on a revenue-received basis. There appears to be no significant difference between the two measures, however.

19. R. 6832-33. All quotations from the record have been corrected for typographical, grammatical, and punctuation errors.

20. Darby and Karni have used the term credence goods to describe goods which "cannot be evaluated in normal use," such as the removal of an appendix or the replacement of a television tube. See M. Darby and E. Karni, "Free Competition and the Optimal Amount of Fraud," *Journal of Law and Economics* 16 (April 1973): 67, 68–69.

21. See R. Kessel, "Price Discrimination in Medicine," *Journal of Law and Economics* 1 (October 1958): 20.

22. Section 5 of the American Medical Association's *Principles of Medical Ethics* states that a physician "should not solicit patients." American Medical Association, *Opinions and Reports of the Judicial Council* (Chicago: American Medical Association, 1971), pp. 30–31. In discussing the advertising prohibition, the AMA's Judicial Council has also made it plain that the ban extends to group practice (Ibid., p. 23):

Many of the questions submitted to the Council involve the subject of solicitation of patients. As is well-known, there is a tendency for physicians to organize themselves into so-called groups under various designations, such as group clinics, diagnostic clinics, group medicine, medical institutes, the medical academy, and similar names. Some of these groups are advertising in a manner that would be considered most reprehensible if done by an individual physician. The Council is unable to see any difference in principle between a group of physicians advertising themselves under whatsoever title they may assume and an individual physician advertising himself.

23. See also Appendix B to the *Brief of the Oregon State Medical Society,* pp. 146–51. . . .

24. R. 6836 (dated June 3, 1936).

* * *

32. R. 7025 (March 14, 1941).

33. R. 7026 (March 19, 1941).

34. R. 7048 (dated Oct. 19, 1938).

35. R. 7011.

36. See notes . . . 34, and 35 and accompanying text. Had insurers continued their cost control efforts, they would undoubtedly have been required to accommodate the many conflicting interests, increase their medical sophistication, and maximize the cost-effectiveness of their methods.

37. See 41 *Fed. Reg.* 13452 (March 30, 1976).

38. See Havighurst and Blumstein, "Coping with Quality/Cost Trade-Offs in Medicare: The Role of PSROs," pp. 52–60.

39. Consumer desires also should dictate that competition among insurance companies would not result in an excessive emphasis on cost control at the expense of desired technological change.

40. In a similar manner, the King County Medical Society in Washington State began to develop a physician-controlled prepaid insurance plan after boycotting the private contract practice plans. See G. Shipman, R. Lampman, and S. Miyamoto, *Medical Service Corporations in the State of Washington,* pp. 22–25 and *Group Health Cooperative of Puget Sound v. King County Medical Soc'y,* 39 Wash. 2d 586, 237 P. 2d 737 (1951).

41. R. 2798 (*Statement of Principles and Procedures for the Control of Contract Practice* adopted by the House of Delegates of the Oregon State Medical Society Oct. 10, 1936).

42. Committee on the Costs of Medical Care, *Medical Care for the American People* (Washington: Department of Health, Education and Welfare, 1970 reprint; originally published 1932), pp. 156–57 (minority report). E. Rayack, *Professional Power and American Medicine* (Cleveland: World Publishing Co., 1967), p. 152.

43. Editorial, "The Committee on the Costs of Medical Care," *Journal of the American Medical Association* 99 (Dec. 3, 1932): 1950–52.

44. R. 3691.

45. R. 3691.

46. R. 3696.

47. R. 3695.

48. The Oregon State Medical Society disapproved of the C.H. Weston Hospital Association in September, 1940, for the stated reason that it was "not owned and controlled by physicians who are members of their local society and the Oregon State Medical Society." R. 3148.

49. R. 5193. As in most other states in which physicians developed their own medical plans, the initial emphasis was on insurance for low-wage groups only. By insuring only low-income groups physicians were able to receive payment from those most likely to default yet still charge their more affluent patients what the market would bear. See R. Kessel, "Price Discrimination in Medicine," pp. 32–42 for a review of the development of physician-sponsored plans and the conflicts with private prepaid plans in Oklahoma, California, Washington, and Illinois. See also Hyde and Wolff, "The American Medical Association: Power, Purpose, and Politics in Organized Medicine," *Yale Law Journal* 63 (1954): 938, 992–94 and H. Somers and A. Somers, *Doctors, Patients and Health Insurance* (Washington: Brookings Institution, 1961), pp. 317–19.

50. R. 3734. By 1940 five medical service bureaus, all of which operated as distinct organizations under the guidance and approval of the Oregon State Medical Society, were formed. According to the *Report of the Oregon Insurance Commissioner,* the five bureaus had 35 percent of the total "hospital association" market. ("Hospital associations," as summarized in the *Report of the Insurance Commissioner* apparently included prepaid medical service bureaus.) See *Report of the Insurance Commissioner,* R. 4818 and R. 5189–5193, for a brief description of the medical service bureaus.

51. R. 5503–04. There is no evidence that Industrial Hospital Association ever accepted the offer.

52. *Journal of American Medical Association* 99 (December 3, 1932): 1951 quoted in E. Rayak, *Professional Power and American Medicine,* p. 155.

53. Ibid., pp. 164–66.

54. Ibid., pp. 172–75.

55. See R. 4460–61 (letter from the Multnomah County Medical Society to Dr. Steagall, Sept. 17, 1936).

56. See R. 2558–60, 2564.

57. R. 2569.

58. R. 2570.

59. See R. 5511–12, 5616, 5708–09, and Defendants' *Opening Statement,* R. 334.

60. See R. 6072 (letter from Oregon State Medical Society, dated April 21, 1938, to physician inquiring about ethical standards of Association). One aspect of medical ethics appears to be a prohibition against solicitation of patients (see R. 5512). Apparently, the initial lack of success of the Association forced it to engage in these commercial tactics.

61. See R. 4208, 4434, 3601 (registration letters dated Dec. 3, 1937, June 7, 1938, and Nov. 29, 1938 from physicians to the Prudential, Pumphrey, and Industrial Hospital Associations).

62. R. 2166–67 (letter from Oregon State Medical Society to Jackson County Medical Society, Dec. 11, 1939).

63. See State of Oregon, *Report of Insurance Commissioner* (1936), R. 4810 and ibid. (1941), R. 3829.

64. See letter from Industrial Hospital Association to Southern Oregon Credit Bureau, January 28, 1939, R. 3575.

65. *United States v. American Medical Association,* 110 F.2d 703 (D.C. Cir. 1940) aff'd. 317 U.S. 519 (1943).

66. 317 U.S. at 528.

67. Compare the differences in medical services bureau plans. R. 2326.

68. Compare with R. Kessel, "Price Discrimination in Medicine," pp. 31–32. Kessel suggests that expulsion from the county medical society is the "most formidable sanction" to control unethical physician behavior such as price cutting. Ibid. at 31. Expulsion from the medical society can mean denial of hospital privileges for physicians. Kessel did not consider, however, the effect that denial of service plan membership would have on physician behavior.

69. R. 2060.

70. R. 2332.

71. R. 3518–22.

72. See "Memorandum of Understanding" between OPS and Physicians of Jackson County, Oregon, August 24, 1942, R. 3470–71.

73. R. 2397.

74. R. 4866.

75. R. 1215.

76. R. 1661.

77. R. 3538–39 (Oct. 1, 1948). It has been suggested to us that OPS may have paid low fees (less than 100 cents on each dollar billed) to physicians in order to offer attractive low-priced premiums to subscribers—a form of predatory or "disciplinary" pricing designed to capture a large enough market share to be effective and to demonstrate to the hospital associations a willingness to compete with them in prices as long as they persisted in their cost-control efforts. However, we found nothing in the record to indicate this directly, nor were we able to compare unambiguously the health benefit premium package of the hospital associations with OPS. See text accompanying note 87 (letter from Dr. Pitman).

78. R. 3520.

79. R. 4371.

80. R. 4866, 4829.

81. See letters from physicians to patients. R. 2121, 2127, and 2157. See also R. 5340, *Pre-Trial Stipulation of Facts.*

82. R. 2154 (dated Dec. 29, 1943), emphasis deleted.

83. R. 2157 (dated May 19, 1944).

84. R. 2121 (dated Apr. 3, 1947).

85. R. 2121 (dated Apr. 3, 1947).

86. R. 6592-93.1. Compare with AMA, *Principles of Medical Ethics.* Advertising by OPS in extolling the benefits of health insurance in general probably had a positive effect on the growth of the entire health insurance industry.

87. R. 1580.

88. R. Ibid.

89. Two of the five associations, Pumphrey and Weston, went out of business by the end of 1940, before the emergence of OPS. See R. 4818, 4829 (*Reports of the Insurance Commissioner of Oregon* for Dec. 31, 1939, and Dec. 31, 1940).

90. T. Hammond, "Corporate and Organizational History of OPS and other Hospital Associations in Oregon," p. 9. In 1974, Blue Shield covered only 16 percent of Oregon's population. See *Blue Cross/Blue Shield Fact Book,* 1975, p. 17.

91. T. Hammond, "Corporate and Organizational History of OPS and other Hospital Associations in Oregon," p. 7.

92. Blue Cross in Oregon also covers physician services and hospitalization and competes with Blue Shield for this insurance. Past Blue Shield attempts to merge with Blue Cross in Oregon ended in failure because of the issue of ultimate control of the combined organization. See R. 3219 and R. 3220.

93. See note 9.

94. *Aetna Dental Claim Procedures* provided by Aetna to one of the authors, December 23, 1976.

95. See, e.g., *Time Magazine,* December 20, 1976, p. 37. See also, Council on Wage and Price Stability, *Labor-Management Innovations In Controlling Cost of Employee Health Care Benefits.*

96. See "Editorial," *Washington Post,* October 1, 1976; and "Aetna Tests Plan to Reduce Unneeded Surgery," *Washington Post,* November 30, 1976, p. 1.

97. Charlotte L. Rosenberg, "He Challenged Aetna's Hard-line Fee Policy—and Won," *Medical Economics* (Sept. 11, 1972): 31.

98. *Ibid.,* p. 34.

99. "Letters to the Editors," *Medical Economics* (Dec. 4, 1972): 27.

100. *Ibid.,* pp. 27–28.

101. *Ibid.,* pp. 28–29.

102. *Aetna Affidavit, Exhibit D. State of Ohio v. Ohio Medical Indemnity, Inc.,* Cir. No. 2-75-473 (S.D. Ohio, filed July 9, 1975).

103. However, Aetna has recently decided in Washington, D.C. to cover the expense of second opinions on "elective" surgery. See "Aetna Test Plan to Reduce Unneeded Surgery," *Washington Post,* November 30, 1976, p. 1.

104. *Aetna Affidavit,* p. 2.

105. Justice Department, *Complaint,* October 18, 1948, Section 32(a) and (i), R. 6–7.

106. Ibid., section 35(a), R. 8.

107. Ibid., *Prayer,* section 3, R. 9–10.

108. *U.S. v. Oregon State Medical Soc'y.,* 95 F. Supp. 103 (D. Ore. 1950)., aff'd. 343 U.S. 326 (1952).

109. Ibid., p. 109. The court quoted from an editorial in a bar association publication. Editorial, *Oregon State Bar Bulletin* (Aug. 1950).

110. 95 F. Supp. p. 109. The court further quoted from the above-cited Editorial that "The trend and drift towards Socialized Medicine should be all the lawyer needs to recognize that Socialized law is but the next step for those dedicated to the socialized-police state." Ibid.

111. Ibid., p. 116.

112. Ibid., p. 107.

113. Ibid.

114. *United States v. Oregon State Medical Society,* 343 U.S. 326 (1952).

115. Ibid., p. 336.

116. The situation in Oregon can be viewed as an attempt by physicians to decrease the elasticity of the demand for health care by eliminating the price conscious element of the market, the hospital association.

1.7 Controlling Health Care Costs: Strengthening the Private Sector's Hand*

CLARK G. HAVIGHURST

The Council on Wage and Price Stability (CWPS) recently has published a series of three highly valuable reports on health care costs.[2] The present essay serves to underscore and elaborate what the second of these CWPS reports, detailing labor-management innovations in cost control, called "the heretofore unappreciated potential of the private sector to combat the problem [of rising health care costs] and possibly exert substantial downward pressure on [them]."[3] The argument here is that the Council's studies have uncovered the key to a needed rethinking of health policy, challenging the prevailing assumptions about the direction in which the nation must move to solve the health sector's undoubted problems. Senator Edward Kennedy has stated the most widely held view as follows:

> The different elements [of the health care system]—employers, employees, doctors, insurance companies, hospitals—all understand what has to be done. But they all say they can't do it. There seems to be only one way to get health care costs under control. The federal government has to become involved.[4]

The insight offered in this essay is that, while federal "involvement" in the health sector is clearly called for, it need not take a form as broad as the intervention contemplated in Senator Kennedy's Health Security proposal.[5] As the CWPS staff suggests,[6] it can appropriately be confined, at least initially, to untying and strengthening the private sector's hands, allowing private decision makers a reasonable chance to determine, and do, "what has to be done."

I. WHAT THE PRIVATE SECTOR IS AND IS NOT DOING

The CWPS September staff report on labor-management cost-control innovations is striking not only for what it shows to be going on in the private sector but also for what it shows is not going on. On the one hand, it reveals a wide variety of serious, imaginative efforts by unions, employers, insurers, and others to solve complex cost-related problems. These creative efforts to reconcile conflicting interests, to assure administrative cost-effectiveness, and to adapt promising ideas to particular circumstances all suggest that there may be no one right answer to the cost problem but that the motivation, flexibility, and experimental capacity of the private sector are valuable resources in the fight, frequently capable of achieving at the grass roots what government, at its level, cannot. The Council's efforts thus have value not only in promoting the exchange of cost-control ideas

*This essay is adapted from testimony delivered before the Council on Wage and Price Stability, Houston, Texas, October 21, 1976. Its preparation was supported by Grant No. HS01539 from the National Center for Health Services Research, DHEW. The counsel of Randall Bovbjerg is gratefully acknowledged.

and experience but also in revealing the importance of diversity in attacking the problem of health care costs. They should cause people to take the private sector seriously as a potential factor in the ultimate solution.

Equally noteworthy is the Council's demonstration that many highly promising approaches to cost control are *not* being pursued. Especially significant is the almost total absence of mechanisms having a direct impact on the providers of services, particularly physicians. Even though it is doctors' treatment and pricing decisions which primarily determine health care costs, the only influence over these decisions that is being achieved by private sector efforts is almost entirely indirect, even incidental. Such cost-containment techniques are thus apt to be both more costly to administer and less effective than more direct measures would be. Several examples of surprising cautiousness in cost control can be drawn from the Council's report:

1. Second opinions prior to elective treatments have been made mandatory only with respect to dental care, not elective surgery.[7]
2. Even when an obligation to obtain a second opinion exists, it appears to fall on the patient, not the dentist,[8] even though a more efficient arrangement would be a direct understanding with individual providers that they would advise the health insurer or plan administrator of their treatment intentions in advance, thus triggering the second-opinion procedure automatically; such an arrangement would permit denial of payment altogether to a provider who violated the understanding and would largely obviate educating, pressuring, and denying indemnification to uncomprehending patients.
3. The only health plans which have obtained individual provider commitments on fee levels and excluded noncomplying providers are those involving opticians and pharmacies; yet there is no good reason why doctors, dentists, and hospitals also could not be put under individually negotiated reimbursement schedules.[9]
4. The predominant response to the excessive hospitalization allegedly induced by insurance covering inpatient but not outpatient care has been to broaden coverage to elim-

inate the bias;[10] yet direct controls on hospital admissions would seem to be an equally logical means of dealing with this problem.
5. Even where such controls on hospitalization do exist, they are administered by professional organizations, not by the parties with a stake in cost control.[11]

The question which the Council's report brings to mind is why the private sector, its motivation clearly strong, nevertheless has neglected certain obvious responses to cost problems, adopting inefficient or less effective means when better arrangements seem available.

These observations suggest that the discovery by the CWPS of the private sector's active interest and effectiveness in controlling health care costs needs to be supplemented by increased understanding of precisely why such efforts have not appeared before, have not prevented our current cost problems from arising, and have been more limited in scope than the magnitude of the problem requires. This essay argues that the private sector's past failings are not the result of any inherent deficiency in the market mechanism and that certain relatively simple policy changes, involving only limited federal intervention in the health services industry, could give the private sector many opportunities it heretofore has lacked to deal with health care costs. If these arguments are correct, then what the CWPS has observed in the way of private cost-control ingenuity is more than a useful anti-inflationary development. It is a cornerstone of an approach to health policy that, if adopted, could prove highly effective in promoting the needed balancing of the benefits and costs of medical care. Such an approach is outlined briefly in this essay in the belief that it is a promising alternative to the more sweeping financing and regulatory proposals currently being considered. Indeed, strengthening the private sector's ability to deal with cost problems could well hasten the day when the federal government could, without fear of setting off another burst of inflation, substantially expand its assistance to those citizens who are now unable to obtain adequate attention to their health needs.

As a practical political matter, there may be little time left for calling appropriate public and congressional attention to the alternative of relying primarily on the private sector to achieve effective and sensitive containment of health care costs. This essay expresses the hope that the important work of the CWPS will stimulate not only private cost-control efforts for their own sake but also policymakers' attention to the possibility that private decisions would be more effective than public decisions in appropriately allocating society's resources to and within the health care sector.

II. THE PROBLEM: THIRD-PARTY PAYMENT WITHOUT COST CONTROLS

What emerged most sharply from the CWPS's April report on rising health care costs was that cost problems stem from Americans' having too much of the wrong kind of financial protection against burdensome medical expenses. It should be stressed, however, that it is not third-party payment alone which has produced our problems but the breadth of its coverage and the absence in the various programs of any significant administrative checks on the price or utilization of services.[12] Indeed, most of the "unique" features of the health care industry that were noted in the April report are merely reflections of the particular financing mechanisms which have evolved. Thus, the central decision-making role of the physician, while obvious,[13] is of major consequence only because, when health insurance was introduced and its coverage expanded, no other accountability for the cost of care was substituted for the doctor's previous fiduciary obligation to look out for his patient's pocketbook as well as his health. Similarly, the ability of hospitals to tolerate inefficiency and to expand their investment in expensive capital equipment and in larger and more highly trained staffs[14] flows directly from the decreasing need, due to automatic third-party cost reimbursement, to keep the cost of care within particular bounds.

While these points were well made in the CWPS April report, that statement might have gone further in tracing the reasons *why* financing mechanisms took the form they did. Were consumers simply perverse in seeking first-dollar ("shallow") coverage and neglecting to protect themselves adequately against unpredictable, catastrophic risks? Was it inevitable that health insurance would leave providers free to spend insurers' money without accountability? If not, why did not financing mechanisms develop in such a way as to assure that services rendered at plan expense were truly needed and that needed care was rendered in the least expensive acceptable way? Did insurance company executives simply not recognize the importance of experimenting with cost controls and different delivery arrangements in order to find acceptable low-cost alternatives? Were consumers not interested in lower-cost arrangements? Such questions make it clear that our current problems stem from history, from long-established practices that only lately have been recognized for what they are—one of the most potent vehicles for systematically misallocating the nation's resources that we have ever seen.

Once third-party payment patterns were established with relatively shallow coverage and without controls initiated by insurers in the consumer's interest, a vicious upward spiral was set in motion as cost increases made possible by insurance necessitated purchase of more insurance protection, in turn stimulating further cost increases and more insurance. Predictably, this spiral eventually reached the plane of political action. The Medicare and Medicaid programs, designed to help particularly vulnerable groups cope with higher costs, were the first response to the emerging crisis; but, being modeled after the privately developed insurance plans which preceded them, these programs simply accelerated the inflationary trend. Now, little more than ten years later, still higher costs have produced pressure for a "national health insurance" program which, it is hoped, will "solve" the cost problem for everyone. The variety of direct and indirect cost controls being implemented by government are simply an attempt to supply belatedly what the private sector did not.

What were the causes of the private sector's failure to control costs without government assistance? Excessive growth of the wrong kinds of financial protection against medical care costs can be traced to just two major causes, neither of which has been widely recognized as the pernicious influence it is: (1) the tax law's treatment of health insurance premiums and (2) provider dictation of the type of insurance plans available to consumers. An understanding of how these influences have distorted (and continue to distort) the provision of health services and the private sector's cost-control efforts points toward policy proposals which would give the private sector the chance it never really has had to assure that consumers get value for money in health care.

III. SOURCES OF THE PROBLEM

A. Tax Treatment of Insurance Premiums

As the CWPS April report observed,[15] the tax treatment of health insurance premiums has substantially weakened the consumer's incentive to self-insure when it would make good sense to do so, and thus has determined in large measure the character of privately purchased health insurance. Quite simply, the tax law has long encouraged employers and employees to buy group insurance with low deductibles—that is, shallow coverage—in order that even routine medical bills could be paid with untaxed rather than after-tax dollars. Economist Martin Feldstein has estimated that a typical wage earner can purchase nearly 50 percent more health care for the same money in this manner.[16] Such shallow coverage invites consumers to seek and providers to give care which would not have seemed worthwhile if paid for out of pocket. Overinsurance against routine expenses has greatly expanded the area in which normal cost constraints do not operate. The growing popularity of dental insurance as a fringe benefit is another manifestation of the tax law's inducement of overinsurance; the tax benefit aside, such plans benefit dentists more than patients.[17]

Change in the tax treatment of health insurance premiums would be one useful step permitting increased reliance on consumer cost-consciousness to discourage overinsurance and to induce the design and purchase of insurance plans or other financing schemes with cost-control features. Outright repeal of favorable tax treatment for premiums is politically impossible, of course, but introduction of an upper limit on the exclusion of employer-paid premiums from income and wages for income and FICA tax purposes might be feasible. Better yet, the present form of subsidy might be dropped and a more straightforward subsidy adopted in the form of a limited credit against the employee's taxes for employer- and employee-paid premiums on his private health insurance. Although the maximum tax credit might be set to continue the subsidy at the current level of approximately $8

billion per year and to avoid both at net tax increase and a serious revenue loss, a switch to tax credits to encourage health insurance coverage could be the occasion for a tax reduction indicated for fiscal reasons. The credit also could bring about other arguably desirable results, such as an increase in Social Security revenues, an overall reduction in the net tax burden of low- and middle-income taxpayers, and a tax increase for persons in higher brackets. Far from being politically impossible, such a package would have some attractions.[18] In addition to ending the disproportionately favorable tax subsidy for individuals in higher brackets, a system of limited tax credits would make it possible to allow larger credits for lower-income taxpayers if they were considered unable to meet additional costs out of pocket. The tax system could easily provide for refundable credits—payments to those persons who had income taxes insufficient to absorb the credit.

Such alterations in the nontaxability of income earmarked for use by the health sector would have important public benefits. The availability of a new tax credit would spur the purchase of basic insurance protection by those persons who are not now covered adequately. But the fixed limit on the credit would mean that people would be spending their own after-tax money for additional coverage and thus would be under normal constraints not to obtain more coverage than they really need. Shallow coverage would almost certainly be reduced as more people sought protection primarily against unpredictable and catastrophic costs. Most employees would find reductions in their current health benefits more than offset by the extra take-home pay made possible by the new tax credit and the lower premiums on less comprehensive insurance.[19] Once consumers and their bargaining representatives came to recognize that their interests no longer lay in taking income in the form of extra health-related fringe benefits, insurers would be pressed to provide optimal protection for the amount of money which people were willing to commit. They would immediately find greater resistance to premium increases, causing them to consider greater use of cost controls as a means of giving more essential coverage for a given price. Thus, some such change in the tax system seems an important step in restoring the private sector's incentive to control health care costs optimally.

A fully worked out health policy also would have to address possibilities for restoring the cost consciousness of beneficiaries of public programs and an expansion of public programs to cover all those in need of more heavily subsidized care. As indicated, the tax system might be adapted to serve these purposes, or a system of vouchers might be used. Price competition for the patronage of otherwise indigent citizens could be encouraged by letting plans, within some limits, pay experience-related dividends or even cash rebates to those who spent their tax credits or their vouchers to enroll.[20] This approach is clearly preferable to requiring the poor to supplement the government subsidy if they want additional coverage or enrollment in a "better" plan. Yet, by allowing people to benefit from their economizing choices, it achieves the desired result of reintroducing constrained consumer choice as the determinant of resource allocation. The proposal of such fundamental changes in the Medicare and Medicaid programs will seem impractical or impolitic to many observers, but nothing less than meaningful price competition will fully serve the objective of appropriate cost control. The other approaches available are distinctly second-best.[21]

The practical problems confronted in changing the tax law and federal health programs to strengthen or reintroduce consumer cost-consciousness are obviously considerable, as are the additional problems of protecting consumers against possible mistakes in their purchasing decisions. Nevertheless, these problems should yield to careful study and seem quite minor when compared to those which would be encountered in controlling costs and the quality of care directly under other national health insurance plans.[22] It is regrettable that so little effort has been expended on rethinking the forms of government subsidy to the health sector as a means of stimulating private decision makers to spend wisely.

B. Provider Resistance to Cost Control.

The second—and probably the more important—major cause of the private sector's failure to establish financing programs which serve consumers' interests is the control which medical care providers have exerted over the design and implementation of such plans. Health insurance was opposed absolutely by the medi-

cal profession for many years. Only when the hospitals and doctors themselves came to sponsor—and control the practices of—third-party payment schemes (Blue Cross and Blue Shield) did they become an accepted medium of financial protection.[23] These plans were designed, however, not only to protect patients but also to assure providers that they could easily collect payment for their services. This emphasis resulted simultaneously in excessive shallow coverage and inadequate protection against the rare but large and unpredictable costs which (without the tax advantage) are the only risks that most rational consumers would elect to insure against.[24] State legislation, enacted largely at the behest of medical care providers, restricted the development of plans which served consumer interests, and the provider-dominated "Blues" were given unique powers to contract with providers directly for the provision of services. Commercial insurers, on the other hand, were barred from any role in supplying and controlling services by the prohibition against the "corporate practice of medicine."[25] Instead, they were relegated to indemnifying patients for bills incurred, a role which greatly impaired their ability to monitor or control provider behavior. At the same time, "ethical" standards of the medical profession and other subtle sanctions were being invoked to prevent doctors from associating with independent health care plans which competed with the uncontrolled system.[26]

Despite the restraints imposed, history has provided occasional glimpses into the private sector's potential for stimulating constructive approaches to cost problems. Prepaid group practice, the forerunner of the health maintenance organization (HMO) movement, has been the only mechanism to achieve any permanence, and it has taken root in only a few places and only after legendary struggles and many compromises with organized medicine.[27] Less well recognized, because uniformity in insurer behavior is mistaken for inevitability, is the role that organized medicine has played in dictating the practices of private health insurers. The most revealing experience, which occurred in Oregon in the 1930s and 1940s, was the subject in the early 1950s of an unsuccessful antitrust suit.[28] The record of that litigation has recently been reexamined by two Federal Trade Commission (FTC) economists for insights into our current problems.[29] They have found that the introduction of a Blue Shield plan in Oregon, coupled with a partial boycott by doctors of allegedly "unethical" insurance plans, halted for all time the insurers' established practice of requiring physicians to justify their expenditure of insurer funds. Under the pressures thus brought to bear, the insurers ceased the practices which the doctors found objectionable but which today seem to be merely rudimentary versions of precisely the kinds of utilization controls which Congress hoped that Professional Standards Review Organizations (PSROs) would be able to impose on medical practice.[30]

The rediscovery of the experience in Oregon reveals two extremely important things. First, it shows that it *can* happen, that relatively direct controls by insurers over physicians' decision making are possible and have been used in a substantial way at least once in our history. Just as the CWPS has revealed the ability of employers and unions to take substantial cost-control initiatives, the Oregon experience demonstrates health insurers' potential for exerting a direct and desirable influence. Second, the Oregon story suggests an answer to the earlier question about why current private-sector efforts are confined to either (1) attempting to influence professional decision making indirectly or (2) relying on professional organizations to supply the controls and set the standards. It was clearly the power of organized medicine and its captive insurance plan which stood in the way of continuing the practices of the Oregon "hospital associations." Similarly today, the medical profession's power to dictate the limits of third-party cost control accounts for many of the inadequacies of current private-sector efforts. Indeed, the CWPS's studies reveal several clear instances of private-sector initiatives which were substantially curtailed because of organized professional resistance.[31] These instances of professional obstructionism were remarked on editorially by the *Washington Post,* which described the Council's September report as "another piece of evidence that health care has gotten too expensive and impersonal to be left completely in the hands of those who provide it."[32]

Organized medicine justifies its concerted resistance to cost-control efforts of others by invoking the "doctor-patient relationship" and arguing that it is improper for anyone to oversee professional decision making unless the organized profession has approved the overseer. For example, while some peer-review mechanisms are now customary, the profession is still uncomfortable with PSROs because they are accountable in some measure to the federal government and not solely to local doctors.[33] Professional groups argue that they are looking out for patient interests, and undoubtedly this is a central feature of their concern. But, even though the professional organizations may be sincere in speaking for patients' health needs, their only legitimate role is that of advocate, not arbiter, because patients have other interests which doctors are not competent to represent—particularly an interest in cost control. Moreover, although admirable in many respects, the medical profession's ethics, in emphasizing the duty to serve health needs to the exclusion of other considerations, stand in the way of introducing cost concerns, reinforcing rather than mitigating the natural desire to do everything humanly possible and to avoid facing the dilemmas created by a need to economize. While serving well as a guide to physician conduct, medical ethics are not ultimately helpful as a guide to private spending or to social policy, which cannot responsibly ignore the existence of benefit/cost tradeoffs in medical care.[34] Finally, doctors' opinions on the value of medical care are likely to be exaggerated[35] and to neglect patients' reasonable preferences for less care, for noninvasion of their persons, for accepting some risk, and, in the extreme case, for death with dignity. There is here an opportunity to give limited effect to the important social and human concerns about oversubmission to doctors that have been expressed recently by such writers as Ivan Illich[36] and Rick Carlson.[37]

So frequently has the doctor-patient relationship been invoked to protect the medical profession's self-interest that it is possible to suspect some disingenuousness;[38] after all, any monopolist values his "relationship" with the customers he exploits. Nevertheless, it is not necessary to view the organized profession as a villain or to impugn its motives in order to deny it the role it has sought to assume.[39] Even if doctors are completely sincere in their belief that they stand between their patients and those who would sacrifice their health merely to save money, it is still necessary to reject them as the final authority because of their flawed perception. It is a commonly held view that all the health industry's deficiencies both in controlling costs and in promoting quality are traceable to a small number of irresponsible physicians whom the profession has a responsibility to catch and control. This formulation of the problems, almost universally accepted by doctors and very much institutionalized in the PSRO program[40] and the law of medical malpractice,[41] is wrong because it implies that customary standards are correct and that nothing fundamental should change in medical practice. Yet, following a generation in which physicians and hospitals have operated under increasingly inadequate cost constraints, there is every reason to believe (and some evidence suggesting[42]) that the prevailing standard or style of medical practice is more costly than what well-informed consumers would choose to purchase if they were spending their own money.[43] For these reasons, organized medicine's views on the value of various medical procedures and treatments should be received only as expert advice and, because conflicts of interests can influence even professional judgments, should be regarded as truly authoritative only when based on scientific evidence of efficacy and cost-effectiveness and not merely on opinion and accepted practice.[44] Because there is no "one right way" to render medical care, privately sponsored departures from customary practice should be insulated from professional pressures and tolerated by the courts if fairly implemented.[45]

In any political debate, the doctors' claim that they speak for their patients and for the quality of care is a powerful weapon. Indeed, this advantage which the medical profession enjoys in political contexts is the chief reason why the private sector may be better able to challenge doctors' judgements than are politically vulnerable agencies charged with cost-control responsibility.[46] Private decision makers with an immediate interest in cost control are less apt to collapse in the face of an unsubstantiated quality-of-care claim than is a public decision maker, who is usually in a position to commit the public's money to keep his conscience clear and protect his political image by resolving all plausible doubts in favor of more and better health services. Although regulatory mechanisms may succeed in arriving at some helpful compromises with the medical establishment, the very necessity for compromise guarantees that significant portions of the public interest will be systemat-

ically sacrificed to accommodate special interests.[47] Private-sector initiatives, on the other hand, are more likely to address the many tradeoffs on their merits and are thus capable of going substantially further than public decision makers in the direction of cost control—if the medical profession is precluded from organizing concerted resistance, either by boycott in the marketplace or by political action in a comprehensively regulated environment.

What emerges from these wide-ranging insights is simply the need to free health insurers and others engaging in aggressive cost-control activities from undue legal restrictions and from the threat of organized resistance by the medical profession. Fortunately, recent clarification of the applicability of the antitrust laws to the organized "learned professions"[48] provides a powerful legal weapon for controlling such objectionable behavior. While further legal clarification is necessary, the FTC and the Antitrust Division have recently shown interest in medical society activities and should soon declare the necessary principles, perhaps initiating litigation to make the point clearer yet. Properly applied, antitrust principles would prohibit medical societies not only from organizing formal boycotts[49] but also from circulating information and opinions calculated to stimulate collective pressure on the initiators of unwanted cost controls.[50] The following recent news report dramatizes the impact which the new awareness of antitrust restrictions is already having on medical society behavior:[51]

> Dr. Sweeny indicated [that the American Medical Association Council on Medical Service, of which he was chairman] had intended to write a strong report criticizing moves by health insurance companies to require second opinions in elective surgery.
> But legal counsel warned that such action might be viewed by the Federal Trade Commission as being restraint of trade, and a new report had to be prepared.
> Now, Dr. Sweeny said, "the council is very disappointed with the report. It isn't what we had intended to do for this association at all."

The legal advice given the AMA was sound, and it is to be hoped that state and local medical societies and other professions are getting the same message.

IV. WHAT THE PRIVATE SECTOR COULD DO

Given only a small amount of encouragement and protection against organized professional resistance, the market for health services financing and delivery could begin fairly quickly to re-structure itself to allow consumers effectively to express their preferences with respect to the cost as well as the quality and style of much of the medical care they receive. Of course, there are several legal developments which would be necessary to permit maximum response. Roughly in descending order of importance, these needed legal changes include alterations in the tax law to strengthen private incentives to economize; comparable changes in public financing programs; adjustment of the PSRO program to weaken professional control over in-novation and to clarify the acceptability of re-sponsible alternative standards and delivery ar-rangements;[52] repeal or invalidation of state-imposed impediments to reputable cost-control efforts and organizational innovations; and judi-cial and regulatory recognition of the validity of contractual arrangements departing from tradi-tional insurance modes and traditional standards of practice. Even without these changes, how-ever, private-sector forces could begin to oper-ate immediately if the need to defer to the pref-erences of organized medicine could be minimized. As experience developed, the need for further legal action could be assessed.

Although there is a great deal that unions, em-ployers, consumer cooperatives, medical group practices, hospitals, HMOs, and others can do about health care costs, private health insurers are the entities in the best position to explore and develop the full range of possible cost-control arrangements which lie between tradi-tional, "hands-off" insurance plans and the total-substitute delivery systems contemplated in the federal HMO legislation.[53] No one can predict with certainty, of course, how insurers would respond to market conditions if they were given a substantially freer hand legally and clear antitrust protection against professional retalia-tion. Because insurers long ago became accus-tomed to the notion that it is not their function to control health care costs, they do not now pos-sess all of the expertise and techniques needed to solve cost problems. Moreover, as the CWPS review of labor-management innovations

sharply reveals, the job of controlling costs is extremely difficult, requiring great sensitivity to patients' interests as well as a willingness to challenge doctors on their spending habits. Given the severe difficulties, it is impressive to learn from the Council's findings and from in-surance industry spokesmen[54] of the great amount that has already been done. There is much more that can be done, however.

Insurer-initiated cost-control measures could take many forms. Various exclusions from coverage are one possibility. Although some ob-servers might object to any departure from "comprehensiveness" of benefits, such exclu-sions have the salutary effect of putting particu-lar consumption decisions back in the hands of the cost-conscious patient and his physician-fiduciary. Exclusions from coverage could be designed so as not to erode essential protection against a medical-financial calamity but nevertheless to reflect the circumstance that many health care expenditures are highly dis-cretionary and dependent as much on personal tastes and circumstances as on medical need. Some examples of how such exclusions might be employed to good cost-control advantage are as follows:

1. *"Major-risk" insurance.* A high-deductible "major risk" insurance plan, endorsed by Martin Feldstein,[55] would put most medi-cal care back in private hands, beginning coverage only when financial catastrophe threatened. Under a tax regime which did not encourage shallow coverage, such in-surance would find many takers among those who recognized the administrative and other avoidable costs of overinsurance and who trusted themselves and their physicians to make sensible purchasing decisions in time of need.[56]
2. *Specific exclusions.* An insurance plan might exclude (or single out for heavier cost sharing) certain specified procedures on the ground that they are discretionary or easily budgetable. Examples are dental care, cosmetic surgery, outpatient psychi-atric care, certain hysterectomies, routine childbirth, and many tonsillectomies. Limits might be placed on the number of x-rays covered for certain conditions, and questionable diagnostic procedures might be excluded.

3. *Exclusion of certain catastrophic treatments.* As a means of offering reasonable but less expensive protection in the exceedingly difficult area of catastrophic disease, a plan might find consumers willing to accept the exclusion from coverage of a number of extremely expensive measures whose value is less than clear and in some measure dependent on the patient's preferences and circumstances.[57] Examples might include coronary bypass surgery, exotic treatments for terminal cancer, some organ transplants, bone marrow replacements, and experimental procedures such as artificial heart implantation (when it comes). Although one would not want patients to waive their rights to beneficial technology, some extravagantly expensive treatments are surely candidates for explicit exclusion from coverage by rational insurance purchasers.

4. *Indemnity plans.* Plans could limit themselves to paying, not incurred costs, but a fixed indemnity based on estimated minimum or average cost, leaving the patient free to spend more for additional increments of perceived quality. An easy example would be a commitment to pay for drugs at the estimated wholesale cost of the generic product, leaving the patient to pay the pharmacist's mark-up and any premium which a brand-name drug might command.[58] This would allow competition to operate not only on the pharmacies but also on the drug companies and those doctors whose prescriptions were more costly to fill. Similar indemnities could be paid for a wide variety of procedures and treatments, including hospital care (on either a per-diem or a spell-of-illness basis).[59]

5. *Utilization review.* Utilization review procedures which insurers might introduce are simply another way of imposing coverage limitations similar to the foregoing. But, because advance specification of limits on hospital stays and use of ancillary services is practically impossible, a case-by-case review is needed to give effect to the plan's policy, which may be liberal or stringent in accordance with the premium charged and the attendant necessity for cost control. It would seem reasonable to require participating physicians to obtain advance approval of some hospital admissions and some costly procedures so that only medically necessary care would be paid for. Obviously the procedures for making such reviews would be of considerable importance, but one cannot reasonably object to the principle of allowing consumers to bind themselves in advance to accept the plan's determinations on the scope of coverage. The surgical second-opinion plans currently being experimented with have so far shrunk from applying this principle so as to make the second opinion or other review binding with respect to the plan's obligation to pay.[60]

The medical profession's criticisms of coverage limits implemented through insurer-initiated second opinions and utilization reviews, or otherwise, should not obscure the fact that the insurer is acting in the interest of the plan subscribers, who, having paid only for essential protection, expect the plan to control expenditures. The patient remains free, of course, to proceed with the surgical treatment at his own expense on his doctor's advice. The same holds true for extra hospital days, extra ancillary services, and so forth, which the plan might refuse to cover because of a finding that such costs are discretionary and should be purchased privately, if at all. In all of this, the plan is engaged in the entirely legitimate business of helping consumers to overcome their ignorance as purchasers of care, of delineating the realm in which self-insurance is the more rational policy, and of minimizing the impact of the "moral hazard"[61] which insurance necessarily involves. As long as it is merely defining coverage, the insurer cannot fairly be said to be engaged in the "corporate practice of medicine" or to be interfering in doctor/patient relationships.[62] Indeed, well designed coverage limits would put physicians in a position to serve their patients more fully, helping them as consumers to spend wisely in areas of significant doubt concerning benefit/cost ratios. With patients paying their own bills for marginally productive care, competition for patients would no longer induce doctors to order more services just because patients expect it but instead would encourage doctors to develop their ability to achieve good results for less, a skill that is not adequately rewarded under present conditions.

Insurers could also serve consumers usefully in strengthening their bargaining position vis-à-vis providers. An individual plan could negotiate fees and charges in advance with individual providers, thus obtaining for its insureds the benefit of competitive pricing. Providers not agreeing would be at a disadvantage in serving plan subscribers and could be excluded altogether from certain types of plans. If insurers did their job well, assurances of reasonable quality would also flow to their insureds. Moreover, in a market featuring several competing plans engaged in negotiating fees and charges, low prices would prevail in those areas having an excess of facilities or manpower, thus contributing powerfully to the redistribution of medical personnel and to deterrence and elimination of unneeded capital investments. Insurers might find it desirable and efficient to gravitate toward sponsoring more tightly organized provider groups as a means of offering a plan with more efficient cost controls, better quality assurance, economies of scale, and better identification in the consumer's mind. Possibilities include using the HMO model, "independent practice associations,"[63] and the new "health alliance" concept.[64] These arrangements may spring up under other auspices as well, but insurers are perhaps best equipped to assess their feasibility and cost-effectiveness in particular localities.

Precisely because of the many complexities and questions surrounding the workability, acceptability, and cost-effectiveness of particular cost-control techniques, development and refinement of cost-control strategies would seem best left to the inherent checks and balances of the competitive marketplace. Insurers competing in cost-control endeavors must satisfy not only consumers and their increasingly sophisticated purchasing agents (unions and employers) but also individual providers, who must be induced to cooperate. This dual responsibility supplies substantial guarantees against abuses while continuously challenging competitors to find the best mix of strategies through experimentation and adaptation to various and changing circumstances in a relatively uncontrolled environment. Under governmentally imposed controls, on the other hand, there would be only limited pressure or opportunity to innovate and only political checks on clumsy, ineffective, or excessively expensive cost-control policies. PSROs, for example, are subject to little over-

sight and to no significant competitive pressure to lower costs,[65] and their transformation into quality-improving agencies, contrary to congressional intent, already has revealed how political forces can weigh heavily against cost control.[66]

Even if insurers cannot gear up overnight to provide this new and important service to their subscribers, it is important to put pressure on them to do as much as they can given the present state of the art. The first step is to establish the legitimacy of insurers' efforts so that they will no longer present a united front in response to their customers' pressure. Once this front is broken, the successful innovators would be able to increase their market shares at the expense of the laggards. With the first olive out of the bottle, the benefits of innovation would spread rapidly and would not long be confined to the large and sophisticated employment groups which provided the initial impetus for change. Obviously, pressure from purchasers to control costs is currently much diluted by tax considerations, and consumers and employers require some education before they will fully recognize the value of insurance coverage which is less than total and automatic. Nevertheless, innovation is already beginning and can be expected to proliferate even if government continues to tolerate obstacles to substantial efforts.

Additional pressure on insurers is already supplied by government, which itself must be viewed by insurers as a potential competitor—indeed as a potential usurper of their role. Health insurers must recognize that there is very little reason to preserve a role for them in the future health care system if they continue to prove unable to do the single thing for which they are clearly better equipped than government—that is, to offer consumers a meaningful range of choice so that consumers' decisions on the relevant tradeoffs rather than providers' or bureaucrats' incentives and preferences can shape the health care delivery system.

If the stimulus to greater insurer efforts supplied by competitive and other pressures were found, or felt, to be inadequate, favorable tax treatment of health insurance premiums could be made contingent on approval of the insurance plan by regulatory authorities who were charged with restoring cost-consciousness and competition as well as with protecting the public and providers against abuses. Traditional "free-choice-of-physician" plans, which are one cornerstone of the medical profession's monopoly power, could even be excluded from the marketplace altogether—if that seemed necessary.[67]

The overriding strategy must be somehow to divide providers into a multiplicity of competing units having both correct incentives and reasonable freedom to agree with consumers on the quantity and quality of care to be provided at a mutually acceptable price. Competing health insurers are in the best position to take the actions needed to introduce correct competitive pressures, thereby bringing about the long-desired "restructuring" of the health care delivery system. In addition to limiting coverage and thereby forcing individual doctors to compete in applying their professional judgment to economizing possibilities, insurers also could facilitate competition among organized physician groups. Doctor groups which found themselves being denied the benefit of their own efficiency because their patients were paying insurance premiums based on community-wide experience could seek to have their patients rated separately for insurance purposes.[68] In response, new groups could be formed, with insurer assistance, by doctors seeking to avoid the loss of patients to these efficient groups. While perhaps more loosely organized and operating from separate offices, these new groups would also seek to control costs and to establish an identity in the consumer's mind. Thus, the new and highly important concept of "health alliances" (closed-panel plans not fitting the HMO Act models) could become a reality without benefit of a special governmental program to nurture them.[69] Competition among such plans would focus, much as it does now, on quality, reputation, amenities, convenience, and patient satisfaction, but also would focus, for the first time, on cost and the necessity for giving value for money.

Given the wide range of promising, even exciting, possibilities for private-sector cost-control initiatives, it is hard to see any reason except the distaste or self-interest of insiders in the medical marketplace why these approaches have not received significant attention before now.

V. HOW THESE IDEAS RELATE TO THE HEALTH POLICY DEBATE

A. Regulation versus Private-Sector Efforts

Obviously, much of the foregoing discussion swims against the tide of the ongoing health policy debate, which deals mostly with how, and how much, to regulate the system and not with the more fundamental issue of whether comprehensive regulation is really the best way to correct the industry's obviously defective performance. While there is almost a consensus that the private sector has failed, there is only poor understanding of why that market failure occurred, most people accepting as conclusive the following propositions: health care is "different" or "unique;" consumer ignorance is the source of the problem because decision making must be delegated to non-cost-conscious doctors; consumers (voters) prefer comprehensive third-party coverage of as many health expenditures as possible; and private third-party payment is synonymous with the absence of effective controls on the cost of care. The foregoing discussion indicates that all of these propositions, while containing some truths, are far too simple.[70] To paraphrase Mark Twain, the report that the market cannot be restored to health is greatly exaggerated.

The inevitability of vastly expanded federal and state regulation of the health care industry is so widely accepted that many persons are now unwilling to consider any alternative. Yet confidence in the efficacy of regulation is not high among policymakers, and recent months have seen an increasing awareness of regulation's shortcomings, in health as well as elsewhere. Academic work has enumerated and documented the many reasons why regulation is likely to be ineffective. Some of this work has emphasized not only the ominous parallels to other regulatory endeavors, which have generated intense inflationary pressures and systematic misallocations of resources,[71] but also the symbolic and other special features of health care and health care regulation which make saying "no" to more or better health services particularly difficult.[72] Confirming the skeptics' predictions, empirical evidence of the ineffectiveness of health planning and certificate-of-need programs is now beginning to appear.[73] In addition, practically no one still believes that

PSROs will make more than a slight difference in controlling costly hospital utilization, and the shift of PSROs' primary mission from cost control to quality improvement presents new dangers of cost escalation.[74] Although doubts about regulation have as yet caused no change in the direction of the drift toward governmental controls, congressional reluctance to enact long-imminent "national health insurance" is traceable to doubts about the efficacy of the controls now in use or in the experimental stage. It seems quite possible that, if a clear and persuasive alternative policy appeared, repressed doubts about regulatory approaches would rise to the surface and a fundamental reappraisal could be launched. Moreover, many of the interest groups affected, particularly those who are paying the excessive costs, might find such an alternative strategy attractive, thus improving its political prospects.

The last previous attempt to present an alternative to comprehensive regulation of the health care industry was the "HMO strategy" launched in 1970.[75] The depressing history of that promising idea, culminating in its virtual destruction at the hands of Congress, need not be recounted here,[76] but many people who rallied to that banner are still believers in the philosophy it represented and the prospect it held out. Moreover, the failure of the HMO Act of 1973 to stimulate major changes in the market for health services was more a failure of regulation than of the market, since it was excessive regulation which caused expectations to be disappointed.[77] Moreover, the HMO story demonstrated once again the power of organized medicine, which concurred with congressional liberals in overburdening HMOs with restrictions.

HMOs are still a good idea and very much a part of the strategy advocated here. It should be noted, however, that this strategy is not just a restatement of the HMO idea. In 1970, when HMOs first appeared in the debate on health policy, many observers made the error of seizing on HMOs as the most politically salable vehicle for introducing privately initiated cost controls and competition in the health services industry.[78] This proved to be a tactical mistake because it depended on Congress to do too much, but it was an understandable mistake. HMOs seemed indeed to be the "wave of the future," and the broader approach of encouraging insurer-initiated cost controls seemed too radical, too

questionable under state legal restrictions, and too easily squelched by professional opposition.[79] Indeed, it seemed that HMO competition was required to trigger significant efforts on the part of insurers, accustomed as they were to serving merely as pass-through mechanisms and providing only actuarial and claims-payment services to their customers. But when Congress failed to embrace the opportunity which HMOs presented (the recent amendments still largely miss the point), those who believed that a market-oriented response could be organized were left pretty much where they began. What seems to be needed, then, if serious attention is to be drawn to nonregulatory solutions to our problems, is a strategy which appears to be wholly new and not just a warmed-over version of the HMO idea, respectable as that was. I believe that such a new campaign can and must be launched and that the discovery by the CWPS of the private sector's capacity to fight the cost battle is a key step in dramatizing the possibilities.

At least three significant new developments observed in this essay make it appropriate to look again at market-oriented approaches to dealing with health care cost problems. These developments are (1) the new consciousness of employers, unions, and the public at large concerning health care costs; (2) commercial insurers' increasing recognition of their own responsibility for cost control;[80] and (3) the new applicability of the antitrust laws to the medical profession and the recognition in the antitrust enforcement agencies and elsewhere of the importance of preventing concerted professional resistance to privately initiated cost-control efforts. When these developments are combined with recognition of the many untried possibilities for cost control, a new and appealing affirmative strategy begins to emerge. What it requires at this critical point, as battle lines for the Ninety-Fifth Congress are being drawn, is not further investigation and subtle elaboration in the academic literature but a solid endorsement—at least as an idea deserving serious and immediate attention—by authoritative groups desirous of heading off government domination of the health services industry and a further narrowing of private choice. A concerted effort to refine the ideas presented in this essay and to develop a concrete policy proposal also should be launched. One important figure in the health policy debate has suggested, not wholly in jest, that what is needed to explore this approach is a "Committee of 101" to rival the Health Security proposal's sponsoring "Committee of 100." I agree, and hope that a responsible movement along this line can be catalyzed soon.

B. Other Values at Stake.

While heavy emphasis on cost concerns is appropriate in the present climate, it is easy, in the campaign to control costs, to neglect other values which are also of great importance. For example, concern about costs has already produced far-reaching regulatory initiatives—the PSRO law, the health planning legislation, and the HMO Act—which generally confirm providers' dominance and weaken the system's ability to innovate and to offer consumers a meaningful range of choice.[81] To have any chance of success in solving problems to the public's satisfaction and, indeed, to have any political appeal at all, market-oriented cost-containment policies cannot simply exalt the market but must be attuned to the other values which health care effects and to the special concerns which it excites. Thus, attention needs to be given not only to how costs are to be contained but to how consumers are to be protected against overreaching and dishonest operators,[82] how the quality of care is to be maintained,[83] how geographic maldistribution of providers will be rectified,[84] how monopolistic hospitals' rates are to be controlled,[85] and so forth. In some respects, it will be necessary to accommodate the strong desire in the health sector to regulate things in order to protect the ignorant unorganized consumer against possible mistakes. Powerfully felt distributive-justice concerns also must be addressed.

A market-oriented strategy can be designed to address such problems and concerns. All that is essential is that the market's basic integrity not be undermined by measures dealing with specific problems. Special emphasis also must be placed on measures to improve the market's functioning and to narrow providers' dominance over its organization, the flow of information, and the range of choices available to consumers. Such measures, even though they do not contemplate increased political control, all would be in keeping with the public's demand for increased provider "accountability" and for a greater part in decision making. Moreover, there

is nothing implicit in the endorsement of a market-oriented strategy which denies the reasonable demands of social justice, and only those who demand the appearance of absolute equality in this symbolic area should find reason to object to the implications of permitting reasonable diversity and relying on constrained private choice.[86] Even if such equality were attainable in reality, which seems most unlikely, it could only be done by giving the disadvantaged costly health benefits which they would prefer to forgo if they could have even a fraction of the savings in cash. It would seem wise to recognize and resist the tug toward a health policy which is more an expensive symbolic gesture than a sensible redistributive scheme.

A market-oriented system would address itself in some ways to the public's reputed new doubts about the capabilities of government as well as to some new themes in the health policy debate. For example, recent repeated emphasis on individuals' personal responsibility for their own health may foreshadow a trend away from shifting total financial responsibility to government and toward acceptance of personal responsibility for selecting a health care plan and for deciding how much of a financial commitment to make. Moreover, the public's emerging suspiciousness toward the medical profession and increasingly bitter resistance to its dominance[88] suggest a desire for more alternatives. Perhaps most important in its implications both for cost control and for an expanded range of constrained choice is another new and increasingly dominant theme in health policy discussions— namely the expression of serious reservations about the ability of health services to make significant contributions to human welfare in many of the cases where great expense is incurred and, more generally, about the benefits obtainable from further increases in society's investment in health services.[89] A corollary of this new skepticism should be a recognition that the apparent range and subjectivity of consumers' preferences in this area, as in others, does not necessarily signify irrationality and that different people can come rationally to different conclusions about what quantity and quality of services to buy. A market system would fit in well with this new awareness by allowing people, many with their purchasing power subsidized, to make their own decisions about how much health care is worth to them. On the other hand, regulatory approaches, by their very nature, threaten to narrow the range of choice and ultimately to define a single standard of care which everyone must accept.

No single standard and style of health care can be appropriate for all Americans, given their widely varied attitudes, tastes, and religious convictions, their other needs, and the necessarily limited resources at their disposal, including the public funds available to some of them. Implementing a single standard would mean either (1) "leveling down," which means denying people the right or opportunity to choose a higher, or different, style or standard even if they are willing to pay the added cost, or (2) "leveling up," which means bringing the entire population up to a level defined primarily by the preferences of the upper-middle-class professionals providing the service. At present, the rhetoric of the policy debate—e.g., "the right to health care"—seems slanted toward leveling up, though some leveling down is implicit in the expressed need to control costs and to "ration" care. A strong dose of leveling down also appears in the Kennedy-Corman Health Security bill and other proposals which seek to make all Americans part of a single "insured" group, with the total aggregate cost fixed politically and with equal, but limited and politically determined, services for all.

What emerges from the new themes in the health policy debate is another basis for reopening consideration of the value of a health care system based primarily on diversity and choice. New awarenesses at long last have focussed primary attention not only on the value of health services in the aggregate, where there can be no real dispute, but also on their highly questionable value at the margin, where benefits are frequently problematic and where personal preferences and alternative uses for resources are apt to be decisive. This new sophistication is at least equivalent in importance to the three new developments mentioned earlier as circumstances warranting the "rediscovery" of the market and private decision making as the appropriate instruments for restoring provider accountability and fiscal prudence to the health sector.

NOTES

1. Council on Wage and Price Stability, *The Complex Puzzle of Rising Health Care Costs: Can the Private Sector Fit It Together?* (Washington: Executive Office of the President, December 1976), pp. 99–100 (hereinafter cited as *CWPS December Report*).

2. Council on Wage and Price Stability, *The Problem of Rising Health Care Costs* (Washington: Executive Office of the President, April 1976), reprinted in *CWPS December Report*, pp. 69–75 (hereinafter cited as *CWPS April Report);* Council on Wage and Price Stability, "Labor and Management Sponsored Innovations in Controlling the Cost of Employee Health Care Benefits," 41 *Federal Register* 40298 (September 17, 1976), reprinted with minor revisions in *CWPS December Report*, pp. 99–177 (hereinafter cited as *CWPS September Report); CWPS December Report.*

3. *CWPS September Report*, p. 98.

4. J. Iglehart, "Health Focus," *National Journal* 8 (May 1, 1976): 598.

5. S.3, 94th Cong., 1st Sess. (1975).

6. See *CWPS December Report*, pp. ii–iv.

7. *CWPS September Report*, pp. 105–18. *See also* Cohn, "Aetna Tests Plan to Reduce Unneeded Surgery," *Washington Post*, November 30, 1976, p. 1.

8. *CWPS September Report*, pp. 115–18.

9. Id., pp. 119–24, 155–56. One union has obtained some doctors' commitment to accept the union's fee schedule. Fee schedules of any kind present antitrust problems but are probably acceptable if competitively arrived at. In other words, competing insurers may use schedules which they develop unilaterally and over which they negotiate with providers individually. It is noteworthy that Blue Shield plans ordinarily negotiate with physicians collectively, not individually. Similarly, Blue Cross plans frequently encounter collective resistance to their cost-control efforts and have seldom been able to break the hospitals' united front. The distinction between competitive individual action by providers and concerted action is most important for present purposes and explains in part why the Blues have not been adequate cost-control vehicles.

10. Id., pp. 165–67. Indeed, there is a general trend to broader coverage amounting to overinsurance. See text accompanying notes 15–16, infra.

11. Id., pp. 132–34, 161–63. Blue Cross and Blue Shield are the main overseers of review processes and are apparently acceptable to providers.

12. In other forms of insurance, "adjusters" prevent claims from exceeding reasonable bounds. Despite the highly discretionary character of many health care expenditures, few comparable controls exist to counter the apparent "moral hazard," as the tendency to exploit an insurance fund is known.

13. *CWPS April Report*, pp. 85–87.

14. Id., pp. 86–88.

15. Id., pp. 84–85.

16. M. Feldstein, "The Medical Economy," *Scientific American* 229 (September 1973): 151; M. Feldstein,

"How Tax Laws Fuel Hospital Costs," *Prism*, January 1976, p. 15, 19. On the tax subsidy to the health sector, see also B. Mitchell and S. Vogel, "Health and Taxes: An Assessment of the Medical Deduction," *Southern Economic Journal* 41 (1975): 660; K. Davis, *National Health Insurance: Benefits, Costs, and Consequences* (Washington: Brookings Institution, 1975), pp. 14–17.

17. Lawyers recently have been favored by legislation making prepaid legal services a tax-free benefit.

18. Some political difficulties undoubtedly would arise, however, because the tax impact would not be uniform within income brackets or graduated perfectly according to income. Lower-income taxpayers would face an increased Social Security tax which those with incomes above the FICA base would not have to pay. On the other hand, workers with elaborate fringe benefits would face a substantial increase in their net income tax as the value of their health benefits became taxable in an amount only partially offset by the new credit. Perhaps there are other "loopholes" which might be closed at the same time to weaken inevitable equity objections to this change, which, though generally desirable from an equity standpoint, is needed primarily for other reasons.

19. There are several reasons why consumers might continue to purchase comprehensive protection. For one thing, they are accustomed to it and may wish not to be under pressure to economize in purchasing health services. Further, they may not be easily educated to the net savings obtainable from shifting to out-of-pocket payments and avoiding the inherent costs of a broad insurance program. On the other hand, certain types of comprehensive plans may be valued for the preventive care they are motivated to provide. But, even more important, comprehensive plans may come to be seen as providing another valuable service, namely help in making wise and cost-effective purchasing decisions. HMOs already supply such a service, and cost controls under insurer-organized plans could well be seen by consumers in the same light—as a reliable check on their personal physicians' possibly self-interested or insufficiently cost-conscious prescriptions.

A more troublesome possibility is that, even with the tax law changed, consumers would continue to obtain inadequate catastrophic protection. This would occur if the current prevalence of shallow coverage reflects in an important degree people's implicit reliance for catastrophic protection, not on insurance or personal savings, but on established mechanisms of public relief to take care of them if disaster strikes. To some extent, such "insurance" is in fact supplied by the Medicaid program, public and Hill-Burton hospitals, and the perceived willingness of the system to provide some critically needed care without charge, and many consumers are rational to count on these mechanisms and not to pay for insurance protection. It

would be a reasonable policy objective, however, to seek to put all or nearly all such care on a more rational basis through subsidized private insurance, and to this end a requirement that the tax credit be used to purchase catastrophic coverage would be justified. A possible strategy might be to allow the maximum credit (say, $200 for a family) to be claimed for either (1) 100 percent of premiums paid for plans providing only approved catastrophic coverage or (2) 33⅓ percent of premiums paid under a comprehensive plan also providing catastrophic protection. The maximum and the latter percentage could be adjusted upward for lower-income people.

20. A variation might be to issue two vouchers annually, one good for, say, $600 of health benefits for a family of four and the other convertible by a health plan either into cash in an amount up to, say, $300 for added coverage supplied by the plan or into a check payable to the beneficiary for two-thirds of whatever portion of the $300 was not taken in health benefits. Plans could then compete within limits by varying coverage and offering rebates. If the beneficiary valued the added health benefits at more than two-thirds of their cash value he would choose them, but he would not be compelled to take them if he had a different preference. The tax system could be employed in the same way.

21. Nonprice competition is not a sufficient substitute for price competition since the added benefits, "quality," and amenities may be valued by consumers at considerably less than their dollar cost—a reflection of the fact that beyond some point more health services are not necessarily what people want most. The probability that preferences would be violated is particularly high in the case of federal programs since the needy individuals being covered are precisely those most likely to have better uses for the money. Moreover, the probable absence of cost sharing for indigents removes the possibility of competitive reductions of deductibles and coinsurance obligations. Further, added benefits would be even more nearly worthless if the mandatory minimum benefit package were already as comprehensive as those under the Health Maintenance Organization Act of 1973, 42 U.S.C. §§300e et seq. (Supp. IV, 1975), as amended, Pub. L. No. 94-460, 90 Stat. 1945 (Oct. 8, 1976), and some national health insurance proposals. Just as nonprice competition produces wasteful spending in other regulated industries—by the airlines, for example—, requiring health plans to dissipate the benefits of their efficiency in providing new uneconomic services is simply to encourage new forms of waste.

Another unfortunate result of prohibiting price competition among health insurers and other plans seeking to serve federal beneficiaries would be to stimulate them to compete for low-risk (or low-consuming) populations and to avoid the neediest patients. Trying to counter these tendencies by open enrollment and nondiscrimination requirements is both costly and oppressively bureaucratic—an attempt to make the best of a bad idea. The Health Maintenance Organization Act provisions are particularly destructive of useful price competition. See Havighurst, Testimony, *Hearings on Competition in the Health Services Market Before the Senate Subcommittee on Antitrust and Monopoly* (May 17, 1974): 1036, 1080.

22. See, for example, C. Havighurst & J. Blumstein, "Coping with Quality/Cost Trade-offs in Medical Care: The Role of PSROs." *Northwestern University Law Review* 70 (March-April 1975): 6, 62–66; C. Havighurst and R. Bovbjerg, "Professional Standards Review Organizations and Health Maintenance Organizations: Are They Compatible?" *Utah Law Review 1975* (Fall, 1975): 381, 411–21.

23. See, for example, H. Somers and A. Somers, *Doctors, Patients, and Health Insurance* (Washington: Brookings Institution, 1961).

24. See note 19 supra.

25. H. Hansen, "Laws Affecting Group Health Plans," *Iowa Law Review* 35 (Winter, 1950): 209, 211–19; J. Laufer, "Ethical and Legal Restrictions on Contract and Corporate Practice of Medicine," *Law and Contemporary Problems* 6 (Autumn, 1939): 516, 522–27. See notes 62–63 infra and accompanying text.

26. See, for example, J. Berlant, *Profession and Monopoly: A Study of Medicine in the United States and Great Britain* (Berkeley: University of California Press, 1975); E. Rayack, *Professional Power and American Medicine* (Cleveland: World Publishing Co., 1967): R. Kessel, "Price Discrimination in Medicine," *Journal of Law & Economics* 1 (October 1958): 20.

27. See American Medical Ass'n v. United States, 317 U.S. 519 (1943); Group Health Cooperative v. King County Medical Society, 39 Wash. 2d 586, 237 P.2d 737 (1951); Note, "The Role of Prepaid Group Practice in Relieving the Medical Care Crisis," *Harvard Law Review* 84 (February 1971): 887, 954–60.

28. United States v. Oregon State Medical Society, 343 U.S. 326 (1952).

29. L. Goldberg and W. Greenberg, "The Effect of Physician-Controlled Health Insurance: U.S. v. Oregon State Medical Society," *Journal of Health Politics, Policy & Law* 2 (Spring, 1977): forthcoming.

30. See Havighurst & Blumstein, pp. 38–60.

31. *CWPS September Report*, pp. 109, 116–17, 120. The profession's resistance to second-opinion plans with more than advisory effect is reported in *Wall Street Journal*, November 24, 1976, p. 14. Another striking demonstration of the ability of organized medicine to maintain its freedom to spend the public's money without restraint occurred a few years ago, when the Aetna Life and Casualty Company undertook to assist its insureds in resisting in court doctors' claims for payment of excessive charges or for unnec-

essary services. Medical societies the country over passed resolutions calling for boycotts of Aetna's patients, and Aetna had to negotiate a change in its policy with the AMA. See Goldberg and Greenberg.

32. Editorial, *Washington Post*, Oct. 1, 1976.

33. Havighurst and Blumstein, pp. 41–51. The prototype for PSROs, the "foundations for medical care," were peer-review mechanisms controlled by the local medical society. See R. Egdahl, "Foundations for Medical Care," *New England Journal of Medicine* 288 (March 8, 1973): 491; C. Havighurst, "Health Maintenance Organizations and the Market for Health Services," *Law and Contemporary Problems* 35 (Autumn, 1970): 716, 769–77.

34. See C. Fried, *Medical Experimentation: Personal Integrity and Social Policy* (Amsterdam: North Holland Publishing Co., 1974).

35. See, for example, A. Cochrane, *Effectiveness and Efficiency: Random Reflections on Health Services* (London: Nuffield Provincial Hospitals Trust, 1972).

36. I. Illich, *Limits to Medicine* (London: Marion Boyars, 1976). This is an enlarged version of the author's *Medical Nemesis* (New York: Pantheon, 1975).

37. R. Carlson, *The End of Medicine* (New York: Wiley, 1975).

38. See, for example, the references cited in note 26.

39. Antitrust prosecutions frequently do not require proof of monopolistic intent, for example.

40. See Havighurst and Blumstein; Havighurst and Bovbjerg.

41. See C. Havighurst, "'Medical Adversity Insurance'—Has Its Time Come?" *Duke Law Journal 1975* (January 1976): 1233, 1237–52; R. Bovbjerg, "The Medical Malpractice Standard of Care: HMOs and Customary Practice," Ibid.: 1375.

42. See, for example, Cochrane; U.S. Public Health Service, *Forward Plan for Health FY 1977–81*, at 144–61 (Washington: Department of Health, Education and Welfare Pub. No. 05-76-50074, 1975); D. Neuhauser, "The Future of Proprietaries in American Health Services," in *Regulating Health Facilities Construction*, ed. C. Havighurst (Washington: American Enterprise Institute, 1974): 233–37; Feldstein, "The Medical Economy." The "evidence" is anecdotal, however, showing only widespread spending of doubtful efficacy.

43. This shorthand way of expressing the social optimum is elaborated in Havighurst and Blumstein, pp. 13–20.

44. See, for example, Cochrane.

45. Contractual alterations of providers' duties, under some circumstances, should supersede the implied obligations enforced by the law of torts. Cf. Bovbjerg.

46. The deficiencies of political processes in this regard are reviewed in Havighurst and Blumstein, pp.

20–45; C. Havighurst, J. Blumstein and R. Bovbjerg, "Strategies in Financing Medical Care for Catastrophic Disease," *Law and Contemporary Problems* 40 (Autumn, 1976): forthcoming.

47. See, for example, C. Havighurst, "Regulation of Health Facilities and Services by 'Certificate of Need,'" *Virginia Law Review* 49 (October 1973): 1143, 1178–88, 1194–1217.

48. Goldfarb v. Virginia State Bar, 421 U.S. 773 (1975).

49. Klor's, Inc. v. Broadway-Hale Stores, Inc., 359 U.S. 207 (1959); Fashion Originators' Guild v. Federal Trade Commission, 312 U.S. 457 (1941); American Medical Ass'n v. United States, 130 F.2d 233, 248–49 (D.C. Cir. 1942), *aff'd*, 317 U.S. 519 (1943).

50. Cf. Eastern States Retail Lumber Dealers' Ass'n v. United States, 234 U.S. 600 (1914).

51. "Second Opinion Statement Weakened," *American Medical News*, Dec. 13, 1976. p. 12, cols. 2–3. This article is one of five on adjoining pages reporting ways in which the AMA is accommodating itself to new antitrust realities.

52. See Havighurst and Bovbjerg.

53. For example, Health Maintenance Organization Act of 1973, 42 U.S.C. §§300e et seq. (Supp. IV, 1975), as amended, Pub. L. No. 94-460, 90 Stat. 1945 (Oct. 8, 1976).

54. For example, M. Miller, "Statement of the Health Insurance Association of America Before the Council on Wage and Price Stability," June 29, 1976; W. Bailey, "Rising Health Care Costs—A Challenge to Insurers," *National Journal* 8 (May 1, 1976): 608.

55. M. Feldstein, "A New Approach to National Health Insurance," *Public Interest* 23 (Spring 1971): 93.

56. See note 19.

57. For a thorough review of cost-control measures in the catastrophic disease area and the conclusion that private decision making is a preferable vehicle for confronting the serious dilemmas presented, see Havighurst, Blumstein and Bovbjerg.

58. Federal "maximum allowable cost" regulations applicable to drug purchases under Medicare and Medicaid provide an interesting comparison, 45 C.F.R. §19 (1976). Federal beneficiaries are denied the option of paying the difference in price between generic and brand-name products.

59. J. Newhouse and V. Taylor, "How Shall We Pay for Hospital Care?" *Public Interest* 23 (Spring, 1971): 78.

60. See notes 7–8 and accompanying text. One dental plan makes its own determinations binding, however.

61. See note 12.

62. See notes 25 and 63. While somewhat subtle, the conceptual point here is both legally and ethically im-

portant. Havighurst and Blumstein (pp. 55–58) argue that PSROs, in reviewing utilization, should not be viewed as "regulating" medical practice and should be seen instead as "rationing only public financing, not health care itself" (id., 55):

> There are two distinct issues which PSROs seem likely to confuse. First, is the care unproductive or even counterproductive? An affirmative judgment by the PSRO reflects adversely on the doctor's professional competence, and it is this implied rebuke which, coupled with the widespread disagreement on the technical issues involved, makes PSROs so threatening to physicians. Second, should the federal government pay? Here, if the distinction is rigidly maintained, there is no possible reflection on the prescribing physician, unless he has failed to prepare his patient for the possibility that self payment will be required. The PSRO program would have had a better chance of successfully addressing quality/cost trade-offs if it had been portrayed as involving the second question primarily. Id., 57, n. 196.

The distinction between actually controlling medical practice and merely defining coverage has received judicial recognition. In *Association of American Physicians & Surgeons v. Weinberger*, 395 F.Supp. 125 (N.D. Ill. 1975), cert. affirmed, 423 U.S. (975), PSROs' utilization reviews were held not to interfere with the physician's right to practice. However, in *American Medical Ass'n v. Weinberger*, 522 F.2d 921, 925 (7th Cir. 1975), the court noted that similar review requirements "may have the effect of directly influencing a doctor's decision on what type of treatment will be provided, thus directly interfering with the practice of medicine." Arguing ethically as well as legally, Havighurst and Blumstein (pp. 57–58) contend that, with PSROs:

> the doctor's professional function is not usurped. What happens instead is that, in the case of certain procedures or treatments, which the PSRO is charged with identifying, a resource constraint is introduced (or reintroduced) into the management of each case—namely the patient's ability and willingness to pay for nonessential care. Although practically all other producers in the society must compete for the consumer's dollar against alternative uses for it, physicians expect the individual physician's production decisions automatically to trigger payment by a complaisant third party. . . . [But, b]y definition, the medical benefit from . . . excluded care is not important enough to be covered by a public program in a society which cannot meet its citizens' every need.

These arguments about the limited implications of insurance-plan coverage limits effectuated by assessments of medical "need" are even stronger when applied to private health insurers. Not only can the patient be deemed to have selected the insurance plan voluntarily and to have accepted the insurer as the enforcer of the bargain struck among the premium payers, but he is much more likely than the typical federal beneficiary to have other resources available to purchase the excluded services if they are desired.

63. Insurers can organize HMOs providing services through "independent practice associations" under the HMO Act of 1973, as amended. But §1311(a), 42 U.S.C. §300e-10(a)(Supp. IV, 1975), in overriding certain restrictive state laws applicable to HMOs, does not clearly exempt "IPAs" so as clearly to allow the formation of closed-panel, cost-controlled plans in every state. Nevertheless, insurers are probably free to enlist doctors' participation in many types of cost-control activity. See note 62.

64. P. Ellwood and W. McClure, "Health Delivery Reform," unpublished paper, InterStudy, October 25, 1976. See text accompanying note 68.

65. Havighurst and Bovbjerg; Havighurst and Blumstein.

66. Id. See also R. Egdahl and P. Gertman, eds., *Quality Assurance in Health Care* (Germantown, Md.: Aspen Systems Corp., 1976): 331.

67. The main regulatory need might be for assurance of adequate catastrophic coverage. See note 19. Otherwise close regulatory specification of offerings might retard change rather than promote it, as it has under the HMO Act. See notes 75–77 and accompanying text.

68. See "The Biggest HMO Advocate Backs Off on Prepayment," *Medical Economics* (August 9, 1976): 29, 40.

69. Ellwood and McClure. The pitfalls in seeking a legislative restructuring of the system are revealed by the HMO Act. See notes 75–77 infra and accompanying text.

70. That health care is "different" cannot be denied, but it is far from clear which way this perception cuts. Sociologist Paul Starr, for example, asks whether health care is more "a technical activity like water supply" or "primarily a social and moral activity like education." P. Starr, "A National Health Program: Organizing Diversity," *Hastings Center Report,* February 1975, p. 11. Concluding that health care is "different" from water supply, Starr argues, very much as I do, that a decentralized system is preferable from a value standpoint (see note 86), though he perhaps has more confidence than I do in government's ability to preside over a system featuring meaningful pluralism. My own work suggests that the symbolic elements in health care make government and professional decision making no more certain to be efficient or accurate than that of the ignorant consumer. See note 46 and accompanying text. Indeed, politicization of health care decision making may yield poorer decisions since it perpetuates a high degree of provider influence, allows rhetoric and symbolism to overwhelm benefit-

cost calculations, and relies on interest-group bargaining to determine outcomes. Many important interests can get lost in this process, as Starr observes. One might conclude that, precisely because health care is important to people and touches fundamental values, government should keep its distance, playing a facilitative but not a dominant role. The argument in this paper is that the private sector is potentially capable of overcoming most of the individual consumer's various disadvantages as a purchaser of health services. (The purchasing power of some must be subsidized, of course.)

71. R. Noll, "The Consequences of Public Utility Regulation of Hospitals," in *Controls on Health Care* (Washington: Institute of Medicine, National Academy of Sciences, 1975): 25; W. McClure, "The Medical Care System Under National Health Insurance: Four Models," *Journal of Health Politics, Policy and Law* 1 (Spring, 1976): 22; Havighurst, "Certificate of Need;" C. Havighurst, "Federal Regulation of the Health Care Delivery System: A Foreword in the Nature of a 'Package Insert,'" *University of Toledo Law Review* 6 (Spring, 1975): 577.

72. See note 46 and accompanying text.

73. For example, F. Hellinger, "The Effect of Certificate of Need Legislation on Hospital Investment," *Inquiry* 13 (June 1976): 187; D. Salkever and T. Bice, "The Impact of Certificate of Need Controls on Hospital Investment," *Milbank Memorial Fund Quarterly* 54 (Spring, 1976): 185; Lewin & Associates, Inc., *Evaluation of the Efficiency and Effectiveness of the Section 1122 Review Process* (1975).

74. See, for example, Havighurst and Blumstein; O. Anderson, "PSROs, the Medical Profession, and the Public Interest," *Milbank Memorial Fund Quarterly* 54 (Summer, 1976): 379; Egdahl & Gertman.

75. P. Ellwood et al., *The Health Maintenance Strategy* (Minneapolis: Institute for Interdisciplinary Studies, 1970), reprinted in *Medical Care* 9 (May–June 1971): 291.

76. See, for example, P. Starr, "The Undelivered Health System," *Public Interest* 42 (Winter, 1976): 66; P. Starr, "The New Medicine: An Experiment Designed to Fail," *New Republic,* April 19, 1975, p. 15.

77. See Havighurst, Testimony; Institute of Medicine, *HMOs: Towards a Fair Market Test* (Washington: Institute of Medicine, National Academy of Sciences, 1974).

78. For example, Havighurst, "Health Maintenance Organizations."

79. See Havighurst, "Speculations on the Market's Future in Health Care," in *Regulating Health Facilities Construction,* p. 249.

80. See note 54.

81. See, for example, Havighurst and Blumstein; Havighurst and Bovbjerg; Havighurst, "Certificate of

Need;" Havighurst, "Foreword;" Havighurst, Testimony.

82. Cf. Havighurst and Bovbjerg, pp. 411–21.

83. Cf. Havighurst, "Medical Adversity Insurance," pp. 1241–52, 1263–73 (discussing an outcomes-oriented incentive program to replace the tort remedy for malpractice).

84. Although a reconstituted market would probably redistribute manpower in time, contractual obligations to practice in underserved areas, voluntarily incurred by prospective medical students, would seem a promising approach. A long enough term of obligated service would weed out those who viewed it as merely an added education cost or a "Peace Corps" stint and attract instead those likely to establish permanent rural or ghetto practices. A bloc of such students should force the medical schools to teach what they need to know for such a career.

85. Some regulation would seem justified on traditional natural-monopoly grounds, but is difficult. A reconstituted market would reduce the need if insurers undertook to bargain with hospitals and hospitals were prohibited under the antitrust laws from combining for bargaining purposes.

86. Embracing on value as well as economic grounds a health system based on "competition under constraint," Paul Starr (p. 15) argues as follows:

Such a system would transfer important decisions from the federal government to a level at which people might have more direct control and a clearer understanding of the consequences. Various religious groups, for example, hold distinct positions on the use of certain medical procedures or on questions like the desirability of prolonging dying patients' lives. Rather than seek a false social consensus, it may be easier and wiser to allow different groups to reach their own conclusions and bear the consequences themselves. Such questions are likely to become progressively more acute as biomedical technology expands our capacity to maintain life after health and to rearrange genetic and physiological processes previously beyond our reach.

87. E.g., J. Knowles, "The Responsibility of the Individual," *Daedalus* 106 (Winter, 1977): 57; U.S. Public Health Service, pp. 97–121 passim.

88. For example, Illich; Carlson; D. Kotelchuk, ed., *Prognosis Negative* (New York: Vintage Books, 1976); Health Policy Advisory Center, *The American Health Empire* (New York: Vintage Books, 1972).

89. For example, Cochrane.

1.8 The Malpractice Experience of Health Maintenance Organizations*

WILLIAM J. CURRAN and GEORGE B. MOSELEY, III

Reprinted by special permission of the Northwestern University Law Review from 70 *Northwestern University Law Review* 68–89 (1975). Copyright © 1975 by Northwestern University School of Law. All rights reserved.

Many health care authorities, governmental officials, and legislators place a great amount of faith in health maintenance organizations (HMOs) and medical care foundations as at least a partial solution to the nation's health care delivery problems. There is considerable activity nationwide studying all aspects of the operation of these programs. Almost coincidental in time with the upsurge of interest in these organizations has been the rapidly escalating problem of medical malpractice and malpractice litigation in this country. So serious was "the crisis in malpractice" considered on the national level that in 1971 President Nixon established a special commission under the Secretary of Health, Education and Welfare to study the matter, hold public hearings, sponsor research and make recommendations to alleviate the crisis.[1] Congress, agreeing fully with the President in assessing the seriousness of the problem,[2] appropriated some $2 million for the work of the Secretary's Commission. Its final report provides a useful assessment of the malpractice problem across the United States, but, unfortunately, no particular attention was given in the report to the special circumstances of malpractice in HMOs.

The purpose of this article is to examine and evaluate the present and anticipated medical malpractice experience of HMOs and relate this experience, as much as practicable, to the quality of medical care given to the member patients of these programs. The intention is to review the level of malpractice claims brought against HMOs, their methods of handling complaints, claims and law suits, and to contrast this experience with the malpractice experience of the surrounding general medical community. Major emphasis will be placed on any variables unique to the philosophy and operation of HMOs which may increase or decrease the probability of malpractice or malpractice claims. Research for this article included a field study of 15 organizations: 12 HMOs and three foundations for medical care were selected with a view to covering the widest variety of institutional types[3] while being careful to include the largest and best known programs.[4] The total group of organizations studied provides health services for over fifty percent of the entire membership served by HMOs and foundations.[5]

Before reviewing the results of this study, however, it will be useful to look at the fundamentals of the malpractice suit as it has developed in recent years. Consequently, attention is first turned to an examination of the case and statutory law which will have a bearing on HMO liability and then, by means of the survey, to an analysis of what some of the existing HMOs have done and may do to alleviate the malpractice risk.

---

*This article is the product of research supported by the Department of Health, Education, and Welfare Grant No. HSM 110-70-390 from the National Center for Health Services Research and Development, Rockville, Md.

HMOs AND THE LAW OF MEDICAL MALPRACTICE

Ingredients of the Malpractice Suit

As the cause of action normally is framed, a claim of medical malpractice is a tort involving negligence.[6] Like other negligence torts, medical malpractice requires three main ingredients: an established standard of care applicable to the provider of medical care, a breach of the standard by the provider, and an injury to the patient resulting proximately from the breach.[7] Claims of medical malpractice have succeeded most often in the past when directed against the physician who performed the acts constituting the malpractice. On those occasions when the malpracticing physician has been an employee of a hospital, the doctrine of respondeat superior has been used to hold the hospital liable for the injuries resulting from the malpractice.[8] This liability has been found regardless of the hospital's actual or prospective ability to control the personnel or factors causing the malpractice.

In recent years, however, the legal bases for medical malpractice liability have been expanded beyond those situations where there is direct involvement in an act of malpractice or a master-servant relationship between a hospital and the malpracticing physician. Hospitals now are incurring malpractice liability in cases where they could or should have had some control over the physician committing the malpractice.[9] Physicians are being held liable for breaches of a "fiduciary" duty based on factors in addition to the doctor's medical competence.[10] In a few, as yet rare, cases physician liability has been based on a finding of a breach of a guarantee of a "cure" by the physician.[11]

Hospital Malpractice Liability: An Analogy to HMO Malpractice Liability

While the law of physician liability for malpractice is well developed and principles governing the liability of hospitals are in a stage of fast moving evolution, the law of medical malpractice for HMOs is virtually nonexistent. Consequently, HMO liability must be analyzed by analogy, most profitably to the legal status of hospitals.

First, however, it is necessary to have a basic understanding of the legal status of HMO as an organization. An HMO typically is a nonprofit corporation which enters into contracts with individual subscribers for the purpose of providing a specific, comprehensive package of health care services[12] for which the member or subscriber promises to pay membership dues at a fixed monthly or quarterly rate. In the most completely integrated HMO the same corporation which employs the physicians who provide medical services also builds or buys hospitals through which it provides hospital services. In the less integrated HMO the corporation simply contracts with a separate group of doctors, organized into a partnership or professional corporation, for the provision of medical services. It might also contract with an existing hospital for use of hospital beds, facilities, and services. The structure of most HMOs falls somewhere between these two models.

Traditionally, hospitals have not been considered insurers of patients' health or safety.[13] However, they are held to a duty of ordinary care for each patient's safety and required to extend reasonable health care as the patient's known condition indicates.[14] They are also responsible for hiring reasonably competent personnel[15] and providing equipment and facilities sufficient to treat the particular conditions of patients.[16] But as far as actual malpractice is concerned, hospital liability has usually been limited to a respondeat superior liability for the malpractice of health professionals employed.[17] If the malpracticing doctor is not an employee, but merely a member of the hospital's medical staff, he has generally been viewed as an "independent contractor" for whom the hospital bears no liability.[18]

Application of these traditional concepts to HMOs which employ some or all of their physicians directly, would logically result in malpractice damage responsibility. Where the malpracticing physician simply serves on an HMO's medical staff pursuant to a formal contract defining an arm's length relationship between the two, the HMO could defend on the ground that the physician, legally and practically, practiced his medicine quite independently of the HMO. Moreover, the typical HMO organizational structure would facilitate this kind of defense. When an HMO has entered into a contract, not with individual physicians, but with a group of physicians having a separate legal status as a partnership or professional corporation, often with a separate private practice as well, it would be difficult to see how the doctors are nevertheless employees of the HMO. The Health Insurance Plan (HIP) of New York relies heavily on this argument on those rare occasions when it is a defendant in a malpractice suit. Among HMOs, HIP probably maintains the greatest legal distance between itself and the several independent physician groups providing medical services to HIP members. In order to emphasize this separation, whenever it is sued for malpractice, HIP automatically crossclaims against the physician group involved for any damages which HIP may suffer.[19]

The law of hospital malpractice liability since 1966, however, has evolved in a way which does not bode well for the potential liability of HMOs. In that year the Supreme Court denied certiorari in the case of *Darling v. Charleston Community Memorial Hospital,*[20] a landmark decision holding that hospitals are liable for a much wider range of factors affecting the quality of care delivered in the hospital, including the competence of non-employee physicians on the hospital's medical staff. The *Darling* court either refused to accept the view that a hospital is no more than a passive facility wherein independent practitioners attempt to meet the medical needs of their patients with little, if any, cooperation from the hospital, or it chose to recognize that the hospital now has become the focus of the total health care delivery procedure, with the attending physician just one of many factors or resources determining the quality or effectiveness of the procedure, over which the hospital has or should have primary control.

A series of cases has since sought to interpret and elaborate upon *Darling*. The hospital's liability there was founded in tort, the court holding that the standard of care by which a hospital's performance would be measured could be found in the hospital's own rules of operation or procedure.[21] Other decisions have gone further to say that a hospital may be found liable for a breach by its medical staff of any rule, regulation, bylaw, or policy formulated by the hospital or some other health care agency which proximately caused injury to a patient.[22] These cases suggest that a hospital's corporate bylaws, rules of operation, official policies, medical staff bylaws, the detailed criteria which a hospital must satisfy to earn the accreditation of the Joint Committee on Accreditation of Hospitals, and

the regulations of a state hospital licensing authority, all could be used in defining the standards of care to which the hospital must adhere in dealing with its patients. Additionally, at least two courts have held that guidelines formulated by other hospitals may be introduced to show the standards of care for a particular hospital.[23]

Several cases have also considered the specific issue of a hospital's relationship with the physicians on its medical staff. Specifically, hospitals have been required to screen and review the members of their medical staffs[24] and have been held responsible for the tortious acts of independently contracting physicians on the sole ground that they were on "inquiry" notice of the malpracticing doctors' tortious propensities.[25] One case has even gone so far as to challenge the validity of the traditional employee/independent contractor distinction.[26]

If, then, hospitals have come to be viewed as "community health centers"[27] for purposes of malpractice liability, the legal ramifications for HMOs should not be difficult to ascertain. With rare exceptions, HMOs have substantial influence over the physicians who provide their medical care. Not only are the physicians often devoting their entire professional energies to the treatment of HMO members, but they typically do so pursuant to a contract which is renegotiated annually with the HMO. The present practice of most HMOs is to leave the discipline of incompetent or malpracticing physicians to the physician group of which they are a member. But, as the scope of their operations expands and their total number grows, and as a history of malpractice suits against HMOs accumulates, courts are likely to view this contractual leverage as evidence of meaningful control and require that it be exercised for the protection of individual members. It is possible, moreover, that the physicians' relationship to HMOs is even more interdependent than their alliance with hospitals for the reason that an HMO must rely upon its doctors to provide the medical services it has promised. Thus the lack of a traditional employee relationship should prove even less of an obstacle for HMO malpractice liability than it has for hospital malpractice liability.

Ironically, the HMO may be in a somewhat better position to defend itself against malpractice suits based on acts committed, not by the HMO doctors, but by the personnel of the hospital through which it obtains services for its members. Except where the HMO actually owns its own hospital facilities, the HMO-hospital relationship usually is based on an arm's length contract between parties of equal bargaining strength. The outcome will probably be different, however, when HMO and hospital are intimately tied. For example, the Kaiser Foundation Health Plan, the largest HMO in the country, contracts with a separate corporation of hospitals, Kaiser Hospitals, Inc., for the provision of hospital services to its members.[28] But, since those hospitals are organized almost exclusively for the purpose of treating Kaiser Plan members, and since there is a virtual identity between the boards of trustees of the Kaiser Foundation Health Plan and Kaiser Hospitals, Inc., potential liability of the Kaiser group for hospital employees seems imminent.

Malpractice Liability Based on Contractual and Fiduciary Relationships

Mention should be made of two other potential bases of HMO liability which either are not available in suits against hospitals or have otherwise been little used. The first is analogous to the formal legal relationship between a patient and his doctor which is contractual in nature and based upon an express or implied agreement.[29] It is thus possible for a patient to sue his physician for breach of that agreement in contract.[30] In addition, a contractual duty is a prerequisite to a malpractice action in tort. Nevertheless, suits against physicians usually are brought in tort, not because of the absence of a contractual relationship, but because the tort action is simpler and provides an easier method for obtaining damages for pain and suffering.[31] Contractual liability, however, seems particularly appropriate in the HMO context. Although there is an express contract between the member patient and the HMO which may not contain specific assurances of high quality care, these terms may usually be implied. The HMO, after all, has agreed to meet the member's every health need up to well defined limitations and to furnish an acceptable physician for these purposes. And, whether that physician is considered an agent of the HMO or the HMO an agent of the physician, it would not be unreasonable for the member to infer a guarantee that high standards of quality will be met.

A final basis for potential HMO liability finds its roots in the nature of the fiduciary duty owed a patient by his physician. A fiduciary relation is said to exist wherever trust and confidence are reposed by one party in the influence or dominance of another,[32] creating in the latter a duty to act with greater diligence and care than that required by a common negligence standard of due care. A doctor is traditionally liable in tort for injuries committed in violation of standards established by "good medical practice."[33] It has increasingly been held, however, that the patient's vulnerability and the physician's role as repository of the patient's trust dispose of the traditional notion that a physician's obligations emanate from, or are limited by, the art and science of medical practice, and, instead, give rise to a fiduciary relationship.[34] The reason given by one court for assigning this new duty to the physician was that[35]

the patient, being unlearned in medical sciences, has an abject dependence upon and trust in his physician for the information upon which he relies during the decisional process, thus raising an obligation in the physician that transcends arm's length transactions.

Another case described the duty more specifically by saying that the fiduciary relationship creates the expectation and duty that the doctor will provide for the patient's total care, including cooperation with the patient in any litigation over an illness or injury treated by the physician.[36]

A persuasive case can be made for the proposition that an HMO member places similar trust and confidence in the HMO in which he enrolls. The significance of this trust is heightened by the fact that the member pays substantial sums of money to the HMO for the dispatch of its duties and by the fact that the member's health, and perhaps life, depend upon the HMO's performance. Moreover, after making promises to the member for the availability of a certain package of health services, it is the HMO which selects the providers who will perform those services. The patient, "being unlearned in medical sciences," has no choice but to trust in the HMO's ability and desire to choose only competent providers. When it appears that this trust has been violated justifiable court action may result.

Implications of PSROs for Malpractice Liability of HMOs

The 1972 Social Security Act Amendments provided for creation of an infrastructure of "professional standards review organizations" (PSROs) to monitor the quantity and quality of health care services delivered through certain federally funded programs beginning in 1975.[37] The professional standards review concept is designed to evaluate health care services on the basis of four criteria: (1) medical necessity, (2) recognized quality, (3) appropriateness of delivery environment, and (4) duration of delivery.[38] As PSROs become operational, their monitoring and review authority will apply only to services provided under the federal Medicare, Medicaid and maternal and child health programs.[39]

The procedures and norms of the quality review performed by the PSROs[40] are critically relevant to HMOs for several reasons. First, many HMOs, particularly those which are just now organizing, depend for large chunks of their initial memberships and revenues upon contracts to provide services to designated Medicaid and Medicare populations. As a result, major portions of many HMOs' health care delivery operations will be immediately subject to PSRO review with the consequence that these programs may be inclined to extend the same level of quality review to the rest of its operations. Second, if Congress enacts some form of national health insurance, as it is expected to do in the next few years, nearly every resident of the country, HMO members included, will have all or part of his health costs reimbursed by a federal program.[41] There is a good chance that Congress will expand PSRO monitoring activities to cover the new federal expenditures. Finally, the federal PSRO legislation may prompt individual states to enact their own regulation, making independent evaluative standards applicable to all government sponsored health care.[42]

It seems fair to say that, as a result of PSRO review, many patients will not receive the kind of medical care they otherwise would have received. Enforcement of a PSRO norm may, for example, result in the administration of a particular treatment in a less costly institution (*e.g.,* an extended care facility rather than a hospital) or on an out-patient basis,[43] or it may mean that a patient admitted to a hospital will be dis-

charged sooner than he otherwise would have been.[44] It should be noted, however, that the only real mandatory effect of an adverse PSRO determination is to remove the possibility of government reimbursement for the costs of care; the patient retains the option of assuming the additional expense himself. But if the patient cannot afford the extra expense, the physician must either terminate treatment or provide his services free of charge. It is at this point that the implications for medical malpractice become ominous.

There is significant case law to the effect that, though a physician may refuse to enter into a contractual relationship for services with a patient who appears unable to pay for his medical care, he cannot discontinue that relationship once it has been initiated.[45] However, for treatment denied pursuant to a PSRO determination, the physician is legally protected. The legislation immunizes from liability both practitioners and other providers acting in compliance with PSRO norms,[46] as well as the PSRO reviewing physicians performing duties and functions under the statute.[47] This immunity, however, is conditioned upon the physician's having exercised[48]

due care in all professional conduct taken or directed by him and reasonably related to, and resulting from, the actions taken in compliance with or in reliance upon such professionally accepted norms of care and treatment.

As a result of this condition, the attending physician will continue subject to common law standards for his treatment of the patient following a negative determination. Thus, even though one mode of treatment has been rejected by the PSRO, the physician is obliged to continue his relationship with the patient, seeking PSRO approval for alternative types of treatment. It is conceivable, of course, that PSRO determinations could close off virtually all plausible courses of treatment and effectively require that the patient-doctor relationship cease. Alternatively, there will be a great many courses of treatment for which norms will not immediately, if ever, be established. In these latter areas the immunity clause does not apply and a doctor's malpractice liability is once again measured by common law standards. It should also be emphasized that the PSRO immunity clause protects the physician who first seeks approval of a PSRO and is denied. Whether this same protection extends to the doctor who simply prescribes the established norm even though believing different care would be appropriate is as yet uncertain.[49]

Hospitals[50] and HMOs, like individual physicians, are similarly liable for the premature discharge of a patient. Thus, where injury results from discharge, the liability immunity clause in the PSRO act again becomes quite important. Hospitals are covered by the express language of the immunity clause referring to "providers" of health services;[51] an HMO will likewise qualify for protection if found sufficiently involved in the delivery of health care to its members to be considered a "provider." Whether hospital or HMO, however, the provider must still observe "due care" in its dealing with the patient. In the context of a discharge from hospitalization, this probably obligates the provider to relocate the patient in an alternative facility under appropriate circumstances.

ACTUAL MALPRACTICE EXPERIENCE OF HMOs

With malpractice liability thus established as a threat to HMOs of even greater consequence than to hospitals, it is now appropriate to examine some of the steps a number of HMOs have taken to cope with the problem. The remainder of this article is thus devoted to a discussion of the findings of the study of actual HMO malpractice claims experience and the implications of recent developments in the law of medical malpractice.[52]

By way of overview, it may be observed that if there is a serious "malpractice crisis" in this country it was not greatly evident in surveying administrators and physicians in the HMOs which were the subject of this study.[53] Five of the 12 HMOs reported that they had made no payments at all on malpractice claims. Admittedly, these were the smaller and newer operations, but almost all have avoided responsibility for large awards, none paying out more than $100,000 on any individual claim, with the exception of one west coast plan.

When asked to compare their malpractice claims levels with those of surrounding medical communities, officials of four organizations

thought their experience better than that in neighboring areas. The remainder thought their incidence of claims and suits about the same as in surrounding communities. These opinions were not, however, based upon verifiable data and may be considered self serving, but little hard evidence is available either way except in Washington State where the Aetna Insurance Company is responsible for about 80 percent of the malpractice insurance sold. For Washington State physicians generally, Aetna paid out $1.45 for every $1.00 in premiums paid in 1972; for every $1.00 paid in 1972 by Group Health Cooperative of Puget Sound, an HMO operating in Seattle, Aetna was called upon to pay out only $.89.[54]

Operational Characteristics of HMOs Affecting the Incidence of Malpractice Claims

Interviews with HMO officials revealed a number of characteristics believed by these officials to have particular bearing upon the incidence of malpractice claims against them. One significant feature, from an overall standpoint, was the widely acclaimed HMO philosophy of offering comprehensive health services, including preventive care, with the goal of maintaining health rather than, and in addition to, merely dealing with sickness. It was suggested that some HMO members would take this philosophy literally and feel that their good health has been guaranteed by the organization. Some HMOs do in fact conduct aggressive enrollment campaigns, including mass advertising; in California, for example, membership has been sold on a door-to-door solicitation basis, a notoriously "hard sell" style of salesmanship.[55]

A more frequently mentioned possible negative factor in malpractice claims provocation, however, was the large organizational character of most HMOs, accompanied by less personal relationships between doctor and patient than exist in private practice. Patients seem more willing to sue "the organization" than they would a private practitioner. Also, there are unavoidable assembly line techniques used in large organizations which would be unnecessary in private, solo practices. A number of the HMOs surveyed make extensive efforts to create an atmosphere of warmth, trust, and intimacy to counteract the impersonality of which HMOs are often accused. Patients, for example, may be assigned their own doctor and encouraged to seek that doctor out on all visits. However, there are often long delays, days or even weeks, in seeing a specific physician and most patients' habits are to wait until they are quite sick before coming into the HMO walk-in services without prior appointment.

A few officials also mentioned the composition of their memberships as perhaps contributing to a higher incidence of malpractice claims. Among characteristics mentioned were higher income levels, college education, and social-political activism. All of these were thought to contribute to suit consciousness and an awareness of legal rights.

On the other hand, many reasons were asserted for a belief that, in overall claims experience, HMOs would prove superior to the general medical community. First named was the "good feeling" of the membership toward the HMO because of its lower cost and its comprehensive high quality medical care. Also it was said that for many HMOs, especially those run as cooperatives, there is a sense of belonging, closeness, and informality between members and staffs. For example, in a California television interview quoted in the *Ribicoff Report* in 1969, Thomas Waterhouse, attorney for the Ross-Loos Group in Los Angeles, spoke of "the type of practice the group has, the loyalty of patients to the group" as a significant factor in Ross-Loos' favorable malpractice experience.[56]

Various methods were cited for obtaining a friendly membership attitude. Election of members to the governing boards was considered highly advantageous. In addition, many HMOs publish regular newsletters and hold frequent membership meetings. In terms of physical atmosphere, one HMO stressed its use of several small waiting rooms rather than one large area for its ambulatory service. Other plans are moving to achieve reductions in size of operations by decentralizing their services in local outpatient clinics.

Five HMOs spoke highly of their efficient and sensitive systems for handling patient complaints as an important preventive of malpractice claims. All 12 HMOs operate formal or informal complaint systems and all reported that these programs are utilized to improve patient-staff relationships and the quality of care.

Also cited on the positive side as reducing the incidence of malpractice claims were more sub-

tle features in HMO operations. The fact that no large bills for service are sent to members immediately after an unfortunate outcome of medical care helps avoid resentment over expenses from provoking a malpractice claim, as often happens in private practice. It was also said that the relative ease of changing doctors in an HMO may contribute to avoiding clashes of personality and other personal animosities which may provoke malpractice claims. Lastly, it was observed that continuity of care, without additional costs, enabled members to keep returning for further care until they were satisfied, thus avoiding possible legal action over a particular outcome.

Handling of Claims and Suits

In most HMOs, formal malpractice claims are handled simply by notifying the malpractice insurance carrier, whose adjusters and attorneys completely take over management of the case. There are two significant alternatives to this approach: self-insurance and binding arbitration. The use of self-insurance carries with it the need to handle all claims and law suits throughout the process. Presently three of the HMOs surveyed employ both self-insurance and binding arbitration. A fourth plan uses arbitration alone and still another uses self-insurance without arbitration. Thus, while the current trend is toward self-insurance, a strong interest has also developed in binding arbitration which can legally be included as a required part of the total package sold to a subscriber.[57] The only outright rejection of binding arbitration in the malpractice context has come from the two programs surveyed which are closely or exclusively related to trade unions, Labor Health Institute in St. Louis and the New Haven Community Health Plan. The reason for rejection, however, was organized labor's opposition to binding arbitration in labor disputes, not specific bad experiences with malpractice arbitration. The Kaiser Foundation in Northern California, which originally rejected arbitration, is now awaiting an evaluation of the experience of the Southern California Region with an experimental arbitration plan. Kaiser has also instituted arbitration in its Hawaii Region where it is employing the services of the American Arbitration Association.

There has been very little actual experience with arbitration hearings in malpractice cases, either in HMOs or elsewhere. For example, the Ross-Loos Medical·Group, which has had binding arbitration as a part of its operation for more than 30 years in that supposed hot-bed of malpractice suit risk, Southern California, has had only five cases go to arbitration in all of this period.[58] Consequently HMO officials and attorneys have been quite sophisticated about the real advantages of arbitration: none has seen it as a panacea to drive away the malpractice claims "menace" or even to reduce the total amount of pay-outs on claims.[59] Indeed, its main advantage is believed to be in earlier settlement of claims and consequent avoidance of legal and other expenses involved in litigation delays and courtroom trials.

Physicians in HMOs react to malpractice suits much like doctors and other professional people, including lawyers, who are sued anywhere else; they feel insulted and personally attacked. They find the experience traumatic and are inclined, at least at first, to fight the suit regardless of how the merits of the claim may be viewed by others. However, membership in an HMO medical group gives them some not inconsiderable advantages in coping with the personal situation. First, they have the close support of other doctors in the group, some of whom may have been subject to similar actions. More important, suit is often against the organization which must defend it directly. The doctor may be only one of several involved in the treatment of the patient and thus may not be subject to pressures he otherwise would feel if the full brunt of the outcome were on his shoulders alone. After some early interviews the physician is very often removed entirely from the matter, with all medical involvement being handled by the clinical director.

The more elaborate system for handling malpractice claims was found at the Kaiser Foundation's Northern California Region, a very large, self-insured operation. On the medical staff of every Kaiser facility is a physician who acts as a medico-legal chief. All subpoenas, other legal documents, and correspondence served upon any doctor in that facility are brought to him; he evaluates the documents, talks with the doctor, and examines the medical records. He also disposes of rudimentary legal problems on the spot, such as testimony, consent for treatment of a minor, blood transfusion problems with Jehovah's Witnesses, and the like. Claims which

jell into suits are passed on to an attorney serving full time in this field in the general counsel's office in the headquarters in Oakland; but the medico-legal chief in the facility continues to function as medical liaison on the case. The attorney, in turn, is assisted by two committees. The first is a medical review committee which meets monthly to evaluate all cases and determine a position to be taken by Kaiser. The second is a professional liability committee which has more specific responsibilities for strategy when a trial is imminent; settlement is discussed and upper limits of payment are established. This latter committee also becomes concerned with overall policy concerning professional liability in the organization.

Measures Employed by HMOs to Control the Quality of Care

Every administrator and physician surveyed expressed the view that the quality of medical practice in their programs was at least equal to that obtainable in their respective geographic areas, and many thought the HMO quality probably superior to that otherwise available to their members. The reasons given were related to the group nature of the practice, with its wide range of services and specialty consultants, and the removal of an economic barrier to comprehensive care. Studies, in fact, indicate that the hospitalization rate of HMO subscribers is less than the general average, though average length of hospitalization is about the same.[60] Many physicians attributed this improvement in care in part to having other doctors "looking over our shoulders" as well as having available ready access to specialty consultants which avoided the problem of attending physicians attempting to go beyond their capacities. A few, however, also pointed to the need for greater efficiency and productivity in HMO practice which requires attending physicians to work faster and spend less time with each patient. Nevertheless, all physicians uniformly observed that their personal relationships with patients were just as warm and meaningful as in private practice, hospitals, or other facilities where they had practiced or been trained.

Defensive medical procedures (that is, treatment administered primarily to forestall law suits or produce an adequate defense to a malpractice claim) undertaken by the HMOs surveyed were generally found to be used to the same extent as in the respective surrounding geographic areas. Generally, these procedures are not of such a nature as to raise significantly the cost to the patient[61] but may have the benefit of protecting the physician if his diagnosis or management is later challenged. Some defensive practices may actually produce better quality medical care. For example, one medical director stated that he was prescribing approximately half the antibiotics he had in private practice but was ordering more x-rays and throat cultures. Recent malpractice decisions in the courts may well accelerate these trends as more American courts find extensive liability for errors in diagnosis.[62]

Perhaps the most important means of assuring quality care in any medical organization, however, is recruitment of well-trained and capable physicians, and installation of effective review procedures over the care rendered by these doctors. The study gave special attention to this area. All of the HMOs visited were found to have quite elaborate programs of physician recruitment. Evaluation of candidates is also quite thorough. At the Group Health Cooperative of Puget Sound the entire medical staff screens prospective candidates while a personnel committee conducts interviews. At Metro Health Plan in Detroit, a candidate may be interviewed by as many as 12 staff physicians. At the Group Health Plan in St. Paul a unique procedure is followed: physician recruits are screened by an independent medical board composed of doctors in no way associated with the HMO. In every program a candidate is interviewed by at least the medical director and the head of the department or specialty to which he is applying.

Officials from each of the 12 HMOs asserted that their medical staffs were composed of all, or nearly all, American Specialty Board certified or eligible doctors. At Kaiser Foundation in Northern California, for example, it was indicated that 90 percent were Board certified, eight percent were Board eligible, and the remaining two percent were employed in emergency room positions. At HIP in New York there was found a greater degree of codification of physician standards than in the other HMOs, due largely to the more arm's length relationship between HIP and its 28 independent medical groups.[63] This HMO, in fact, has published a 24-page booklet outlining professional standards for medical groups and medical group centers. The booklet specifies procedures for appointment to staff with HIP central office approval through a "medical control board" composed of 18 physicians from the community at large as well as HIP groups, general principles of group operation, organization and composition of groups, basic specialties to be included, and services to be provided.[64]

Physicians can expect to serve a probationary period of from one to three years in all but one of the programs. Also, a periodic assessment of the performance of all doctors on the staff is usually conducted. The Puget Sound group has a particularly thorough and organized system for evaluating new physicians. During a two year probation they are assigned to a preceptor and are evaluated semi-annually by a panel drawn from the probationer's own department or specialty and from other fields. General practitioners are included in the evaluation of specialists, and vice versa. Evaluative questionnaires are even sent to the Cooperative's chief clinic nurse, hospital and nursing administrators, and patient-appointments personnel. If a doctor is to remain with the group after the two years, a two-thirds vote of the medical executive committee and the entire medical staff must be obtained. Under this procedure, there has been a fifteen percent dropout rate during, or at the conclusion of, the probationary period.

Dismissal or severe discipline of physicians for malpractice is generally uncommon, however. Most dismissals (or failures to be appointed to the regular staff) on the ground of incompetence take place in the probationary period. Dismissal for low standards of practice becomes less likely, and more difficult legally, the longer the doctor serves on the staff.[65] In malpractice situations involving a regular staff member, if a pattern of incompetence is found, the physician's work is reviewed by the medical director and other medical staff and rehabilitation plans are devised which may include a required rotation through certain departments or a series of post-graduate educational courses. Failure to cooperate with the suggested plan and to improve in practice can lead to separation from the staff, usually by resignation.

As to formal quality control mechanisms among the programs, they vary considerably and no real pattern is visible. Chart review mechanisms are employed in only about five organizations. Other methods in use include grand rounds, joint hospital review committees, tumor boards, continuing education requirements, and member attitude surveys. Peer review for utilization control is growing as a practice in HMOs and will continue to grow with recent federal legislation imposing further standards and procedures in this area.

Malpractice Insurance Coverage

Eight of the 12 HMOs surveyed carry medical malpractice insurance with independent insurance companies while four are self-insured up to very high limits. Over recent years the tendency to self-insure has grown. Annual premiums paid in 1972 to insurance companies varied from a low in a newer, smaller east coast plan of $6,943 for its basic coverage and its $5 million umbrella policy, to $143,000 in an urban based midwestern HMO for its basic coverage and a $2 million umbrella policy. Most of the HMOs have umbrella coverage in the $1 million to $5 million range, but one large west coast group had umbrella coverage over its self-insurance running to $40 million. None, however, receives a special experience rating by its insurance carrier due to the fact it is an HMO. One east coast plan, which paid the lowest annual premium of all surveyed, was able to achieve this favorable position by persuading its carrier to rate it in the same category as its affiliated, university medical center. Another has received a special rate for its physicians but not for its hospital operations.

The absence of an insurance industry practice of special experience ratings for HMOs was confirmed in a series of interviews with officials of leading major national carriers of malpractice insurance.[66] None of these officials was aware of any data specially collected by the insurance industry on the overall malpractice claims experience of HMOs nor of any especially favorable ratings. Each was also asked whether a favorable rating was justified by the fact that by employing a group of doctors, HMOs might be able to organize more effective loss control programs.[67] Most of the respondents rejected this idea because significant economies were derived in groups primarily from the lower cost of acquiring the premium volume and servicing the insured doctors, not from loss control programs.

It must be noted, however, that insurance carriers do calculate total annual premiums for HMOs by taking into account a number of specific features of the particular HMO, such as the number of physicians employed, their specialties, and whether they are full or part time with the HMO, the size of the enrollment and volume of patient visits annually, whether the HMO owns and operates its own hospitals, geographic location of the organization, and the actual malpractice claims experience of the HMO in the past. These, though, are not considered special features of an HMO operation but are merely an accumulation of factors bearing on risk as measured by all casualty insurance underwriters.[68]

CONCLUSION

By way of overall assessment, the large and well-operated HMOs which were the subject of this study were found generally to deal quite well with the operational aspects of medical malpractice. They tended to take advantage of their size and administrative structure to set up efficient, though often informal, patient complaint systems and malpractice claims processing. They acted responsibly toward their members and the public in carrying more than adequate insurance coverage, again a virtue of their size and ability to buy group policies and to spread the premium cost widely among the membership. The quality of care delivered also was very good, due largely to efficient grouping of manpower, facilities, and services around the organizational goal of health maintenance. Personnel methods were effectively used to select competent physicians and monitor their performance periodically.

Nevertheless, none of these 12 operations identified constant improvement of quality in all aspects of medical care delivery as a deliberate management goal of the organization. The lack of a clear position in this area may be explained in part by the functional separation in most of the projects between "plan" management and the professional medical group which provides the care. As discussed earlier, this same type of separation of responsibility exists in most hospitals between the administration of the hospital and the organized medical staff. Court cases like *Darling v. Charleston Community Memorial Hospital*[69] and, more recently, *Purcell v. Zimbelman*,[70] evidence judicial movement toward corporate responsibility for quality of care in the governing bodies of all hospitals. A few states have adopted this position by statute.[71]

Variations in organizational structure of HMOs across the country and within individual states has militated against establishment of any consistent legal position on HMO responsibility for quality of care and consequent malpractice. In the long run, however, a movement to corporate responsibility on the part of all HMOs for the quality of care rendered, and for all forms of malpractice committed by physicians and other personnel regardless of the intricacies of a particular structural organization, seems highly likely in view of other trends in the field. There is already a movement toward "institutional licensing" whereunder a medical care facility or organization would have authority to utilize its personnel in accordance with its own determination of functions and without the necessity of conforming to rigid professional categories established by state licensure boards.[72] The recent HMO legislation passed by Congress is similarly intended to remove state legal barriers to the organization of HMOs and to their utilization of personnel.[73] The objective of such laws is to centralize responsibility for personnel utilization. However, with removal of licensure law barriers built on the theory of controlling quality of care by controlling categories of professional staff, there must be substituted some other reliable measure or measures of the quality of care delivered. On the national level, the most commonly discussed method is outcome measurement where actual successes or failures in patient management for particular illnesses are evaluated. Senator Kennedy's proposed HMO bill[74] of the last session included establishment of a Medical Care Commission which would have measured quality largely on this outcome basis. At least two of the HMOs surveyed are also investigating establishment of outcome indices for the quality of care rendered to their members.

Malpractice litigation is essentially based upon an outcome measurement.[75] Achieving a bad result raises the question of possible negligence by the attending physician or other personnel. If HMOs are clothed by law with extensive power over their medical personnel, including doctors, and are judged on the basis of outcome in the results of the medical care they deliver, then it seems inevitable that they will be held to answer malpractice claims concerning

that care. In response, HMO membership contracts may well move toward providing malpractice protection for members directly against the central plan which provides the care, either on traditional legal theories of negligence and the court system, or through HMO-organized arbitration schemes, perhaps with a no-fault system of liability. Such a movement would seem to be in the interests of patients who would thereby have greater certainty in collecting fair money damages for legitimate claims. Such a movement would also have salutory effects in encouraging HMO establishment of firm and effective management policies to establish, monitor, and constantly improve the quality of medical care they deliver.

NOTES

1. DEPARTMENT OF HEALTH, EDUCATION, AND WELFARE, REPORT OF THE SECRETARY'S COMMISSION ON MEDICAL MALPRACTICE xvi (HEW Pub. No. (OS) 73–88, 1973) [hereinafter cited as MALPRACTICE COMMISSION REPORT].

2. SENATE SUBCOMM. ON EXECUTIVE REORGANIZATION, 91st Cong., 1st Sess., MEDICAL MALPRACTICE: THE PATIENT VERSUS THE PHYSICIAN 1–2 (Comm. Print 1969) [hereinafter cited as RIBICOFF REPORT].

3. The HMOs included were Family Health Program of Southern California, Long Beach, California; Kaiser Foundation Health Plan, Northern California Region, Oakland, California; Ross-Loos Medical Group of Los Angeles, California; Group Health Association, Washington, D.C.; New Haven Community Health Care Plan, New Haven, Connecticut; Harvard Community Health Plan, Boston, Massachusetts; Group Health Plan, St. Paul, Minnesota; Labor Health Institute, St. Louis, Missouri; Health Insurance Plan of Greater New York, New York City; Group Health Cooperative of Puget Sound, Seattle, Washington; Marshfield Clinic, Marshfield, Wisconsin; and Metro Health Plan, Detroit, Michigan.

The foundations studied were Maricopa Foundation for Medical Care, Phoenix, Arizona; San Joaquin Medical Foundation, Stockton, California; and Physician's Association of Clackamus County, Gladstone, Oregon.

4. Each of the organizations was visited and information was gathered through structured interviews conducted with key personnel. An attempt was made and was usually successful in including, in each site visited, interviews with the executive director, medical director, legal counsel, and member complaints secretary. In many visits, conversations were also conducted with other administrative staff and with physi-

cians actually rendering medical care to members. No clinical or administrative records of patients or of individual malpractice claims were requested and none were examined.

5. The medical foundations are excluded from the discussion below because none of the three contacted engage in any way in handling malpractice claims or securing insurance coverage for member physicians, and all three believed that they had no liability for malpractice committed by those physicians. Nevertheless, it should be noted that the peer review programs of the foundations can have an effect in reducing the incidence of malpractice by their physicians.

6. As discussed below, however, with more threatening overtones for HMOs, there also is the possibility that the cause of action will lie in contract.

7. W. PROSSER, LAW OF TORTS §30 (4th ed. 1971).

8. *See, e.g.,* Bernardi v. Community Hosp. Ass'n, 160 Colo. 280, 443 P.2d 708 (1968) (hospital held liable for malpractice of nurse acting out of the presence of the doctor). *See* text accompanying notes 12–18 *infra.*

9. *See, e.g.,* Darling v. Charleston Community Mem. Hosp., 33 Ill. 2d 326, 211 N.E.2d 253 (1965), *cert. denied,* 383 U.S. 946 (1966). *See also* text accompanying notes 20–26 *infra.*

10. Canterbury v. Spence, 464 F.2d 772, 782 (D.C. Cir. 1972); Cobbs v. Grant, 8 Cal. 3d 229, 242, 502 P.2d 1, 9, 104 Cal. Rptr. 505, 513 (1972).

11. Guilmet v. Campbell, 385 Mich. 57, 188 N.W.2d 601 (1971). *See also* Gault v. Sideman, 42 Ill. App. 2d 96, 191 N.E.2d 436 (1963); Hawkins v. McGee, 84 N.H. 114, 146 A. 641 (1929).

12. This is in contrast with Blue Cross/Blue Shield organizations which promise only to provide reimbursement for the cost of health care services which the enrollees have obtained on their own.

13. *See* Wood v. Samaritan Institution, 26 Cal. 2d 847, 851–52, 161 P.2d 556, 558 (1945); DeMartini v. Alexander Sanitarium, Inc., 192 Cal. App. 2d 442, 13 Cal. Rptr. 564 (1961); Gray v. Carter, 100 Cal. App. 2d 642, 224 P.2d 28 (1950).

14. *See* Vistica v. Presbyterian Hosp., 67 Cal. 2d 465, 432 P.2d 193, 62 Cal. Rptr. 577 (1967); Wood v. Samaritan Institution, 26 Cal. 2d 847, 161 P.2d 556 (1945). Both these cases concerned the hospitals' liability for injuries suffered by a patient with a known mental incapacity. In these earlier cases, no attempt was made to explore the full depth of a hospital's potential liability for a patient while on the hospital's premises.

15. *See* Rice v. California Lutheran Hosp., 27 Cal. 2d 296, 163 P.2d 860 (1945); Thomas v. Seaside Mem. Hosp., 80 Cal. App. 2d 841, 183 P.2d 288 (1947).

16. *See* Carrasco v. Bankoff, 220 Cal. App. 2d 230, 33 Cal. Rptr. 673 (1963).

17. *See* Bernardi v. Community Hosp. Ass'n, 160 Colo. 280, 443 P.2d 708 (1968); Bing v. Thunig, 2 N.Y.2d 656, 143 N.E.2d 3, 163 N.Y.S.2d 3 (1957).

18. *See* Moon v. Mercy Hosp., 150 Colo. 430, 373 P.2d 944 (1962); Emory University v. Porter, 103 Ga. App. 752, 120 S.E.2d 668 (1961); Bradshaw v. Iowa Lutheran Hosp., 251 Iowa 375, 101 N.W.2d 167 (1960).

19. Interview with Allan Kornfeld, President, Health Insurance Plan of New York, in New York City, May, 1973.

20. 33 Ill. 2d 326, 211 N.E.2d 253 (1965), *cert. denied,* 383 U.S. 946 (1966).

21. *Id.* at 332–34, 211 N.E.2d at 257–58.

22. *See* Penn Tanker Co. v. United States, 310 F. Supp. 613, 618 (S.D. Tex. 1970); Steeves v. United States, 294 F. Supp. 446, 455 (D.S.C. 1968); Kapuschinsky v. United States, 248 F. Supp. 732, 748 (D.S.C. 1966); Pederson v. Dumouchel, 72 Wash. 2d 73, 80, 431 P.2d 973, 978 (1967); Duling v. Bluefield Sanitarium, Inc., 149 W. Va. 567, 583, 142 S.E.2d 754, 764–65 (1965).

23. *See* Foley v. Bishop Clarkson Mem. Hosp., 185 Neb. 89, 173 N.W.2d 881 (1970); *cf.* Tonsic v. Wagner, 220 Pa. Super. 468, 289 A.2d 138 (1972) (dissenting opinion) (attack upon hospital's failure to formulate an adequate rule for the protection of its patients).

24. *See* Purcell v. Zimbelman, 18 Ariz. App. 75, 500 P.2d 335 (1972); Mitchell County Hosp. Authority v. Joiner, 229 Ga. 140, 189 S.E.2d 412 (1972); Pederson v. Dumouchel, 72 Wash. 2d 73, 431 P.2d 973 (1967).

25. *See* Purcell v. Zimbelman, 18 Ariz. App. 75, 500 P.2d 335 (1972); Mitchell County Hosp. Authority v. Joiner, 229 Ga. 140, 189 S.E.2d 412 (1972); Foley v. Bishop Clarkson Mem. Hosp., 185 Neb. 89, 173 N.W.2d 881 (1970); Fiorentino v. Wenger, 19 N.Y.2d 407, 227 N.E.2d 296, 280 N.Y.S.2d 373 (1967). *But see* Hull v. North Valley Hosp., 159 Mont. 375, 498 P.2d 136 (1972). The line of reasoning in these cases is best expressed in the following language from the interim opinion in a California case:

> The hospital has a duty to protect its patients from malpractice by members of its medical staff when it knows or should have known that malpractice was likely to be committed upon them. Mercy Hospital had no actual knowledge of Dr. Nork's propensity to commit malpractice, but it was negligent in not knowing, because it did not have a system of acquiring knowledge available to it properly; it failed to investigate the Freer case, which would have given it knowledge; and it cannot excuse itself on the ground that its medical staff did not inform it.

Gonzales v. Nork, Civ. No. 228566 (Sacramento Super. Ct. Nov. 27, 1973).

26. Rucker v. High Point Mem. Hosp., Inc., 20 N.C. App. 650, 202 S.E.2d 610, *aff'd,* 285 N.C. 519, 206

S.E.2d 196 (1974) (contract between hospital and physician held to create an employment relationship). Not only are hospitals being forced to screen out and dismiss incompetent or potentially malpracticing physicians, but they are also under pressure to observe certain procedures in disciplining doctors. A large body of case law defines the rights of a physician as a member of a hospital medical staff and the procedures which must be followed in removing him. They can be summarized by saying that medical staff privileges are generally considered a property right as well as a personal right, Edwards v. Fresno County Hosp., 38 Cal. App. 3d 702, 113 Cal. Rptr. 579 (1974), of the physician which may not be terminated without full compliance with the requirements of due process. Poe v. Charlotte Mem. Hosp., Inc., 374 F. Supp. 1302 (D.N.C. 1974). *See* note 65 *infra.*

27. Moore v. Board of Trustees of Carson-Tahon Hosp., 88 Nev. 207, 495 P.2d 605 (1972).

28. *See* Valentine v. Kaiser Foundation Hospitals, 194 Cal. App. 2d 282, 15 Cal. Rptr. 26 (1961).

29. *See* Raner v. Grossman, 31 Cal. App. 3d 539, 543, 107 Cal. Rptr. 469, 471 (1973); Agnew v. Parks, 172 Cal. App. 2d 756, 764, 343 P.2d 118, 123 (1959); Miller, *The Contractual Liability of Physicians and Surgeons,* 1953 WASH. U.L.Q. 413 [hereinafter cited as Miller].

30. *See* Scott v. Simpson, 46 Ga. App. 479, 167 S.E. 920 (1933); Miller, *supra* note 29, at 413.

31. W. PROSSER, LAW OF TORTS §32, at 162 (4th ed. 1971); RESTATEMENT (FIRST) OF CONTRACTS §314, Illus. 7, at 467 (1932). Miller, *supra* note 29, at 424.

32. Twomey v. Mitchum, Jones & Templeton, Inc., 262 Cal. App. 2d 690, 708, 69 Cal. Rptr. 222, 235 (1968); Lappas v. Barker, 375 S.W.2d 248, 251 (Ky. 1964).

33. W. PROSSER, LAW OF TORTS §32, at 165 (4th ed. 1971). *See* Langford v. Kosterlitz, 107 Cal. App. 175, 290 P. 80 (1930).

34. *See* Canterbury v. Spence, 464 F.2d 772, 782 (D.C. Cir. 1972); Cobbs v. Grant, 8 Cal. 3d 229, 242, 502 P.2d 1, 9, 104 Cal. Rptr. 505, 513 (1972).

35. Cobbs v. Grant, 8 Cal. 3d 229, 242, 502 P.2d 1, 9, 104 Cal. Rptr. 505, 513 (1972).

36. Alexander v. Knight, 197 Pa. Super. 79, 177 A.2d 142, 146 (1962).

37. 42 U.S.C. §§1320c-1 to -19 (Supp. II, 1972).

38. *Id.* §§1320c-4(a)(1)(A) to (C), 5(d) respectively.

39. *Id.* §1320c.

40. Under the legislation the Secretary of Health, Education and Welfare has divided the country into over 200 service or catchment areas. 42 U.S.C. §1320c-1(a) (Supp. II, 1972). For each one of these areas, he has begun designating organized groups of practicing physicians, generally sponsored by the local medical societies, as PSROs. *Id.* §1320c-1(b). Briefly, the legislation gives PSROs responsibility for applying

established norms in reviewing certain types of patient treatment proposed to them by attending physicians. *Id.* §1320c-5(a). Those norms are formulated by a national council of physicians, *id.* §1320c-5(c)(1), which recommends appropriate durations of hospitals stays, *id.* §1320c-5(d), as well as other types of limitations upon particular treatments for particular health conditions, *id.* §1320c-4(a)(2)(B), 5(b)(1). Prior to elective hospital admissions and extended or costly courses of treatment, PSROs review types of cases specified by the Secretary of HEW. *Id.* §1320c-4(a)(3), 5(b). At designated times after a patient has been properly admitted to a hospital, the PSRO must review a certification by the attending physician that there is a continuing medical need for further hospitalization. *Id.* §1320c-5(d).

The law provides for application of certain sanctions against doctors who resist compliance with a PSRO's decisions or determinations. In individual cases of non-compliance there will be no federal reimbursement for care going beyond the established norms. *Id.* §1320c-7(a). A physician who consistently refuses to comply may be suspended or permanently excluded from further participation in the affected federal health programs. *Id.* §1320c-9(b).

41. B. DECKER & P. BONNER, PSRO: ORGANIZATION FOR REGIONAL PEER REVIEW 11, 68 (1973). *See, e.g.,* S. 2970, 93d Cong., 1st Sess. (1973) (Administration bill); S. 3286, 93d Cong., 2d Sess. (1974) (Kennedy-Mills bill); S. 2513, 93d Cong., 1st Sess. (1973) (Long-Ribicoff bill).

42. Two years ago, for example, the Arizona state legislature imposed on all hospitals in that state the obligation of establishing committees of doctors to review the quality of the medicine practiced within the hospital. ARIZ. REV. STAT. ANN. §36–445 (1974).

43. *Id.* §§1320c-4(a)(1)(C), 4(a)(2), 5(b)(2).

44. *Id.* §1320c-5(d).

45. Becker v. Janinski, 15 N.Y.S. 675, 677 (C.P.N.Y. 1891). *See, e.g.,* Ricks v. Budge, 91 Utah 307, 64 P.2d 208 (1937). *Ricks,* however, is not entirely representative since the doctor refused to continue treatment at a time when the patient was virtually in the operating room in immediate need of surgical care.

46. 42 U.S.C. §1320c-16(c) (Supp. II, 1972). The statutory language refers to liability "on account of any action taken . . . in compliance with or reliance upon professionally developed norms of care and treatment applied by a [PSRO] . . . ." *Id.*

47. *Id.* §1320c-16(b).

48. *Id.* §1320c-16(c)(2). The term due care is not defined in the statute and it is likely that the common law will have to be consulted for an interpretation. As for the physician reviewer, a common law doctrine provides that a doctor giving a "second opinion" on a patient's diagnosis and treatment owes that patient a higher than normal degree of diligence in arriving at a

diagnosis and prescribing treatment when his assessment of the patient's condition conflicts with that of the original attending physician. Steeves v. United States, 294 F. Supp. 446 (D.S.C. 1968). One might be tempted to draw an analogy between such a "second opinion" and a PSRO's review determination, but difficulty lies in deciding whether there is a true patient-doctor relationship between the patient and the reviewing physician justifying a higher standard of care. The effect of imposing such a standard upon the reviewer would be greater weight given to the judgment and recommendations of the attending physician. *Cf.* 42 U.S.C. §§1395f(a)(6)-(7) (Supp. II, 1972); 20 C.F.R. §405.1035 (1974). The PSRO law is silent on the weight to be given the attending doctor's recommendations, but each PSRO has the opportunity to require such emphasis when it formulates its own review procedures. 42 U.S.C. §§1320c-4(b) to (c) (Supp. II, 1972).

49. *See* Comment, *PSRO: Malpractice and Liability and the Civil Immunity Clause,* 42 GEO. L.J. 1499 (1974).

50. LeJeune Road Hosp. v. Watson, 171 So. 2d 202 (Fla. 1965); Meiselman v. Crown Heights Hosp., 285 N.Y. 389, 34 N.E.2d 367 (1941).

51. 42 U.S.C. §1320c-16(c) (Supp. II, 1972).

52. A major frustration in this study, as in all efforts to explore what the Secretary's Commission called "the malpractice problem," has been the lack of reliable and complete data on actual claims and suits in the medical field on an overall national, or any geographic, or functional basis.

The information available is pitifully slight for any given time period and is virtually nonexistent over any length of time wherein trends could be assessed. The Ribicoff Committee Report in 1969 concluded that there was "a surprising lack of information" in the area and "few statistics." It also noted a lack of "basic literature in the field." RIBICOFF REPORT, *supra* note 2, at 1. This situation was somewhat improved by the Malpractice Commission through its very useful closed-claims file study for 1970 and a few excellent research studies sponsored by the Commission. *See* MALPRACTICE COMMISSION REPORT, *supra* note 1, at Appendix 1-836 [hereinafter cited as Appendix]. But, in general, only crude statistical methods could be used to compare HMO malpractice experience in recent years with the general medical community. *See, e.g.,* note 54 *infra.*

53. *See* note 3 *supra.*

54. This information is based on an interview with Dr. Harold Newman, Executive Director, Group Health Cooperative of Puget Sound in Seattle, Wash., June, 1973.

The only other available means of comparing HMO malpractice claims experience with the general community was in the national picture provided by the Secretary's Commission on Medical Practice. There were 12,600 claims filed in 1970, providing approximately one claim for every 16,700 persons in the United States. MALPRACTICE COMMISSION REPORT, *supra* note 1, at 5–6. The incidence of claims for the 12 HMOs in this study in 1972 was one for 11,400 persons. For a number of reasons, however, this ratio is conservatively low. Some HMOs kept records only on actual malpractice actions filed in court, thereby excluding claims on which no action was brought and which may have been settled with a money payment. Also, at least one group, Health Insurance Plan of Greater New York, keeps no records on claims or suits against its independent medical groups. It was reported by the Secretary's Commission, moreover, that approximately 40 percent of actual claims (excluding mere warnings) in 1970 resulted in any payment to claimants. APPENDIX, *supra* note 52, at 20. In contrast, these HMOs in 1972 made payments in 55 percent of all claims. Finally, based upon the national figures of the Secretary's Commission, HMOs seem to have paid out larger average awards and settlements. The median national payment in 1970 was approximately $2000. *Id.* at 21. Payments by HMOs in 1972 were, on the average for the different groups, between $5,000 and $10,000 with a median of $8,000.

The fact that the HMO figures are for the year 1972 may similarly make any comparison with the 1970 national averages invalid, since both national and HMO ratios can well be assumed to be rising annually. However, there are no available national figures for any years before or after 1970 and data from all of the 12 HMOs were not available for earlier years. Also, most HMOs are concentrated in urban areas where numbers of claims and amounts of payments are most probably higher than the national average in any recent year.

55. *See* Schneider & Stern, *Health Maintenance Organizations and the Poor: Problems and Prospects,* 70 Nw. U.L. REV. 90 (1975) (this issue).

56. RIBICOFF REPORT, *supra* note 2, at 428.

57. *See* Henderson, *Contractual Problems in the Enforcement of Agreements to Arbitrate Medical Malpractice,* 58 VA. L. REV. 947 (1972).

58. Interview with Tom Waterhouse, Attorney for Ross-Loos Medical Group of Los Angeles (Pasadena, Cal., June, 1973). *See also* MALPRACTICE COMMISSION REPORT, *supra* note 1, Appendix at 425, 424–50.

59. Series of interviews of attorneys and officials of the HMOs in this study, May-June, 1973.

60. Greenlick, *The Impact of Prepaid Group Practice on American Medical Care: A Critical Evaluation,* 399 ANNALS 100, 112 (1972).

61. *But cf.* Havighurst & Blumstein, *Coping with Quality/Cost Trade-Offs in Medical Care,* 70 Nw. U.L. REV. 6 (1975) (this issue).

62. *See* Freese v. Lemmon, 210 N.W.2d 576 (Iowa 1973); Helling v. Carey, 83 Wash. 2d 514, 519 P.2d 981 (1974); Curran, *Glaucoma and Streptoccal Phasyngitis:*

Diagnostic Practices and Malpractice Liability, 291 N. ENGL. J. MED. 508 (1974).

63. *See* text accompanying note 19 *supra.*

64. D. LOGSDON & H. BASS, PROFESSIONAL STANDARDS (1975).

65. *See* Ludlam, *Physician-Hospital Relations: The Role of Staff Privileges*, 35 LAW & CONTEMP. PROB. 879 (1970).

66. *See* R. MILLS & J. ROGERS, HEALTH MAINTENANCE ORGANIZATIONS: MEDICAL MALPRACTICE INSURANCE PROBLEMS (supplement A, final report, contract no. HSM-100-70-390 (1970)). The companies surveyed were Aetna Casualty and Surety Company, American Mutual Liability Company, Employers Mutual Insurance Company of Wausaw, Hartford Insurance Company, Medical Protective Company, North American Reinsurance Company, Reliance Insurance Company, and St. Paul Fire & Marine Insurance Company.

67. Two recent law review articles suggested that lower group ratings for medical society sponsored malpractice policies were negotiated because of cooperative loss control programs. *See* Brant, *Medical Malpractice Insurance: The Disease and How to Cure It*, 6 VAL. U.L. REV. 152, 161 (1972); Uhthoff, *Medical Malpractice—The Insurance Scene*, 43 ST. JOHN L. REV. 578, 597–98 (1969).

68. This information is based upon an interview with Norman Zolot, General Counsel for the New Haven Community Health Plan, in New Haven, Conn., May, 1973.

69. 33 Ill. 2d 326, 211 N.E.2d 253 (1965), *cert. denied*, 383 U.S. 946 (1966).

70. 18 Ariz. App. 75, 500 P.2d 335 (1972).

71. A 1968 Michigan law states:

The governing body of each hospital shall be responsible for the operation of the hospital, the selection of the medical staff, and for the quality of care rendered in the hospital.

MICH. STAT. ANN. §14.1179 (12) (1969). A 1971 Indiana law declares that the hospital board is the "supreme authority" in the institution and makes the hospital medical staff responsible to the board for its clinical work and for reviewing professional practices in the hospital. IND. ANN. STAT §16-10-1-6.5 (1973).

72. H. COHEN & L. MIIKE, DEVELOPMENTS IN HEALTH MANPOWER LICENSURE (HEW Pub. No. (HRA) 74-3101, 1973).

73. *See* 42 U.S.C. §1395mm (Supp. II, 1972).

74. S. 3327, 92d Cong., 2d Sess. (1972) (passed in Senate).

75. Expert testimony is required to establish the general average of medical care standards applicable to the case at hand. But an absence of such testimony in cases where malpractice by someone seems obvious to the court can result in application of the doctrine of res ipsa loquitur under which an outcome measurement is allowed to stand alone as enough to convict a doctor of malpractice. *See* R. MORRIS & A. MORITZ, DOCTOR AND PATIENT AND THE LAW 403-04 (5th ed. 1971).

ISSUES FOR CONSIDERATION AND SUGGESTIONS FOR FURTHER READING

To what extent should the costs of health care be assumed as a public burden? How should this be done? What types of checks should regulate the rising costs of health care?

In the past, certain medical conditions (e.g., end-stage renal disease) have received special legislative and economic consideration (e.g., through the provision of kidney transplants and dialysis at reduced or no cost). What priorities, if any, should determine public health care expenditures? Students may wish to examine these questions against the backdrop of the economic articles in this chapter and the following articles: Rettig, "Valuing Lives: The Policy Debate on Patient Care Financing for Victims of End-Stage Renal Disease," 40 *Law & Contemp. Prob.* 196 (1976); and Havighurst, Blumstein, and Bovbjerg, "Strategies in Underwriting the Costs of Catastrophic Disease," 40 *Law & Contemp. Prob.* 122 (1976).

Other approaches to the problems considered in this chapter are suggested by Enthoven, "Consumer-Choice Health Plan," 298 *New Eng. J. of Med.* 650, 709 (Mar. 23, 1979; Mar. 30, 1979), a proposal to replace the present fee-for-service system of health care delivery with a new national health insurance designed to induce voluntary changes that would foster competition. The Enthoven proposal is modeled on the Federal Employees Health Benefits Program. An interesting review is set forth in Mechanic, "Approaches to Controlling the Costs of Medical Care: Short-Range and Long-Range Alternatives," 298 *New Eng. J. of Med.* 249 (Feb. 2, 1978).

Three symposiums on health contain articles that students should find rich sources for additional study in this area: 35 *Law & Contemporary Problems* 229 (part 1), 667 (part 2) (1970); 40 *Law & Contemporary Problems* 46 (No. 4, 1976); and 6 *Univ. of Toledo L. Rev.* 577 (1975).

For a discussion of peer review through Professional Standard Review Organizations (PSROs) as a cost/quality control device, you may wish to begin with Gosfield, "Medical Necessity in Medicare and Medicaid: The Implications of Professional Standards Review Organizations," 51 *Temple Law Quarterly* 229 (1978).

CHAPTER 2

THE REGULATION OF HEALTH CARE DELIVERY: ADMINISTRATIVE ISSUES

OVERVIEW

The articles in this chapter explore several interrelated issues about the delivery of health care. Who is entitled to health care, and, in particular, who will pay for the care extended to those who cannot pay? The articles by Schwartz and Rose explore the possibilities for securing health care through the imaginative use of the Hill-Burton Act.

A related question is, Who shall provide health care? The licensing of health profession-als is a topic that could have as easily been treated from an economic perspective in the preceding chapter because of the restrictive impact of licensure provisions on entry into the medical services marketplace. But it is included here, under administrative issues, to illustrate the role that state and federal laws play in controlling practitioners by defining the nature and scope of their functions. A related issue—the effort to meet the demand for more physicians with foreign medical graduates (FMGs) and physician extenders or substitutes—is also considered.

2.1 Access for Minorities into Mainstream Hospital Care

MARILYN G. ROSE

Reprinted with permission of the Legal Services Corporation, from 13 *Clearinghouse Review* 83–86 (June 1979). Copyright © 1979 by the Legal Services Corporation. All rights reserved.

On March 19, 1979, administrative hearings under Title VI of the Civil Rights Act of 1964 (42 U.S.C. §2000d) opened against three nonprofit hospitals in New Orleans.[1] The issues to be adjudicated at that hearing offer great potential for legal services attorneys across the country to aid their clients who have problems in obtaining access to quality and unsegregated medical care.

BACKGROUND

The current hearing is the latest of the legal proceedings which were spawned by *Cook v. Ochsner,* 319 F. Supp. 603 (E.D. La. 1970). The initial complaint in *Cook* alleged that 10 New Orleans area hospitals had violated their obligations to provide uncompensated services under the Hill-Burton Act, 42 U.S.C. §§291 *et seq.,* and not to discriminate on the basis of race under Title VI. In early 1971, the Department of Health, Education, and Welfare (HEW) was named as an additional party-defendant and charged with a failure to enforce the obligations under both acts. In March 1972, the Hill-Burton causes were severed for separate trial, which resulted in a consent agreement with the hospitals in 1972 and a court order against HEW in 1973 (61 F.R.D. 354 (May 1973)), modified regulations under the Hill-Burton Act (42 C.F.R. §§53.111 and 53.113; *see also* 43 Fed. Reg. 49954-5, 49954-2, 4916102), a contempt action against six of the hospitals in 1974, and two decisions by the Fifth Circuit in 1977 (559 F.2d 270 and 559 F.2d 968).

In December 1974, the civil rights causes were the subject of a consent agreement between plaintiffs and HEW, in which HEW agreed to conduct a compliance review of 18 New Orleans area hospitals and,

... if warranted, take steps necessary either to ensure that the hospitals under review, including defendant hospitals, are in compliance with Title VI of the Civil Rights Act of 1964 or are terminated from Federal financial assistance.

The district court approved the agreement in February 1975.

During the ensuing investigation, two of the hospitals (Southern Baptist and Mercy) refused to give HEW data and challenged the Title VI jurisdiction of HEW, claiming that the only federal monies which they received were Medicare payments (42 U.S.C. §§1395 *et seq.*) and that those monies did not constitute federal financial assistance within the meaning of Title VI. That contention ripened into motions for summary judgment by those hospitals against plaintiffs, and a cross-claim and motion for summary judgment by the United States (representing defendant HEW) against the two hospitals. In September 1976, the district court denied the hospitals' motions and granted HEW's motion.

In July 1977, HEW issued letters of finding against four of the original defendant hospitals and commenced negotiations seeking to secure voluntary compliance.[2] The efforts with respect to three of the hospitals failed, and in May 1978, HEW issued notices of opportunity for hearing against them. The three hospitals thereafter attempted to enjoin the administrative proceeding, raising again the "Medicare is not federal financial assistance" claim as well as challenging the administrative action as *ultra vires,* both because HEW had allegedly not engaged in "good faith" negotiations and because HEW was advancing an invalid legal theory. In February 1979, the district court denied the motions for injunction.[3] In December 1978, the administrative law judge granted the motion of one of the original plaintiffs to intervene in the administrative proceeding but granted only *amicus* status to a community organization which had not been a plaintiff in *Cook.*

LEGAL ISSUES

There are three major theses upon which plaintiff-intervenor and HEW are proceeding. First, they claim that the defendant hospitals have a past history of racial discrimination, and Title VI requires that recipients of federal financial assistance take affirmative steps to overcome the effects of prior discrimination. Even when such past discriminatory practices have been formally abandoned, if the consequences of these practices continue to impede full availability of the services of a recipient of federal financial assistance to the beneficiaries, then the recipient must take additional steps to eliminate those "present effects." These affirmative action requirements are set forth in HEW's civil rights regulations (45 C.F.R. §§80.3(b)(6)(i) and 80.5(i)).

The regulations and theory have support in well-established precedents. For example, in *Green v. County School Board of New Kent County,* 391 U.S. 430 (1968), the Supreme Court made it clear that school authorities not only had an obligation under the fourteenth amendment to end prior discriminatory policies and practices, but they were required to take appropriate remedial steps to eliminate all vestiges of discrimination "root and branch."

Second, intervenor and HEW claim that whether or not these particular hospitals have a history of official discrimination, the statistical evidence establishes a prima facie case of racial discrimination, and the hospitals have the burden of going forward to rebut that evidence. The use of statistical evidence to establish a prima facie case of racial discrimination under Title VI was approved by the Supreme Court in *Teamsters v. United States,* 431 U.S. 324 (1977). Although acknowledging that there was sufficient evidence of specific acts of discrimination to bring "the cold numbers convincingly to life," the Court went on to state that statistical evidence has long been held sufficient to demonstrate a prima facie case. (*Id.* at 339–40). In the instant case, the particular hospitals are located in a city which is 45 percent black. Prior to the mid or late 1960's, two of the hospitals had no black in-patients and the third, at best, served only a token number. The deviation between the population of the area which the hospitals serve and the patient census is enormous. A statistical expert shall testify at the hearing that the probability of such a deviation existing by random selection is virtually zero.

Added to the statistical disparity is the fact that all the hospitals signed assurances to comply with the HEW civil rights regulations and guidelines. Since the commencement of the Title VI program, the HEW guidelines have required that where there is a significant variation between the racial composition in the patient census of a hospital and the racial composition of the service area or potential service area, the hospital has a responsibility to determine the reason for the variation and to take corrective action. While these hospitals have long been aware of the guidelines and their responsibility under them, they have not taken actions to ameliorate the disparity. Plaintiffs-intervenors and HEW will also introduce testimony of past discriminatory conduct, giving life to the "cold statistics." The total context, just as in *Teamsters,* shall clearly shift the burden to the hospitals to explain the reason for the disparity on non-discriminatory grounds.

The third legal claim is that while under the above two theories the moving parties would establish a prima facie case of *intentional* discrimination, Title VI requires only that they establish a prima facie case of *discriminatory effect.* In this regard the Title VI regulations provide:

A   recipient . . . may   not . . . utilize criteria or methods of administration which have the effect of subjecting individuals to discrimination because of their race, color, or national origin, or which have the effect of substantially impairing accomplishment of the objectives of the program as respect individuals of a particular race, color, or national origin. 45 C.F.R. §80.3(b)(2)

These hospitals provide regular inpatient services only to the patients of private physicans who have been granted staff privileges. Whatever the reason,[4] a disproportionately low number of blacks have private physicians, and most of the physicians on the staffs of these hospitals have few, if any, black patients. Plaintiff-intervenor and HEW contend that the method of administration of these hospitals thus has the effect of denying them access to federally-funded services and benefits in violation of Title VI.

This theory, and indeed this particular regulation (45 C.F.R. §80.3(b)(2)), was approved by the Supreme Court in *Lau v. Nichols*, 414 U.S. 563 (1964). Similar legal principles of discriminatory effect have been upheld in the areas of employment and housing discrimination under Titles VII and VIII.[5] The Third Circuit, in the *Rizzo* case, stated that where discriminatory effect is established, a violation of Title VIII is established unless the defendant shows:

> . . . a justification which serves a legitimate interest . . . and that there is no alternative course of action which could be adopted that would enable that interest to be served with less discriminatory impact.[6]

Intervenor and HEW contend that a similar standard should be applied under Title VI.

APPLICATION ELSEWHERE

While all three theories have potential applicability across the country, the first two theories have more limited applicability than the third theory. In particular, the first theory, dependent upon a history of overt past discrimination, might be limited to particular areas of the country. The third theory, however, does not depend upon either a history of intentional discrimination or a rebuttable presumption of inten-

tional discrimination. Congress, in providing the terms on which federal money should be spent, can proscribe the results. In *Lau v. Nichols*, 414 U.S. 563 (1974), the Supreme Court stated just that:

> The Federal Government has power to fix the terms on which its money allotments to the States shall be dispersed. Whatever may be the limits of that power they have not been reached here. Senator Humphrey, during the floor debates on the Civil Rights Act of 1974, said:
>> "Simple justice requires that public funds, to which all taxpayers of all races contribute, not be spent in any fashion which encourages, entrenches, subsidizes, or result in racial discrimination." 110 Cong. Reg. 6543 (1964).

Nor do the multiple opinions of the Supreme Court in *Regents of University of California v. Bakke*, 98 S.Ct. 2733 (1978), undermine the discriminatory effect theory. *Bakke* involved the use of explicit racial criteria to favor certain racial groups (blacks and Asians) over whites. The case under discussion does not involve the permissibility of explicit racial criteria to establish a preference. It involves an indictment of methods of administration which prevent minorities from gaining access to federally-funded services, and the administrative judgment of a federal agency, as set forth in regulations and guidelines to proscribe that result.

Each of the three major opinions in *Bakke* is entirely consistent with the proposition that an administrative agency may indict methods of administration which have the effect of discriminatorily excluding minorities from federally-funded services and benefits.[7] Further, there would appear no rationale for treating Title VI cases differently from Title VII and Title VIII cases, and the same Supreme Court has approved the "discriminatory effect" standard under the latter two titles.[8] In any event, the issue may be considered again by the Supreme Court. Recently the Court granted certiorari to a Second Circuit affirmance of the discriminatory effect standard in cases arising under the Emergency School Aid Act in an opinion asserting that *Bakke* did not eliminate the discriminatory effect standard in Title VI cases.[9]

OTHER LEGAL SUPPORT

The discriminatory effect theory also has support in the very litigation out of which the current administrative proceeding arose. In *Cook v. Ochsner*, 61 F.R.D. 354 (E.D. La. 1973), the plaintiffs and HEW filed cross motions for summary judgment on two issues: (1) whether a hospital policy requiring admission only through a private physician violated the "community services" obligation of the Hill-Burton Act, and (2) whether a hospital policy of refusing to participate in the Medicaid program violated the "community services" obligation of the Hill-Burton Act. The district court found the record on the former issue inadequate to determine summary judgment, indicating that the matter should be resolved only after an evidentiary hearing or after stipulation of relevant facts (*Id.* at 359). However, with respect to the Medicaid issue, the district court found that the refusal to participate in Medicaid effectively excluded the 100,000 beneficiaries of that program in the New Orleans metropolitan area from the Hill-Burton hospitals and constituted discrimination against them in violation of the community service requirements of that Act (*Id.* at 360).

Most recently the two issues which were separated in *Cook* have been reunited. In October, HEW proposed new regulations implementing the uncompensated and community service obligations. In the proposed regulations,[10] HEW provides, *inter alia:*

§124.603. In order to comply with its assurance that it would provide a community service, an applicant must: (a) Make the services . . . available . . . without discrimination on the ground of race, color, national origin, creed, or any other ground unrelated to an individual's need for the service or the availability of the needed service in the facility . . . An applicant will be considered to be out of compliance with this requirement if it adopts an admissions policy which has the effect of excluding persons on a ground other than those permitted under the preceding sentence.[11]

In the preamble to the proposed regulation, HEW explicitly states that this proposed regulation arises from its concern that "some medical facility admission policies (such as preadmission deposit requirements and admission only through physicians with staff privileges) have served to limit access to those facilities by persons in need of their services. . . ."[12]

In March 1979, the Massachusetts Department of Public Health (a state Hill-Burton agency) acted on a complaint filed by Medicaid beneficiaries who could not receive ophthalmology services at their local hospital because all but one ophthalmologist with staff privileges at the hospital refused to treat Medicaid patients.[13] The agency held that the hospital was in violation of its community service obligation under the Hill-Burton Act:

Where, as was the case here, access to certain services is predicated upon admission by physicians who do not treat Medicaid patients, access to these hospital services by Medicaid patients is unlawfully limited. Although the hospital may not intend to discriminate against Medicaid recipients in the provision of these services, its policies and practices will run afoul of the Community Services Regulations if they have the effect of excluding Medicaid or Medicare patients, or of limiting their access to a hospital service.[14]

The potential for making mainstream hospital care more available, and accessible, for minorities and the poor may be increased by the progeny of *Cook v. Ochsner.*[15]

Copies of relevant pleadings are available from the Clearinghouse.

NOTES

1. In the matter of Mercy Hospital, Southern Baptist Hospital, Hotel Dieu Hospital, HUD Docket Nos. EO-75-4 and EO-78-5 and HEW Docket Nos. 78-VI-7, 78-VI-8, and 78-VI-9. Title VI provides that:
No person in the United States shall, on the ground of race, color, or national origin, be excluded from participation in, be denied the benefits of, or be subjected to discrimination under any program or activity receiving Federal financial assistance.
Plaintiff-Intervenor is represented by the author, and by Jack M. Stolier and Theon Wilson, New Orleans Legal Services Corporation. Available from the Clearinghouse, No. 26,336.

2. Title VI requires that the federal funding agencies, prior to taking any enforcement action, whether fund

termination administrative hearings or enforcement actions in federal court (upon referral to the Department of Justice), must attempt first to secure voluntary compliance. *See* 42 U.S.C. §2000d-1.

3. With respect to the "Medicare" issue, the district court referred back to its earlier decision of September 1976, which was issued orally, from the bench. The court held that the three hospitals, which signed assurances of compliance with Title VI at the time they came into the Medicare program (and in order to qualify for the Medicare program), were estopped from challenging the applicability of Title VI to that program. The court did not specifically reach the issues briefed by plaintiff-intervenor and HEW on both occasions that Medicare payments constitute federal financial assistance and that they do not come within the language of Title VI excluding "contracts of insurance or guaranty."

4. In New Orleans, the historic pattern was to direct poor blacks into the charity hospital system and middle class blacks (or those covered by private health insurance) into the one "black" hospital. The advent of Medicare and Medicaid largely did not change that pattern. While some middle class blacks increasingly obtained service from a few "white" hospitals in the community, these particular hospitals continue to provide limited service to the black community. Their Medicare and Medicaid patient enrollments are disproportionately white, albeit the production of the population covered by those programs is black, *e.g.,* in 1974, Southern Baptist rendered service to 4262 Medicare patients with only 74 (1.7%) of those being black, although 33% of the population covered by Medicare in the New Orleans metropolitan area is black.

5. *See* Griggs v. Duke Power Co., 401 U.S. 424 (1971); Albermarle Paper Co. v. Moody, 422 U.S. 405 (1972); Metropolitan Housing Development Corporation v. Village of Arlington Heights, 558 F.2d 1283 (7th Cir. 1977); and Resident Advisory Board v. Rizzo, 564 F.2d 126, 147 (3rd Cir. 1978).

6. Resident Advisory Board v. Rizzo, 564 F.2d 126, 149 (3rd Cir. 1978).

7. Justice Powell would permit affirmative action to give a preference to minorities, even in the absence of an explicit finding of past intentional discrimination, "where a legislative or administrative body charged with the responsibility made determinations of past

discrimination." 98 Sup. Ct. at 2754. Justices Brennan, White, Marshall, and Blackmun would permit racial preferences to minorities where broad societal discrimination had resulted in the exclusion of minorities from the benefits of federally-funded programs at a particular institution. 98 Sup. Ct. 2776, 2789. Justices Stevens, Burger, Stewart, and Rehnquist would give Title VI a broader reading than simply that of "a constitutional appendage." 98 Sup. Ct. at 2814.

8. In Washington v. Davis, 426 U.S. 229 (1976), the Supreme Court, while holding that discriminatory effect does not per se violate the equal protection clause of the fourteenth amendment, said that under Title VII of the Civil Rights Act of 1964, 42 U.S.C. §2000e, when hiring and promotion practices disqualify substantially disproportionate numbers of blacks, discriminatory purpose need not be proved. Similarly, in Village of Arlington Heights v. Metropolitan Housing Development, 427 U.S. 252 (1977), the Supreme Court, while invalidating the finding of an equal protection violation from the racially disparate impact of zoning requirements, remanded the case for consideration of whether Title VIII, 42 U.S.C. §3601 et seq., was violated. On remand, the Seventh Circuit found that the decision left the discriminatory effect standard intact under Title VII (*see* 558 F.2d 1283), a conclusion with which the Third Circuit agreed (Resident Advisory Board v. Rizzo, 564 F.2d 126, 147 (1978)).

9. *See,* New York Board of Education v. Califano, 584 F.2d 576, (1978), *cert. granted,* 47 U.S.L.W. 3543 (1979).

10. 43 Fed. Reg. 49954 *et seq.*

11. *Id.* at 49968.

12. *Id.* at 49962.

13. Perry v. Cape Cod Hospital (Mass. Dep't of Public Health, March 14, 1979). Available from the Clearinghouse, No. 22,735C.

14. *Id.* at p. 5.

15. To assist legal services workers in identifying and remedying civil rights violations by providers, Jack Mark Stolier of the New Orleans Legal Assistance Corporation has prepared *A Health Advocate's Guide to Title VI of the 1964 Civil Rights Act and Section 504 of the Vocational Rehabilitation Act of 1973* (January 1979). It is available from the Clearinghouse, No. 26,587.

2.2 Opening the Doors of the Non-Profit Hospital to the Poor

JEFFREY SCHWARTZ and MARILYN ROSE

Reprinted with permission of the Legal Services Corporation, from 7 *Clearinghouse Review* 655–658 (March 1974). Copyright © 1974 by the Legal Services Corporation. All rights reserved.

One of the focal points of the National Health Law Program's work during its first years was the problem of access of the poor to the nation's mainstream hospital system, that is, the non-profit, voluntary or charitable hospitals which comprise over 60 percent of the general, acute-service hospital beds in the country. Although historically open to the poor through the rendering of charitable service (many of these hospitals were founded by religious and beneficial organizations), the increasing costs of medical care have resulted in the elimination of certain services, including out-patient clinics for the poor and free in-patient service. At the same time the public hospitals, which are increasingly the primary or only health facilities available to the poor, have become more overcrowded, under-staffed, under-financed and under-equipped, intensifying the need to keep the non-profit hospital open to some portion of the poor.

These non-profit hospitals, privately-owned and operated by self-perpetuating boards, have received large federal subsidies in the form of direct grants under the Hill-Burton Act[1] and indirect grants in the form of charitable status under the Internal Revenue Code.[2] The use of these federal subsidies has provided the legal justification by which the rights of the poor to receive treatment at non-profit hospitals have been pursued by Legal Services attorneys and the National Health Law Program.[3]

I. TAX-EXEMPT HOSPITALS MUST SERVE THE POOR

In December 1973 the District Court for the District of Columbia issued a Memorandum Decision on cross-motions for summary judgment in the case of *Eastern Kentucky Welfare Rights Organization v. Shultz*.[4] The court held that non-profit hospitals must not deny service to persons unable to pay if they are to retain tax exempt status under Section 501(c)(3) of the Internal Revenue Code and their donors are to be able to deduct contributions under Section 170(c). This decision came in the course of holding invalid a 1969 ruling of the Internal Revenue Service which eliminated the previous requirement (Rev. Ruling 56-185) that tax-exempt hospitals must give free and below-cost services to the poor. The court ordered the federal defendants to refrain from following that policy and from granting Section 501(c)(3) and 170(a)-(c) status to non-profit hospitals until and unless such hospitals:

a. Satisfy the requirements found in Revenue Ruling 56-185, in particular, that they:
(1) be operated, to the extent of their financial ability, for those not able to pay for services and not exclusively for those who are able and expected to

pay; (2) furnish the above 'charitable' services on a reduced rate and below cost or no charge basis; (3) not refuse patients in need of hospital care who cannot pay.

b. Conspicuously post, in appropriate accessible public areas, notice, to be prepared by the defendants and subject to Court approval, which shall include:

(1) That the hospital has applied for or has been granted tax exempt status under 501(c)(3) of the Code; (2) An intelligible recitation of the previously mentioned provisions of Revenue Ruling 56–185.[5]

This decision presents a tremendous opportunity for poor people across the country to establish their rights against individual hospitals which claim tax-exempt status. According to the IRS, there are over 11,000 hospitals and nursing homes exempt under these provisions of the Code. In view of the fact that for the past four years the Internal Revenue Service has not required free service to the poor, it is to be assumed that many of these facilities currently are not providing such care. It should be noted also that the court did not negate that aspect of IRS policy that Section 501(c)(3) hospitals must provide a community benefit by participating in Medicaid and other public programs and by operating emergency service.

The *EKWRO* decision may also be useful as a defense to collection actions by hospitals against the poor, in the same manner as the Hill-Burton obligations are used.[6]

Of broader utility is the court's holding that poor people's organizations and the individual poor denied service at non-profit hospitals have standing to proceed, and that the administrative action taken by the Internal Revenue Service is subject to court review. The decision on both of these points should be useful in other poverty law cases. One broad issue the court refrained from reaching involved whether the action of IRS violated the rule-making requirements of the Administrative Procedure Act. Consequently, the court did not determine whether plaintiffs had standing as persons denied their right to comment upon proposed regulations under Section 553 of the Administrative Procedure Act.

One other item should be noted. Although hospitals claim that they are financially unable to provide "free service," it should be noted that studies on the subject indicate that the financial position and net income of hospitals increased substantially in the period from 1961 to 1971.

II. HILL-BURTON HOSPITALS MUST TREAT MEDICAID BENEFICIARIES

In *Cook v. Ochsner*,[8] the federal district court ruled that Hill-Burton hospitals violated their obligations to provide a "community service" by not participating in the Medicaid program, thus denying access to what amounted to eleven percent of the metropolitan New Orleans population, which had no other means to pay for such service, and that HEW violated its obligations by not enforcing this requirement. In January 1974, in response to this finding (and the order that ran with it) HEW issued proposed regulations that Hill-Burton facilities, in order to comply with their community service obligation must:

Make administrative arrangements, if eligible to do so, for reimbursement for services with those principal third-party payors (private and governmental) which offer reimbursement for services that is not less than the reasonable cost of such services, and . . . Take such additional steps as may be necessary to ensure that the services which it offers are not categorically denied to all persons having a specific source of payment which provides reimbursement at not less than the reasonable cost of such services.[9]

In the preface to the proposed regulation HEW avoids mentioning the court order in *Cook*, but relates the development of this proposed regulation to suggestions received in connection with the development of the "free service" regulation that Hill-Burton hospitals be required to participate in the Medicaid program.[10]

Although nationwide information is not available as to the number of hospitals which exclude Medicaid beneficiaries, the experience in New Orleans would indicate that it is substantial. In New Orleans, seven of the nine Hill-Burton hospitals discriminated against Medicaid beneficiaries, with four hospitals not even qualifying as Medicaid providers. Consequently, this regulation, when final, may provide a good opportunity to ensure that each of the Hill-Burton hospitals (approximately 3800) do in fact extend their services to all Medicaid and Medicare patients on an equal basis with all other patients.

One problem should be noted. The proposed regulation is limited to programs paying "reasonable cost." One of the October 1972 amendments to the Social Security Act changed the basis for reimbursement to "reasonable cost or customary charges," whichever is lower. Obviously the objective was to prevent hospitals from charging public programs more than the private insurance programs. If this is not dealt with in the final regulation, it may create a problem for enforcement against those hospitals where that is the situation. We do not believe that that is the intention of the court order in *Cook,* nor a logical result of congressional intent as expressed in the 1972 Social Security Act Amendments.

III. HILL-BURTON HOSPITALS MAY NOT SEND BILLS FOR SERVICES TO THE POOR

In the proposed "free service" regulation of April 1972, HEW provided that the only services which would qualify toward a hospital meeting its obligations were those for which a prior written determination would be made (with exceptions for emergency situations and similar circumstances). The interim and final regulations were amended to permit hospitals to count services for which no collection efforts other than the rendering of bills was pursued. The Health Law Project strongly opposed that change, because it would allow a hospital to defer a decision beyond the admission process, keeping the poor, who could not pay deposits, out of the hospital, and it would also allow the transfer of old bad debts to the free service to the poor program. The District Court for the Southern District of New York recently agreed with that position in *Corum v. Beth Israel Hospital.*[11] The court said:

It is fully understandable that hospitals wish to count towards their Hill-Burton requirement all services for which collection proves difficult. The statute, however, does not contemplate this convenient result. Rather, the only services for which the statutory assurance is received are those

provided to persons who are *'unable,'* not merely unwilling to pay. Bad debts incurred by the hospitals from persons not covered by the statute are an expense of operating which they must bear themselves.[12]

Plaintiffs in *Corum* also challenged the legality of other provisions of the regulation: the limitation of its applicability to twenty years after the facility which received the grant opened; and the maximum limitation of free service to the lesser of three percent of cost of operations or ten percent of the grant. In addition, plaintiffs challenged the statutory delegation of regulation-making power to the Federal Hospital Council by virtue of its veto power over regulations proposed by the Secretary. The court found that these provisions were not illegal. An appeal is being considered concerning those portions of the decision in which the court held against plaintiffs. The Health Law Project believes that those provisions are appropriately subject to challenge.

In dealing with problems raised by the regulation provision limiting a Hill-Burton hospital's obligation to a twenty-year time period, it should be noted that in *Corum* the facility constructed with the grant had just opened, and the court contemplated that the hospital would give a significant amount of free service over the twenty-year period. However, a hospital which never gave any free services during the many years of its operations as a Hill-Burton facility would stand in a different posture. To the extent that such a hospital is defending its current lack of free service by its now expired obligation, the twenty-year limitation is of questionable validity and should be attacked.[13] (It should be noted that at least one state (Colorado) has chosen to delete the twenty-year restrictions from its State Plan, and HEW has taken the position that this is acceptable.)

In a subsequent decision, rendered January 29, 1974,[14] the *Corum* court reiterated its previous decision that a Hill-Burton grantee could not unilaterally decide what type of services would satisfy the "reasonable volume" requirement but then decided that the doctrine of "primary jurisdiction" dictates that the scheme set forth in the "free service" regulation must first be followed. In the latter respect the court noted that the regulation requires the Hill-Burton grantee to file an annual statement, which provides plaintiffs with the opportunity to participate. The complaint was dismissed, with the proviso that the hospital file its annual statement immediately and with the court stating that if such is not done, plaintiffs shall have an opportunity to bring an injunctive action enforcing this obligation. In the course of its decision the court reiterated that the state agency has an obligation to decide the *kind* as well as the *amount* of services, taking cognizance of the provision in the regulation that sets forth criteria, including the *nature* of services provided by the applicant, the *need* of the population, and the *extent and nature* of joint or cooperative programs with other facilities.[15]

Note that this decision on primary jurisdiction is distinguishable in a number of circumstances: first, where states have refused to *adopt* free service plans (see below); second, where the state has adopted a plan and set a level, but the hospital has refused to comply and an individual complaint is filed. In the latter case the individual cannot trigger a hearing, and it would appear that the Supreme Court decision in *Rosado v. Wyman*,[16] finding no primary jurisdiction problem, is applicable.

IV. COST-OF-LIVING COUNCIL STATES THAT FREE SERVICE MUST BE TRULY FREE

Of a similar mind with plaintiffs and Judge Lasker in the *Corum* case, the Cost-of-Living Council defines "free care" as "health care services and property furnished to patients who are not billed and for whose care third party payors are not billed." This definition appears in the Federal Register, Vol. 39, No. 16 (Jan. 23, 1974) in the Final Phase IV Regulations for the health care industry

V. CONFORMITY ACTION

Although the "free service" regulation of the Hill-Burton Act has been in effect since November 1972, reports from Legal Services attorneys across the country indicate that most states have not amended their State Plans to comport with the requirements of that regulation, and that other states, while adopting a "free service" plan, have included clearly illegal provisions and are not enforcing the provisions

which they have adopted. Along the lines of conformity suits brought in the welfare area, action against the state agencies would appear to be in order. Ironically, the states themselves have sued HEW for the impoundment of Hill-Burton funds,[17] but there is some question whether they would be able to spend those funds if they do not have legally acceptable State Plans.

VI. A WASTE OF POVERTY FUNDS

In 1970, Congress amended the Hill-Burton Act to provide a greater emphasis on outpatient services, permitting, for the first time, non-hospital-connected ambulatory operations (such as Neighborhood Health Centers) to obtain Hill-Burton funds. At the same time, Congress established a priority for urban and rural poverty areas to obtain these funds. However, at HEW and the majority of state agencies, it has been "business as usual." In mid-1971, HEW sent a memorandum to the state agencies advising them to ignore the poverty priority because the Census Bureau had not released its economic data. Several months of pressure finally resulted in a repeal of that memorandum and an admission that it was erroneously premised, but did not result in a repeal of the award of a vast portion of fiscal year 1971 and 1972 funds without regard to the poverty priority. A lawsuit[18] has been filed by a number of consumer organizations seeking the restoration of the money illegally spent; in addition, impoundment counts are included for fiscal year 1973 and 1974 funds. At an average of $70 million per year, this amounts to $280 million for the four years, only a small portion of which has gone to ambulatory facilities serving the poor in those states which did obey the law despite the HEW directive.

This article has covered a number of areas in which the courts have held that poor people have rights of access into otherwise "private" hospitals. These court decisions will only be meaningful if they are enforced at the local level. In the Hill-Burton area, local action includes pressing state agencies to enforce the commitments, with judicial enforcement following the failure of the state agencies to take action. It also includes local community action—all Hill-Burton hospitals have had to inform the states agencies as to which of the presumptive compliance guidelines they have chosen. Evidence indicates that in many places they have chosen the "certification that they would not turn anyone away" on the belief (we hope mistaken) that they would never be required to live up to that commitment. In the tax area, local action includes enforcing the "posting" requirement of the *EKWRO* order, and local monitoring by the IRS of hospital compliance with rendering free care. The potential is enormous, but only if local action is forthcoming.[19]

NOTES

1. 42 U.S.C. §291.

2. 26 U.S.C. §§501(c)(3) and 170(a)-(c).

3. With respect to Hill-Burton as a legal tool, *see* Rose. *Hospital Admission of the Poor and the Hill-Burton Act,* 3 CLEARINGHOUSE REV. 185 (December 1969); Rose, *The Duty of Publicly-Funded Hospitals to Provide Service to the Medically Indigent,* 3 CLEARINGHOUSE REV. 254 (February 1970); Rose, *The Hill-Burton Act—The Interim Regulation and Service to the Poor: A Study in Public Interest Litigation,* 6 CLEARINGHOUSE REV. 310 (October 1972); Comment, *Provision of Free Medical Services by Hill-Burton Hospitals,* 8 HARV. CIV. RIGHTS-CIV. LIB. L. REV. 351 (March 1973); Rose, *Recent Gains for the Poor in Obtaining Access into Hill-Burton Hospitals,* 7 CLEARINGHOUSE REV. 145 (July 1973).

With respect to the "charitable" tax status of hospitals, *see* Rose, *The Implications of the Charitable Deduction and Exemption Provisions of the Internal Revenue Code upon the Service Required of a Voluntary Hospital to Treat the Poor,* 4 CLEARINGHOUSE REV. 183 (August-September 1970); Rose, *The Internal Revenue Service's "Contribution" to the Health Problems of the Poor,* 21 CATH. U.L. REV. 35 (Fall 1971); Schwartz, *Expanding the Quantity of Medical Services Available to the Poor—Suing the "Private" Hospitals under the Internal Revenue Code,* 7 CLEARINGHOUSE REV. 587 (February 1974).

4. No. 1378–71 (D. D.C., Dec. 20, 1973) (slip opinion). Available from the Clearinghouse, Clearinghouse No. 6118C (28pp.).

5. *Id.* (D. D.C., Jan. 28, 1974) (order & judgment). Available from the Clearinghouse, Clearinghouse No. 6118E (3pp.).

6. *See* Burlington County Memorial Hospital v. Smith, No. 68480 (N.J. Dist. Ct., Burlington County, Sept. 21, 1973) (stipulated dismissal), for an example of a Hill-Burton defense which may be adapted for the 501(c)(3) defense. Available from the Clearinghouse, Clearinghouse No. 12,059B Answer and Counterclaim

(5pp.); 12,059E Amended Answer (2pp.); 12,059F Defendant's First Set of Interrogatories (37pp.).

7. *See* Davis, *Net Income of Hospitals,* 1961–1969 (Staff Paper No. 6), ORS, SSA, 1971; Pettengill, *The Financial Position of Private Community Hospitals,* 1961–1971, Social Security Bulletin, Nov. 1973, Vol. 36, No. 11.

8. No. 70–1969 (E.D. La., May 29, 1973). Available from the Clearinghouse, Clearinghouse No. 3973Q Opinion—Memo of Reasons (12pp.).

9. 39 Fed. Reg. 1446, 1447 (February 9, 1974).

10. A Draft Analysis of the proposed regulation, prepared by the authors and Joseph Onek from the Center on Social Welfare Policy and Law, is available from the Clearinghouse, Clearinghouse No. 12,058 (6pp.).

11. No. 72 Civ. 2654 MEL (S.D.N.Y., Jan. 17, 1974) (slip opinion). Available from the Clearinghouse, Clearinghouse No. 8363U Memo and Opinion (21pp.).

12. *Id.* at 17.

13. The *Corum* court implied that if the circumstances were different, it might decide differently. It stated: "We do not possess sufficient information to know with certainty that under all circumstances application of the presumptive compliance guideline would yield results in accordance with the Act. However, we can say that its application to Beth Israel Medical Center, the facility of concern to us in this case, is reasonable, a conclusion which renders further analysis unnecessary. Because Beth Israel Medical Center is large and its Hill-Burton grant comparatively small, the lesser of three percent of operating costs or ten percent of the grant will always be the latter. Accordingly, since the obligation will run for twenty years from completion of the funded construction (42 CFR §53.111(a)(1)), Beth Israel Medical Center can be required under the regulation to provide services equal to twice the amount of the grant. Such a requirement appears to satisfy amply the reasonable volume assurance contemplated by the statute, and the presumptive compliance guideline, as applied in this case, is valid and consistent with the Act," (Slip Op. at 13).

And with respect to the twenty year provision, the court said: "We do reiterate, however, that, in the particular circumstances of this case, a combination of the presumptive compliance guideline (in this instance ten percent of the grant annually) with the twenty-year term produces a result which is reasonable given the size of the grant," (Slip Op. at 15).

14. No. 72 Civ. 2654 MEL (S.D. N.Y., Jan. 29, 1974). Clearinghouse No. 8363V Opinion (13pp.).

15. 42 C.F.R. 53.111(h)(2).

16. 397 U.S. 397 (1971).

17. Florida v. Weinberger, No. 2151–73 (D. D.C. filed 1973).

18. National Association of Neighborhood Health Centers v. Weinberger, No. 74–52 (D. D.C., filed

January 1974). Available from the Clearinghouse, Clearinghouse No. 12,060A Complaint (17pp.).

19. For specific litigation approaches under tax exempt theories, *see* Schwartz, *Expanding the Quantity of Medical Services Available to the Poor—Suing the "Private" Hospitals Under the Internal Revenue Code,* 7 CLEARINGHOUSE REV. 587 (February 1974).

2.3 Professional Licensure, Organizational Behavior, and the Public Interest

HARRIS S. COHEN

The past few years have witnessed a growing sensitivity to the problems associated with state licensure of health practitioners. Numerous articles have been written critical of one or another facet in licensure (Hershey, 1971; Forgotson, Roemer, and Newman, 1967; Carlson, 1970; Akers, 1968; Grimm, 1972; Cohen, 1973; Sadler and Sadler, 1971). States, professional associations, and health organizations are seriously addressing the issues of licensing and credentialing. In 1971, the Department of Health, Education, and Welfare submitted to the Congress a comprehensive report on the subject (U.S. Department of Health, Education, and Welfare, 1971). However, despite the broad interest in these issues, they are rarely examined in a context in which the major legislative struggles of "to license or not to license"—to borrow an expression of William Curran's (1970)—as well as the specific jurisdictional boundaries that are defined (or left undefined) in the practice acts might be more meaningfully analyzed. This paper will attempt to develop a conceptual framework of licensure as a political process critical to the organizational autonomy and self-regulation of the health professions.

THE PROFESSIONS AND THE LICENSING PROCESS

A view that is gaining wide acceptance in the sociology of professions is that professional status results from an interactive process based upon the profession's claims to specialized competence. As Bucher and Stelling (1969: 4) note, the professional "claims that he, uniquely, possesses the knowledge and skills to define problems, set the means for solving them, and judge the success of particular courses of action within his area of competence. To the extent that others accept these claims, the professional is accorded the license and mandate that Hughes has written of as being central to being professional." Freidson (1970: 137), too, describes the autonomy and special privilege accorded professions as predicated upon three claims: "First, the claim is that there is such an unusual degree of skill and knowledge involved in professional work that nonprofessionals are not equipped to evaluate or regulate it. Second, it is claimed that professionals are responsible—that they may be trusted to work conscientiously without supervision. Third, the claim is that the profession, itself, may be trusted to undertake the proper regulatory action on those rare occasions when an individual does not perform his work competently or ethically."

The profession's autonomy is critically linked to the credentialing system, wherein the basic prerequisites and standards of competence are established for professional practice. This system includes—but is by no means limited to: (1) *licensing* by the state, (2) *certification* by the professional association, and (3) the *accreditation* of educational programs. The professions traditionally have sought exclusive control of each component in the credentialing system; and they have succeeded in many instances in forging the three processes of licensure, certification, and accreditation—and other processes as well—into "one comprehensive health-manpower credentialing system" Grimm, 1972: I1). Thus graduating from a program approved by the profession's accrediting arm is often a prerequisite for taking the certification or licensure examinations.

Autonomy in the credentialing system is tantamount to self-regulation, as reflected in most of the health practice acts in this country which delegate authority to the licensed profession to regulate itself. To quote Freidson (1970: 44), "the state uses the profession as its source of guidance, exercising its power in such a way as to support the profession's standards and create a sociopolitical environment in which the profession is free from serious competition from rival practitioners and firmly in control of auxiliary workers. Within that state-protected environment, the profession has sufficient power of its own to control virtually all facets of its work without serious interference from any lay group."

Professional Autonomy

In analyzing professional autonomy, it is important to emphasize that the individual health professions possess *varying* degrees of autonomy even when their members are credentialed by the licensure process. The literature on professions and professional behavior tends to focus upon the specific, and in some ways unique, role played by organized medicine—as exemplified by the American Medical Association and state medical societies—without calling attention to dramatic differences in the degree of autonomy possessed by other professions. In the final analysis, the measure of a profession's control and self-regulation in the licensure process will depend on its relative political strength vis-à-vis other professional and interested groups in the state. Thus, the literature on professions tends to describe "ideal types," modeled on the status and authority already accorded by the state to *certain* health professions to regulate their own professional practice. Other health professions will tend to pattern

their credentialing procedures upon the older and more established professions.

The disparate statutory composition of licensing boards in the health field illustrates this variability. Practice acts in most health disciplines require either that all or a majority of board members be licensed practitioners in the respective licensed category. Other categories—including dental hygienists, nurse midwives, and, in some states, practical nurses—are regulated by boards that do not include a single member of the particular licensed category, but rather are dominated by members of another related profession (Pennell and Stewart, 1968). Thus, while the character of the board is in essence the same in both instances with the majority of membership "having direct professional and economic interests in the areas regulated by the boards" Grimm, 1972: I18), the relative autonomy of the *licensed* profession is rather varied.

Another aspect of professional autonomy in the licensing process relates to the basic motivation behind the establishment of state licensure. In 1972, legislative bills were introduced in 30 states to consider the merits of licensing one or more of 14 categories of health personnel that were not previously licensed.[1] Some of this legislative activity may have been initiated by essentially external sources, such as in the case of ambulance attendants and emergency medical technicians, with the primary motivation being the protection of the public safety. These bills generally vest the licensing authority in departments of health or other state agencies, and only rarely provide for the establishment of a specialized board of examiners. This pattern, however, is relatively uncommon in the licensure of health personnel. More often than not, the professional associations themselves are the key actors in generating licensing legislation. There are even instances in which state associations were founded for the express purpose of promoting such legislation, although (Akers, 1968: 465) "sometimes in a defensive move to prevent other, already established, professions from regulating them."[2] As Moore (1970: 125) has pointed out, professions have sought governmental licensure (1) as a means of public recognition, (2) as protection from competition by the relatively untrained, and (3) "to establish a preemptive jurisdiction over services that may in fact be in considerable and justified jurisdictional dispute.''

As noted above (U.S. Department of Health, Education, and Welfare, 1971: 28), licensure also fulfills the ''fundamental role of establishing minimum standards to protect the health and safety of the public.'' However, there has yet to be developed an objective measure of the range of health services that pose substantial threat to the public safety to warrant governmental licensure. Certainly an argument could be made for licensing all health practitioners without exception, insofar as the health of the public is at stake. But this would mean the possible licensing of scores of different occupational categories which, of course, would be untenable on numerous grounds. The issue of public safety, remaining as it is a very imprecise and ambiguous concept, is often secondary to other considerations, such as profession's desire for autonomy and self-regulation. Thus, while numerous practice acts are formally justified in terms of protecting the public safety, the actual factors accounting for the promotion of such legislation may have had more to do with the above sociopolitical considerations than with the profession's concern for protecting the public from the charlatan or undertrained practitioner.[3]

Another facet of professional autonomy in the credentialing process is evident in the close collaboration between the professional association and the governmental agency charged with administering the practice act, particularly when the agency is a specialized board of examiners (Akers, 1968: 470–472). As with the initiation and promotion of the practice acts, the professions themselves generally were the driving force behind legislation to establish specialized boards. David Truman (1951: 418) has noted that when groups have sought regulation, such as in the licensing of occupations, the independent examining board or commission has typically been regarded as the most appropriate form for their purposes, because it assures privileged access for the initiating group. The tendency of regulatory agencies to become the ally or public sponsor of the regulated interest has been noted even when the demand for government regulation originated from outside the profession. As Truman (1951: 418) remarks, ''Experience indicates . . . that the regulated groups will have more cohesion than those demanding regulation, that they can therefore keep close track of the

work of the commission, and that consequently little will be done by a commission beyond what is acceptable to the regulated groups.''[4]

Professional Associations

The associations' access to the examining boards is facilitated in those states and professions where board members are appointed by the governor from a list of nominations submitted by the professional associations, or, as in medicine, where the laws of 23 states provide that the medical society shall have a *direct* voice in the appointment of board members (Derbyshire, 1972: 161). Commenting on the latter method of board appointment, Derbyshire points out that ''politics is theoretically removed from the board in that the members of the medical society are in a better position to judge the qualifications of the doctors than is the governor.'' *Medical politics,* however, is hardly eliminated in the process. Again quoting Derbyshire (1972: 161), ''the medical societies are by no means always likely to recommend the most highly qualified people for appointment. All too frequently, they ignore professional and educational attributes, endorsing some faithful political stalwart who has worked his way up in the councils of the medical society.''

The organization's ability to nominate or appoint members to the examining boards—who, in most cases, will constitute the majority discipline on the board—is clearly another means of perpetuating the profession's autonomy and self-regulation. Conversely, in cases where this is lacking and the profession is either not represented on the board at all or comprises a minority of the board, the regulated profession will tend to be apprehensive of a process in which decisions related to quality are determined by groups external to the profession. In a recent article, examining the pros and cons of licensing in the field of occupational therapy, one author (Crampton, 1971: 207) cited the composition of the examining boards ''which, by law, may turn out not to be comprised in whole or in part of the professionals for whom the law was enacted,'' as a major problem facing the profession.

The association's interaction and influence with the examining board does not cease at the point of selecting board members; in conjunction with the boards, the associations initiate moves for new legislation, decide what provisions should be added, deleted, or changed to correct inadequacies in existing laws, and work for the passage or defeat of bills that relate to the profession's jurisdictional boundaries and credentialing mechanisms (Akers, 1968: 467; Gilb, 1966: 151–153). Similarly, the associations participate in the formulation of the administrative rules and regulations that govern the conduct and practice both of the boards and of individual practitioners licensed in the state. In fact, some of the major political struggles in the area of manpower licensure continue well after the debate and controversy have been resolved in the legislative branch only to be resumed with equal or greater vigor in the administrative branch in determining the meaning and effect of the enacted legislation.

RECENT PROPOSALS FOR CHANGE

Several recent proposals have been made that would introduce countervailing interests in the governance of licensing boards. This is not to imply that the professions typically function in such a way that the interest of the general public is ignored. Certainly, as indicated by Kaplin (1972: J33), when the profession applies "its special expertise in order to protect the public from professional incompetence, its decision may benefit rather than harm society."

However, there has been deep concern for some time with the effects of specific group biases in limiting the social responsiveness and accountability of professional associations. As Robert MacIver (1966: 53) wrote, in a paper first published in 1922: "The possibility that there may still be an inclusive professional interest—generally but not always an economic one—that at significant points is not harmonized with the community interest is nowhere adequately recognized. The problem of professional ethics, viewed as the task of coordinating responsibilities, of finding, as it were, a common center for the various circles of interest, wider and narrower, is full of difficulty and far from being completely solved. The magnitude and the social significance of this task appear if we analyze on the one hand the character of the professional interest and on the other the relation of that interest to the general welfare."[5] This concern is reflected in some of the current literature which describes professional credentialing as a sociopolitical process dealing not only "with

narrow, clear-cut questions of professional competency but also with issues of broad social concern." Consequently, as Grimm (1972: I19; see also U.S. Department of Health, Education, and Welfare, 1971: chapter 1) points out, "the infusion of ideas from the community would help to combat the natural insularity of the boards."

The Public and Licensure

One approach to credentialing that is receiving considerable attention is to expand the composition of licensing boards to include public members with interests outside the respective fields being licensed. A leading proponent of this approach, William Selden (1970: 125; see also Grimm, 1972: I18–I20), suggests that the addition of nonmembers of the professions on licensing boards "would provide greater and more consistent assurance that the public welfare is the overriding criterion on which its decisions are made." The Department of Health, Education, and Welfare (1971: 76), in its recent report on licensure, went even further to recommend that several interests be added to the boards which might be representative of: consumers; other health professions; various modalities of health care delivery, such as group practice and public institutions; educators; and others in policy-making positions in health care.

As a direct response to these proposals, numerous bills have been introduced within the past year to amend certain practice acts for the purpose of adding public members to the boards. This certainly has important potential in the direction of infusing greater public accountability in the licensure process. However, the effect of such changes in board composition will ultimately depend on a number of factors, including the status and autonomy of the public members; the extent to which public members are permitted to challenge decisions made by professional members of the boards; the extent to which they accept the responsibility of challenging such decisions; and the availability of an organized constituency or power base from which to exert leverage on other board members when it is felt that they are not acting in the public interest. In light of these considerations, a recent Labor Department report (Shimberg et al., 1972: 379–381) recommended the inclusion on licensing boards of a technically competent representative of a state government agency instead of a nonprofessional public member.

Another critical factor that should be considered with regard to lay representation is the *number* of positions to be designated for public members. Some proponents of public representation on licensing boards are urging (Derbyshire, 1972: 161) that a single position be granted to a public member. Indeed, a good number of the legislative bills recently introduced for the purpose of restructuring board composition would expand the present boards by adding *one* or *two* public members to the total board membership. The net effects of such token structural change would probably not be very far-reaching, especially in boards that traditionally have been dominated by the licensed profession. Other commentators (Selden, 1970: 124) are quite emphatic in urging that a *substantial* number of public members be placed on the boards. It would appear that unless board composition were to be *dramatically* altered, the considerable influence of professional associations on the governance and decision making of licensing boards would continue unchecked by other interests. What is suggested, therefore, is a means of introducing greater pluralism in the credentialing system.

Reorganization of Licensing Boards

A related proposal aimed at broadening the perspective of licensing boards and enhancing their potential accountability to the public would centralize the licensing function within a single departmental unit, such as a state health or education department. In the words of a recent monograph (U.S. Department of Labor, 1969: 3), "With administration centralized, occupational groups can continue to be major forces in establishing and enforcing regulatory policies, but through a state agency which can reconcile the interest of the general public with those of the private associations." (See also Shimberg et al., 1972: 372–373.) In this connection, William Selden proposes a single state licensure board for all of the health professions that would be organized with subcommittees for each of the professions. The subcommittees, with majority membership from the licensed profession and including members from related professions and the general public, "would be charged with responsibility for developing policies regarding

licensure for their respective professions, subject to the approval of the state board" (Selden, 1970: 126; see also Carlson, 1970: 871–872). As we pointed out elsewhere, however, this form of reorganization might prove ineffective in regulating the professions or even in mandating coordination or joint planning. State licensing boards tend to have considerably stronger links to their respective professional associations than to other public agencies—even when these boards are located within state departments of health or education (U.S. Department of Health, Education, and Welfare, 1971: 30).[6]

An alternative model of board restructuring would establish a single licensing board with but *one* representative of each licensed profession. Thus, instead of perpetuating the profession's autonomy and influence by delegating major policy responsibility to subcommittees—which for all practical purposes would probably function as boards—this approach would alter very dramatically the pattern of professional self-regulation that has developed in the health field. We are not suggesting that this approach is politically feasible; it does, however, provide an alternative that at least merits public consideration in weighing the pros and cons of the state-protected environment that presently characterizes licensure in the health professions.

Institutional Licensure

A third proposal, that has been labeled "institutional licensure," and is currently receiving much attention, would introduce a clearly interdisciplinary character to licensing. The implications of a system that delegated the responsibility for competence and quality of practitioners to institutions have been critically examined from several perspectives, including (1) the opportunity for greater legal and administrative flexibility in allocating responsibilities within institutions, and (2) the effects that such a system might have on the present status of the health professions. These issues are largely unresolved at this time and are certainly well-deserving of the discussion that has been generated by both the Department of Health, Education, and Welfare recommendation calling for the further study and demonstration of institutional licensure (U.S. Department of Health, Education, and Welfare, 1971: 77), and the treatment of this concept in the literature (Hershey, 1969a:

71–74; Hershey, 1969b: 951–956; Carlson, 1970: 872–878; Roemer, 1971: 50–51; Tancredi and Woods, 1972: 103).

A point that is sometimes underemphasized is that institutional licensure conceivably could provide the opportunity and impetus for greater interprofessional coordination. Ideally, the basic credentialing policies in such a system would emanate not from any one discipline, but rather from a representative committee or commission that would reflect the views of several disciplines—including medicine, nursing, hospital administration, allied health, labor unions, and other interests in personnel credentialing. Such an approach might lessen the autonomy of certain or all of the professional associations (depending on how broadly one conceives of institutional licensure)[7] in regulating the professions. But it might also increase the scope of professional policy making, insofar as individual professions would be afforded the opportunity of contributing meaningful inputs in defining the scope of other related professions—an end product that could be extremely valuable to the public, but that is probably unattainable under the present system of licensure. Thus, the "team approach" to licensure may be viewed not only as a means of providing for flexibility within the health care institution, but also as a means of introducing countervailing interests to the existing system wherein professional associations control their respective credentialing systems (Roemer, 1971: 51).

Joint Regulation

Legislation recently enacted in a few states is consistent with the above proposal and its implications for interprofessional coordination and policy making. These laws mandate the responsibility for promulgating scope of practice regulations for emerging fields and expanded roles, such as the case of nurse practitioners, to *both* the medical and nursing boards of examiners.[8] While it is too soon to evaluate the net effects of such cooperative efforts in credentialing, a rather strong argument can be made to justify this approach as being responsive to the cracks that are beginning to appear in the present system of licensure. The joint regulation approach may also be viewed as a prototype of joint boards or some variation on the theme of board restructuring, as examined above. There is,

however, some indication that when jurisdictional issues are at stake, professional associations may prefer a private approach rather than resorting to statutory or administrative definitions of jurisdiction which "may fence the profession in as well as others out." As Gilb points out, "some professions, such as psychologists in some states, have found it so difficult to arrive at an enforceable definition of their work that they have had to forgo licensing and rely on registration, certification, or the licensing of use of a title, with no clear-cut definition of the work it describes" (Gilb, 1966: 182; Moore, 1970: 124–125).

In sum, these four approaches—public representation, reorganization of boards, institutional licensure, and jointly promulgated regulations—would provide a system of professional checks and balances in the states' regulation of health practitioners. The fundamental issues in credentialing would be addressed from a perspective broader than that of a single interested profession. The pros and cons of these alternatives will undoubtedly continue to be debated both within and among the professions. This is natural; credentialing traditionally has been, and continues to be, of central concern to the professions. As the professional associations and the public become more cognizant of the imposing public responsibilities that have been granted the professions by the state, measures to infuse greater pluralism and public accountability may need to be adopted, by both the public and private sectors, to ensure the public safety as well as the continued contribution and viability of the professions.

NOTES

1. This information is based upon a study by this writer of the response by professional organizations and states to a recommended moratorium on the further licensure of health occupations. (See U.S. Department of Health, Education, and Welfare, 1971: 73–74.) The following are the categories of personnel considered in 1972 for licensure: ambulance attendants and emergency medical workers, chiropractors, dental technicians, directors of clinical laboratories, EEG technicians, medical technologists and technicians, naturopaths, nurse anesthetists, opticians, physical therapy assistants, psychologists, psychotherapists, radiology technicians, and speech pathologists and audiologists.

2. See also Stevens (1971: 105). These statutes, at first "permissive," i.e., persons may work in the field

without being licensed but may not use the protected title, and later, as the profession becomes more established, "mandatory," i.e., only persons licensed may practice at all, have been dubbed "friendly" licensing laws. See Forgotson and Roemer (1968: 347).

3. The language in two recently introduced bills illustrates the use to which the element of public safety is put in justifying legislation:

AN ACT . . . to provide for the licensing and regulation of psychotherapists, to impose a penalty on persons practicing psychotherapy without a license, and generally related to psychotherapists and the practice of psychotherapy.

WHEREAS, Individuals with mental and emotional problems from time to time have sought the help of certain persons conducting either individual psychotherapy or group psychotherapy; and

WHEREAS, Some of the individuals operating as psychotherapists lack the training and experience necessary to recognize existing and developing mental illness, or to recognize when the methods and techniques which they use are having harmful effects on the personality structure or the emotional or mental health of the individual; and

WHEREAS, The State, in the interest of the public health, safety, and welfare, wishes to protect individuals from psychotherapy which endangers their emotional and mental health; and

WHEREAS, it is realized that some persons operating as psychotherapists, although they do not have an academic background in psychology or psychiatry and although they employ heterodox methods, can perform necessary and needed services for the residents of this State, and

WHEREAS, It is not in the interest of the State or its citizens to limit the practice of psychotherapy entirely to persons of certain academic backgrounds, but only to assure that persons with existing or developing mental or emotional disorders be protected from destructive psychotherapeutic methods and techniques and be referred to appropriate psychotherapists; now therefore . . .

Maryland House Bill No. 1068 (1972)

AN ACT Providing for a Board of Registration of Radiologic Technologists.

It is declared to be the policy of the Commonwealth of Massachusetts that the health and safety of the people of the state must be protected against the harmful effects of excessive and improper exposure to ionizing radiation. Such protection can, in some major measure, be accomplished by requiring adequate training and experience of persons operating ionizing radiation equipment in each particular case under the specific direction of licensed practitioners as defined herein. It is the purpose of this article to establish standards of education, training and experience and to require the examination and certification of operators of ionizing radiation equipment.

Massachusetts House Bill No. 4099 (1972)

4. In this respect, the state licensing agency has much in common with other forms of regulatory agencies. See Krislov and Musolf (1964: chapters 3 and 4).

5. For another early, but still timely, critique of professional self-regulation, see Fesler (1942: 46–60).

6. This writer was co-author of the Report on Licensure.

7. For a discussion of institutional licensure, see U.S. Department of Health, Education, and Welfare (1971: chapter 10).

8. See Idaho Code, sec. 54–1413 (1971), "An Act . . . authorizing a professional nurse to perform acts recognized as appropriate according to rules and regulations promulgated by the Idaho State Board of Medicine and the Idaho Board of Nursing"; and Maryland House Bill No. 468 (enacted May 31, 1972), "An Act . . . to exempt individuals to whom duties are delegated by licensed physicians from the necessity of obtaining a license to practice medicine."

REFERENCES

Akers, Ronald L.
1968 "The professional association and the legal regulation of practice." Law and Society Review 2 (May): 463–482.
Bucher, Rue *and* Joan Stelling
1969 "Characteristics of professional organizations." Journal of Health and Social Behavior 10 (March): 3–15.
Carlson, Rick J.
1970 "Health manpower licensing and emerging institutional responsibility for the quality of care." Law and Contemporary Problems 35 (Autumn): 849–878.
Cohen, Harris S.
1973 "State licensing boards and quality assurance: A new approach to an old problem." Pp. 49–65 in U.S. Department of Health, Education, and Welfare. Quality Assurance of Medical Care. Washington, D.C.: U.S. Government Printing Office.
Crampton, Marion W.
1971 "Licensing of occupational therapists." American Journal of Occupational Therapy 25 (May–June): 206–209.
Curran, William J.
1970 "New paramedical personnel—To license or not to license?" New England Journal of Medicine 282 (May 7): 1085–1086.

Derbyshire, Robert C.
1972 "Better licensure laws for better patient care." Hospital Practice 7 (September): 152–164.

Fesler, James W.
1942 The Independence of State Regulatory Agencies. Chicago: Public Administration Service.

Forgotson, Edward H. *and* Ruth Roemer
1968 "Government licensure and voluntary standards for health personnel and facilities." Medical Care 6 (September–October): 345–354.

Forgotson, Edward H., Ruth Roemer, *and* Roger W. Newman
1967 "Legal regulation of health personnel in the United States." Pp. 279–541 in Report of the National Advisory Commission on Health Manpower, II. Washington: U.S. Government Printing Office.

Freidson, Eliot
1970 Profession of Medicine. New York: Dodd, Mead.

Freidson, Eliot *and* Buford Rhea
1965 "Knowledge and judgment in professional evaluations." Administrative Science Quarterly 10 (June): 107–124.

Gilb, Corinne Lathrop
1966 Hidden Hierarchies: The Professions and Government. New York: Harper and Row.

Grimm, Karen L.
1972 "The relationship of accreditation to voluntary certification and state licensure." SASHEP Staff Working Papers, II., I1–I42. Washington: National Commission on Accrediting.

Hershey, Nathan
1969a "An alternative to mandatory licensure of health professionals." Hospital Progress 50 (March): 71–74.

1969b "The inhibiting effect upon innovation of the prevailing licensure system." Annals of the New York Academy of Science 166 (December): 951–956.

1971 "New directions in licensure of health personnel." Economic and Business Bulletin 24 (Fall): 22–35.

Kaplin, William A.
1972 "The law's view of professional power: Courts and the health professional associations." SASHEP Staff Working Papers, II. J1–J37. Washington: National Commission on Accrediting.

Krislov, Samuel *and* Lloyd D. Musolf (eds.)
1964 The Politics of Regulation. Boston: Houghton-Mifflin.

MacIver, Robert M.
1966 "Professional groups and cultural norms." P. 53 in Howard M. Vollmer and Donald L. Mills (ed.), Professionalization. Englewood Cliffs, New Jersey: Prentice-Hall.

Moore, Wilbert E.
1970 The Professions: Roles and Rules. New York: Russell Sage Foundation.

Pennell, Maryland *and* Paula A. Stewart
1968 State Licensing of Health Occupations, Washington: U.S. Government Printing Office.

Roemer, Ruth
1971 "Licensing and regulation of medical and medical-related practitioners in health service teams." Medical Care 9 (January–February): 42–54.

Sadler, Alfred M. *and* Blair L. Sadler
1971 "Recent developments in the law relating to the physician's assistant." Vanderbilt Law Review 24: 1193–1212.

Selden, William K.
1970 "Licensing boards are archaic." American Journal of Nursing 70 (January): 124–126.

Shimberg, Benjamin, Barbara F. Esser, *and* Daniel H. Kruger
1972 Occupational Licensing and Public Policy, Report to U.S. Department of Labor. Princeton: Educational Testing Service.

Stevens, Rosemary
1971 American Medicine and the Public Interest. New Haven: Yale University Press.

Tancredi, Lawrence R. *and* John Woods
1972 "The social control of medical practice: Licensure versus output monitoring." Milbank Memorial Fund Quarterly 50 (January): 99–125.

Truman, David R.
1951 The Governmental Process: Political Interests and Public Opinion. New York: Knopf.

U.S. Department of Health, Education, and Welfare
1971 Report on Licensure and Related Health Personnel Credentialing. Washington: U.S. Government Printing Office.

U.S. Department of Labor
1969 Occupational Licensing and the Supply of Nonprofessional Manpower, Manpower Research Monograph No. 11. Washington: U.S. Government Printing Office.

2.4 Comments

ROBERT C. DERBYSHIRE

Dr. Cohen has produced a well-documented review of some current attitudes toward licensing and accreditation procedures for medical personnel. Possibly his desire to be objective made it difficult for me at times to separate his opinions from those of the authorities he quoted. At any rate, I shall comment on the article as a whole.

Inescapable is the conclusion that all is not well in the field of licensure of many professions, medicine included. In reading Dr. Cohen's article, I soon concluded that I must try to answer at least three questions:

1. Is the situation as bad as he would have us believe?
2. Is there not at present a system of "checks and balances" of which many people are unaware?
3. Doesn't the recommendation of institutional licensing ignore the lessons of history?

I shall address myself to these questions after making some general comments on trends in licensure and discipline.

But first, a brief historical note is in order. Several methods of licensing physicians have been tried and found wanting. At various times, physicians have been licensed by their preceptors, by non-medical boards, by medical schools (many of which were diploma mills), and by the state medical associations. Serious flaws soon appeared in each system.

As early as 1798, the Maryland legislature established a board of medical examiners which, because of apparent citizen disenchantment, it repudiated in 1838, allowing anyone to practice medicine without restrictions. This policy remained in effect until 1892, when the legislature passed a new practice act providing for two boards, one representing the Medical and Chirurgical Faculty, the other the State Homeopathic Society. This is only one example of the many political compromises which pervade the whole history of licensure.

In 1873, Texas passed the first modern medical practice act. But boards of medical examiners did not attain firm legal standing until 1889, when the Supreme Court of the United States upheld the West Virginia statute.

For the last 100 years, the practice of medicine has been regulated by the individual states whose widely varying laws and regulations have made the builders of the Tower of Babel models of orderly conduct by comparison. Improvement was all but imperceptible until five years ago, when a uniform licensing examination was offered to the states.

Ever since 1873, boards of medical examiners have been composed exclusively of physicians, mainly because of their claim that the highly specialized functions of the profession cannot be evaluated by outsiders; hence the process of licensing must, of necessity, rest solely in the hands of the profession. This concept has naturally spread to other professions. Similarly, and certainly with less justification, physicians claim that they should be the sole judges in disciplinary actions because they are the only ones who can understand the ethical standards of medical practice. Only recently has a state legislature, that of California, required the inclusion of a representative of the general public on the board of medical examiners.

Regardless of their manner of appointment and their possible lack of qualifications, board members are truly public servants in that they contribute much time and energy to the work of the boards with little or no remuneration. That these dedicated public servants do not always adequately carry out their duties is evidenced by the fact that socioeconomic considerations and political factors often govern their decisions. In certain states the boards for all practical purposes, establish quotas for the admission of new physicians.

But the citation of Freidson (Cohen, 1973) that "the profession has sufficient power of its own to control all facets of its work without serious interference from any lay group" is untrue. Today, lay groups are regulating the medical profession as never before. The work of physicians is constantly reviewed by hospital officials, boards of trustees, and government agencies as well as by representatives of the profession. Even the treasured peer review is often subject to supervision by another agency.

Certainly anyone who has worked with a state legislature on revisions of medical practice laws is acutely aware of the fact that the legislators, not the physicians, make the final decisions. Moreover, disciplinary actions of the boards in all states are subject to review by the courts. So the boards and the medical associations by no means govern every aspect of medical practice. Indeed, they should not, and the public should be informed that systems of checks and balances are not completely lacking.

The influence of the professional associations in appointing board members is not entirely healthy. In the first place, it might be construed as a usurpation of the appointive prerogatives of the executive. (This point of view has not yet been challenged legally.) In the second place, it prevents the governor from appointing able people who might not choose to belong to the associations. Nevertheless, self-regulation of a profession is not entirely bad if it is accompanied by adequate restraints.

Dr. Cohen (1973) asserts, "The associations' interaction and influence with the examining board does not cease at the point of selecting board members; in conjunction with the boards, the associations initiate moves for new legislation," etc. This is not entirely correct since the boards, once their members have been appointed, are agents of the state and are accountable to the executive. Furthermore, although this is not widely known, the public has a voice equal to that of the profession in the establishment of regulations. This applies to the majority of states which have specific laws governing the rule-making power of agencies.

To many members of medical boards as well as to the medical association, my advocacy of the inclusion of a nonmedical member on boards is nothing short of heresy. My point is that the primary function of the boards is to protect the public. They are public bodies and should have public representation. Dr. Cohen refers to my suggestion as tokenism which would mean little. I disagree. A single, highly qualified, nonmedical person can perform a real service in representing the public. Some members of the medical profession express distaste for this because they think of it as policing. If this is necessary, so be it! I am unable to understand, however, how more than one or two public members could contribute much to a board with such highly technical functions.

The recommendation that single licensure boards be established for all of the health professions has not been favorably received by authorities on the subject. They contend that it would lead to the rise of another top-heavy bureaucracy which would not improve the licensing procedure. Physicians also fear that a lay administrator with dubious qualifications could veto actions of boards through ignorance or political pressure.

Whoever proposed "institutional licensure" must indeed have ignored the lessons of history. This procedure could prove even worse than the early system whereby a preceptor of inferior quality granted licenses. Under such a plan, there would be an irresistible tendency for institutions to grant licenses to suit their convenience and needs rather than on the basis of quality of applicants. In one state, for example, a hospital board undertook to license its own doctors in defiance of the law. Although their experience was limited only by the time required to obtain an attorney general's opinion, the chairman of the board exposed his ignorance by appointing a grossly unqualified physician as medical director and chief surgeon. The chairman possessed neither the intelligence nor the background to permit him to make such judgments.

The suggestion of licensure by a committee is completely unsound. Committees can not practice medicine, and the individual responsibility traditionally held by the physician must be maintained. The term "team approach" to the practice of medicine has become a worn cliché embraced by many people today. Practice of medicine by a team undoubtedly has advantages. But such an approach reminds me of the sign which the late President Truman had on his desk reading, "The buck stops here." Someone must have final responsibility in the practice of medicine, and this must continue to be the doctor. When the going is difficult, the members of the "health care team" have a tendency to disappear, pointing to the physician as the "captain of the ship."

I conclude my commentary by answering the questions raised in the second paragraph:

1. The licensing process is far from ideal, but it is not quite as bad as Dr. Cohen would have us believe.

2. There is a system of checks and balances in the form of hospital review committees, boards of trustees, legislatures, and the courts. Moreover, citizens can enter into the rule-making procedures of the boards. The public should be informed of the means available for checking on the performance of the boards. Although few people may choose to exercise this prerogative, the knowledge that it exists would tend to restore confidence.

3. Institutional licensure for health professionals would indeed be a giant step backward, and those who advocate it should heed the lessons of history.

Despite my several points of disagreement, I believe Dr. Cohen has performed a service by presenting this review of current attitudes toward licensure and accreditation. Only as a result of such documented studies can we hope to improve the procedures.

REFERENCE

Cohen, Harris S.
1973 Professional licensure, organizational behavior, and the public interest. Milbank Memorial Fund Quarterly/Health and Society 51 (Winter): 73–88.

2.5 Licensure of Foreign Medical Graduates: An Historical Perspective*

IRENE BUTTER AND REBECCA G. SWEET

Reprinted with permission of the Milbank Memorial Fund, from 55 *MMFQ/Health and Society* 315–340 (1977). Copyright © 1977 by the Milbank Memorial Fund. All rights reserved.

Although it has been demonstrated elsewhere that the progressive liberalization of immigration policy has attracted large numbers of foreign medical graduates (FMGs) to the U.S. health care system (Stevens and Vermeulen, 1975), the current debate over FMGs has largely neglected the corresponding developments in state licensure policies as they have affected the entry of FMGs into this country's medical profession. It is essential to understand that the fluctuations in the nation's immigration policies and the response of the states through their licensure policies reflect broad historical pressures.

These pressures date back to the 1920s, when the world center for medical education shifted from Germany to the United States. At this time, many foreign physicians, despite the restrictive immigration quotas of the period, came to America seeking a higher level of training. These foreign physicians received official support in 1926 from both the Council on Medical Education and the American Medical Association, which opposed restrictions on FMGs desiring graduate medical education in this country. But this receptiveness diminished in the 1930s when the financial hardship of the Depression made

American physicians resent the influx of foreign doctors. In 1938 the AMA House of Delegates passed a resolution declaring that U.S. citizenship should be required of all FMGs (Stevens and Vermeulen, 1975), and many state boards adopted this requirement in an attempt to limit the licensing of foreign physicians.

In contrast to these restrictive licensure policies of the states, the federal government began, after World War II, to implement a set of immigration policies favorable to foreigners seeking advanced education in this country. Before this time, an FMG who wished to stay in the U.S. for more than a brief visit could enter the country only as immigration quotas permitted. But, in 1948, the Smith-Mundt Act extended the Fulbright exchange program to include FMGs and created the exchange visitor visa (J visa) to allow FMGs to remain in the U.S. until completion of their studies, thus providing a much more accessible alternative to immigration. This visa became FMGs' major vehicle for entry into the U.S., to the extent that, in the 1960s, approximately two-thirds of the FMG inflow consisted of exchange visitors. The recognition of physician shortages after the Second World War and the Korean War resulted in the further easing of U.S. immigration laws for FMGs. In 1965, Congress amended the Immigration Act by abolishing the quota system for countries, establishing ceilings on immigration which favored immigrants from the Eastern Hemisphere, and allowing preference to be given to professionals in occupations with manpower shortages in this country. Because a U.S. physician shortage was

*We wish to thank Diane Tasca and Karen Klingensmith for their research and editorial assistance.

Research for preparation of this article was supported by the U.S. Department of Health, Education, and Welfare, Health Resources Administration, under contract number HRA-106-74-68 and The Robert Wood Johnson Foundation.

declared by the Department of Labor, the 1965 revision of the Immigration Act gave FMGs a distinct advantage over other potential immigrants.

The law was liberalized still further in 1970 by legislation which facilitated the conversion of exchange visas into immigrant visas. Previously, most exchange visitors who wished to alter their status had been required to leave the U.S. for two years before applying for immigrant status. This policy was changed to allow the prospective immigrant to remain in the U.S. during the conversion process if his application for an immigrant visa had been approved.[1] The number of FMGs taking advantage of this opportunity has grown significantly: in 1970, before the law took effect, 890 foreign physicians were approved for conversion, whereas by 1973, the number had increased to 4,140 (Stevens et al., 1975). The overall effect of these changes has been a dramatic flow of foreign medical graduates into this country over the past twenty years; since 1953, the number of FMGs in the U.S. has increased sixfold, and, at the present time, one out of every five physicians practicing in the U.S. was educated abroad (Stevens and Vermeulen, 1975).

Although these immigration policies have undoubtedly been viewed by the federal government as at least partial solutions to perceived physician shortages in the U.S., their success in that regard has largely been determined by state governments whose jurisdiction encompasses the crucial matter of licensure. At this point, it must be noted that in discussing the licensure policies of the states one is actually talking about two different sets of policies for each state: the first concerns full licensure, which allows the physician the full scope of independent medical practice; the second covers what we will refer to as "less-than-full" licensure which is the system of different licenses authorizing limited and/or temporary practice within the state. The relationship between these two licensure systems will be treated more fully later in this discussion, but it should be noted at this point that both the full and less-than-full licensure systems of the states have changed in response to the large influx of FMGs over the last few decades.

In 1935, ten states did not under any circumstances grant full licenses to graduates of foreign institutions. Through the next ten years this number declined steadily, leaving only Arkansas, Louisiana, and Nevada in 1962; in 1968, Louisiana began to license FMGs, followed by Arkansas and Nevada in 1971. During this time the states generally modified their full licensure systems by gradually eliminating requirements unrelated to the competency of physicians and by developing more uniform qualification standards for licensure. An even more obvious receptiveness to FMGs has manifested itself in the less-than-full licensure systems. The tremendous expansion of less-than-full licensure in the last two decades is at least partially attributable to the growing presence of FMGs in this country's health care system, a correlation which is strengthened by the fact that FMGs use less-than-full licenses to a much greater extent than USMGs do.

In this analysis of trends in the development of both full and less-than-full licensure systems during the last two decades, we have drawn on the following major sources of information: for the period between 1953 and 1973, data from *Medical Licensure Statistics*, published annually in *JAMA*, were used; data for 1974 and 1975 were taken from a report which was prepared for the Department of Health, Education, and Welfare entitled *State Policies on the Limited and Temporary Licensure of Foreign Medical Graduates* (NTIS No. PB-253073).[2] For the purpose of establishing a basis for detecting changes in the full licensure system, we have dealt principally with the five basic requirements for full licensure and the policies regarding licensure endorsement that exist in the fifty states and the District of Columbia. These requirements concern citizenship and visa status, the basic science examination, postgraduate training, certification by the Educational Commission for Foreign Medical Graduates (ECFMG), and the Federation of State Medical Boards' Licensing Examination (FLEX). In the case of trends in less-than-full licensure, the only information consistently available in *JAMA* refers to the number and types of less-than-full licenses authorized by different states at different times. Because *JAMA* tables did not yield sufficient data to describe the changes in requirements for and durations of less-than-full licenses during the past two decades, an historical perspective could not be developed, and the presentation of these aspects of less-than-full licensure had to be limited to the information gathered in 1974 and 1975 from the medical boards.

FULL LICENSURE OF FMGs: 1953–1975

1. Citizenship and Visa Status

During the past two decades, the states have frequently altered their requirements concerning the citizenship and visa status of FMG applicants for full licensure. Although the fluctuation in state policies has been considerable, there has been a clear tendency among the states since the late 1960s to relax their citizenship and visa requirements. Such requirements involve either an immigrant visa, a declaration of intent to become a citizen, or naturalized citizenship. The most stringent of these requirements is naturalized citizenship since the attainment of this status requires an immigrant visa and five years of U.S. residence; the requirement of the immigrant visa alone is obviously a less stringent prerequisite for licensure. Although the states report that they regard the declaration of intent as a more stringent requirement than the immigrant visa, it seems more realistic to treat these as essentially the same requirement, since anyone with an immigrant visa can easily file a declaration of intent with the Immigration and Naturalization Service, and the declaration itself has not even been required for citizenship since 1952.

The states' imposition of these requirements changed dramatically in the late 1960s, as Fig. 2.5.1 indicates. For every year between 1953 and 1968, at least twenty states required naturalized citizenship of FMGs seeking full licensure, while only a handful of states did not impose any citizenship-related requirements. During this time, a steadily increasing number of states adopted the requirement of the immigrant visa or the declaration of intent as a kind of middle ground between no requirement at all and the requirement of full citizenship. But in 1969 the number of states requiring naturalization of FMG candidates for full licensure dropped to sixteen and in 1970 dropped to ten. This sharp decrease continued; in 1975 only five states,[3] Montana, New Hampshire, South Carolina, Wisconsin, and Wyoming, required that FMG applicants for full licensure become U.S. citizens.

Between 1967 and 1970 the number of states requiring the immigrant visa or declaration of intent rose dramatically, apparently in response to the concurrent decline in the number of states requiring citizenship. However, after reaching a peak of twenty-eight in 1970, the number of states electing this middle ground dropped sharply and has leveled off in the last few years at eighteen. But the most significant change has occurred in the number of states which do not explicitly impose any visa or citizenship related requirement upon foreign applicants for full licensure. Whereas no more than six states licensed FMGs regardless of citizenship status in any year between 1953 and 1970, since then this number has risen, at first gradually, and then very rapidly, to the present total of twenty-eight. In short, between 1953 and 1975, twenty-eight states lessened their citizenship-related requirements, while only two states increased them.

It is difficult to completely account for the pattern which emerges from these figures, that is, the tendency of the states since 1969 to drop the requirement of full citizenship, frequently by first substituting the less stringent requirement of the immigrant visa or declaration of intent, and then abolishing citizenship and visa requirements altogether. The rapid disappearance of the naturalization requirement can, to a large degree, be explained by recent legal decisions which affirm the equal protection of the laws under the Fourteenth Amendment, and which hold the requirement of citizenship for licensure as an unconstitutional denial of this right.[4] It is likely that the increasing number of such court decisions also accounts for the decline in the number of states imposing any requirement related to citizenship or visa status. In any case, elimination of citizenship and visa requirements for licensure can be viewed as one aspect of the general tendency of the states to do away with requirements which bear little relation to the competency of physicians.

2. Basic Science

In the past twenty-two years, the number of states requiring FMGs seeking full licensure to pass a special basic science examination has decreased significantly, from seventeen in 1953 to seven in 1975. The tendency to eliminate the basic science requirement is further underscored by the fact that six of the seven states presently requiring a basic science examination will waive the requirement under certain circumstances. This development can be partially traced to the nearly universal adoption by the states of

Figure 2.5.1   Citizenship and Visa Status Requirements for Full Licensure of FMGs, 1953–1975.

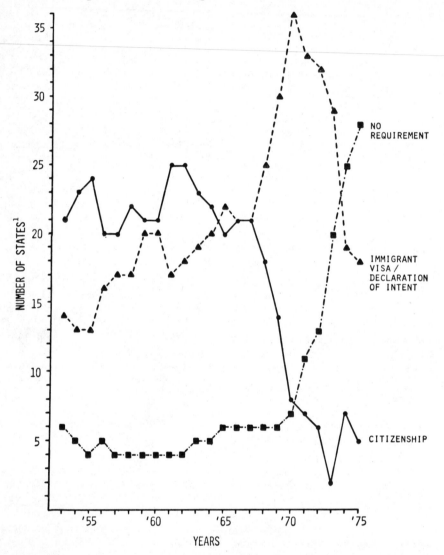

[1]States which did not grant licenses to FMGs in a given year were not included in the totals for that year.

FLEX, which by administering its own basic science test has made another basic science examination superfluous. Indeed, three of the states still maintaining a basic science requirement will waive it if the candidate has passed the basic science portion of FLEX. The claim that FLEX has hastened the demise of the basic science requirement is further supported by the fact that the states have been dropping basic science at a faster rate since the advent of FLEX in 1968: thirteen states eliminated the requirement be-

tween 1968 and 1975, while only ten states had abolished it during the fifteen years prior to the introduction of FLEX.

The seven states[5] still requiring the basic science examination are Arkansas, Colorado, Kansas, South Dakota, Tennessee, Texas, and Washington. The basic science substitutions currently available in these states include FLEX, academic background in the basic sciences and differing amounts of medical practice in this country.[6] Only one state, Colorado, will not waive the examination under any circumstances. During the period under consideration, twenty-five states made no changes at all with respect to the basic science requirement, other than arranging for waivers. Four of these states (Colorado, South Dakota, Tennessee, and Washington) have consistently required a basic science examination, while twenty-one states have never had a basic science requirement during this period.

3. Postgraduate Training

The fact that an FMG has graduated from a foreign medical school recognized by the U.S. and has acquired basic medical skills does not guarantee that he will function adequately within the American medical profession. Exposure to American medical procedures and technology, as well as an understanding of the various social and cultural patterns of American life, appears to be a further prerequisite for competent participation in the American health care system. In recognition of the fact that important preliminary experience is most commonly obtained through postgraduate training in American hospitals, a growing number of states have made postgraduate training a prerequisite for full licensure, and have stipulated that this training be pursued in AMA-approved programs.

This attitude represents a change of emphasis for the states. Up until the late 1950s it appears that more importance was attached to assessing the quality of the FMG's undergraduate medical background. Requirements for licensure aimed at assuring the quality of this background varied greatly from state to state and were not nearly so clear cut as the present requirement of participation in AMA-approved programs. Up until 1963, in an attempt to screen out unqualified FMGs, some state licensure boards imposed additional standards upon the qualifications of foreign physicians for licensure, such as the requirement in seven states that FMGs spend an additional year in an approved U.S. medical school after graduating from an approved foreign institution, or the stipulation in five states that the FMG's school of medical education be either equivalent to schools within these states or subject to board approval. In a similar vein, in 1950 the Council on Medical Education (CME) of the AMA and the Executive Council of the Association of American Medical Colleges (AAMC)

began to compile a list of foreign schools which met with their approval, and, as of 1956, nineteen states had made graduation from a school on this list a prerequisite for the licensure of foreign physicians. The list was limited in a number of ways; chiefly, it was incomplete and contained a disproportionate number of European schools, therefore restricting the licensure of non-Europeans. During this period, several states also required National Board certification of FMGs seeking licensure; however, since graduates of foreign schools had been barred from taking the National Boards since 1952, this stipulation represented a thinly disguised means of excluding FMGs from licensure. Though these requirements may have reflected the understandable desire of the state boards to assure the competence of FMGs, they also perpetuated the FMG-USMG dichotomy in licensure standards, and some of them actually excluded FMGs from full licensure altogether.

Accompanying the trend of the 1960s away from such idiosyncratic and exclusionary training requirements[7] has been a modest increase in the amount of AMA-approved postgraduate training required by the states, as is shown in Fig. 2.5.2. Between 1953 and 1975, only four states decreased the amount of postgraduate training required of FMG applicants for full licensure, while twenty-five states maintained the same requirements throughout the period, and thirteen states increased their requirements. It must be noted, however, that because the postgraduate training of U.S. physicians has become lengthier and has emphasized specialty programs more than was the case in the early fifties, the moderate increase in the amount of postgraduate training required of FMGs may also reflect the generally increased emphasis upon specialization in the American medical profession.[8] But, whatever the reason, these increases in postgraduate training requirements parallel the trend noted above toward more concrete, equitable, and organized measures for assuring the competence of foreign graduates and integrating them into this country's health care system.

4. ECFMG Certification

One of the earliest products of the trend toward more systematic review of FMG qualifications was the examination administered

Figure 2.5.2 Postgraduate Training Requirements for Full Licensure of FMGs, 1953–1975.

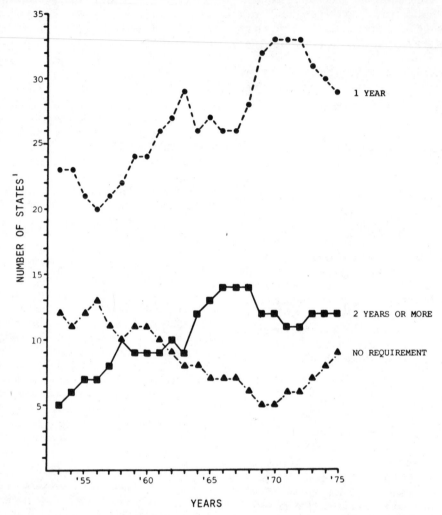

YEARS

[1]States which did not grant licenses to FMGs in a given year were not included in the totals for that year. California's postgraduate training requirement involves a number of different options which made it impossible to include California in any one category; for this reason, California was not included in the totals for any year.

worldwide by the Educational Commission for Foreign Medical Graduates (ECFMG). Since its introduction in 1957, this examination has become the primary method for screening foreign applicants to U.S. postgraduate training programs, and is required for entrance into all training programs approved by the Liaison Committee on Graduate Medical Education of the American Medical Association. In replacing the list of foreign medical schools approved by the Council on Medical Education of the AMA and the Executive Council of the Association of American Medical Colleges, ECFMG has contributed greatly to the standardization of licensure requirements and has also made full licensure more accessible to qualified FMGs throughout the country.

During the period between 1957 and 1975, a steadily increasing number of states adopted the requirement of ECFMG certification for full licensure (ECFMG certification is a two-part process consisting of approval of foreign credentials and a written examination). Within a year of its introduction, fifteen states had opted for

ECFMG over the CME-AAMC list of approved foreign schools, while seven states continued to use the list alone, and ten more states required both ECFMG certification and graduation from an approved foreign institution. After 1958, *JAMA* tables no longer listed graduation from a CME-AAMC-approved foreign school as a separate requirement for full licensure. As of 1975, forty-six states required that FMG applicants for full licensure be certified by ECFMG; two of the states which do not explicitly require ECFMG certification for licensure do demand a specified amount of postgraduate training in an AMA-approved program, for which ECFMG certification is a universal prerequisite.[9]

In spite of the trend between 1957 and 1975 toward standardization of licensure requirements through the use of ECFMG, we have identified several instances in which the ECFMG examination may be circumvented. Of these, potentially the most significant substitution has been authorized by the Commission itself: in February 1972 it began certifying FMGs who have passed FLEX, even if they have not taken ECFMG's examination. As of this writing, few FMGs have actually taken advantage of this provision, but its potential effect is great, inasmuch as twelve states currently allow FMGs who have not taken ECFMG to sit for FLEX, and twenty-seven of those states which do require ECFMG certification as a prerequisite for FLEX will accept a FLEX score obtained in another state. In other words, an FMG could, conceivably, apply for licensure in a state requiring ECFMG, sit for FLEX in a state which does not demand ECFMG as a prerequisite, obtain ECFMG certification on the basis of a passing FLEX score, and receive a full license in the original state without having taken the ECFMG examination. But, although opportunities do exist to circumvent ECFMG, it must be pointed out that such substitutions do not grant easier access to licensure (since FLEX is by no means less difficult than ECFMG), and ECFMG, as a prerequisite to FLEX and AMA-approved postgraduate training, as well as a licensure requirement in its own right, remains the principal means of channeling foreign medical graduates into the American health care system.

5. FLEX

The nearly universal adoption of FLEX throughout the United States epitomizes the trends we have been discussing and has hastened their progress immeasurably. Among the original aims of the Federation of State Medical Boards in creating FLEX were the standardization and improvement of licensing examinations and the normalization of the endorsement process. These goals must be recognized as having been at least partially achieved by the almost national acceptance of FLEX as the single licensing examination for foreign medical graduates. The introduction of FLEX in 1968 was itself the nucleus of the gradual standardization of licensure policies and the movement toward adopting a uniform standard for physician competency. As has been previously mentioned, there is undoubtedly a connection between the use of FLEX and the accelerated disappearance of the basic science requirement. Similarly, FLEX has simplified the endorsement process and made it somewhat more equitable and accessible to FMGs.

The adoption of FLEX by the states has progressed at nearly a constant rate since its inception. In 1968, when the Federation first offered FLEX, eight states used the new examination in lieu of the individual state board examinations. They were joined by nine more states in 1969, eight in 1970, nine in 1971, six plus the District of Columbia in 1972, eight in 1973, and one in 1975. Only Florida has not yet adopted FLEX as its licensing examination, a situation which the Florida licensing board expects to change in the near future.

One aspect of FLEX, however, does seem to run counter to the intended effect of the examination. FLEX itself is a three-day examination with a standard passing score set by the Federation, consisting of a weighted average obtained by weighting scores from the three days as 1/6, 1/3, and 1/2 of the total score; however, the states impose differing policies with regard to the attainment of this weighted average. It was not possible to determine how long the present scoring policies have been in effect, but, as of 1975, twenty-seven states stipulate that FMGs applying for licensure obtain a FLEX weighted average of 75 percent at *one* three-day examination period, while twenty-three states allow FMGs to combine scores from different examination trials. Such policies seem to make it somewhat easier for FMGs to pass FLEX in the states allowing combinations than in the states demanding that candidates for licensure retake the entire examination every time they fail. Variations also exist in that several states require FMGs to obtain various minimum day and/or subject scores over and above the passing score designated by the Federation. At this point, it is hard to assess the effects of these different scoring policies upon the licensure of FMGs; however, there is some indication that the more stringent scoring policies may somewhat inhibit the licensure of foreign physicians.[10] To the extent that they do, these scoring policies qualify the degree to which FLEX has equalized the licensure requirements of the states.

ENDORSEMENT

Only in the last several years have the majority of the states expanded their licensure policies to include provisions for the endorsement of FMGs' out-of-state U.S. licenses. As is indicated in Fig. 2.5.3, only eight states would endorse licenses which FMGs had obtained from other states in 1953, and it was not until 1974 that all the states and Washington, D.C., had established endorsement provisions for FMGs. One important explanation for the rather belated development of FMG endorsement lies in the changes wrought by FLEX upon the endorsement process as a whole. Until the nationwide adoption of the Federation's standardized licensing examination, each state administered its own unique examination for licensure, thus precluding any uniform standard for endorsement of out-of-state licenses. Before FLEX, the endorsement policies of several states consisted of a series of reciprocal agreements with other states, whereby two states would officially establish the equivalence of their standards for licensure and agree to endorse each other's licenses.

The complexity of these individualized endorsement systems led the states to seek less cumbersome alternatives. A major reason for the establishment of FLEX by the Federation of State Medical Boards was to "create a rational basis for interstate endorsement" and to promote the uniformity of endorsement policies (Derbyshire, 1969). As a direct result of the adoption of FLEX by the states, a growing number of FMGs have received full licenses through endorsement. In 1967, before FLEX was introduced, nineteen states endorsed the out-of-state licenses of 1,083 foreign medical

graduates; by 1973, when most states were using FLEX, the number of FMG endorsees had quadrupled, with thirty-eight states licensing 4,359 foreign medical graduates through endorsement.

Although the advent of FLEX has greatly simplified the endorsement process for FMGs, there still exist legal opportunities for states to impede the geographic mobility of foreign medical graduates. Because most states officially require that foreign candidates for endorsement meet the same standards demanded of FMGs obtaining their initial U.S. licenses through examination, the endorsement process is significantly affected by variations in the FLEX scoring policies of the states (discussed above). States which do not accept the combinations of day or subject scores from their own candidates for initial licensure usually will not endorse licenses based upon passing averages obtained through score combinations. A similar barrier arises between the states which demand that FMGs obtain certain minimum scores on FLEX in addition to the Federation's passing score, and those states which accept the Federation's standard. Another obstacle to uniform endorsement throughout the country is a carry-over from the pre-FLEX era. The variability among the individual state licensing examinations was so great that many FMGs licensed by state board examinations during the last two decades may not now be eligible for licensure by endorsement in some states without taking FLEX. For example, today Georgia still will not endorse a license based on the pre-FLEX New York State Board Examination.

Of course, irregularities in endorsing standards also arise from differences in leniency that exist between states. Several states have endorsed FMG credentials other than FLEX, for example, foreign and Canadian licenses, and American Specialty Board certification, and states vary with respect to their standards for the documentation of an FMG's credentials.[11] It is impossible to determine the net effect of the various barriers and easements to endorsement outlined here. Some states make it possible to circumvent the licensure requirements of other states, while some states inhibit interstate mobility by imposing stricter standards. All that can be said to summarize the historical development of endorsement with respect to foreign medical graduates is that the states made provisions to

Figure 2.5.3 Number of States Granting Full Licenses to FMGs by Endorsement, 1953–1975.

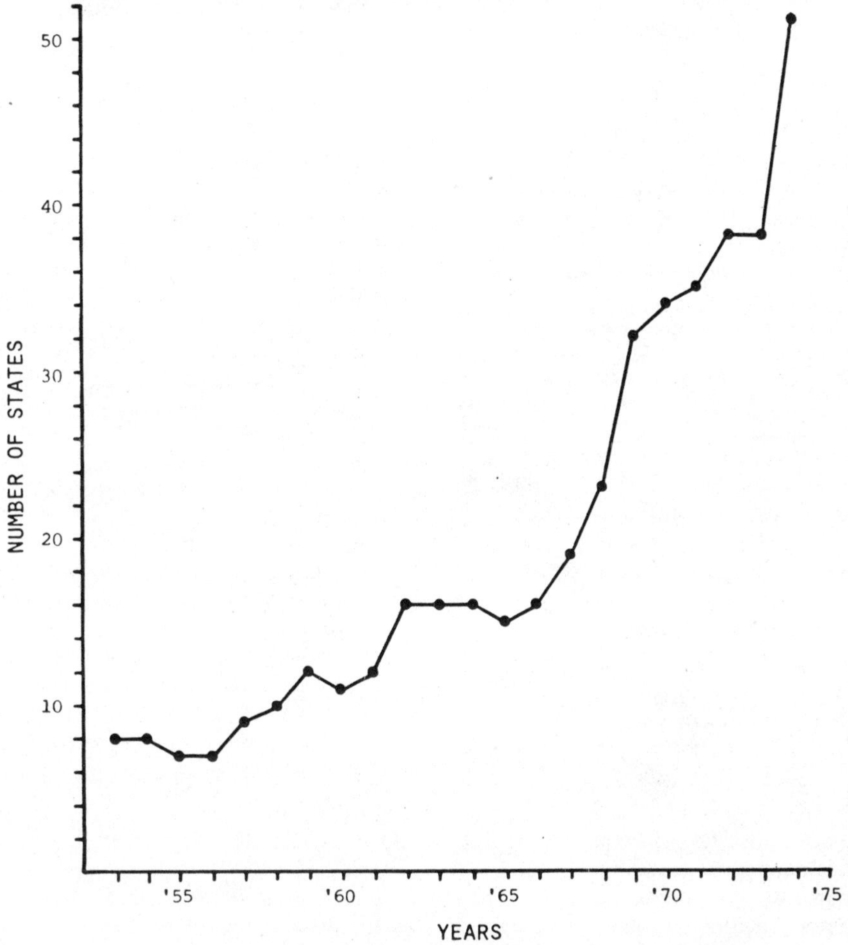

endorse FMGs only gradually until the advent of FLEX; once a uniform nationwide licensing examination broke down the idiosyncratic differences between the states' individual licensing examinations, many states quickly joined the ranks of those endorsing FMGs. At the present time, all states will license FMGs through endorsement, and many of these endorsement policies have been modified to ease the process; however, states could go still further in promoting uniform licensure standards, thereby eliminating the remaining barriers to the interstate mobility of foreign medical graduates.

LESS-THAN-FULL LICENSURE

Less-than-full licenses can be viewed either as intermediate steps or as distinct alternatives to

the full licensure system. With the development of specialization in medicine in recent years, educational less-than-full licenses have proliferated as preliminaries to the full license, allowing a physician to practice in a limited sphere and under supervision until completion of postgraduate training. On the other hand, governmental, faculty and shortage area less-than-full licenses represent alternatives to full licensure for those physicians who either have no need for full licenses or are unable to obtain them.

Of the nine types of less-than-full licenses presently available to physicians throughout the U.S., we have chosen to limit our discussion to the five less-than-full licenses most relevant to FMGs during the period between 1953 and 1975. They are the licenses which authorize practice in educational settings (i.e., postgraduate training programs); in government institutions under state, county, or municipal control; in medically underserved areas as designated by the state boards; in faculty positions in medical schools; and in any situation, including that of private practice, until naturalized citizenship is attained, at which time full licensure is conferred.

Four other types of less-than-full licenses have been excluded from our study because they were of little interest to foreign medical graduates: the *locum tenens* license permitting a physician possessing an out-of-state license to assume responsibility for the private practice of a licensed physician during his or her absence; two licenses allowing practice during an emergency, or in a camp or school, for which FMGs are not usually eligible; and the license authorizing practice for a short time until the medical board meets to confer full licenses.

Data on less-than-full licenses for the years 1953 to 1973 were limited in that only those less-than-full licenses which are formally issued by medical boards were recorded in *JAMA*. Provisions for simple registration of physicians and exemptions from the medical practice acts for various situations were not covered in the *JAMA* tables through 1973 and so could not be included in this discussion. This is unfortunate since exemptions have been largely ignored in other literature, although they are especially important: besides permitting practice without a full license, they usually exclude the board from controlling the eligibility requirements of the physicians practicing in the exempted situations, and often the board does not even know the location or number of such practitioners.

Even when the survey is limited to the five types of less-than-full licenses described above, it is obvious that there has been a dramatic increase in the number of states offering less-than-full licenses to FMGs during the last two decades. In 1953, only two types of less-than-full licenses were available to FMGs in only twelve states: these were the educational and governmental licenses. During the next twenty years, the shortage area, faculty, and citizenship licenses appeared for the first time, and the number of states authorizing the educational and governmental licenses doubled. The license allowing practice in postgraduate training programs was the most widely used less-than-full license throughout the period (Fig. 2.5.4). This educational license was available in ten states in

1953 and in twenty-seven states in 1975, and, when the educational exemptions are also counted, a total of forty-six states today have made provisions for practice in educational settings. As is noted above, the greatly increased use of this license appears to be related to the increased specialization of physicians in the United States, which has necessitated longer periods of postgraduate training. Because a greater number of physicians who were practicing in lengthy training programs were not yet eligible for full licensure, or planned to practice in a state only for the duration of their training, boards recognized the need to provide legal status for these trainees through the use of the educational less-than-full license.

Use of the governmental license has also grown significantly during the last two decades. Such use may have expanded because the governmental license authorizes limited practice in the institutional settings which are less appealing to U.S. medical graduates; in the last few years some of these institutions have come to depend heavily for their supply of physician manpower upon the growing population of foreign medical graduates. In addition, the governmental license in many of the states allows the FMG to practice while attempting to pass FLEX. For these reasons, we suggest that the growth of the governmental less-than-full license in the last twenty-two years has corresponded to the inflow of FMGs during this period. As is shown in Fig. 2.5.4, in 1953 only three states had provided for less-than-full practice in governmental institutions, whereas, by 1975, eighteen more states had established a governmental less-than-full license, and, when exemptions are included, a total of twenty-four states currently authorize less-than-full practice in government institutions.

The other three less-than-full licenses available to FMGs appeared more recently and have been used much more selectively than the educational and governmental licenses. The shortage area license first appeared in 1959 (Fig. 2.5.5). It was used by only one state in any given year between 1959 and 1969 (the state varied from year to year); however, the number of states granting this license increased to six by 1975. Despite its limited usage, it is clear that this license offers much potential as a remedy for the current problems of physician supply in underserved areas throughout the country. The

Figure 2.5.4 Number of States Granting Educational or Government Less-Than-Full Licenses, 1953–1975.

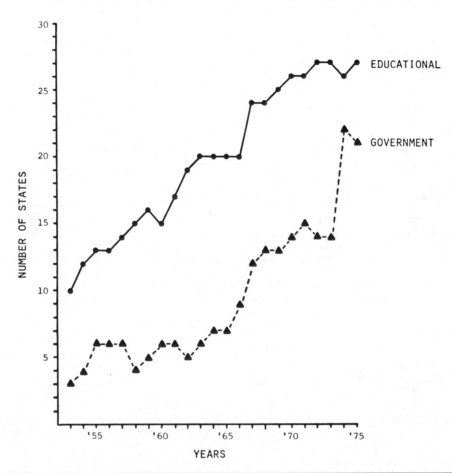

license which allows an FMG to practice while waiting to become a naturalized citizen has been authorized by a smaller number of states than those actually requiring such naturalization for full licensure (Fig. 2.5.5). In the early 1960s, naturalized citizenship was required by twenty-two states for full licensure, but only two of these states permitted FMGs to practice under the special citizenship license, which authorized practice under more liberal terms than those of any other less-than-full license. At the present time, however, each of the states requiring citizenship for full licensure authorizes this license. Finally, the faculty less-than-full license was available in only one state until 1961, after which time it was dropped for a while and was not used by any state until 1967 when an increasing number of states began to offer it (Fig. 2.5.5).

This license is designed specifically for those outstanding foreign physicians with short-term medical school appointments who do not intend to become fully licensed in the U.S. In 1974, fourteen states had made provisions for faculty less-than-full licenses in their medical practice acts and six more states exempt such physicians from board regulation.

The available information does not give rise to definitive statements regarding the development of state policies with respect to the eligibility, duration, and renewal standards for limited and temporary licenses during the period between 1953 and 1975.[12] In general, however, we learned from licensing board members and hospital administrators that a growing number of states have consistently imposed at least the requirement of ECFMG certification for less-

Figure 2.5.5   Number of States Granting Shortage Area, Citizenship, and Faculty[1] Less-Than-Full
Licenses, 1953–1975.

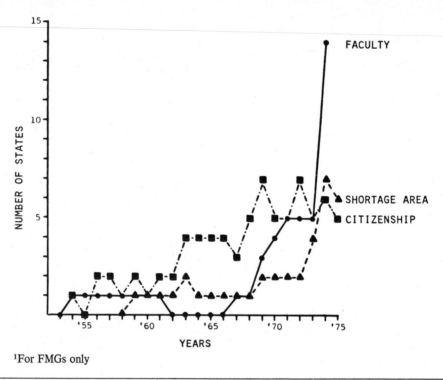

[1]For FMGs only

than-full licensure. In the last several years, most states have established methods for introducing the ECFMG requirement into their less-than-full licensure systems. In fact, by 1975, forty-eight states required at least ECFMG certification for all their less-than-full licenses, while only two states specified no requirements for their licenses and one state reported minimal requirements (a reputedly easy examination).[13] The ranges of requirements and durations which the states have established for their less-than-full licensure systems as of 1975 are summarized below.

Educational licenses usually require only ECFMG certification, and permit practice until the completion of postgraduate training, although sometimes the duration of this license is open-ended. Occasionally, the ECFMG requirement is not imposed by the board, but is maintained by the training institution, in order to guarantee the accreditation of the training program. The educational less-than-full licenses of most states are renewable annually: fourteen states specified a maximum duration of from two to five years for this license, while fifteen states allow the trainee to practice for the duration of his program.

In contrast to these fairly consistent policies regarding the educational license, governmental less-than-full licenses run the gamut of requirements and durations. The requirements for this license can include ECFMG, postgraduate training, FLEX, or any combination of these. In a few cases, a full license is required; in fewer cases, virtually no requirements are specified. The variety of the requirements for the governmental less-than-full license throughout the states indicates that the states may be using this license rather flexibly as a mechanism to alleviate manpower shortages. Hawaii, obviously a popular state in which to reside, demands that the physicians working in its state institutions meet the rather stringent requirement of three years of approved postgraduate training, while a relatively less attractive state for physicians such as Mississippi specifies no requirements for its governmental license whatsoever. Another, though narrower, opportunity for states to regulate their licenses according to their needs is afforded by duration/renewal policies. Ten of the twenty-one states offering governmental licenses in 1975 implied that, theoretically at least, their licenses could be renewed annually for an unlimited number of times, provided that all of the states' requirements and conditions are continually met by the licensee. A representative from one state admitted that his state's governmental license is issued only once and can continue in perpetuity. Other states have established more specific maximum durations for their less-than-full governmental licenses, usually ranging from one to five years, with annual renewals.

Both the shortage area license and the citizenship license resemble the full license in the stringency of their qualification standards. The shortage area license usually requires at least ECFMG and several years of postgraduate training, and often FLEX or a U.S. license is required in addition. Physicians may practice under such licenses from one year to an indefinite period of time. The citizenship license is usually granted after the FMG has met all the requirements for full licensure except naturalization, and allows the FMG virtually the full scope of practice while fulfilling the residence requirement for U.S. citizenship. This lack of restriction most likely reflects the prevalent attitude that citizenship is a requirement which has no bearing upon a physician's competence. These licenses usually last a maximum of six to eight years, and are renewed annually. The faculty license also confers a full scope of practice, but limits the FMG to the confines of the teaching hospital and to the duties of a professor. Probably because the physician to whom the license is granted is an internationally eminent member of the medical profession, the explicit requirements for this license are minimal, and usually include only ECFMG. Since this license is designed for visiting faculty, it generally lasts for only one year, the length of the FMG's temporary faculty appointment.

In summary, the less-than-full licensure systems of the states reveal an increase in both the types of licenses and the availability of these licenses throughout the country. Given the growing variety of less-than-full licenses for FMGs and the growing number of states making provisions during the last two decades for FMGs to practice in some capacity, it appears that the less-than-full licensure system has become significantly more accessible to foreign medical graduates since 1953.

DISCUSSION

In 1953, the states were generally less receptive to foreign medical graduates than they are today. At that time they were considerably more restrictive with regard to full licensure than is presently the case: a number of states employed rigid approval mechanisms for foreign medical schools, or used idiosyncratic screening methods, while others simply excluded all FMGs from full licensure. These policies have relaxed considerably since the middle 1960s, and states are moving toward more standardized screening systems and more uniform qualification procedures. A persistent trend has been to eliminate licensure requirements that are unrelated to physician competency, such as naturalization and visa status. In place of these requirements, ECFMG certification, postgraduate training, and FLEX constitute an interrelated set of requirements with the double potential of indicating physician competence and resolving the more disturbing aspects of interstate differences in the treatment of FMGs.

Although the states have made steady progress in establishing more standardized procedures for competency appraisal, there is potential for even greater consistency. Further progress by the states in reassessing and eliminating the differences in FLEX scoring policies, in endorsement policies, and in the length of postgraduate training requirements could substantially contribute to even greater uniformity in minimum qualification standards, while also enhancing the geographic mobility of FMGs within the nation.

Despite a clear and persistent trend toward national uniformity in competence appraisal procedures, the survey has uncovered little information to suggest that, over time, competency assurance has become more effective. For example, measurement of physician competence remains focused on examination performance even though the evidence demonstrating the validity of the tests in predicting aptitude for competent patient care is limited. Moreover, for the purpose of full licensure, assessment of physician qualifications continues to be confined to a single point in time: the point of career entry.

Periodic reevaluation of physician capabilities is only now beginning to enter policy-related discussion.

The past two decades have also seen a substantial growth both in the variety of less-than-full licenses available to FMGs and in the number of states authorizing less-than-full practice for FMGs. The survey documents a rising trend both in preliminary and alternative types of less-than-full licenses. Unfortunately, the perspective provided on less-than-full licensure is, of necessity, rather narrow because of the lack of documentation on prerequisites, qualification standards, and durations of these more restricted types of licenses. Based on information collected by the authors in 1975–76, it is evident that compared with full licensure, the less-than-full licensure policies of the states contain appreciably greater variability with regard to qualification standards, durations, and types of less-than-full licenses issued. When this fact is considered in light of the varying manpower supplies and deficits confronting the states, it raises the question of whether nationally uniform less-than-full licensure standards constitute a desirable goal. An answer to this query lies beyond the scope of this paper, but has been attempted by the authors in a previously cited study (Butter, 1976).

With regard to the effectiveness of competence assurance, it is our view that the less-than-full licensure system has the potential for serving as a useful adjunct to full licensure in that it can direct physicians of different and changing levels of demonstrated competence into appropriately structured practice situations. By recognizing differing levels of initial competency among physicians, and by acknowledging the function of periodic reassessment of physician capabilities, the states can avail themselves of more options in meeting manpower requirements, while at the same time strengthening their role in competence appraisal.

Admittedly, widespread reform will be required before less-than-full licensure can effectively serve to expand and complement the existing procedures of competence appraisal. During the past two decades the states have demonstrated the ability to coordinate and standardize licensure qualification procedures. Based on their success in this regard, a new commitment by the states to increasing the effectiveness of competence assurance, for FMGs and USMGs

alike, appears to lie within their realm of capability and constitutes a logical and promising direction for the future.

NOTES

1. Exceptions to this policy were exchange visitors financed by their own governments or by the U.S. government, and those whose country of last permanent residence has declared a need for the exchange visitor's skills as indicated on the "skills list" prepared by the State Department.

2. The HEW report was based on three partially interrelated and overlapping surveys: the first was a comparative tabulation of statutes and rules and regulations in the fifty states and the District of Columbia; the second, a telephone survey of these fifty-one licensure boards, was a follow-up to the first survey to determine actual practice in the administration of the laws; and the third was a detailed on-site investigation of twelve states selected because of their varying dependencies on FMGs. A substantial number of discrepancies existed between the *JAMA* data and the findings compiled for the HEW report. In cases of disagreement, it was assumed that the information elicited directly from the licensure boards in the surveys was more accurate and the *JAMA* data were revised accordingly; unfortunately, nothing could be done to corroborate the *JAMA* data from 1953 to 1973. For a more comprehensive discussion of the *present* state of both the full and less-than-full licensure systems, see Butter (1976).

3. This total includes Wisconsin which eliminated all citizenship and visa-related requirements for full licensure in June 1976. Ohio and California offer FMGs two paths to full licensure, two alternate sets of requirements, and in each state, one of these sets includes the requirement of full citizenship. However, these states were not counted among the states requiring citizenship for licensure since more FMGs in these states choose the other path, which couples a lesser visa-related requirement with increased postgraduate training.

4. Two recent opinions of the Office of the Attorney General in Michigan (OAG 1971–1972, No. 4755 and OAG 1972–1973, No. 4776) struck down the state's requirement of citizenship for licensure, citing US Const., AM XIV, § 1, and *In re Griffiths,* 406 US 966 (1973), *Graham v. Richardson,* 403 US 365 (1971), and *Truax v. Raich,* 239 US 33 (1915) among other cases.

5. This total does not include Utah, which does not normally impose a basic science requirement, but which does examine physicians in the basic sciences if they are requesting Utah to endorse an out-of-state license based on a state board examination (not FLEX) taken within the last three years.

6. Kansas, South Dakota, and Washington will waive the basic science exam for those FMGs who have

passed FLEX; South Dakota, in addition to its FLEX substitution, will waive the examination for applicants who have practiced five years or more in the U.S. Arkansas allows ten years of U.S. practice to substitute for its basic science test; Texas will waive the requirement if the applicant's academic background shows sufficient strength in the basic sciences, and Tennessee does not impose the requirement upon FMGs seeking endorsement of out-of-state licenses if they have lived in the U.S. for two years.

7. In 1975, Illinois and New York continued to use lists to determine the amount of postgraduate training to be required of FMGs from various countries. Illinois has been designated here as requiring one year of training of most FMGs while New York has been counted as a two-year state because it requires two years of postgraduate training of FMGs from most non-European countries.

8. Along these lines, the AMA has recently recommended that two years of approved postgraduate training be required both of USMGs and FMGs who are seeking full licensure (see *American Medical News,* American Medical Association, December 8, 1975, p. 3).

9. California, Connecticut, Illinois, Indiana, and Tennessee do not explicitly require ECFMG for full licensure; however, Illinois and Indiana do require AMA-approved postgraduate training. California requires its own special oral clinical examination instead of ECFMG.

10. The relationship between FLEX scoring policies and the numbers of FMGs obtaining licenses in different states is discussed with the aid of statistical indicators by Butter (1976).

11. At present, only the District of Columbia at the Board's discretion will endorse a foreign license, but, at one time, as many as thirteen states gave their boards statutory authority to endorse licenses from foreign countries. Today, twenty-five states (and occasionally Rhode Island) will endorse a Canadian license issued by the Licentiate Medical Council of Canada (LMCC), and New York will accept a Canadian license for endorsement when it is accompanied by Specialty Board Certification or a passing score on Day 1 of FLEX. Information regarding the endorsement of Specialty Board Certification was not available before 1974, so that it was impossible to trace trends in this endorsement option. At the present time,

West Virginia, Massachusetts, and Virginia will issue full licenses by endorsement to Specialty Board diplomates, and New York will endorse certain foreign specialty board certificates. With respect to the documentation of credentials, the Maine licensure board reports that FMGs who possessed only copies of their medical school diplomas, and were therefore unable to obtain initial licenses in other states requiring the original document, were obtaining full licenses in Maine, which will substitute an ECFMG certificate for the diploma, and then seeking endorsement of the Maine license elsewhere.

12. A comprehensive survey and analysis of requirements, durations, and renewal procedures of states' less-than-full licensure policies in 1975 is presented in Butter (1976).

13. Although ECFMG certification is officially required of FMGs in most less-than-full practice situations in the U.S., the requirement is not always enforced. A large number of FMGs exist in a "medical underground"; uncertified by ECFMG, they have still found employment in hospitals (many of them government institutions) and work "with a high degree of independence . . . in physician roles despite the lack of adequate United States credentials" (Weiss et al., 1974).

REFERENCES

Butter, I. 1976. *Foreign Medical Graduates: A Comparative Study of State Licensure Policies.* U.S. Dept. of Health, Education, and Welfare, Washington, D.C., Publication No. (HRA) 77-3166.

Derbyshire, R.C. 1969. *Medical Licensure and Discipline in the United States.* Baltimore: The Johns Hopkins Press. p. 52.

Stevens, R.; Goodman, L.W.; Mick, S.S.; Darge, J.G. 1975. Physician Migration Reexamined, *Science* 190 (October): 440, Table 3.

Stevens, R., and Vermeulen, J. 1975 *Foreign Trained Physicians and American Medicine.* U.S. Dept. of Health, Education, and Welfare, Washington, D.C., Publication No. (NIH) 73-325. p. xiv.

Weiss, R.; Kleinman, J.; Brandt, U.; Feldman, J.; and McGuinness, A. 1974. Foreign Medical Graduates and the Medical Underground, *New England Journal of Medicine* 290:1408–1413.

2.6 To Practice or Not To Practice: Developing State Law and Policy on Physician Assistants*

HARRIS S. COHEN and WINSTON J. DEAN

Reprinted with permission of the Milbank Memorial Fund, from 52 *MMFQ/Health and Society* 349–376 (1974). Copyright © 1974 by the Milbank Memorial Fund. All rights reserved.

The recent advent of the physician assistant phenomenon—in which a specially trained non-physician practices medicine under the supervision of a physician—has generated extraordinary interest and conjecture. While physician assistants are still relatively few in number, the concept represents a bold departure from traditional medical education and practice, as well as a potential solution to the problem of physician maldistribution. One area of particular interest and concern has to do with the legal and public policy issues centering on the practice of medicine (albeit a limited and circumscribed degree of medicine) by a non-physician. Recognizing that health manpower roles and responsibilities, generally, are in large measure determined by the numerous state laws that define the scopes of practice in the health professions, it is not surprising that the legal issues in this area have gained such prominence in the ensuing discussion and deliberations on the physician assistant.

This paper provides a current analysis of the law and policy that have developed in the states in reponse to the physician assistant (hereafter, PA) concept. In contrast to earlier studies (Curran, 1970a; Willig, 1971; Ballenger, 1971; George-

town Law Journal, 1971; Sadler and Sadler, 1971; Pratt, 1972; Dean, 1973; Howard and Ball, 1973; Barkin, 1974) that were based almost exclusively upon the *statutory* law relating to PAs and the need for statutory recognition of the PA, this paper will focus on a later point in the evolution of state policy, i.e., the adoption of administrative rules and regulations. Thus the present study contributes to the previous work in this area not only a more current analysis of public policy, but also a more realistic appraisal, based upon the state regulations, of what the PA may or may not do.

It should be pointed out that we are still not able to speak very concretely about the states' actual *implementation* of their PA laws and regulations. We are dealing, of course, with a very current and fluid policy issue, and one with potential for substantial administrative discretion. Generally, the greater prominence of discretionary action over formal rules in administrative behavior is due to the fact that in a large number of policy issues either "no one knows how to formulate rules," or "discretion is preferred to any rules that might be formulated" (Davis, 1969:15). Certainly this is the case with regard to state policy on PAs. Notwithstanding the detail provided in some of the statutes and regulations, a great deal of discretion is afforded to each of the parties involved in the state's regulation of the PA. Subsequent studies of PA law will need to address systematically the actual implementation of such policy, and attempt to evaluate the impact of specific regulatory provisions.

---

*This is a revised version of a paper presented at the Conference on State Mid-Level Health Worker Planning, sponsored by the Health Manpower Policy Study Group, School of Public Health, University of Michigan, May 13, 1974. The views expressed in the paper are those of the authors.

As mentioned above, writers on this subject have pointed out the need for statutory recognition of the PA so that both he and his supervising physician (hereinafter, SP) would be accorded legal protection from charges of practicing medicine without a license or aiding and abetting the illegal practice of medicine. Thirty-seven states have enacted legislation permitting PAs to practice under the supervision and direction of a physician. Although specific details of the PA statutes vary considerably, they take two basic forms: One form of PA law, the *general-delegatory model,* is an amendment to the medical practice act that gives the physician authority to utilize a PA under his direction and supervision. No other formal requirements are provided, and the SP is thus accorded the widest latitude in selection and utilization of the PA. Seven states have enacted this type of amendment to the medical practice act, which is exemplified by the language of the Connecticut statute:

> The provisions of this chapter (Medical Practice Act) shall not apply to . . . any person rendering service as a physician's trained assistant, a registered nurse, or licensed practical nurse if such service is rendered under the supervision, control, and responsibility of a licensed physician.

Some of the pros and cons of this type of statutory approach have been discussed previously (see Dean, 1973) and, therefore, will not be repeated in this paper. The second form of PA law, the *regulatory-authority model,* authorizes a state agency, generally the state board of medical examiners, to develop and implement rules and regulations governing the education and practice of PAs. To date, 30 states have enacted this form of legislation. Note that Colorado has both a general-delegatory statute as well as the unique Child Health Associate Law which, for purposes of this paper, will not be considered a PA statute (Curran, 1970b; Silver, 1971; Cohen and Miike, 1973:4–5).

The analysis contained in this paper is based upon the most current PA statutes and regulations obtained from state agencies. Of the 30 states with regulatory-authority statutes, 10 states (Alaska, Hawaii, Iowa, Maryland, Massachusetts, Michigan, Nevada, South Carolina, South Dakota, and Wisconsin) had not yet issued PA rules and regulations at the time this information was collected, in early 1974. In most instances, the statutes in these states had been enacted only within the last year or so, thereby not permitting adequate time for the formulation of rules and regulations.

In compiling the current laws and regulations on PAs, the authors also addressed two questions to each of the state agencies responsible for approving PAs. One dealt with the number of PAs that already had been approved in each state. This information is included in the following table. Approximately 650 PAs have been approved for practice, including PAs employed in states with general-delegatory statutes. Although the total number of approved PAs appears small when compared to membership of other health occupations, it should be stressed that most PAs have been approved only within the last three years, and that educational programs are just now reaching the point where sizable numbers of PAs are being trained. Therefore, one may expect that the number of PAs will increase dramatically within the next several years, especially with increased federal support of PA training. The number of approved PA applicants, as listed in the table, also gives some indication of the administrative burden placed on various state regulatory agencies, an issue that is discussed again later in the paper. Our survey, incidentally, also confirmed one of the features of the general-delegatory statute discussed elsewhere (Dean, 1973:6); i.e., without state involvement in the PA approval process, data on the number and location of PAs practicing in the state are not usually available. We were also interested in obtaining information from the states on any litigation involving PAs since enactment of the PA statute, but no such litigation was reported.

REGULATING THE EDUCATION AND TRAINING PROCESS

While most of the state regulations require that the PA complete an approved training program, there is substantial variability in the specific approaches taken in regulating the education and training process. In many respects, this particular area of regulation is characterized by an even greater range or continuum of regulatory authority than the regulation of the individual

Table 2.6.1 Physician Assistants Approved by States (As of March 1, 1974)

State	Number of Approved PAs	State	Number of Approved PAs
Alabama	23	Nebraska	2
Alaska	26	Nevada	0
Arizona	5	New Hampshire	24
Arkansas	5[a]	New Mexico	6
California	10	New York	128
Colorado	NA[b,c]	North Carolina	75
Connecticut	NA	Oklahoma	19
Delaware	NA	Oregon	58
Florida	30	South Carolina	NA
Georgia	48	South Dakota	NA
Hawaii	NA	Tennessee	NA
Idaho	13	Utah	19
Iowa	12[d]	Vermont	9
Kansas	NA	Virginia	50[e]
Maine	NA	Washington	57
Maryland	NA	West Virginia	28
Massachusetts	NA	Wisconsin	NA
Michigan	NA	Wyoming	6
Montana	2[a]		
		Total	655

[a]In some states with general-delegatory statutes, such as Arkansas and Montana, accurate information on the number of PAs practicing in the state is not available and the number reported pertains to those PAs in practice who are known to the agency reporting.

[b]Not available

[c]The number of PAs practicing under the Colorado general-delegatory statute is not available. However, it was reported that there are 23 approved "child health associates."

[d]Iowa is permitting PAs to practice pending promulgation of regulations.

[e]Includes both nurse practitioners and physician assistants. No breakdown available regarding the number of physician assistants.

PA. At the one extreme, some states are completely silent about the educational training process (although in addressing the PA's qualifications for state certification there may be some reference to his completing a PA training program, which is generally a minimum of two academic years). At the other extreme, states have assumed control over virtually *every* aspect of the PA educational program. Between these two poles, one finds a sweeping range of requirements that give the states control over the establishment, recognition, and functioning of PA training programs.

Medical School or University Sponsorship

A number of states stipulate that the education and training of PAs must be linked to the medical

education system in order to be approved by the state. Alabama, for example, requires that the PA "training program must be sponsored by a four year medical college or university with appropriate arrangements for the clinical training of its students, such as a hospital maintaining a teaching program." To be sure, this approach provides the opportunity to conduct PA training in close proximity to the training of physicians which may serve to enhance the level of sophistication and breadth of a PA training program.

But there are also potential drawbacks associated with medical school or university-hospital sponsorship that need to be considered. One is that it might preclude recognition of alternative training modalities capable of producing a significant supply of competent PAs in a given state. The military corpsmen, recognized in one state, for example, as eligible to take the

RN licensure examination, certainly represent a potential source of PA manpower. In addition, the community colleges could conceivably train large numbers of competent PAs but probably would not be approved in states requiring medical school or university-hospital sponsorship of PA training. Furthermore, by placing PA training within the medical education structure, the state regulations may have added to the PA credentialing process a new and potent actor, the medical school. Conceivably, some medical schools may consider the rapid development and growth of PAs as not being in the best interests of the medical profession. Thus, placing such training programs within the medical education system may be viewed as one means of checking the development of this occupational category.

Required State or National Accreditation of the PA Program

A number of states require that the PA training program be accredited by a national organization such as the Council on Medical Education of the American Medical Association in order to be approved by the state. Other agencies whose approval of a training program will satisfy a state's accreditation requirements include: the American Association of Medical Colleges, the American Osteopathic Association, the National Commission on Accrediting, the Department of Health, Education, and Welfare, the Department of Defense, and, at the state level, the department of education or board of medical examiners.

In delegating control of the *accreditation* process to national medical organizations, some states appear to have placed PA training and credentialing very heavily within the medical education system. In light of the recommendations by the Study of Accreditation of Selected Health Educational Programs (National Commission on Accrediting, 1972), urging adoption of a more broadly representative accrediting body for the allied health professions than the AMA's Council on Medical Education, some will surely question whether this same organization should be given such vast authority in the accrediting of PA programs as well. One must remember, of course, that in almost every instance, the administrative regulations for PAs were formulated by state boards of medical examiners. Thus the developing policy with respect to PAs is very much influenced by the same considerations of self-regulation and autonomy that characterize the role of professions in the licensure process (Cohen, 1973a).

Qualifications and Responsibility of Teaching Staff

Only a few of the states with regulatory authority in the area of PA training have specific requirements for preceptors and other teaching staff in the training programs. In these instances, the preceptor must be a licensed physician and generally must be present at the site of the training program. In some states, there appears to be sufficient flexibility in the requisite supervision of PA trainees in much the same way that the SP's supervision of the *practicing* PA is governed by the rule of "reasonable proximity to the physician."

In Vermont, the instructing physician must also certify to the department of health that a training plan was undertaken that includes specific skill objectives, performance standards expected of both parties involved, and a method of evaluation. This statement must be jointly signed by the PA and the teaching physician. Wyoming requires physicians involved in the training of PAs to register with the state and to provide the names of the PA trainees. This practice would appear to depart from that of other state-approved manpower categories.

Periodic Reports to the State

A number of states require the PA training programs to provide periodic evaluative reports on various aspects of the program. The Alabama regulations stipulate, for example, that in order to retain recognition, the training program must make available to the board of medical examiners annual summaries of case loads and educational activities including volume of outpatient visits, number of inpatients, and the operating budget, as well as a satisfactory record of the entrance qualifications and evaluations of all work done by each student. In addition, it must notify the board in writing of any major changes in the curriculum or a change in the directorship of the program.

Periodic Renewal of Program Approval

Approval of the PA training program in several states must be renewed periodically. In some instances, this is merely implied in the requirement of the program to report periodically to the state. Thus, if a program were to report major shifts in curriculum, directorship, or supervision, it is reasonable to expect that the state might rescind its approval of the program. It should be noted that the present disparity among the states with regard to approval of PA training programs may be due for some change. The AMA's recently published essentials (American Medical Association, 1974), dealing with curriculum, preceptorship, advisory committees, clinical instruction, and facilities of PA training programs, may bring about much greater uniformity in the states' regulation of PA training.

EQUIVALENCY AND PROFICIENCY ALTERNATIVES

The education and training of the PA is certainly a critical requirement in most of the regulations and, as pointed out above, is spelled out in considerable detail in several instances. But, as in other categories of health manpower, there are several alternative pathways that the PA applicant may present in lieu of the generally prescribed educational program. Such equivalency measures are extremely important in the area of PA credentialing for at least two reasons: First, this may facilitate the deployment into needed civilian positions of military corpsmen who otherwise might not qualify because of the educational requirements for state approval. Second, the PA concept is so new and dynamic that alternative options must be provided that recognize quality training of a different structure than that formalized in any given state. As noted by Cohen and Miike (1973:33–37), there is a growing acceptance in other health fields, as well, of educational equivalency designed to promote the more efficient utilization of manpower.

Several different approaches related to equivalency are found in the PA regulations. Vermont requires that candidates for PA registration shall have completed one of the following (a) a recognized PA program, (b) two years of

nursing school, (c) one year of medical school or school of osteopathy and one year of experience and training under a physician, or (d) two years of experience and training under a physician. In the latter two alternatives, the PA must have been trained to perform certain services listed in the regulations as the requisite PA skills. Vermont appears to be the only state that goes so far with the equivalency approach as to approve the PA without *any* didactic training—which would be the case if the candidate presented two years of experience under a physician as the basis of his PA training. In contrast, California permits full academic credit through equivalency measures, but provides that no student shall be graduated unless a minimum period of one year is spent in residence in full-time clinical training with direct patient contact.

The Georgia regulations require graduation from an approved PA program "or satisfactory completion of a formal course of study in the health field combined with actual work experience related to the program of study such that the total of these two segments would cover at least four years, provided that the combined study and experience of such applicant is consistent with the job description contained in the application." Equivalency in this case is interpreted almost in a "compensatory" fashion, with the applicant needing *four* years of substitute training instead of the two-year, formal PA program. In New York, the state health commissioner has the discretion of accepting—in lieu of all or part of an approved PA training program—evidence of an extensive health-oriented education and of appropriate experience and training. He may also require the applicant to pass a proficiency examination, which will be discussed below, and to make up deficiencies in his education or experience prior to registration. And, in Wyoming, the applicant may take an equivalency *examination* in lieu of completing a PA training program (although it is not clear whether the examination may be substituted for all or just part of the requisite didactic training).

The issue of educational equivalency also comes up in relationship to interstate reciprocity. Needless to say, an approved PA who moves across state lines may be faced with a different set of state requirements for PA approval. In the few state regulations that explicitly address the question of reciprocity, e.g., California and New York, PA applicants approved in other states must demonstrate that they have met equivalent educational requirements. But even in the majority of states that are silent on the issue of reciprocity, it is probably reasonable to infer such policy if the applicant can successfully demonstrate that his training was equivalent to the requirements of the new state.

With regard to proficiency testing, or the measurement of an individual's competency to perform at a certain job level (U.S. Department of Health, Education, and Welfare, 1971:53), five states (Alabama, New York, Oklahoma, Virginia, and Wyoming) authorize the use of proficiency testing, although the precise standards and the types of examinations are not spelled out. Maine and New Mexico permit PAs to practice if they have passed the national examination for assistants to the primary care physician developed by the National Board of Medical Examiners (NBME). In Nebraska, PAs may be approved who have been certified "under a national certification program of the American Medical Association's Council on Medical Education as 'program equivalent trained persons'; provided some measure of competency testing is utilized by the Council of Medical Education, such as the test developed by the National Board of Medical Examiners." In this connection, it is of interest to note that the states have been urged to adopt these certification measures, particularly the NBME examination, to satisfy the state requirements for professional competence of the PA (Casterline, 1974:119; Todd, 1972:566).

Although the number of PAs who have been approved by means of proficiency or equivalency mechanisms is not known at this time, it is clear that the laws and regulations, for the most part, provide relatively broad latitude for employing such mechanisms. The major obstacles to utilization of these mechanisms will probably not be posed by the presence of legal restrictions, as is the case in other health manpower categories, but by the operational complexity of developing reliable tests for measuring competency and in defining what constitutes an appropriate substitution for PA training.

According to Casterline (1974:120), evaluation of the PA's on-the-job training and experience will ultimately require validation by the SP, who is subject to regulation by his own state board of medical examiners. This assumes, of course,

that the medical boards are viable and effective monitors of the professional competence of practicing physicians. However, as we point out below with regard to board discipline and sanctions, this assumption rests on very shaky ground.

JOB DESCRIPTION

Among the several provisions incorporated in the PA statutes and regulations to afford suitable protection for the public is the requirement that a job description be submitted together with the application to the state for PA approval. Seventeen states (Alabama, California, Florida, Georgia, Idaho, Iowa, Nebraska, New Hampshire, North Carolina, Oklahoma, Oregon, South Dakota, Vermont, Virginia, Washington, West Virginia, and Wyoming) require such job descriptions which typically must list in detail all tasks that the SP might delegate to the PA. The PA must also indicate that he has sufficient training and ability to perform the functions listed in the job description. Generally, the state regulatory body is also authorized to require that the PA demonstrate his competence, if this is deemed necessary to make a thorough evaluation of the PA's qualifications.

In some states (Alabama, California, New Hampshire, Vermont, Virginia, and Wyoming), the regulations contain a *detailed* list of tasks that may be performed by the PA. Notwithstanding the inclusion of such lists in the regulations, *elastic* clauses may be found that permit the PA to perform additional duties, provided his competency to assume greater responsibility is appropriately demonstrated to the regulatory body. This suggests, therefore, that the PA regulatory agencies have substantial discretion in approving the roles and duties that can be assumed by a particular PA. In states where job descriptions are required, the PA has the option of demonstrating advanced or specialized skills and, thereby, to receive approval to practice in accordance with his unique training and skills. Where the regulations do not require a job description or provide a detailed task list, there is an implied authority for the PA to perform, under the direction and supervision of a physician, those tasks that he is competent to perform.

Job descriptions may provide a useful mechanism for regulatory agencies to determine how a

PA will be utilized by a physician. This is especially important in light of the fact that PA training programs remain diversified in terms of content and that no single standard for PA competency has been agreed upon. Nevertheless, there are several potential disadvantages to the job description requirement. Administratively, it places upon the regulatory agency the burden of reviewing each application on an individual basis. Each application must be reviewed to compare the training and experience of the PA to the proposed list of functions that he will perform. In cases where questions are raised about the capability of the PA to perform certain tasks, an effort must be made to determine the PA's qualifications by means of interviews, examinations, or some other method. In some states, the regulatory agency is required to interview both the PA and the SP. Needless to say, this is an extremely time-consuming process and may seriously strain the resources of the regulatory agency if a large number of applications are received. This is particularly the case in those states where the members of the regulatory agency serve on a volunteer basis and have but modest staff resources.

Another potential difficulty relates to liability of the PA and SP in the event that the PA does not adhere to the approved job description. It would appear that in most states this could result in withdrawing the SP's right to employ a PA, as well as the PA's right to practice. Additionally, an injured patient in a malpractice action might receive the benefit of a legal inference of negligence if it can be shown that the injury occurred while the PA was functioning beyond the limitations of his job description. This possibility clearly underlines the need for both the PA and the SP to stay within the bounds of the job description. As the PA acquires the skill to perform additional procedures, the job description should be amended before new duties are assigned.

STATE APPROVAL OF THE SP

The fact that PAs or, in many instances, the PA training programs, must be approved by the state is not at all unique, and resembles the same fundamental approaches found in the credentialing requirements of other categories of health manpower. However, what is unique with respect to the state's regulation of PAs is the re-

quirement in a number of states that not only the PA be approved but the SP as well. This opens up a new avenue of controls not generally found in other areas of state manpower regulation. Casterline (1974:120–121) justifies the need for this approach:

A substantial number of statutory exemptions in many licensing jurisdictions allow physician's assistants *to practice medicine* under the direct supervision of a physician. In such cases, the physician must have more than a casual relationship with his PA. Often an employment contract stipulates the responsibility of the physician and his assistant and the duties the PA will be authorized to perform. Such a contract and "job description" when filed with a board of medical examiners then becomes documentation relating to the continued licensure of the physician as well as the registration of the PA. Therefore, . . . it is important for state medical boards to assume the responsibility of approving, in essence, the physician-mentor to serve in that role.

Another commentator (Howard, 1972:102) notes that the early thinking on PA legislation was largely based on the notion that "because the physician's assistant works in close relationship with the physician, the physician is in the best position to know the extent of his competence and should be relied on as the primary regulator of his activity."

In the case of California the SP must provide the state board of medical examiners with detailed information on his own qualifications to supervise the PA. Specifically, the California regulations require the SP to submit the following information:

The professional background and specialty of the proposed Supervising Physician, information pertaining to the medical education, internship and residency of said physician, enrollment in continuing educational programs by said physician, membership or eligibility therefor in American Boards in any of the recognized areas of medical specialty by said physician, hospitals where staff privileges have been granted, the number of said physician's certificate to practice medicine and surgery in the State of California, and such other information the Board deems necessary. Participation by the proposed Supervising Physician as a preceptor in an approved educational program for an Assistant to the Primary Care or Specialist Physician should be indicated and whether the proposed Physician's Assistant was supervised by said physician pursuant to such preceptorship program. The application should indicate the number of other Physician's Assistants supervised by the proposed Supervising Physician and whether any other applications to supervise a Physician's Assistant have been filed with the Board which are then pending. A description by the physician of his practice, including the nature thereof and the location and the way in which the Assistant is to be utilized.

In addition, the California regulations include as one of the grounds for either denying approval initially to supervise a PA or subsequently revoking, suspending, or placing on probation such approval "the failure of the Supervising Physician to participate in and meet the minimum requirements of a continuing education program satisfactory to the Board." It should be noted that this requirement is inconsistent with the state's present licensure requirements of other physicians who do not supervise PAs (where the state does not now require continuing education as a condition to practice medicine). Given this disparity between the regulation of SPs on the one hand and the general physician population on the other, one would anticipate a "chilling" effect from such a provision that discourages widespread utilization of PAs by California physicians. Similar comments will be made below on some of the other provisions of California's PA policy.

Other examples of controls on the SP are the requirement in Nebraska of a signed statement by the SP that he will not delegate or authorize any PA to engage in any of the health professions, other than medicine or surgery, unless such PA has the proper license therefor. And in Alabama the SP must have been in practice for at least five years (three years for a board-certified specialist) to be eligible to supervise a PA.

While in most cases the regulations do not specifically require the approval of the SP, such authority is at least implied in the large number of states that require the SP to provide the state with a job description for the proposed PA. Certainly, it can be argued that if a proposed job description revealed a fundamental lack of understanding on the part of the SP as to the tasks that a PA was capable or incapable of performing, the situation would be scrutinized, and possibly result in rejection of the application. It should also be noted, with respect to approval of the SP, that in some states the applicant for PA approval is the SP acting in behalf of the PA (and in a number of instances it is the SP who must pay the application fees and not the PA).

SUPERVISION

Although the statutory language with regard to supervision may vary, each of the state laws and regulations indicates that the PA is to function in a *dependent* or agency relationship to his SP. A relationship of this type obviously suggests that the SP must assume responsibility for the proper supervision of his PA, and, to this end, the statutes and regulations governing this supervisory requirement take several forms. To ensure that no SP employs more PAs than he is theoretically capable of supervising, most of the statutes and regulations limit the number of PAs that can be employed. Seven states (Alabama, Arizona, Colorado, Idaho, Nevada, Oregon, and Washington) allow only one PA per physician, while 14 states (California, Florida, Georgia, Iowa, Maine, Massachusetts, Nebraska, New Hampshire, New Mexico, New York, North Carolina, Oklahoma, Virginia, and Wyoming) allow two PAs per physician. The remaining 16 states with PA laws have not addressed this issue, either statutorily or in the administrative regulations. Clearly, this type of limitation does not *guarantee* that the physician will provide adequate supervision of the PA, but it does prevent one potential abuse of the PA concept by physicians who might be willing to incur risks of civil liability by employing large numbers of PAs in order to enhance the scope and potential profitability of their practices.

For the most part, the PA statutes do not provide the specific requirements for PA supervision; most of the laws simply declare that the PA must practice under the "supervision and control" of the physician. Responsibility, however, for defining the level and type of requisite supervision is delegated to the state administrative agency that must approve PAs. In response to this authority, these agencies have developed a variety of definitions and requirements for supervision. Most PA regulations do not require direct, over-the-shoulder supervision of the PA by the physician. The North Carolina regulations exemplify this approach:

> The assistant must generally function in reasonable proximity to the physician. If he is to perform duties away from the responsible physician, such physician must clearly specify to the Board those circumstances which would justify this action and the written policies established to protect the patient.

A similar provision appears in the regulations of five other states (Alabama, Florida, Virginia, West Virginia, and Wyoming).

Although this type of language presents some interpretative problems such as what is meant by the terms "reasonable proximity" or "perform duties away from the responsible physician," it does allow for flexibility so that the regulatory body can meet unique problems that may arise. For example, if a physician in an isolated rural area were to seek permission to utilize a PA outside of the office setting and without personal, direct supervision, the state body would have an opportunity to review all aspects of the matter, including medical care needs in the area and PA qualifications, and then make a decision on the merits of the individual case. Obviously, this type of regulatory approach vests a great deal of discretionary power in the hands of the regulatory agency—which, incidentally, poses a number of administrative law issues. Operationally, it means that the agency may have to spend a considerable amount of time making decisions on a case-by-case basis.

In three states (Maine, New York, and Oklahoma), the SP is not required to be physically present when the PA is providing services, but neither is there any further clarification or specification concerning standards of supervision. Unless there is some provision in the regulations to furnish guidance on this point, the burden seems to fall on the SP to determine how he will supervise his PA. This ambiguity is removed to some extent in Oklahoma by the requirement there that the SP submit a job description outlining how he intends to utilize the PA.

The question of over-the-shoulder supervision is approached in another way by Georgia, Nebraska, and Washington. These states stipulate that the SP need not be physically present when the PA is performing his delegated tasks so long as the PA is functioning in the office or normal place of practice of the SP. Georgia also allows the PA to make house calls, hospital rounds, serve as an ambulance attendant, or perform functions normally performed by the SP, if the PA is qualified. Here, again, the amount and type of supervision required when the PA performs these functions is not spelled out.

Nebraska further liberalizes its supervision requirement by stating that personal presence of the SP is not required if the PA functions in a licensed hospital where his SP is a member of the medical staff and where the hospital board has given its approval. The PA may also deliver care outside of the office or hospital setting (a) if the patients are specifically named and designated on a daily basis, and (b) if the geographical location of such PA functions is identical to the places of primary practice of the SP. The state of Washington permits certain types of well-qualified PAs to practice in remote areas away from the SP provided that approval is obtained from the state's board of medical examiners. The regulations, however, require that the SP review at least weekly all patient care provided by the PA if such care is rendered without direct consultation of the SP. The SP is also required to countersign all notes made by the PA.

In Arizona and Oregon, another approach to supervision is taken. The regulations in these states stipulate that a PA shall not exercise independent judgment in making a diagnosis or prescribing treatment except in life-threatening emergencies. The PA is required to report the results of his examination to the SP who then makes the diagnosis and prescribes the treatment. An even more restrictive approach governing the method of PA performance is found in the California and New Hampshire regulations:

> Supervision of an Assistant to the Primary Care Physician . . . refers to the responsibility of the Primary Care Physician to review findings of the history and physical

examination . . . and all follow-up physical examinations with said Assistant together with the patient at the time of completion of such history and physical examination and to consult with said assistant and patient before and after the rendering of routine laboratory and screening techniques and therapeutic procedures . . . , excepting where the rendering of routine laboratory and screening techniques are part of the history and physical examination or follow-up examination performed.

These regulations do point out, however, that the presence of the SP is not required when the PA attends chronically ill patients at home, in nursing homes, or in extended-care facilities if such activity is for the sole purpose of collecting data for the SP.

The relatively strict approach to PA supervision evident in the Arizona, Oregon, California, and New Hampshire regulations poses a serious question as to whether PAs in these states will be able to fully utilize their training and experience. Advocates of the PA concept maintain that one of the primary objectives of this new category of health manpower is to relieve the physician of time-consuming, routine duties so that he may concentrate greater effort on more complex and demanding medical problems. Theoretically, the PA, with his special training and clinical experience, would be capable of examining patients, making some determination about the severity of their illnesses, referring to the physician those cases beyond his competence, and treating those problems that are within his competence. This *modus operandi,* if followed, implies that the PA must make some independent diagnostic and treatment decisions.

In barring the PA from making independent judgments relating to diagnosis and treatment, the Arizona and Oregon regulations have relegated the PA to a much more restricted role than is probably necessary, and have taken a markedly different approach from the majority of states with PA regulations. If the regulations are rigidly adhered to by physicians and PAs in these two states, the PA role may evolve into that of a technician responsible for conducting examinations, tests, and certain routine treatment procedures without being above to exercise any form of independent judgment. This requirement, by its very nature, would mean

that the PA must function near the physician. Accordingly, opportunities for utilizing the PA's skills in remote settings may not be available. It should be pointed out that these restrictions apparently have not curtailed PA registration in Oregon. As of March 1, 1974, the Oregon Board of Medical Examiners had approved 58 PAs, which represents one of the largest number of approvals among states with regulatory-authority statutes. Arizona had approved five PAs as of the same date, but the Arizona PA law was not enacted until 1972—a year after the Oregon law.

The supervision requirements promulgated in both California and New Hampshire also raise certain questions as to whether the PA might not be a potential liability to the physician. According to the regulations, the SP must consult with the PA after completion of a history and physical examination, and with *both* the patient and the PA before and after rendering treatment procedures. Such strict requirements for physician consultation and supervision involving all treatment procedures would dictate that the physician spend an inordinate amount of time consulting with patients and PAs, and may result in confining the PA's role to physical examinations only. This would certainly negate many of the advantages of PA employment altogether.

From a practical standpoint, the requirement that the PA practice in *reasonable* proximity to the physician unless otherwise authorized by the regulatory agency is probably the most prudent approach to take at the present time. This policy, along with a required position description, a limitation on the number of PAs per physician, and the statement that the SP in all cases is responsible for the acts of the PA, would appear to provide (a) the necessary flexibility to determine how PAs can be employed most effectively and efficiently, and (b) a reasonable degree of protection for the public.

PATIENT CONSENT

Three states (California, Virginia, and Washington) require consent of the patient before services may be rendered by a PA. The Washington regulations merely stipulate that informed consent will be required. California and Virginia, however, mandate that the patient must give prior written consent to the PA's performing medical services on an annual basis or as often as the patient is treated by a new PA. The requirement for patient consent appears to be unique to PAs, and it is conceivable that this, too, will cause a "chilling" effect on patient response inasmuch as patients may question why consent is needed for PA services when it is not required for other health workers. Physicians, too, are likely to regard the consent requirement as an unnecessary and unreasonable administrative burden, considering the attention that must be given to maintaining current, signed consent forms. In most states, PAs are also required to wear name tags or display appropriate certificates which clearly identify them as being a physician assistant. This name-tag requirement may serve the same purpose as patient consent for PA services because the PA is clearly identifiable. If the patient objects to being cared for by the PA, he can inform the SP.

REQUIREMENTS FOR ASSISTANTS TO THE SPECIALIST PHYSICIAN

Only a small number of PA laws and regulations address the situation of PAs working under the supervision of *specialist* physicians. The New York law authorizes the use of PAs by specialist physicians, and regulations for the orthopedic and urologic assistant are now being prepared by that state's commissioner of health and commissioner of education, who have joint responsibility for promulgating PA rules. California, too, has developed regulations for the assistant to the orthopedic surgeon and the assistant to the emergency care physician, in addition to its detailed requirements for the assistant to the primary care physician. The South Dakota law permits the assistant to the specialist physician to perform some of the same duties as the assistant to the primary care physician as well as any other specialized tasks for which training and proficiency can be demonstrated. (no PA regulations have as yet been developed in South Dakota.) In contrast, the Washington regulations, patterned after the typology advanced by the National Academy of Sciences (1970), suggest that the assistant to the specialist physician is *less* skilled and is qualified to perform only certain specialized tasks because he *lacks* the more general training and experience attributed to the assistant to the primary care physician.

Although not addressed either in the PA laws or regulations in most other states, it is certainly arguable that under their broad mandate to sanction PAs, state regulatory agencies have the authority to approve assistants to specialist physicians. This may be accomplished administratively in most states by requiring the PA and specialist SP to prepare a description of duties to be performed by the PA. This job description could then be evaluated with regard to the PA's *specialized* training and experience.

CONTINUED COMPETENCE

Although about half of the PA regulations explicitly require renewal of the PA's approval on an annual basis, most of these provisions merely stipulate payment of a renewal fee. Thus, as generally the case with other state-regulated categories of health manpower, re-registration is but a *pro forma* and routine process that does not involve any substantive review of the applicant's competence or performance. Inasmuch as state regulation of PAs is such a recent phenomenon, this is even more disturbing because it fails to take into account the growing concern for assurance of *continued* competence as opposed to *one-time*, initial entry competence. At a time when many of the older and more established health professions, e.g., medicine, dentistry, and nursing, are being required by states to satisfy certain basic, albeit tentative, measures of continued competence, such as continuing education, it would have been opportune for the states and, specifically, the medical profession to build into the PA credentialing process the rudiments of a meaningful renewal process that incorporated a review of the PA's performance, development, and continued capacity to function.

In this context, it is of interest to point out five different approaches to this problem that suggest at least some concern in the states with the issue of continued competence. The California regulations require that evidence be provided in the initial application for PA approval that both the SP and the PA are involved in a continuing education program approved by the state board of medical examiners. Oklahoma requires that prior to renewal of a PA's approval, there must be a review of the PA and the SP and his practice. An important component of the Vermont renewal process is the required certification by the SP that the previous year's performance of the PA was satisfactory. In Arizona and Oregon, upon termination of employment of a PA, the SP is required to submit a summary of reasons for, and circumstances of, termination of the PA's employment. This suggests an interest on the part of the state to examine the actual performance of the PA, and presumably this information would be utilized in any subsequent approval of that particular PA.

Arizona and Oregon also have provisions that require the SP to furnish reports, as required by the board, on the performance of the PA. It is not clear, however, if this report is to be submitted on a periodic basis or if the provision even extends to all SPs, or only to those SPs of whom the board specifically makes such request.

In Washington, the SP must submit together with the renewal application a current statement of utilization, skills, and supervision of the PA. In addition, the Washington regulations contain the provision "that the board will grant specific approval for tasks which may be performed by the assistant based upon the curriculum of the program from which the assistant graduated." However, requests for approval of newly acquired skills may be considered at any regular meeting of the board of medical examiners. Thus, any request by the SP for approval of additional task delegation would probably initiate a re-examination of the PA's qualifications. Moreover, in the event that a currently registered PA, in Washington, desires to become associated with another physician, such transfer may be accomplished administratively with approval of the chairman of the board of medical examiners, providing that the new SP is licensed and in good standing in the state and that evidence is submitted to document the continued competence of the PA.

Thus, while only a handful of states have provisions in their regulations that address the continued competence of PAs, there are at least a few good examples of this concern in the state regulations. These approaches should be evaluated, however, to determine whether they do, in fact, guarantee a minimum standard of competence. In this way, those approaches to continued assurance of PA competence that appear to have the greatest impact upon quality should be adopted by the other states. Clearly, this is an area of evaluative research that might have very

dramatic results on the developing credentialing policy on physician assistants.

DISCIPLINARY AUTHORITY

Disciplinary action can be taken against either the PA or his SP. Most of the regulations list all or most of the following grounds for revoking, suspending, or placing on probation PA approval: representing himself or permitting another to represent him as a physician; practicing beyond the scope of his authority or job description; habitually using intoxicants or drugs to the extent that he is unable to safely perform his duties; being convicted of a felony or criminal offense involving moral turpitude; suffering from a mental condition which makes him incapable of safely performing his duties; or failing to comply with the laws and regulations pertaining to PAs.

Although most of the PA regulations do not specifically address the question of what constitutes grounds for discipline of the SP with respect to his employment and supervision of the PA, state boards of medical examiners apparently have ample authority under the medical practice acts to take disciplinary action against the SP if he were to be found guilty of illegal or unethical conduct relating to employment and utilization of the PA. Several recent reports and studies, however, have argued, on the basis of the scant number of disciplinary actions reported, that agencies responsible for discipline of physicians and other health professionals have not discharged this responsibility very effectively (U.S. Department of Health, Education, and Welfare, 1971: 31–33; Cohen, 1973b; Derbyshire, 1974). The diverse educational backgrounds, experience, and employment settings of PAs coupled with the current lack of appropriate information about their effect on the health care system would make it imperative that state regulatory agencies fully discharge their monitoring and disciplinary functions pertaining to PAs and SPs in order to provide adequate protection of the consumer.

Several of the PA regulations contain unique grounds for disciplinary action. For example, the Alabama regulations provide that a physician may have his right to employ a PA withdrawn if he "has done or caused to be done any act which brings discredit to the medical profession and/or the 'Assistants to the Physicians' Program.'' This provision certainly follows the tradition noted by Cohen (1973b:53–54), of incorporating unusually vague and ambiguous terminology in the disciplinary requirements of professional practice acts. Another unique ground for disciplinary action is the California provision mandating that the SP and PA meet certain continuing education requirements; otherwise, the state may withdraw its approval of the PA to practice and of the SP to employ an assistant.

CONCLUSIONS

Although there is no agreement on the precise role of the PA in delivery of health services, recent studies (Nelson et al., 1974) suggest that patient acceptance of PAs is quite favorable. Such consumer reaction, if sustained, as well as the growth of federal assistance for PA training as one of several strategies to address the problem of medically underserved areas, will probably result in a significant increase in the production and utilization of PAs. Accordingly, regulatory agencies may face growing pressure to promulgate rules that will permit the most effective use of this new category of health manpower. The major pattern of PA legislation has been the granting of regulatory power to state boards of medical examiners, which would suggest continued reliance upon the customary regulatory mechanisms of health manpower. However, our analysis of the regulations already formulated by these agencies indicates very little consensus on the best model of quality assurance. In fact, the diverse nature of present PA regulations exemplifies the generally pluralistic system of state policy in the absence of federal legislation.

The diversity of PA regulatory policy among states raises an important question—should a national credentialing program be established? Given the significant maldistribution of health manpower in the country and the great variability in the training and utilization of PAs, it is appropriate that state agencies continue to have primary responsibility for PA approval. This type of decentralized control would facilitate the continued demonstration of expanding PA roles and competencies, especially in remote settings where direct supervision is impractical. Flexibility, therefore, must be the basic premise of any PA regulatory system.

While it is difficult to point to any of the PA regulatory schemes already developed as a model or ideal-type for regulating PA performance, given the unique and changing scope of this discipline, there are certain elements which, in our opinion, should be adopted universally: First, provision should be made to accept an application for approval from anyone who has passed the national certification examination developed by the NBME. This is based upon our expectation that the examination will undergo continual study and revision to reflect changes in the training and utilization of the PA.

Second, the employing physician should be required to provide a job description for the PA. This description of PA duties, similar in many respects to a contract, can then be reviewed in terms of the training and qualifications of both the PA and his SP as well as the type of medical practice involved. This approach offers a flexible and realistic means of regulating the PA. The SP, after all, bears the ultimate onus of responsibility in the event of any errors of omission or commission, and can be expected to exhibit appropriate care in preparing the job description for review by the state regulatory agency.

Third, the PA supervisory requirements should remain flexible and should be dependent upon the unique qualifications of the individual PA and the setting in which he works. There are numerous places in the country where it is necessary and appropriate to have PAs practicing in remote settings without direct, over-the-shoulder supervision. State regulations should permit such activity where proper safeguards are provided.

Finally, PAs should be required to demonstrate their continued competence on an annual basis, through performance ratings by their employing physicians, examinations, or some other evaluative mechanism that addresses the PA's performance.

These requirements, which are being implemented in a number of states, undoubtedly will place a growing burden on the present resources of state regulatory agencies. If these agencies are to perform their legislatively mandated functions, they must receive adequate financial support. Unfortunately, in some states, these responsibilities have been imposed upon the boards without any additional resources. This situation is inconsistent with the notion of accountability and responsibility inherent in any public agency, and certainly in a state board of medical examiners with its dramatic impact on the health and safety of the public. This brings us full circle to the issue of implementation touched upon at the outset of the paper. Without the necessary resources to administer a PA regulatory program, even the most elaborate administrative rules may have little bearing on the *actual* pattern of implementation.

REFERENCES

American Medical Association
1974   Guidelines for Educational Programs for the Assistant to the Primary Care Physician. Chicago: American Medical Association.

Ballenger, Martha D.
1971   "The physician's assistant: legal considerations." Hospitals, Journal of the American Hospital Association 45 (June 1):58–61.

Barkin, Roger M.
1974   "Need for statutory legitimation of the roles of physician's assistants." Health Services Reports 89 (January-February):31–36.

Casterline, Ray L.
1974   "Who should certify and/or register the physician's assistant?" Federation Bulletin 61 (April):117–122.

Cohen, Harris S.
1973a "Professional licensure, organizational behavior, and the public interest." Milbank Memorial Fund Quarterly/Health and Society 51 (Winter):73–88.
1973b "State licensing boards and quality assurance: a new approach to an old problem." Pp. 49–64 in U.S. Department of Health, Education, and Welfare, Quality Assurance of Medical Care. Washington, D.C.: U.S. Government Printing Office.

Cohen, Harris S., and Lawrence H. Miike
1973   Developments in Health Manpower Licensure. Washington, D.C.: U.S. Government Printing Office.

Curran, William J.
1970a "The California 'physicians' assistants' law." New England Journal of Medicine 283 (December 3):1274–1275.
1970b "New paramedical personnel—to license or not to license?" New England Journal of Medicine 282 (May 7):1085–1086.

Davis, Kenneth C.
1969   Discretionary Justice: A Preliminary Inquiry. Baton Rouge: Louisiana State University Press.

Dean, Winston J.
1973   "State legislation for physician's assistants: a review and analysis." Health Services Reports 88 (January):3–12.

Derbyshire, Robert C.
1974   "Medical ethics and discipline." Journal of the American Medical Association 228 (April 1):59–63.

Georgetown Law Journal
1971   "Paramedics and the medical manpower shortage: the case for statutory legitimization." Georgetown Law Journal 60:157–184.

Howard, D. Robert
1972   "The physician's assistant and national regulation." Federation Bulletin 59 (March):90–106.

Howard, D. Robert, and John R. Ball
1973   "The legal and professional recognition of physician's assistants." Federation Bulletin 60 (January):7–21.

National Academy of Sciences
1970   New Members of the Physician's Health Team: Physician's Assistants. Washington, D.C., National Academy of Sciences.

National Commission on Accrediting
1972   Study of Accreditation of Selected Health Educational Programs, Commission Report. Washington, D.C.: National Commission on Accrediting.

Nelson, Eugene C., Arthur R. Jacobs, and Kenneth G. Johnson
1974   "Patients' acceptance of physician's assistants." Journal of the American Medical Association 228 (April 1):63–67.

Pratt, Ralph D.
1972   "Determining legal sanctions for the p.a." Physician's Associate 2 (April 1):47–49.

Sadler, Alfred M., and Blair L. Sadler
1971   "Recent developments in the law relating to the physician's assistant." Vanderbilt Law Review 24:1193–1212.

Silver, Henry K.
1971   "New allied health professionals: implications of the Colorado Child Health Associate Law." New England Journal of Medicine 284 (February 11):304–307.

Todd, Malcolm C.
1972   "National certification of physicians' assistants by uniform examinations." Journal of the American Medical Association 222 (October 30):563–566.

U.S. Department of Health, Education, and Welfare
1971   Report on Licensure and Related Health Personnel Credentialing. Washington, D.C.: U.S. Government Printing Office.

Willig, Sidney H.
1971   "The medical board's role in physician assistancy." Federation Bulletin 58 (April):126–159; (May):167–201.

ISSUES FOR CONSIDERATION AND SUGGESTIONS FOR FURTHER READING

How should the poor be accommodated in hospitals?

Should physician's assistants be assigned greater roles in providing health care? Should they function with close supervision, limited supervision, no supervision? What does your state's law provide with respect to physician's assistants?

For a thorough discussion of the impact of the Health Professionals Educational Assistance Act of 1976 (P.L. 94–484) on the entry of FMGs into the United States, see Kaye, Danilou, and McDonald, "Alien Physicians and Their Admis-sion into the United States," 16 *San Diago L. Rev.* 61 (1978).

To what extent should the delivery of health care and the availability of health care person-nel, particularly physicians, depend on emigra-tion policy? Is this a proper way in which to address these issues?

In view of the proportion of public resources required to train health professionals in other, often less developed, countries, is it appropriate to lure foreign professionals to the United States with higher salaries and other benefits?

CHAPTER 3

THE ROLE OF LAW IN PROTECTING THE PUBLIC'S HEALTH

OVERVIEW

The articles included in this chapter explore various aspects of the role of law in the protection of public health. The provocative examinations by Wecht and Fielding of the controversial swine flu immunization program review many of the issues inherent in mass immunization. The legal status of compulsory immunization laws at the state level has been long upheld.[1]

The excerpt from Doniger's article on the regulation of the carcinogen vinyl chloride is intended only as an introduction to the complexities of identifying and regulating new environmental hazards as well as fixing regulatory responsibility on the part of competing governmental agencies.

Environmental law is a varied field, and the article by Altschuler tells succinctly an involved yet interesting tale of the pitfalls of regulation as applied to lead paint. The specifics of her story are detailed in the cases noted at the end of this chapter. The *Dunson* case is included as a recent state court decision dealing with the lead paint problem from the perspective of private (tort law) remedy. It involves an action by a tenant/father whose children ingested paint chips containing lead; he seeks redress from his landlord for negligence in failing to remove the dangerous paint.

NOTE

1. Jacobson v. Massachusetts, 197 U.S. 11 (1905).

lated. Although believed to be the same, it was the 1933 virus to which personnel at the CDC were comparing the Fort Dix Virus, so they could not be positive that the Fort Dix virus and the 1918–1919 virus were the same organisms. Second, conditions for a pandemic were ripe in 1918–1919. Massive troop movements facilitated the rapid spread of the virus, and no antibiotics existed at that time to combat the secondary infections that frequently were the actual cause of death. In 1976, neither of those situations existed. Third, the experiments already discussed strongly suggest that swine flu by itself is fairly harmless. The bacillus that seems necessary to produce serious swine flu results was not isolated from the Fort Dix throat swabs. Fourth, the Sergeant who resuscitated Private Lewis did not become ill, suggesting that the virus Lewis carried might not have been especially prone to pass from human to human. This possibility seems plausible in light of the low number of confirmed cases of swine flu at Fort Dix. Fifth, as Colonel Bartley has speculated, Private Lewis might not have died if he had not gone on the march.[5] Sixth, as to the FDA's theory that the swine flu virus was harbored in hogs and was waiting to strike humans, one must ask the obvious question—why now? The majority of the American public had not had immunity to swine flu for many years. Why should the swine flu virus pick 1976–1977 to reappear?

Clearly, in view of the *possibly* grave significance of the Fort Dix flu outbreak, public health officials should have reacted with concern and should have proceeded cautiously. Unfortunately, they instead reacted with alarm and proceeded headlong. On February 20, 1976, while the CDC was still involved in a search throughout the country for swine flu cases—a search that was yielding undefinitive results—the FDA's Bureau of Biologics held a workshop aimed at getting representatives of government, industry, and universities to begin preparations for undertaking a vaccination campaign should one be instituted.[6] During that meeting, the date of April 1, 1976 was suggested as the latest time at which a "go, no go" decision could be made and still leave sufficient lead time for the necessary preparations. Next, on March 10, 1976, a meeting of the CDC's Advisory Committee on Immunization Practices convened. This group generally recommends to the CDC Director— Dr. David Sencer, at that time—whether, and, if

so, precisely what type of, an immunization program should be undertaken by the federal government in response to a particular situation. It took the position that the government should stockpile a vaccine for swine flu and develop plans for administering it, but it did not make any statement as to whether the government should actually proceed yet with a mass vaccination program.[7]

A decision to stockpile and wait was made by the appropriate Committee. How, then, did we end up with a Swine Flu Immunization Program? Immediately following the Advisory Committee Meeting, Dr. Sencer prepared an "action memo" recommending a full-blown immunization program. The memo suggested the strong possibility of a swine flu pandemic and noted that ". . . the Administration can tolerate unnecessary health expenditures better than unnecessary death and illness. . . ."[8] After the memo began to make its way through the HEW bureaucracy, Dr. Sencer contacted the Advisory Committee members and asked them if they agreed with it. According to Dr. Sencer, the majority did. The memo traveled to the White House rapidly. President Ford's reaction was to appoint a blue ribbon panel to meet, on 48 hours notice, to consider Dr. Sencer's proposal. That Committee met on March 24, and recommended that the President go ahead with an immunization program. Minutes after the meeting ended, President Ford appeared on national television and called for the vaccination against swine flu of every man, woman, and child in the United States.

There probably were two main reasons why the majority of the members of the Advisory Committee on Immunization Practices supported Dr. Sencer's memo. First, even though they may have felt that the possibility of a pandemic was slight, the members must have known that upper-level federal bureaucrats already had the memo, and the members may have felt that it was better to agree and protect themselves than to disagree and leave themselves open to attack from above should a pandemic actually occur. A second probable reason for their assent is suggested by a candid comment made by Harry Meyers, Director of the Bureau of Biologics. He has been quoted as saying, after the Bureau's February 20 workshop, "In the world I deal with every day, there are so many things you do that are not terribly interesting. . . . To have a challenge of something that is a real public health interest is really stimulating."[9] Perhaps this comment reflected an atmosphere in the public health community that was highly receptive to a major public health challenge—whether the catastrophic threat to the health of the American public was real or imagined.

Dr. Sencer's memo moved quickly through the bureaucracy because of the fear it produced in laymen with such ominous phrases as "strong possibility [of a pandemic]" and "unnecessary death and illness."[10] President Ford did not have sufficient specialized knowledge to doubt Dr. Sencer. Furthermore, by this time, wild rumors concerning an imminent epidemic were circulating around Washington. The upcoming election doubtlessly caused President Ford to be very receptive to the Swine Flu Immunization Program. It was a natural headline grabber. If a 1977 swine flu pandemic had occurred, but Americans had been spared due to the efforts of President Ford, he might have emerged as a national hero.

The members of the blue ribbon panel really had no other choice but to recommend as they did. On 48 hours notice, they had no time to research the situation. The scientists on the panel were chosen by those proposing the program. Besides, by the time the question reached the panel, it had such political momentum that the decision was for all practical purposes already made. If the Committee *had* been free to explore the situation, hopefully it would have taken cognizance of two very important facts: (1) the supposed outbreak of swine flu at Fort Dix had limited itself to the military installation (not one case had been reported elsewhere); and (2) not a single case of swine flu had been reported in the six weeks since Private Lewis died at Fort Dix. These facts alone were sufficient to require limiting the decision to beginning the process of stockpiling and of planning a method for implementation of an immunization program if one later appeared essential. There was simply no indication that the Fort Dix virus had the potential to cause a pandemic.

Upon analyzing the governmental decision-making process that led to the commitment of 135 million tax dollars, it becomes apparent that no attempt was made to utilize a formal decision-making model. Yet such a model would have been relatively easy to develop. For example, subsequent to the March 24 decision, three experts from Harvard University developed a formal model that rationally and objectively evaluated the desirability of the Swine Flu Immunization Program; and they did it in less time (three weeks) than the actual decision took (February 20, 1976 to March 24, 1976).[11] By identifying various components of the program, any one of which would have changed the decision, they established that the Swine Flu Program would have been desirable only if: (1) the vaccine was highly effective; (2) the cost per vaccination was below $50; (3) there was a minimum of 59 percent population participation; and (4) there was a high probability of dealing with a pandemic strain of virus. Although information sufficient for reaching a decision through examination of all of these factors was not available when the decision was made, using a comparable model drawing on such information as *was* available would have lent order, reason, and credibility to the decision.[12] Instead, the decision was haphazard, emotional, and questionable in the public eye. It was strong-armed into being and had a political taint.

IV. THE GOVERNMENT'S FAILURE TO REEVALUATE THE PROGRAM

The Swine Flu Immunization Program was plagued with problems even before the first inoculation was given. Shortly after the March 24 decision was made, one of the four manufacturers selected to produce the swine flu vaccine produced two million doses of the wrong vaccine.[13] The CDC had supplied the manufacturers with the wrong virus.

Once the proper vaccine began to be produced, more serious problems occurred. First, testing to determine the proper dosage ran into trouble. If enough vaccine was used to produce sufficient antibodies to the flu virus, the reaction to inoculation was too common and too great. On the other hand, a dosage that did not produce so much reaction produced insufficient antibodies to be effective.

When a relatively acceptable dosage was finally found, it still produced considerable adverse reactions. Studies showed that 1 to 5 percent of those inoculated could expect to develop a fever of 100 degrees F. or higher; 20 to 40 percent could expect swelling, tenderness, and redness at the point of inoculation; and 20 percent could expect systemic reactions such as headache and general malaise.[14] As testing continued, a minimum of 1.9 percent of the inoculated individuals experienced severe reactions to the vaccine.[15]

When this last figure came to light, the Swine Flu Program hit its toughest preliminary snag. The insurance companies carrying the manufacturers' liability insurance refused to underwrite production and sale of the vaccine. Insurance representatives based their decisions on three factors, which, along with the insurers' fears attributable to the sheer magnitude of the program, made their nonparticipation inevitable. First, the companies had limited experience with large scale single disease vaccination programs, and none on the scale projected for the Swine Flu Program. Thus, they found it impossible to come up with a reasonably accurate prediction of what premiums they should charge.

Second, the companies estimated that even if the 1.9 percent severe reaction rate found in the preliminary studies held true in the general populace, and if the affected 1.9 percent were the only claimants, and if they based their claims only on strict liability (excluding negligence, etc.), the insurers' costs still could run as high as $5 billion. Premiums to cover such a possibility would be close to $341 million, or 2½ times the cost of the program itself.

Third, the insurance companies greatly feared strict liability. A recent case, *Reyes v. Wyeth Laboratories,*[16] clearly illustrates the companies' predicament. In that case, a child received standard trivalent polio vaccine, and subsequently developed polio. In a suit brought by the child's father against the manufacturer of the vaccine, a jury found that the vaccine had caused the child's polio, and reached a verdict against the manufacturer. The U.S. Court of Appeals, Fifth Circuit, in affirming the verdict, stated that the vaccine, although not "unreasonably dangerous" per se, was "unreasonably dangerous" as marketed, because the manufacturer had not met its duty to warn the child's parents of the risks of the vaccine. Insurance representatives felt the swine flu vaccine was unreasonably dangerous (that is, in the *Reyes* court's words, "dangerous beyond the contemplation of the ordinary consumer") on at least one, and perhaps two, counts. First, without a doubt the vaccine was unreasonably dangerous because the experts themselves were not sure about its effects. Second, if the reaction rate was as predicted, it may also have qualified as unreasonably dangerous.

The pullout by those who make a living at studying risks should have been enough by itself to make the government pause. By late July, there should have been a reevaluation of the program. But additional facts, even more persuasive, should have militated against continuing the program. Not one case of swine flu had been reported in the five months since the Fort Dix episode. As a result, many early proponents of the immunization program, the eminent Dr. Albert Sabin of polio fame among them, were calling for stockpiling the vaccine and waiting, rather than proceeding with the actual inoculation program.[17] Additionally, an experiment had been performed wherein the virus from Fort Dix was injected into monkeys at a laboratory in Fort Detrick. The clinical reaction had been negligible.[18]

Tragically, a reevaluation did not occur. President Ford and HEW apparently were too committed to turn back. For them, it probably had become a basic matter of politics and saving face. The fear used as one of the devices to push the program through had been capitalized upon. What can only be described as propaganda had elicited such pervasive fear of swine flu that the public demanded the program. Had President Ford backed out in the heat of his election campaign, he might well have sunk his political ship. If viewed in this light, his decision to expend extraordinary effort to salvage the Swine Flu Program would not be difficult to understand.

V. THE FEDERAL SWINE FLU STATUTE: ADDING INSULT TO INJURY

President Ford's response to the liability dilemma, and apparently to any doubts he may have had about the inoculation program's value and safety, was to promote legislation whereby the federal government not only would finance the manufacturing of vaccine and administer the inoculation program, but in addition would act, in essence, as its own insurance and reinsurance carrier against future claims and lawsuits. His swine flu bill immediately met opposition for the same reasons that *ought* to have sparked a reevaluation. Primarily, legislators were skeptical because of the lack of reappearance of the swine flu. The bill stalled in committee and almost died until the Philadelphia Legionnaires' Disease hit the press. Many people thought that Legionnaires' Disease and Swine Flu were the same thing; therefore the demand for the Swine Flu Program intensified. President Ford met privately with several Congressional leaders to make a pitch for his swine flu bill. They agreed that there was a need and rewrote the original bill. The new edition was pushed through Congress through informal routes in record time; on August 12, 1976, President Ford signed into law P.L. 94-380, the National Swine Flu Immunization Program of 1976.[19]

The thrust of the statute was that the federal government became the liability insurer for the program. Vaccine manufacturers were relieved of liability for claims not based upon negligence. Although the consumers' sole remedy was against the government, the government could subrogate claims caused by any participant's negligence.[20]

The most unfortunate aspect of the statute was that it underwrote only those physicians and other providers who participated in the program free of charge. This, of course, tended to discourage private physicians' participation. Patients, therefore, frequently did not even consult their personal physicians because they knew the physicians would not administer the vaccine. If private physicians had been underwritten, more patients, especially high risk patients, probably would have consulted their personal physicians. Many of the untoward results could, thus, have been obviated, because most private physicians simply were not recommending the vaccine. Public physicians were.

Recent cases concerning required warnings and informed consent "appeared" in the statute in the form of a provision requiring[21]

[the] development, in consultation with the National Commission for the Protection of Human Subjects of Biomedical and Behavioral Research, and implementation of a written informed consent form and procedures for assuring that the risks and benefits from the swine flu vaccine are fully explained to each individual to whom such vaccine is to be administered. . . . Such procedures shall include the information necessary to advice [sic] individuals with respect to their rights and remedies arising out of the administration of such vaccine.

Millions of consent forms were printed pursuant to these requirements; however, they did not meet even minimal ethical, let alone legal, requirements.[22] The CDC itself did a survey which revealed that up to 13 percent (4.5 million) of the people who were vaccinated were not informed at all as to the possible side effects of the vaccine or as to their legal remedies.[23]

It is important to realize that the swine flu statute differed significantly from other legislation dealing with remedies against the government. The Federal Tort Claims Act,[24] for example, limits liability of the United States to situations involving negligent acts of employees, and specifically excludes claims arising from acts or omissions of parties exercising due care. The swine flu statute specifically allowed claims based upon any theory in tort, including strict liability and breach of warranty. The result is that once a claimant establishes a causative link between the swine flu vaccine and his damages, the government is practically defenseless. It was for this very reason that insurance companies backed away from the program. Much more thought should have been given to this aspect of the statute because, as will be seen later, the insurers' $5 billion cost estimate is turning out to be less far-fetched than it may once have seemed.

VI. EXAMPLES OF GOVERNMENT DISTORTIONS

Despite some last-minute administrative problems,[25] on October 1, 1976, the Swine Flu Immunization Program began, largely because of the government's distortions and omissions of information. Had the news media lived up to their excellent showing in reporting the Watergate affair, perhaps these tactics could have been unmasked in time. Unfortunately, the media let the public down. At a recent meeting of the American College of Physicians, two New York University researchers blasted the media for their coverage of the Swine Flu Program.[26] The researchers charged that pertinent questions involving attendant risks of the program were not asked. There was never a report on what swine flu is, or if and how the vaccine works.

Adversary reporting was minimal; that is, no one seemed to question the Ford Administration's motives. The conclusion of the researchers was that the reporters lacked sufficient medical knowledge to explore what was happening. They merely reported the events and information given to them, thus playing into the hands of the CDC.

For example, in late summer and fall of 1976, two very important studies were made which had the potential to cause the public to question the Swine Flu Program. Neither study was widely publicized by the CDC. Jerome C. Schulman and Peter Palesé, physicians who were located at the Mt. Sinai School of Medicine, concluded that the A/New Jersey flu virus was not a recombinant derived from current human strains of flu virus. Applying a widely accepted theory that recombination of human and animal strains of virus is necessary to produce a flu virus with pandemic potential, these two experts asserted that the Fort Dix virus probably could not cause a pandemic.[27] Their conclusion was corroborated by the most significant study carried out during the entire swine flu era. Drs. A.S. Beare and J.W. Craig of the Common Cold Research Unit at Salisbury, England imported some isolates of the A/New Jersey flu virus. They vaccinated six volunteers with the virus. Of the six, only four became ill. Their symptoms were mild. The other two volunteers never got sick, even though they were always in close proximity to the four ill volunteers. The conclusion of the study was that the A/New Jersey virus was not especially contagious, and that its effects were much more mild than the currently common A-Victoria flu.[28]

The CDC did not stop at omission; it apparently utilized some distortions as well. For example, in July, a public health booklet released in Pennsylvania contained the following report made by the CDC: "We now have adequate data to demonstrate that a *safe and effective* vaccine can be produced for adults. All products tested provided satisfactory immunity levels with only minimal side effects."[29] A similar release made in an FDA drug bulletin in August stated that ". . . clinical trials . . . have demonstrated that new monovalent swine flu vaccines produce significant antibody levels. . . ."[30] Yet, as already stated, researchers in fact were having difficulty finding an effective, yet safe, dosage, and they knew that

the side effects were not so minimal. Dr. Sabin recently stated that only one of the four manufacturers was producing a vaccine that provided an acceptable level of immunity, and that the effective vaccine worked in only a segment of the test population. Moreover, Dr. Sabin claims that the CDC was aware of this situation.[31]

The most pronounced misuse of the media by officials in charge of the program occurred on December 6, 1976. Two weeks after the inoculation program began, three deaths occurred in Pittsburgh, Pennsylvania. The three victims had received swine flu vaccine within an hour of one another at the same clinic and all three had died within the following six hours. The CDC "investigated" and concluded that the vaccinations were not the cause of the deaths. However, the Pittsburgh deaths caused the entire program to lag seriously. Then on December 6, 1976, Missouri public health officials and a CDC spokesman announced that a confirmed case of swine flu had occurred. A few days later, government spokesmen indicated that a mistake had been made. The patient in question did not have a confirmed case of swine flu. A number of officials remarked that they had not intended that the case be reported as a confirmed case of swine flu.

Why were these government actions objectionable? The reporting of the Missouri case by the CDC coincided exactly with a massive advertising campaign intended to bolster the diminished participation in the vaccination program. And although federal health officials knew a "mistake" had been made, they made no move to correct it. It was only after outside pressure was brought to bear that the "mistake" came to light. The only reasonable conclusion that can be drawn from the incident is that the release was at best a case of government capitalizing on a known prior program mistake and was at worst a deliberate hoax promulgated to assist the advertising campaign.

Also glaringly omitted from the swine flu literature was the fact that an excellent alternative to mass vaccination existed: the therapeutic administration, following diagnosis of the disease, of the drug Amantadine. Vaccines have a number of drawbacks. First, they must be specifically formulated for each new flu strain. Second, because they require two to three weeks to take effect, they must be administered in advance of an epidemic. (The result of these two facts is a sort of epidemiological roulette. Scientists must guess what the upcoming flu strain will be and then formulate a vaccine. If the actual flu strain differs enough from that which was anticipated the vaccine will be ineffective). Third, vaccines are totally ineffective after exposure to a virus. Fourth, they produce relatively severe side effects and generally have a low rate of effectiveness. Amantadine was a drug that had been extensively tested for more than ten years and had received FDA approval at just about the time the swine flu decision was being made in the Spring of 1976. Amantadine suffers none of the drawbacks of vaccine mentioned above. In addition, Amantadine has important plusses: (1) it is not specific for any flu virus—that is, it is equally effective against all strains; and (2) it is therapeutic, usually reducing flu symptoms within 48 hours. When all the facts are considered, Amantadine shows itself to be far superior to vaccines. Its low incidence of mild side effects make it especially appropriate for high-risk groups such as the chronically ill, the aged, and the very young. Amantadine's only apparent drawback is that it must be ingested daily. However, since it needs no lead time, the period during which it must be taken can be limited.[32]

A review of the information made available, and not made available, by the CDC shows just how unprincipled the agency's actions apparently were. Half-truths and omissions seemed to come in a steady stream throughout the immunization program. Even demonstrable distortions occurred. By fall, certain key federal public health agencies had become more than misguided; they had begun what appears from a distance to have been a concerted effort to cover up the failings of the program by manipulating the media and duping the public.

VII. THE "INVESTIGATION" OF THE PITTSBURGH DEATHS

In the entire swine flu episode, never was the federal government's abuse of the public trust more obvious than during the "investigation" of the three deaths that occurred in Pittsburgh during the first two weeks of the immunization program. This author, as Allegheny County Coroner, was directly involved in this "investigation."

Here is what happened. During a one hour period at a single clinic, five elderly inoculees suffered serious symptoms immediately following their swine flu vaccination. Three suffered reactions sufficiently severe to necessitate immediate hospitalization. Of those, one died within an hour of arrival at the hospital. Two others suffered side effects at the clinic, but were able to go home. They both died within approximately six hours. All five of the patients suffered the same symptoms: weakness, loss of color, dizziness, and difficulty in breathing. Autopsy findings at the Allegheny County Coroner's Office indicated that heart and lung problems caused the three deaths.

Thereupon, the Swine Flu Program was halted nationally during a whirlwind investigation of the deaths by CDC officials. First, the investigators conducted a telephone survey of local hospitals which revealed that no other persons with side effects from the vaccine had been admitted. Next, they turned to the clinic. They reported that it was well-organized, and was staffed by competent personnel who were using accepted procedures. That was essentially the extent of the investigation. Based upon it, the CDC purportedly cleared the vaccine as the cause of death, and the immunization program was resumed.

Although time was of the essence, the scope of the Swine Flu Program, and therefore of its potential consequences, demanded a much more in-depth investigation than that conducted. The evidence strongly suggested that there was a common thread among the deaths: five people with the same symptoms, all inoculated at the same clinic within an hour, including three sudden deaths from the same causes. The odds against such an occurrence being natural would seem astronomical. The CDC investigators pegged the possibility of three deaths occurring in this manner as only 1 in 50. One exhaustive statistical study has concluded that the probability was more on the order of 1 in 500,000.[33] Robert J. Armstrong, Chief of Mortality Statistics at the National Center for Health Statistics, has been reported as stating he had a gut feeling that the coincidental occurrence of three such deaths would be ". . . an extremely rare event—a tremendous longshot."[34]

The attitude in Pittsburgh of Allegheny County and Pennsylvania health officials was much like that of the President's blue ribbon panel. The investigators hardly could have been expected to be objective; after all, they were sponsoring the program. Furthermore, the investigators uniformly ignored or dismissed various theories presented by highly respected experts. This author, acting in his capacity as Coroner of Allegheny County, suggested that stress from standing in line and exposure to adverse weather conditions for hours may have been a factor. His theory was brushed aside. Not one month later, this author has learned, Dr. Hans Selye, widely regarded as the world's leading expert on human stress, commented that aged persons and chronically ill persons are particularly predisposed to have certain types of stress reactions, such as heart failure, following inoculations.

Two other possibilities suggested by this author also were dismissed lightly by investigators. One was the possible interaction between the vaccine and certain drugs that the deceased had been taking for various illnesses (*e.g.*, heart disease, hypertension, diabetes). The investigators could not imagine how such a possibility could occur; yet, no tests were performed. This author's suggestion that the vaccine might have been inadvertently injected into the victims' veins met a similar fate. Existing studies were similarly ignored—for example, reports in 1975 by several Russian scientists in three separate articles that they had found a relationship between myocarditis and vaccines.[35]

Perhaps the most obvious possibility of all was never investigated by the CDC. It was widely known that the swine flu vaccine was the first flu vaccine ever produced not containing the enzyme neuraminidase. The role that the enzyme's absence might have played in the Pittsburgh deaths should have been explored immediately.

The lack of in-depth investigation into the deaths of the three people in Pittsburgh was appalling. It was nothing short of a whitewash. The deaths highlighted how little was known about the swine flu vaccine in particular, and about mass inoculation programs in general.

VIII. THE PROGRAM ENDS: WHY NOT SOONER?

Ironically, it was the CDC itself that finally called a halt to the Swine Flu Immunization Program.

Through its "watchdog" activities, the CDC began to notice an unusually high incidence of Guillain-Barré Syndrome in inoculees. This rather rare disease causes varying degrees of temporary or sometimes permanent paralysis. It also occasionally affects the involuntary muscles of the heart and lungs, causing death. Although no definite link between the Swine Flu Program and Guillain-Barré Syndrome was established, there was enough evidence to justify calling a halt to the program.[36] It seems unlikely that the possibility (and that is all it was at the time) of Guillain-Barré Syndrome resulting from the vaccine was the principal and sole reason for calling off the program. As shown throughout this Article, the proponents of the program had been proceeding all along in the face of much more damaging evidence. Rather, the program collapsed of its own weight. All the negative factors taken together had finally become too much for Dr. Sencer and his colleagues to ignore any longer. In all likelihood, the "eye fake" created by the focus of national attention on Guillain-Barré Syndrome simply provided the CDC leadership with a convenient means of escape from an unconscionable situation.

To fully appreciate just how incredible it was that the Swine Flu Immunization Program got as far as it did, it is necessary to examine some adverse opinions expressed by medical experts during and after the vaccine campaign. For example, Dr. Martin Goldfield, the man who isolated the Fort Dix virus, and Colonel Joseph Bartley, M.D., Chief of Preventive Medicine at Fort Dix, both opposed the program.[37] They saw no evidence that swine flu was even as serious as A/Victoria flu. More importantly, they recognized that the risk to the public created by a mass vaccination program was unacceptable, and that the probability of a pandemic was small.

Dr. Albert Sabin, an early proponent of the Swine Flu Program, soon noticed the bizarre course the program was taking. Shortly after the March 24 announcement by President Ford, Dr. Sabin evaluated the current epidemiology of swine flu. There was none. Later, in April of 1977, he observed that once the program began no notice was taken of the significant shortage of reported swine flu cases. Dr. Sabin feels that the strategy used for the Swine Flu Program would be useless in the face of a real epidemic.[38]

Dr. J. Anthony Morris thinks that flu vaccines may even be of no value. He had been doing extensive research on flu vaccines for the FDA when the Fort Dix outbreak occurred. Although not conclusive, Dr. Morris' research indicated that not only were vaccines ineffective against flu, they promoted flu. He bases his belief on statistics from the Hong Kong flu pandemic in the late 1960s, which he interprets as demonstrating that those countries employing flu vaccine actually suffered more widespread and more serious cases of the flu. Dr. Morris objected to the Swine Flu Program on other grounds. Early on, he objected to the incomplete testing of the vaccine, and argued that the government should not inoculate every man, woman, and child in the country with a vaccine about which little was known. During the testing to determine dosage, Dr. Morris noted (and his findings were corroborated by Dr. Robert Waldman, a leading virologist) that the proposed dosage of two hundred units was insufficient to produce immunity in most people. In fact, Dr. Morris told this author that the dosage was below government standards.

Dr. Morris finally was fired from the FDA because, he believes, of his outspoken criticism of the Swine Flu Program. In a recent interview with this author, Dr. Morris specifically criticized Dr. Sencer, and Dr. Edward Kilbourne of the Mt. Sinai School of Medicine (a key proponent of the program whose influence on it is discussed below), for engaging in excessive "medical politics," and for pushing the program in spite of such overwhelming circumstances opposing it as the following. First, the lack of infection in the sergeant who gave Private Lewis mouth-to-mouth resuscitation suggested that the Private's illness was not very contagious. Second, the British tests on humans mentioned earlier also showed lack of contagiousness. Third, the tests at Fort Detrick included injecting monkeys with isolates of the Fort Dix virus; most of the monkeys did not get sick and even those that did showed negligible clinical symptoms. Fourth, the CDC reported only nine cases of swine flu from February to December of 1976, none of which caused an outbreak of the disease.

A brief examination of the possible motives of Dr. Kilbourne may provide insight into the direction of the program. Dr. Kilbourne has spent the bulk of his professional life studying vaccines, vaccination programs, and flu viruses. He is a leading authority on mass immunization in the Armed Forces. Dr. Kilbourne repeatedly has proposed that mass immunization of general populations would be just as effective as it seems to be for the troops. He may have seen the opportunity to test this theory when the Fort Dix situation occurred. This supposition is supported by Dr. Kilbourne himself; in January 1976, he published a book in which he stated that he thinks that national, even global, vaccination against type A flu may eradicate it.[39]

Dr. Kilbourne was in the unique position of having substantial influence upon the Director of the agency conducting the immunization campaign.[40] According to Dr. Morris, it was in fact Dr. Kilbourne who was the motivating force behind the immunization program. Just how committed Dr. Kilbourne was to the program was amply illustrated by his comments concerning the Guillain-Barré Syndrome. Twenty-four hours after the program was discontinued, Dr. Kilbourne, on national television, flatly denied any link between the Guillain-Barré Syndrome and flu vaccines.[41] Could he really have investigated that possibility thoroughly in so short a time? Was he aware of a study published in the *Archives of Internal Medicine* in 1966 that noted an association between various vaccines and Guillain-Barré?[42]

Motives of participants in such a complex situation are, of course, difficult to assess. But, given the many factors that ought to have halted the program, is it unfair to speculate that Dr. Kilbourne may have sought to test his theories concerning influenza through his involvement in the Swine Flu Program, and that Dr. Sencer may have allowed himself to be influenced excessively by Dr. Kilbourne? Is it not reasonable to speculate that professional enthusiasm on their part, combined with political ambition on President Ford's part, contributed in great part to the swine flu debacle?

IX. THE PROGRAM'S HUMAN AND FINANCIAL COSTS

The final results of the Swine Flu Immunization Program may never be known. But this author's recent investigation of the current status of the aftermath shows many adverse sequellae and high costs. Recently, a CDC employee unhesitatingly answered "yes" when this author asked the question, "Is there a link between Guillain-Barré Syndrome and the Swine Flu Immunization Program?" He asserted that the

CDC has established a definite statistical relationship between the two: one can expect an incidence of 10 cases of Guillain-Barré Syndrome per one million inoculees; 5 to 10 percent of those permanently affected with paralysis by the Syndrome die; and to date, there are 500–600 cases of Guillain-Barré Syndrome statistically associated with the Swine Flu Immunization Program.

The number of deaths acknowledged to have resulted from the program is not known; however, already 52 wrongful death claims have been filed with the Department of Justice. An additional 22 lawsuits also based on wrongful death have been filed in various courts around the country. A May 1977 decision by the United States District Court in Oklahoma, *Sparks v. Wyeth Laboratories, Inc.,*[43] determined that the Swine Flu Act of 1976 is constitutional. Therefore, the requirement that any lawsuits be preceded by an administrative claim filed with the Department of Justice will in all likelihood cause the above 22 suits filed with courts to be dismissed; but they can still be filed as administrative claims.

The money spent on the Swine Flu Program itself was $135 million. This is only a fraction of what the final costs will be. Plaintiffs in the mentioned wrongful death actions are claiming $1,023,139,657 in damages; in the 22 civil suits they are demanding $287,590,529; and in personal injury claims filed with the Justice Department they are demanding $260,070,134. The grand total from all the claims is $1,675,800,320, a figure that does not include the salaries and incidental costs of the special Justice Department task force assigned to handle swine-flu-related claims. Furthermore, the three attorneys, three secretaries, and assorted part-time help of the task force have received 3,000 inquiries into claim procedures. It is beginning to look as if the insurance carriers' $5 billion estimate of the likely dollar value of claims that might be paid because of the program is not totally out of line.

Furthermore, the ultimate dollar costs may be continuous. The federal government set a dangerous precedent by underwriting the immunization program. If it becomes necessary to underwrite all programs of this nature, the costs will be never-ending; and if the federal government refuses to underwrite future immunization programs, they may never become available.

Unfortunately, the dollar costs of the program may not be its most "expensive" result. Tragically, the diverting of our limited vaccine manufacturing capacity to the swine flu effort has caused a serious depletion in supplies of other vaccines. In May of 1977, the National Immunization Conference stated that we have a rapidly increasing need for mass polio, measles, and other inoculations that cannot be met. Vaccine is just not available because the swine flu effort diverted limited manufacturing capacity, thus preventing a buildup of other vaccines.[44] Even if the vaccines were available, the general public is now fearful—due to the swine flu debacle—of even the most proven vaccines, and might not use them. We may, as a result, be facing very serious related public health problems in the near future.

X. LESSONS FOR THE FUTURE

Hopefully, our swine flu experience has not been a total loss. First, experts in preventive medicine should take note that vaccines often cause untoward results in many persons and may not be particularly effective. A reevaluation of vaccines in general, and flu vaccines specifically, is in order. Second, public health officials should now realize that any kind of vaccination program on a national scale demands objective, sophisticated planning, utilizing rational decision-making models. We cannot again afford to overreact emotionally to a potential public health hazard. For instance, in 1976 the situation just was not similar to that during the 1918–1919 flu pandemic. There were no large troop movements, and we have developed various effective antibiotics to help flu victims cope with flu virus's bacterial sidekicks. Given these facts, we can afford to be calm and objective next time around. Third, people, especially high-risk individuals, must not be treated like cattle. The scenario of elderly persons standing in long lines in adverse weather for hours waiting to be vaccinated must not be repeated. Fourth, alternatives to a specific program must be built into any plan. The Swine Flu Program clearly showed us that a vaccine that is harmless to some persons may cause a catastrophe in others. Most importantly, the federal government must recognize its appropriate role in protecting the public health and must adhere to it with scientific caution. The government should limit itself to facilitating public programs. Employing high-pressure sales tactics like Madison Avenue mass media promoters to push a program is not commensurate with this objective. Certainly, when people's lives are at stake, cheap politics has no place.

In concluding, the author must point out that although the five objectives above are desirable and reasonable, experience tells us that none of them will be achieved unless there is sufficient prodding. We must rely on the news media to investigate, to probe, and to catalyze appropriate action. They must seek out and provide objective, constructive criticism for officials and the public to consider so that we will make better decisions in the future and avoid a repeat of the swine flu travesty.

NOTES

1. This background information is based upon historical material provided in Sabin, *Swine Flu: What Happened? The Sciences,* March/April 1977, at 14.

2. This description of the Fort Dix incident is based upon the account provided in Boffey, *Anatomy of a Decision: How the Nation Declared War on Swine Flu,* 192 SCIENCE 636 (1976).

3. Marwick, *Swine Flu Immunization: 'Go' at Last,* MEDICAL WORLD NEWS, Sept. 6, 1976, at 60, 62.

4. FDA DRUG BULLETIN, August/October 1976, at 3.

5. Boffey, *supra* note 2, at 638.

6. The description, in the remainder of this Part, of the events leading up to the decision to immunize—although not necessarily the interpretation of those events—is based upon the account provided in Boffey, *supra* note 2.

7. Although the decision to stockpile was preferable to what later occurred, it was terribly unrealistic. The strategy was to wait and see if vaccination would be necessary. Vaccines, however, are not effective immediately. Therefore, by the time a plan for implementation could have been completed and implemented, the results undoubtedly would have fallen far short of the need.

8. *Quoted at* Boffey, *supra* note 2, at 640.

9. *Quoted at id.* at 638.

10. *Quoted at id.* at 640.

11. Schoenbaum, McNeil, and Kavett, *Swine Flu Decision,* 295 NEW ENG. J. MED. 759 (1976).

12. The Schoenbaum model itself could have been utilized—but was not—later in the program, when the

necessary information became available, as an aid in deciding whether to continue the program.

13. *The Latest Victim of Murphy's Law—Flu Vaccine Program,* AM. MEDICAL NEWS, Jan. 17, 1977, at 20.

14. Marwick, *supra* note 3, at 64.

15. Zimmerly, *Legislative Boost for Swine Flu Program,* J. LEGAL MED., Oct. 1976, at 20.

16. 498 F.2d 1264 (1977). The manufacturer argued that under the "prescription drug" exception, it had no duty to warn the ultimate consumer of the risks of the vaccine and that it had satisfied its duty to warn because it had described those risks in a package insert that was sent with the vaccine to the health center that was carrying out the vaccination program. The court said, however, that the prescription drug exception did not apply in this case, because the manufacturer should have known that the vaccine would not be administered as a prescription drug—specifically, there would be no physician present who could explain the risks to the consumer.

17. *Lessons of the Swine Flu Debacle,* MEDICAL WORLD NEWS, March 7, 1977, at 33, 34.

18. This information was supplied by Dr. J. Anthony Morris, who, as noted in Part VIII of this Article, was studying flu vaccines at the FDA at the time of the Fort Dix outbreak.

19. 42 U.S.C.A. §247b(j).

20. Some of the stated objectives of the statute were: (1) to develop a safe and effective swine flu vaccine; (2) to facilitate the vaccination of the population of the United States; (3) to research the nature, cause, and effect of swine flu; (4) to research the nature and effect of the vaccine; and (5) to determine the cost and effectiveness of the immunization program. It is interesting to note how closely these objectives resemble the decision-making model mentioned earlier. If numbers 1, 3, 4, or 5 had been handled as the bill ordered, the program might never have gotten off the ground.

21. 42 U.S.C.A. §247b(j)(1)(F).

22. Hines, *Small Things Build into Swine Flu Fiasco,* The Pittsburgh Press, Sept. 12, 1976, at 1-B.

23. *Flu Shot Illegalities Reported,* The Pittsburgh Press, Dec. 15, 1976, at 39.

24. 28 U.S.C. §§1346(b), 2671 (1970).

25. For example, on August 27, 1976, the manufacturers announced that instead of September 1, the intended date for beginning to inoculate, they would have no vaccine ready until October 1; and that even then, only 25 percent of what they had promised would be available. *The Latest Victim of Murphy's Law—Flu Vaccine Program,* AM. MEDICAL NEWS, Jan. 17, 1977, at 20.

26. *See Media Blasted for Coverage of Swine Flu Program,* AM. MEDICAL NEWS, May 2, 1977, at 13.

27. *Lessons of the Swine Flu Debacle,* MEDICAL WORLD NEWS, March 7, 1977, at 33.

28. Beare and Craig, *Virulence for Man of a Human Influenza-A Virus Antigenically Similar to "Classical" Swine Viruses,* 1976 LANCET (VOL. II) 4 (1976).

29. *Swine Flu Update,* PENNSYLVANIA HEALTH, Summer 1976, at 3 (emphasis added).

30. FDA DRUG BULLETIN, August/October 1976.

31. Sabin, *supra* note 1, at 27.

32. *See* Chanin, *Influenza: Vaccines or Amantadine?* 237 J. AM. MED. ASS'N 1445 (1977).

33. *See* Gail, *Mass Vaccination: Probability of Three Sudden Deaths,* 195 SCIENCE 934 (1977).

34. Boffey, *Swine Flu: Were the Three Deaths in Pittsburgh a Coincidence?* 194 SCIENCE 590, 648 (1976).

35. *See* Pavleev, *Myocardial Damage Syndrome in Allergic States,* KARDIOLOGIA, Nov. 1975, at 27; Semyonovich and Samoylova, *Allergic Injuries of the Myocardium with Drug Intolerance, id.* at 23; Yevleva, *Infectious Allergic Myocarditis and Rheumatic Carditis, id.* at 30.

36. *Paralysis Cases Shut Flu Clinics Across Nation,* The Pittsburgh Press, Dec. 17, 1976, at 1.

37. *See* Randal, *Medical Politics Killed Swine Flu Effort,* The Miami Herald, Dec. 23, 1976, at 7-A.

38. Sabin, *supra* note 1, at 30 (1977).

39. Kilbourne, *The Influenza Viruses and Influenza* 530, 531 (1975).

40. *See* Randal, *supra* note 37.

41. *See id.*

42. Leneman, *The Guillain-Barré Syndrome,* 118 ARCH. INTERNAL MED. 139, 142 (Table 2) (1966).

43. 431 F. Supp. 411 (1977).

44. *See Immunization Experts Foresee Problems,* MEDICAL WORLD NEWS, May 2, 1977, at 31.

3.2 Managing Public Health Risks: The Swine Flu Immunization Program Revisited

JONATHAN E. FIELDING, M.D., M.P.H.

Reprinted with permission of the American Society of Law & Medicine, Inc. and the Massachusetts Institute of Technology, from 4 *American Journal of Law & Medicine* 35–43 (1978). Copyright © 1978 by the American Society of Law & Medicine, Inc. and the Massachusetts Institute of Technology. All rights reserved.

I. INTRODUCTION

Why can't administrators of health programs and of health institutions make greater use of analysis of costs versus benefits in making important decisions? This question is asked frequently by businessmen and consultants called in to advise government agencies on how to become more efficient. Reacting to outside criticism and to pressure from those paying the bills, many administrators have in fact moved toward a more businesslike approach. For example, hospitals employ techniques borrowed from business to increase their market share, to make optimal use of staff, to schedule appointments, to improve billing and collections, and to lay out space.[1] Federal and state Life Safety Code requirements for nursing homes and for hospitals are undergoing reexamination to determine whether the expenditure of billions of dollars to comply with them is justified in terms of the benefits of such compliance.[2] Routine medical examinations and screening for medical conditions are under increased scrutiny to decide whether their cost is justified by the quantum of related improvement in the health status of patients in whom problems are identified.[3] A consensus is growing that introduction of new technologies and procedures should be preceded by careful evaluation of their true contribution to improvements in therapy, health status, and patient comfort.[4]

In theory, estimation of benefits to be derived from public health programs requires factoring in the risk of adverse effects on the health of the target population if the program is not undertaken. Yet, the public is rarely inclined to oppose a new program if there is any chance it can improve health. Thus, when the American public learns that public health administrators are preparing to make a decision regarding expenditures to control a disease that is feared and known to occur in epidemic form, it will tolerate little risk taking. Every decision will be news, and even technically sound decisions will have far-reaching political ramifications. Such a situation occurred with the announcement in January 1976 that a soldier at Fort Dix, New Jersey, had died of an influenza virus that shared characteristics with a flu strain thought to have caused the 1918–19 influenza pandemic that killed more than 500,000 Americans. In this case, responsibility for the management of a potentially serious public health problem rested squarely on the shoulders of the federal Center for Disease Control (CDC) in Atlanta, an agency of HEW that has enjoyed a longstanding and deserved reputation for technical excellence in developing programs to combat serious communicable diseases. The roles played by the CDC, by various other federal entities, by at least one prominent virologist, and by President Gerald R. Ford in the creation and continuation of the Swine Flu Immunization Program were sharply criticized recently by Cyril H. Wecht, M.D., an internationally known medicolegal scholar, writing in the *American Journal of Law & Medicine*.[5]

The following brief discussion responds to Dr. Wecht's critique, makes a series of recommendations on how the nation can better prepare for future swine-flu-type situations, and assesses some of the long-range problems stemming from the Swine Flu Program that our nation must resolve in the years ahead.

II. AN ASSESSMENT OF THE WECHT CRITIQUE

Dr. Wecht's Article chronicles a scary tale of how the decision was made in 1976 to inaugurate a massive immunization campaign against the possible "killer" swine flu. According to Dr. Wecht's scenario, the decision-making process was closed. Both the CDC's Advisory Committee on Immunization Practices and the blue ribbon panel convened to advise President Ford were controlled by the CDC Director and by one outside expert. Dr. Wecht speculates that the key decision makers were motivated more by political expediency, theoretical bias, or excessive professional enthusiasm than by public interest. The politics of a hotly contested presidential campaign, he suggests, locked HEW into a premature commitment to, and subsequent continuation of, a full scale inoculation program despite information that militated (1) against a headlong attack, and (2) for a complete reexamination of the program once it was under way. Dr. Wecht's script has Congress stampeded into legislating federal assumption of responsibility for liability claims that might be brought by inoculees. Further, he contends that "half-truths and omissions seemed to come in a steady stream"[6] from the CDC and that the federal investigation of three deaths in Pittsburgh temporally associated with swine flu inoculation was "nothing short of a whitewash."[7] He hopes for a change to calm, objective, and apolitical administration of federal vaccine programs in the future.

In contrast, proponents of the Swine Flu Program contend that an early decision to undertake a mass immunization campaign was required by the lead time necessary to manufacture vaccine, by the serious potential for an epidemic caused by an unusually virulent strain of influenza, and by the probable ineffectiveness of a crash vaccine program triggered only by the appearance of additional human cases of swine flu during the usual flu season. They maintain that sound public policy demands an aggressive approach to a largely preventable illness with high morbidity

and mortality. Furthermore, proponents contend that the decision-making process, including the meetings of the Advisory Committee in Immunization Practices, was remarkably open and they insist that both this standby committee and the blue ribbon panel were free to express their views and to disagree with the CDC's recommendations. To charges of misleading the public comes the retort that never before has a public health program been so fully covered by the media; thus any distortion or misinformation reflects inaccurate reporting, not "bureaucratic smoke." For the first time, carefully worded consent forms were required, informing the public about the known risks of immunization better than in any previous immunization program.

Dr. Wecht's analysis of the Swine Flu Program articulates some widely shared doubts and offers some provocative new perspectives. Indeed, certain of his more valid criticisms stimulated the recommendations presented in Part III below. But Dr. Wecht overstates his case, and some of his assumptions, arguments, and conclusions are particularly questionable. For example, his contention that the great influenza pandemic of 1918–19 only killed people afflicted with a concomitant bacterial superinfection[8] is hard to square with Weinstein's observation that many victims died within 24 hours of original symptoms.[9] Dr. Wecht asserts that the federal government ignored the fact that by late July no clinical case of swine flu had been reported outside Fort Dix, and he leads us to believe that the absence of reported cases meant that swine flu was not a major threat.[10] Yet flu experts suspect that new strains responsible for flu epidemics foreshadow their appearance during flu season with sporadic and usually undiagnosed or unreported clinical and subclinical cases. Some well respected scientists agreed that the A/New Jersey strain isolation probably represented the expected new strain and that the CDC had happened upon a group of seed cases that foreboded a serious epidemic in a largely unprotected population.

Dr. Wecht's analysis has other weaknesses. He gives the impression that the rate of adverse short-term reactions to the swine flu vaccine was unusually high.[11] However, in the final testing, the rate of reactions such as fever, local swelling, general malaise, and/or headache, was typical for other influenza vaccines in general.[12] Furthermore, his Article states that by the end of summer 1976 "most private physicians simply were not recommending the vaccine."[13] In reality, many private physicians did support inoculation, especially for high-risk groups because those groups received the bivalent vaccine, which also conferred protection against A/Victoria flu, a strain that most experts believed would continue to be with us in the winter of 1976–77. Finally, Dr. Wecht unnecessarily characterizes a number of program proponents' actions and motivations in the most stark and unflattering of terms. He feels a "review of the information made available, and not made available, by the CDC shows just how unprincipled the agency's actions apparently were."[14] Dr. Wecht speculates that Dr. David Sencer, who in 1976 was the Director of the CDC, may have been excessively influenced by Dr. Edward Kilbourne, who Dr. Wecht believes (1) had an inside track to Dr. Sencer and (2) may have utilized the Swine Flu Program as a means of testing his theories about vaccines. Both men, Dr. Wecht suggests, may have allowed their "professional enthusiasm" to interfere with the making of judicious decisions based on facts.[15] A serious problem with such opinions is that the hard information on which they presumably were based is not presented in sufficient detail to allow the reader to make an independent judgment. Likewise, statements alleging willful deception by agencies in charge of the program[16] are insufficiently substantiated in his Article.

III. PREPARING FOR FUTURE PUBLIC HEALTH CHALLENGES

Although many public health managers probably would take issue with at least some of Dr. Wecht's conclusions, it is hard to find defenders of the Swine Flu Immunization Program. Nor do many feel that it added to the credibility of public health efforts. Many of Dr. Wecht's allegations of program failings are in fact quite correct; such failings must be avoided when public health dilemmas similar to those presented by swine flu arise in the future. Several suggestions can be made.

First, careful and more businesslike planning is necessary, aimed at developing the ability to immunize a major segment of the population within a period of several weeks. This capability is essential if we are to respond effectively to any epidemic in a nonimmune or only partially immune population, whether the threat is influenza, polio, diphtheria, measles, rubella (German measles), mumps, or some new pathogen. The immunization plan must include mechanisms to coordinate and to logistically support the activities of state and local health departments and practicing physicians in such situations.

Second, while all major decisions on possible national health emergencies include political judgments, strong efforts should be made to keep these decisions in the hands of those (1) who have the ability to understand fully the nature of the problem, (2) who are aware of previous experiences in past similar situations, (3) who can weigh short- and long-term implications of alternative decisions, and (4) who can anticipate the majority of organizational and logistical problems. An advisory group to the Assistant Secretary for Health, composed of technical experts and public health officials with differing philosophical attitudes concerning how the federal government should respond to potential epidemics of serious illness, should be constituted as soon as possible, assigned to long terms of service, and convened immediately when a public health dilemma similar to the swine flu situation occurs again.

The advisory group's mandate should not be to achieve consensus; rather it should be (1) to be sure that all options have been fully explored from a technical point of view, and (2) to suggest methods of reducing the probability of an unnecessary or unsuccessful program. If such an advisory group had been available to the swine flu proponents, it might have suggested, for example, that the virulence of the swine flu was a major unanswered question and proposed trying to find volunteers willing to be exposed to the virus. It might also have proposed that, for the time period during which the swine flu's virulence remained uncertain, the immunization program should first be geared to providing bivalent vaccine (against both swine and Victoria strains of A flu) to the traditional high risk group (over 65 or chronically ill) and then sufficient vaccine should be stockpiled to service the needs of 80 percent of the remaining population.

Third, there must be flexibility in program administration. Of course, in the last days of March 1976, few decision makers would have opted against proceeding with manufacture of swine flu vaccine—even though available information on the nature of the virus was inadequate and the possible similarity to the pandemic strain required further investigation—because vaccine manufacturers claimed that without a firm commitment by April 1, they couldn't produce sufficient vaccine for use when needed. But as Dr. Wecht correctly points out, by late July no new cases of swine flu had been reported anywhere in the world,[17] and monkeys inoculated with the A/New Jersey strain had exhibited negligible clinical reactions.[18] In addition, insurance companies had refused to underwrite vaccine production. It is likely that if the decision had been made de novo at that time, a crash campaign to immunize every man, woman, and child would have been hard to justify. Additional evidence against proceeding with a full scale campaign came from the inoculation of six human volunteers with the Fort Dix virus, resulting in four mild clinical cases of flu, with no clinical symptoms in two volunteers.[19]

Why, then, did reconsideration of the program not take place? Unfortunately, Dr. Wecht's contention that reconsideration was politically untenable and might have led to loss of face is plausible. Yet, such pressures must not be allowed to prevent the development of procedures under which any major public health decision made under conditions of uncertainty will be reconsidered in light of new evidence. The proposed advisory committee should be reconvened when appropriate, to advise not only on technical aspects of vaccine administration, but on whether the existing facts warrant continuation of the existing programmatic approach. HEW officials to whom the CDC reports should require frequent updatings of information and make it clear that they support changes in program direction—even in midstream—if new information mandates the switch.

Fourth, public officials should not oversell immunization programs. The above-described inflexibility in the Swine Flu Program was created in part by the overselling of the program to the American people. A combination of federal government pronouncements and extensive media coverage created the impression that a swine flu epidemic would strike in the Fall, that it was the same flu that killed half a million people earlier in this century, and that inoculation of the entire population was mandatory. A better approach by those attempting to sell flu vaccine programs would be to characterize flu

vaccination as insurance. People buy insurance to protect themselves against the financial impact of a catastrophe, but they rarely expect that the event that could precipitate such a catastrophe will occur. Why not explain to the public that getting a flu shot is a form of insurance that protects them to a large extent against the dangers of exposure to disease (exposure that may or may not occur)? The cost of the insurance is the inoculation fee (if the inoculation is not administered by a public agency) plus associated discomfort, plus an X percent chance of the much more serious and occasionally fatal Guillain-Barré syndrome that has been associated statistically with various vaccines. If the insurance pitch had been used in the Swine Flu Program, the public probably could have accepted a reduced program much more easily.

Fifth, there must be public education providing people with sufficient information to make their own informed decision as to whether they should be inoculated. Although information about influenza can be complicated, especially given the occurrence of changing flu strains and the possibility that cases attributable to several different strains will occur during a single flu season, nevertheless, most people can absorb enough relevant information to make a personal decision. Given the many variables involved—the difficulty of accurately predicting epidemics, the short-term morbidity often associated with flu inoculations, the development of protection in only about 70 percent of inoculees, and the small but definable risk of contracting Guillain-Barré Syndrome—the government has a responsibility to inform the public about the relevant probabilities, benefits, and costs. Where a cost benefit model reveals clear aggregate benefit for any group (e.g., those over 65) based on pessimistic assumptions regarding risk of epidemic, the government should recommend vaccination, but without instilling inappropriate fear in persons not inclined to participate. In the Swine Flu Program, the CDC placed considerable pressure on state health authorities to follow the CDC's strong recommendations, even after questions whether those recommendations were based on the latest information became almost unavoidable.

Sixth, federal immunization programs must set realistic goals. The expressed goal of immunizing 100 percent of the American population against swine flu was unrealistic and out of step with the results of previous large-scale immunization efforts. Setting an impossible goal for the Swine Flu Program ensured that it would appear unsuccessful even if it worked as well as the polio immunization programs, and it put state and local health officers in the difficult position of explaining why national goals could not be met in their areas.

IV. THE SWINE FLU PROGRAM'S AFTERMATH

Some of the untoward effects of the Swine Flu Program are still being felt. Largely unmentioned in articles examining the program's impact has been the diversion of state and local health department resources to the Swine Flu Program. Federal money given to most states was insufficient to assist them in developing the capacity to provide mass inoculation; but even had funds been available to states, the need for personnel skilled in immunization programs would have required temporarily transferring people out of other immunization activities to work on the Swine Flu Program. As a result, many states temporarily diminished their efforts to ensure full protection against the more serious and preventable pathogens affecting primarily children. Their immunization rates dropped. HEW has become sufficiently alarmed about the growing risk of epidemics of preventable infectious diseases that it recommended that the Congress should appropriate $23 million for fiscal 1978 to beef up state childhood immunization programs. Congress acted favorably on this request, and the Carter Administration has requested $35 million for the same purpose for fiscal 1979.

Another untoward result has been public confusion about what swine flu is and whether it should be feared. Some people have assumed that because little is heard about swine flu today as compared to 1976, they probably don't have to be concerned about getting a flu shot. Worst and hardest to correct of the program results is a growing distrust of public health programs in general, especially immunization programs. Many people feel that the Swine Flu Program was a fabrication to help President Ford secure reelection, and that HEW and the CDC acquiesced to political pressures. A public turned to cynicism and distrust by the Swine Flu Program may exaggerate the negative in asking itself such questions as the following: "Why did this virus that was seen as a great enough threat to justify spending $135,000,000 on vaccine and incurring liability claims of over $1 billion not show up during flu season?" "If the initiation of the Swine Flu Program was 'politically motivated,' what other public health programs are launched for political rather than technical reasons?" "How can we as citizens believe our public officials or know what is going on?" These and similar questions can only be precluded by renewed confidence in our public health institutions, reinforced by successful programs and by an absence of obvious political overtones in making decisions. This will take time. Meanwhile, the effectiveness of immunization programs and other public health programs may be affected by the legacy of the swine flu affair.

NOTES

1. For a discussion of the marketing issue, see Clarke, *Marketing Health Care: Problems in Implementation,* HEALTH CARE MANAGEMENT REVIEW, Winter 1978, at 21.

2. *See* Feeley, Walsh, & Fielding, *Structural Codes and Patient Safety: Does Strict Compliance Make Sense?* 3 AM. J.L. & MED. 447 (1977–78).

3. *See* Spitzer & Brown, *Unanswered Questions About the Periodic Health Examination,* 83 ANN. INTERN. MED. 257 (1975).

4. *See* Hiatt, *Protecting the Medical Commons: Who Is Responsible?* 293 NEW ENGLAND J. MED. 235 (1975).

5. Wecht, *The Swine Flu Immunization Program: Scientific Venture or Political Folly?* 3 AM. J.L. & MED. 425 (1977–78) [hereinafter cited as Wecht].

6. *Id.* at 438.

7. *Id.* at 440.

8. *Id.* at 427.

9. Weinstein, *Influenza—1918, A Revisit?* 294 NEW ENGLAND J. MED. 1058, 1059 (1976) (editorial).

10. Wecht, *supra* note 5, at 433.

11. *Id.* at 432.

12. *See* Parkman, Galasso, Top, & Noble, *Summary of Clinical Trials of Influenza Vaccines,* 134 J. INFECT. DIS. 100 (1976).

13. Wecht, *supra* note 5, at 435.

14. *Id.* at 438.

15. *Id.* at 443.

16. *Id.* at 438.

17. *Id.* at 433.

18. *Id.*

19. *Id.* at 436–37.

3.3 Federal Regulation of Vinyl Chloride: A Short Course in the Law and Policy of Toxic Substances Control*

DAVID D. DONIGER

Reprinted with permission from 7 *Ecology Law Quarterly* 500–521 (1978). Copyright © 1978 by the *Ecology Law Quarterly*. All rights reserved.

INTRODUCTION

On January 22, 1974, the B.F. Goodrich Company revealed that three workers at its plant in Louisville, Kentucky, recently had died of angiosarcoma of the liver, an extremely rare and incurable cancer, and that a fourth had died of the same illness five years before.[1] The plant converts vinyl chloride, a petrochemical gas, into polyvinyl chloride, the second most widely used plastic in the United States.[2] The grouping of these rare cancers at this plant immediately raised the suspicion that vinyl chloride was the cause. This suspicion was soon confirmed by reports from other companies that some of their workers exposed to the chemical had developed the same cancer, and by disclosures that since 1970 vinyl chloride had induced a wide variety of cancers in experimental animals.[3]

Within a week of the Goodrich disclosure, the Occupational Safety and Health Administration and the National Institute for Occupational Safety and Health began preparing a workplace standard for vinyl chloride.[4] This marked the beginning of the still incomplete regulation of this pervasive chemical, an endeavor that has involved five major federal agencies operating under 15 separate health and environmental statutes.

This Article examines the federal regulation of vinyl chloride, and through that experience, the complex law and policy of toxic substances control in the United States. Attempts to control toxic substances were begun seriously only in the 1970s. The law and policy in this area are in rapid growth and transition and are still deeply disorganized. The vinyl chloride problem is one of several chemical crises that has strongly influenced the growth of the field.[5]

Vinyl chloride gas (VC) and polyvinyl chloride plastic (PVC) permeate modern American living. PVC has hundreds of widely different uses, some very important and others completely frivolous. PVC is a major construction material, used in products such as water pipe, floor tile, and exterior siding. It is a major food packaging material. PVC is used to make consumer products ranging from household furniture to auto interiors, from credit cards to baby pants. Ironically, it provides a valuable coating for pollution control equipment, due to its resistance to corrosion. VC gas itself has been used as an aerosol propellant and a refrigerant. It was once even tested for use as a general anaesthetic.[6]

Hundreds of thousands of people are exposed to VC at their places of work. Millions are exposed to VC from living and working near the factories where it is made and processed, and near the routes over which it is transported between factories. VC leaches from many of the

*An earlier draft of this paper won first prize in the 1977 Ellis J. Harmon Environmental Law Writing Competition. The author would like to thank Richard H. Cowart and Karl E. Geier for their invaluable editorial assistance. He would also like to express his gratitude to the Editors of Volumes 6 and 7 for their support during the production of this Article.

PVC products with which the consumer is in contact daily—from packaging into food, from pipe into drinking water, from latex paint into indoor air, and from many other sources.[7]

The primary threat from VC is to the workers. To date there have been at least 68 known cases of liver angiosarcoma among roughly 30,000 workers most heavily exposed to the chemical in the three decades prior to 1974. The illness is occurring in these workers at a rate as much as 3,000 times higher than in the general population. VC is also suspected of causing an equivalent number of more common cancers in these workers. Moreover, many other workers are expected to develop liver angiosarcoma and other cancers as a result of their exposure in the 1950s, 1960s, and early 1970s.[8]

Most of the victims known to date have been exposed to VC at levels far higher than those experienced by most workers, consumers, and others. But even low doses of a carcinogen are a matter of serious concern. Presently, it is not possible to identify safe levels of exposure to carcinogens, and some scientists believe that as little as a single molecule of such a chemical, interacting with the appropriate portion of the genetic material of a susceptible cell, can cause a fatal cancer many years later.[9]

The adverse effects of VC are not limited to cancer. At relatively high doses it causes a variety of degenerative symptoms. At low doses it may cause birth defects and mutations.[10]

Unfortunately, VC is not an oddity. It is representative of thousands of chemicals that are capable of causing cancer, other long-term illnesses, and many subtle adverse environmental effects. Like VC, many of these chemicals were once thought to be safe, are important components of significant industries, and are manufactured, transported, consumed, and discarded in vast quantities. Nearly everyone is exposed to them in complex, possibly interactive combinations; nearly everyone is at some degree of risk.[11]

These hazardous substances are only a fraction of the estimated 65,000 chemicals in commerce and the more than four million chemicals that are known.[12] But in absolute terms toxic substances are large in number, and they are responsible for a substantial portion of the illnesses, deaths, and environmental insults experienced today.[13] The vast number of chemicals to be tested, evaluated, and regulated makes toxic

substances control in many respects the major challenge of the health and environmental movement.

One focus of this Article is the staggering complexity and fragmentation of the federal programs to control these toxic substances. About 20 separate health and environmental statutes empower five major agencies to regulate such substances. (See Table 3.3.1.) The patchwork of statutes grew incrementally, mostly over the last two decades, as Congress perceived additional, relatively narrowly defined needs for controls. Together the laws cover virtually all the avenues through which people can be exposed to dangerous chemicals, and most of the avenues through which such substances can harm natural systems.[14]

But although the coverage of these statutes, taken together, is nearly complete, it is highly fragmented. As noted above, to address all of the sources of human exposure to VC would require action by all five agencies acting under 15 of the statutes. Few chemicals are as widely used as VC, and therefore few will fall under so many authorities. Nonetheless, there are already more than 20 chemicals undergoing regulation by two or more agencies.[15] This is likely to be the rule rather than the exception, at least for chemicals currently well established in commerce.[16]

A serious problem is that in many cases the boundaries between agencies' jurisdictions are not clear. Sometimes authorities overlap, empowering two agencies to regulate a given source of exposure.[17] In some areas where two agencies have abutting jurisdiction—i.e., where together their statutes cover a type of hazard without overlap—the dividing line is uncertain, and it is uncertain into which bailiwick a particular source falls.[18] Jurisdictional complexity and confusion often discourage agencies from stepping forward to deal with a problem; each waits for another to act.

Even when jurisdictional issues are resolved, the fragmented system discourages comprehensive assessment and balancing of all of a substance's risks and benefits. No agency has the responsibility to consider the net social gain or loss from different levels of control. Such a holistic consideration might yield a different result than the sum of partial analyses. Moreover, in the case of VC, some risks have been seriously understated and some control costs seri-

Table 3.3.1. Federal Authority over Vinyl Chloride Exposure

Agency Statute	Year Enacted	Uses or Sources of Exposure Covered
Occupational Safety and Health Administration		
Occupational Safety and Health Act	1970	Exposure in factories and in transportation (workers only)
Environmental Protection Agency		
Clean Air Act	1970	Factory emissions
Federal Environmental Pesticide Control Act	1972	Insecticide aerosols
Federal Water Pollution Control Act	1972	VC discharges to water
Safe Drinking Water Act	1974	VC in drinking water, PVC water pipe
Resource Conservation and Recovery Act	1976	PVC sludge wastes
Toxic Substances Control Act	1976	Possible to use in lieu of multiple separate actions under other laws
Food and Drug Administration		
Food, Drug, and Cosmetic Act	1938	Cosmetic aerosols, PVC cosmetic packaging
Food Additives Amendment	1958	PVC food packaging, PVC water pipe
New Drug Amendments	1962	Drug aerosols, PVC drug packaging
Medical Device Amendments	1976	PVC medical devices
Consumer Product Safety Commission		
Federal Hazardous Substances Act	1966	Household aerosols, household plastics and paints
Department of Transportation		
Hazardous Materials Transportation Act	1975	Rail and truck tank vehicles
Federal Rail Safety Act	1970	Rail tank cars and roadbed
Ports and Waterways Safety Act	1972	Barges and tank vessels
Dangerous Cargo Act	1940	

ously exaggerated because of the fragmentation of assessment of both hazards and economic benefits.[19]

The final drawback to the current balkanized system is the duplication of decision making. Many separate, essentially identical proceedings must be held. The duplication wastes the resources of all concerned—government, regulated industries, and health and environmental groups. Some industries may prefer the fragmentation because it slows the speed with which the government places controls on the profitable use and sale of hazardous substances. But in many cases uncertainty over the ultimate scope of regulation probably outweighs the industries' advantages in delay.

In response to problems encountered in the control of VC and several other substances through this fragmented system, the agencies recently have begun efforts to coordinate their many programs and to increase the consistency of their actions. The promise and pitfalls of these efforts are surveyed at the end of the Article, on the basis of the lessons of the VC experience.[20]

The second focus of this Article is how agencies cope with problems of uncertainty and competing, dissimilar interests that are inherent in toxic substances control decisions. As is explored in Part I, the regulation of any of these substances involves complex decision making under uncertainty and controversial value judgments concerning the weighing of health and environmental values against economic interests. The VC case study permits one to see how the many statutes and agencies approach these problems, in a relatively constant scientific, technological, and economic context.

Part II, the case study, makes up the major portion of this Article. It begins with a survey of the uses of VC and PVC, the technology and economics of associated industries, and what is known of VC's toxicity. This is the factual background for all the regulatory proceedings; additional data peculiar to individual areas is given in those discussions.

The next three sections in Part II analyze in depth the actions taken to date respecting three of the major sources of VC exposure. The first section considers the development of a standard for workplace exposure by the Occupational Safety and Health Administration (OSHA). The second addresses standard setting for emissions from factories to the surrounding air, by the Environmental Protection Agency (EPA). The third considers the proposal by the Food and Drug Administration (FDA) to regulate the use of PVC food packaging. Each of these sections illustrates central legal and policy problems in toxic substances control and a range of responses by agencies and interested parties. Considered together, the OSHA and EPA actions also illustrate the underweighting of risks that can result from jurisdictional fragmentation.

The extremes of jurisdictional complexity are illustrated in the next two sections, on VC-propelled aerosol products and the transportation of VC between factories. Authority over aerosols is divided among three agencies: FDA, EPA, and the Consumer Product Safety Commission (CPSC). Authority over hazardous material transportation is divided among OSHA and three agencies within the Department of Transportation (DOT). Because very small economic interests were at stake over aerosols, regulation proceeded relatively smoothly. However, the aerosol episode reveals the potential for serious jurisdictional conflict in those future cases when more money is at stake, when decisions are more difficult, and when the results for a given product might depend on which statute and agency it falls under. In the transportation area the economic interests are greater and the balancing of risk and benefit is more difficult. The jurisdictional lines also are unclear. Moreover, historically none of the agencies concerned has regulated the movement of carcinogens and other substances with long-term or subtle effects. Each is reluctant to assert its authority vigorously and is content to wait for another to step forward.

The last section of the case study briefly surveys the authorities for controlling the remaining sources of VC exposure. Principally, these are exposure routes connected with water, consumer products, packaging other than for food,

and medical devices. The agencies involved are EPA, FDA, and CPSC. No controls of these exposure sources have yet moved beyond the proposal stage. The control of these sources leads to several more examples of jurisdictional overlap, of underweighting of risks, and of conflicting statutory responsibilities.

The final section also considers how the Toxic Substances Control Act,[21] administered by EPA, relates to the control of VC and to future instances in which authority over a dangerous chemical is seriously fragmented. The Act was passed only in 1976, after some standards for VC already had been set under prior laws or had been proposed, and therefore it is of minimal use to control this chemical. But EPA might use the Act in the future to reduce the number of separate, fragmented actions that are needed to regulate similar substances.

Part III of this Article has two purposes. First, in light of the VC episode and similar experiences, it surveys past and ongoing efforts to deal with jurisdictional fragmentation and to coordinate federal action and policy on toxic substances control. It discusses the agencies' internal coordination efforts, interagency agreements, cooperative regulation of particular substances, and two new interagency groups created to foster broader forms of cooperation. Serious coordination efforts are only just beginning.

Second, Part III of the Article confronts the capacity of certain characteristics of the legal framework for toxic substances regulation to deal with the other central policy problems noted above: decision making under uncertainty and balancing of dissimilar, competing interests. The statutory formulations, which are analyzed individually in detail in the appropriate sections of the case study, are considered here in general terms.

From the case study it becomes clear that in view of the problems of factual uncertainty and conflicting values, each agency faces a wide range of rational choices in setting exposure limits and other standards, but no one choice can be said to be objectively "correct." Each agency must make judgments about what to assume when the true facts are uncertain and about which interests to favor among competing ones. The policies or norms that drive these judgments are difficult to state clearly and difficult to apply precisely to the circumstances at hand.

The statutes that delegate responsibility to the agencies for making these judgments provide certain limitations, along with some measure of guidance for decision making. The statutory formulations differ in many particulars, but certain themes and basic alternatives emerge clearly.

First, virtually all the statutes are precautionary; *i.e.,* they direct the agencies to act on the basis of uncertain, suggestive indications that a substance is dangerous. Because many substances can be shown definitively to be harmful only after serious harms have already occurred, these statutes reject the view that control measures must await proof of actual, past harm.

On the balancing problem there is substantial division among the statutes. Most of the statutes require agencies to weigh health and environmental concerns against economic considerations, but several statutes prohibit agencies from considering anything but health factors. Depending upon which approach is used, the results of regulation will differ dramatically. Because of the severe results of the health-only rule, the prohibition is acknowledged more often in the breach than in the observance.

The toxic substances control statutes also differ in the allocation of the burden of persuasion. Most place the burden of showing that a substance should be regulated on the government. Several important statutes, however, place the burden of showing that a substance should be allowed in commerce on the proponent of use. The difference in the burden of persuasion can affect fine judgments at the margin, such as where an agency is deciding between alternative levels of exposure.

Finally, the statutes call for searching judicial review of agency decisions, although ultimately they leave to the agencies a large measure of discretion. Although the statutory formulations regarding standards of judicial review vary, the courts are developing consistent principles for scrutinizing decisions.

Through these devices the statutes give some guidance and offer some control, but they leave the agencies a wide range of legitimate choices. This Article contends that these legal tools are not instruments of finely-tuned control, and that the agencies and advocates waste considerable

energy in unproductive attempts to draw from the statutory differences fine distinctions in the agencies' obligations. Ultimately, regulations emerge from the interplay of available facts, the advocacy of interested parties and the predispositions of the agencies. The dynamics of this process are best seen in operation, as in the VC case study. Before analyzing the actions of the agencies in the regulation of VC, it is necessary to examine the central policy problems of uncertainty and balancing that the agencies have had to face. These problems are considered in the next section.

I. BASIC POLICY PROBLEMS IN TOXIC SUBSTANCES CONTROL: DECIDING UNDER UNCERTAINTY AND BALANCING INCOMMENSURABLE INTERESTS

Two cardinal problems are endemic to any scheme for regulating substances that cause cancer or other long-term, serious health or environmental effects of relatively low probability. First, all decisions must be made under substantial uncertainty about the medical and ecological risks, technological difficulties, and economic costs associated with different degrees of exposure. Second, all decisions involve trade-offs among groups with interests that are not readily comparable. These two problems form serious "boundaries of analysis" that prevent regulatory agencies from making exact, objective, and noncontroversial decisions.[22] This section explores the problems of uncertainty and balancing generally, as a preface to the exploration of agency response to the VC hazard, and to the discussion of the legal framework within which the agencies make decisions.

Cancer is the primary adverse effect of VC, and the disease is the chemical hazard most on the public mind. For these reasons, this section explores the nature of scientific uncertainty in the management of hazardous substances through the example of cancer risk assessment. This section also discusses the technological and economic uncertainties of estimating the difficulty and cost of toxic substances control. Finally, the section examines the difficulty of determining what risk-benefit trade-offs are acceptable to individuals and to the society as a whole. Only with an understanding of the boundaries of our scientific, technological, economic, and ethical knowledge is it possible to evaluate fairly the analytical efforts and normative choices of the agencies that have regulated VC.

A. The Limits of Cancer Risk Assessment

Cancer is a group of illnesses characterized by the unrestrained multiplication of cells that somehow have lost an essential self-regulatory mechanism.[23] The uncontrolled growth of these cells eventually threatens the life of the host organism. Presently, cancer is the second leading cause of death in the United States.[24] One American in four is expected to contract some type of cancer,[25] and one American in five is expected to die of it.[26]

Most forms of cancer are difficult or impossible to cure; less than one-half of all cancer patients survive longer than five years from the discovery of their illness.[27] The elusiveness of cures largely is due to the fact that cancer's basic biological mechanisms at the cellular level are not well understood.[28]

The causes of cancer are, however, somewhat better understood than the cures. Studies of cancer incidence in particular groups have shown strong statistical connections between exposure to certain chemical substances and particular cancers. The connection between tobacco smoke and lung cancer is the most widely known.[29] Markedly elevated cancer rates are also found among certain occupational groups in the United States and in other highly industrialized countries.[30] Cancer rates are elevated where air and drinking water are contaminated with industrial organic chemicals.[31] In general, cancer rates are higher than average in American urbanized areas.[32] From comparisons of different rates of different cancers throughout the world, the World Health Organization and other prominent institutions and individual experts have concluded that 60 to 90 percent of all human cancers are caused by exposure to chemical substances (and, to a lesser extent, radiation) present in our air, workplaces, food, water, and the rest of our environment.[33]

The causal relationships underlying the statistical connections observed in humans have been confirmed for many substances by controlled experiments on animals. With one possible exception, all substances related to cancer in humans have been shown to cause cancer in animals.[34] In addition, animal experiments have implicated 1,500–2,000 other chemical substances as potential human carcinogens.[35] Many of these substances are synthetic organic chemicals that have been in commercial use only since the 1930s. Because cancer is a latent disease that typically manifests itself only 15 to 40 years after exposure begins, it is too early to know the effects of chemicals that have been in widespread use for only this short period.

This evidence suggests that cancer rates could be cut significantly by reducing human exposure to the disease's chemical causes. Even though it may be quite expensive, preventing human exposure to carcinogens often is a more effective and economically efficient method of reducing cancer rates than attempts to cure patients who already have the disease.[36] In order to make the best use of the resources available to prevent cancer, precise data on which substances are carcinogenic and on how dangerous they are at various levels of exposure would be helpful. Unfortunately, the causal relationship between a chemical and cancer is often difficult to establish. Even where a qualitative relationship is visible, precise quantitative estimates of risks to humans cannot be made reliably, particularly for low risks on the order of one case in 10,000 or more subjects.[37]

In the first place, not enough is known about how chemical carcinogens operate, especially at the cellular level. There is general agreement that the substances cause changes in the genetic material of an individual cell or in the mechanisms through which the genetic material controls a cell's behavior, inducing it to multiply wildly.[38] There is uncertainty and disagreement on whether only one such "hit" need occur or whether a certain sequence of independent hits by the same or different substances is needed.[39] Further uncertainty stems from the complexity of cellular metabolism—the system of chemical and physical processes that occur within a living organism. Opinions differ on whether there are chemical reactions that detoxify certain amounts of a carcinogen by converting it into a harmless substance, or that repair genetic changes after they have occurred.[40] The metabolic "pathway" of a substance from its point of entry (e.g., lungs, skin, or digestive system) to its point of damage is also often uncertain.[41]

Whether or not there are defense or repair mechanisms has profound implications for strategies for cancer prevention. If the "one-hit" model is accurate, and if there are no detoxification, repair, or other defense mechanisms, then as little as one molecule of a carcinogenic substance, interacting with the appropriate portion of the susceptible cell, can cause an irreversible cancer. If multiple hits by different substances are needed, any one substance alone may not be carcinogenic (or may be only weakly so) but together these substances may be potent causes of the disease. If detoxification or repair mechanisms or other defenses exist, there may be safe doses—"thresholds"—below which no cancers will be caused. More important than the question of whether a threshold exists is the question of what risks to expect from a range of doses. Different propositions about cancer causation lead to different conclusions about the rate of cancer to expect from each dose.[42]

The second major source of uncertainty is a result of the limitations of available research techniques. Current methods for investigating the carcinogenicity of substances do not permit the verification or disproof of alternative theories of cancer causation. The methods are themselves also the subject of great controversy. Observation from direct human experiences is of limited utility. Purposeful experimentation on humans is ethically unacceptable, since the results often would be fatal. Human evidence of carcinogenesis usually comes from observation of occupational groups exposed, often unwittingly, to chemicals in the industrial economy.[43] Some connections can be drawn in the general population, but for the most part humans are exposed to too many different substances at unknown doses for unknown periods to permit statistically reliable conclusions to be drawn.[44] Moreover, there are synergistic and antagonistic interactions between chemicals that drastically complicate drawing conclusions about the effects of each chemical. Finally, because latency periods run 15 to 40 years or longer, definitive studies of effects on humans are impracticable.[45]

Studies on rodents are the major source of data on the carcinogenicity of chemicals.[46] Their response characteristics are considered essentially similar to those of humans, so that a substance carcinogenic to one is likely to be carcinogenic to the other.[47] But although the qualitative inferences are quite sound, there are limitations on the ability of the animal tests to indicate the magnitude of human risks. It is difficult

both to detect small risks in test animals and to translate risks for animals into risks for humans.

The difficulty in detecting small risks is statistical in nature. For practical and financial reasons, nearly all experiments on animals involve small numbers of subjects, usually no more than a few hundred.[48] In so small a group, a chemical must cause an effect at a relatively high rate for the relationship to be confidently distinguished from random occurrences of the same event.[49] The dose of a substance that induces cancer at rates detectable in such tests is often far higher than most people experience.[50] The critical question is whether lower doses cause cancer, and at what rates. An effect occurring at a very low rate stands a good chance of not being observed in so small a test group, so that the failure to observe an effect in such a test is not a reliable indication of the substance's safety for a larger population.[51] Thus, no test has confirmed the existence of any threshold or detoxification mechanism or resolved any other basic aspect of the theoretical controversies discussed above.[52]

To investigate the effects of low doses directly would require experiments involving enormous numbers of animals. To demonstrate with 95 percent confidence that a given low dose of just one substance causes fewer than one cancer in a million subjects would require a test involving at least *six million* animals. Such "mega-mouse" experiments generally are considered impracticably expensive and vulnerable to laboratory errors that can destroy the statistical reliability of the results.[53]

Limited to observations at unrealistically high doses in unrealistically low numbers, the scientist's recourse is to use mathematical models of dose-response relationships to extrapolate from experimental results downward to the effects of low doses. However, like the theories on which they are based, the models yield widely divergent estimates of the risk associated with each low dose. The extent of the differences is astounding. For example, the major models differ by a factor of *100,000* on the size of the dose that creates a risk of one cancer in a million subjects.[54] The models do provide credible outer limits for the risk associated with each dose,[55] and they do permit the ranking of carcinogens in rough order of their potency. But they cannot provide the regulator with precise estimates of the risks of low doses.

More uncertainty is added to risk estimates by our ignorance of how to translate dose-response data across species lines. There simply is not enough known to determine if humans are more or less sensitive to a given dose of a carcinogen than the test-animals.[56]

Several new techniques for assessing carcinogenicity are developing, but these do not yet hold out the promise of yielding quantitative risk estimates or of answering the basic questions about how cancer is caused. There are "quick" tests—such as the Ames test—of chemicals' abilities to mutate bacteria or other single-celled organisms. There is a high correlation between the ability to cause such mutations and carcinogenicity.[57] Currently, however, the value of the "quick" tests is primarily qualitative; they may be able to distinguish strong from weak carcinogens, but cannot give more precise risk estimates.

One important consequence of the uncertainty about the size of small risks is that a regulator agency does not know the *marginal* risk at each dose; that is, the agency does not know how great a difference in risk is caused by small changes in dose. If there is a large difference, then small increments in the allowable exposure will have a significant impact on human health and must be considered carefully. If the difference is small, the increments are not so important, and extensive efforts to obtain compliance with a small change in a standard might not be worthwhile.

Purely scientific problems of risk assessment are aggravated to some degree for regulatory agencies by their incomplete access to information. Most toxicological research is carried out or sponsored by the industries that make or market the substances being evaluated; industrial researchers have incentives to withhold negative information or to perform poorly designed and executed experiments incapable of revealing negative information.[58] To some extent, this behavior can be controlled by the use of standard test protocols and other means.[59] The problem of unequal access to data and of incentives to misinform or misrepresent is more serious with regard to the assessment of costs.[60]

In sum, because the nature of chemical carcinogenesis is unknown, and because available research techniques are limited in their ability to predict human risks from exposure to carcinogens, the only conclusion that may be drawn

with complete certainty is that no level of exposure to a chemical that causes cancer in animals is sure to be safe. Neither experimental nor theoretical analysis can give the agencies precise estimates of the risks associated with low doses of substances that are known to cause cancer in humans or animals at higher doses. Nor can regulators be sure how sensitive risks are to changes in dose. At present, the best available techniques produce only broad estimates of the outer limits of risk.

B. The Limits of Economic and Technological Assessment

The costs of controlling exposure to a toxic substance are shrouded in as much uncertainty as the risks of the exposure. The difficulty of determining the costs of regulation arises from several compounded problems. At the simplest level, it is difficult to predict the technological problems and direct economic costs of meeting exposure limitations that may be only a fraction of the levels once thought to be safe. It is a more complex task to assess the wider economic consequences of changes in the price or availability of a substance. Finally, it is difficult to know whether the use of substitute products and other secondary responses to regulation will themselves harm health or the environment.[61]

As a general rule, as the degree of exposure control increases, the marginal costs of each additional increment of control increase.[62] Simple and inexpensive measures to reduce exposure will be taken before complicated and costly ones. Of equal importance in the regulation of toxic substances, as the degree of control increases, the cost of control grows more uncertain; the range of effects becomes more difficult even to identify, let alone quantify.[63] Additional improvements will require research and development of new control techniques; it will be uncertain what results can be achieved, how long the research and development process will take, and how much the new controls will cost to develop, install, and operate. In the extreme case, the necessary control means may defy invention, and until some completely unpredictable technological advance occurs, compliance will be impossible without closing the factory.

An increase in the cost of producing a regulated substance will have secondary economic consequences, depending on the profit margins of the producers, the degree of economic concentration of the industry, and the availability of substitute products. The evaluation of costs and benefits in the regulation of toxic chemicals is complicated by uncertainty as to the magnitude of these secondary effects in any given case. If close substitutes are available at prices nearly equal to a substance's preregulation price, producers will not be able to raise prices significantly to recoup the costs of compliance.[64] In such cases the producers' profit margins will decrease, or production will decline. In other cases, the product may have unique and valuable features, and consumers may be willing to pay prices that reflect most or all of the cost increases. Finally, in some situations, human exposure to a toxic substance may be an intentional or unavoidable event, not reducible to safe levels without banning the substance. For such regulations, there is not much uncertainty as to the costs and technological means of control. There remains, however, the difficulty of determining the economic loss to society as a whole, including the adverse impacts of the use of substitutes.[65]

The last major element of uncertainty in the assessment of the costs of regulation is whether any of the substitute responses to regulation will themselves have an adverse health or environmental impact. If the substitutes are readily forseeable, something may be known of their toxicity. On the other hand, their effects may not yet be known,[66] and the effects of substitutes not yet identified cannot be predicted. This dimension of uncertainty, like those discussed above, becomes more significant as regulation becomes more severe, because increasingly stringent regulations will be more likely to result in substantial substitutions taking place.

The uncertainty in estimates of the costs of regulation is compounded by the fact that the regulated industries, the government, and other interested parties have unequal access to data and different incentives governing their approaches to estimation. To begin with, the parties tend to disagree on the emphasis to be placed on short-term, as opposed to long-term effects. Consumers require some time to react to price increases or diminished supply of the regulated substance; the location and utilization of substitutes cannot take place immediately. Plant shutdowns and production cutbacks may cause localized increases in unemployment in the short

term, but this may be compensated for by increases in production and employment in the manufacture of substitute products. Thus, emphasis on the short-term "dislocation costs" of a regulation will commonly overestimate the regulation's long-term impact. At the same time, the long-term effects are much more difficult to estimate, particularly if potential technological advances in the production of substitutes are not known at the time regulation of a particular product is proposed.

The problem of uncertainty is further aggravated by the fact that often the parties with the most accurate information on the costs and effects of regulation have an incentive to withhold or misinterpret that information. In general, the regulated industries have better access to information and more expertise concerning the technological difficulties and direct costs of exposure control than do the regulatory agencies, the unions, or the consumer and environmental groups.[67] To some extent, the industries also have the same advantage regarding the economic value of their substances.[68] The industries also have strong economic and institutional incentives to exaggerate the difficulties and costs of a potential regulation, with the hope of limiting its strength. Subsequent experience often reveals the industries' predictions to have been inflated in this manner.[69]

The imbalance is difficult to rectify. Whereas toxicological research can be regularized and made more reliable by the use of standard test protocols and evaluative techniques, no standard protocols for economic assessments have yet been developed or agreed upon. Governmental agencies are developing analytic capabilities of their own,[70] and they can compel industries to submit necessary data. These capabilities, however, require larger staffs and budgets, and significant legal barriers remain to obtaining the necessary information.[71]

Another means of coping with the imbalance is to discount the industries' representations as to the difficulties and costs of control and as to the economic value of the regulated substance. The shortcoming of this rule is that it does not encourage an end to exaggeration, and it may in fact lead industries to "cry wolf" all the more.[72] On the assumption, however, that industries will continue to overstate their problems under any rule, this rule is an effective way to improve the government's bargaining position.

In sum, the regulatory agency's data concerning the costs of regulation are as imprecise as its information about risks. The technological limits to present control capabilities are uncertain, and the limits to future capabilities are even more so. Only the costs of the readily forseeable controls can be calculated with much confidence. The wider economic and health consequences of regulation are difficult to identify in advance, especially if the regulated substance is in widespread use and if the regulation is stringent. As the agencies approach the task of balancing competing health and economic interests, they have only limited knowledge of the relative economic values at stake.

C. The Balancing Problem: Dilemmas of "Socially Acceptable Risk"

The greatest difficulties in the toxic substances area are in the selection of a level of risk that is somehow acceptable in light of its economic benefits. Even if risks and costs are known with certainty, they still are not fully comparable. Lives cannot be fully valued in dollars, and no satisfactory method exists for expressing one in terms of the other. Furthermore, as the people exposed to harm are not identical to those who bear the costs of control, any control measures transfer resources from the former to the latter. Both of these problems raise value-laden questions of fairness.

Several approaches to the problem of comparing health interests with economic interests have been suggested. One view is that no price can be put on a human life and that no economic benefit justifies causing a person's death. This view does not comport with everyday human behavior, however; people routinely drive automobiles, for example, placing their own and others' lives at risk.[73] Concluding that some trade-off between health and economic interests is socially and ethically acceptable, some theorists have attempted to derive economic values for individual human lives. For example, the "human capital" approach sets the value of a life at the individual's future earnings, or at the individual's net future contribution to the economy.[74] This technique has the obvious disadvantage of failing to value those aspects of life and personality that are not rewarded in the marketplace.

The approach currently in favor among economists and policy analysts focuses on the fact that while people are unwilling to name a dollar sum worth their own death, they apparently are willing to trade economic benefits for increases or decreases in the risk of death for each individual in a large group. A number of studies have examined individuals' "willingness-to-pay" for changes in the risk of death, particularly in hazardous categories of employment.[75] Some have asserted that risk-benefit combinations can be derived from these studies that are socially acceptable and that should be used as benchmarks for legislative, regulatory, and judicial policy making about toxic substances.[76]

Yet there are problems with the basic premise that socially acceptable risk-benefit relationships can be derived in this manner. It is questionable whether *observed* risk-benefit relationships of this kind should be treated as *norms* for toxic substances control or other programs of safety and health protection. For one thing, it is unlikely that the subjects of such employment risk studies were fully informed about their risks, at least not precisely enough to make subtle distinctions that can be extrapolated to larger populations. Second, it is possible that employees in hazardous industries are less adverse to taking risks than the general population. Finally, workers in most hazardous job categories may not have sufficient alternative employment opportunities or sufficient bargaining power to be able to insist on risk premiums that accurately reflect the perceived value of increased risks to their health and safety.

The problems of balancing health and economic values are compounded by the distributional impact of any toxic substances control measures. Although there may be no sharp division between the class of people who obtain the economic benefit of chemical use and the class of people who bear the health risks, some people gain or lose more than others. The employee exposed to vinyl chloride or other toxic substances in the workplace runs greater risks than the investor who never enters the plant. The farmworker exposed to dangerous pesticides bears a higher risk than food-company investors or the consumers of food. One who lives near a plant that emits toxic chemicals to the air or drinking water bears greater risks than another living far away. Which groups are subsidizing which others is often a matter of one's point of view and political values.[77]

A similar distributional issue exists because of the delayed impacts of many toxic substances. In the use of toxic chemicals, the economic benefits accrue quickly, but the adverse health and environmental effects are often delayed by many years. It may be tolerable for one generation to subject itself to future harms in exchange for present benefits, but severe equity problems are raised if the adverse effects span generations.[78]

D. Summing Up the Decision Problem

Toxic substances regulation, as we have seen, is characterized by ubiquitous problems of technological, medical, and economic uncertainty and by the difficulty of balancing incommensurable interests in standard-setting. It might seem, therefore, that factual analysis is a waste of resources for agencies and other parties affected by regulation. In reality, this is not so. First, although there is a wide range of decisions that an agency may make without being clearly wrong on a factual basis,[79] medical, technological, and economic research serves to eliminate relatively quickly a great number of clearly unsupportable regulatory possibilities. In addition, rough estimates of the health threats and economic significance of a number of chemicals, even though they may be uncertain, permit an agency to set priorities for regulation. Finally, continued pressure for more effective and precise information will continue to stimulate advances in the state of knowledge on these subjects.

Public debate on questions of acceptable risk has been markedly unsophisticated. Some commentators and some statutes call for absolute freedom from exposure to carcinogens regardless of cost.[80] Others emphasize the economic costs of environmental regulation, discounting impacts on health and the environment. For the most part, however, the toxic substances statutes represent a national political judgment that a middle ground should be reached. Those statutes establish "rule of reason" balancing tests that will support agency decisions favoring health interests over the economic interests that would result from an unregulated market.[80a] These standards, however, give virtually no guidance on the relative weight to be accorded health and environmental interests in comparison to economic ones, and to date, the agencies' actions reflect Congress's lack of consensus on the issue of acceptable risk.

A measure of guidance to decision makers in the face of uncertainty and lack of consensus is provided by the observation that regulatory decisions involve moral as well as economic values. We may begin with the observation that the sacrifice of an individual for the benefit of a group is acceptable if the benefit served is the group's survival or the fulfillment of some other basic need. The sacrifice is morally unacceptable, however, if it is for no more important benefit than the provision of the luxuries of our consuming society. That some must die so that all can eat is one thing; that some must die so that all can have see-through food packaging is another.[80b] Particularly where non-essential products are concerned, the long-term goal of toxic substances control and the long-term effect of each regulation should be to channel economic growth away from industries hazardous to health and towards safer products and forms of employment.

* * *

NOTES

1. These events are summarized in Occupational Safety and Health Administration, *Standard for Exposure to Vinyl Chloride*, 39 Fed. Reg. 35,890, 35,890–91 (1974) [hereinafter cited as *OSHA Permanent Standard for VC*]. See also Hearings on Dangers of Vinyl Chloride before the Subcomm. on Environment of the Senate Comm. on Commerce, 93d Cong., 2d Sess. 39–42 (1974) (testimony of Dr. Marcus Key, Director, National Institute for Occupational Safety and Health) [hereinafter cited as *VC Hearings*].

2. See text accompanying notes 81–82 *infra*. [*Text and notes omitted.*]

3. See text accompanying notes 124–129, 139–141 *infra*. [*Text and notes omitted.*]

4. Dep't of Labor, *Possible Hazards of Vinyl Chloride Manufacture and Use, Request for Information and Notice of Fact-Finding Hearing*, 39 Fed. Reg. 3874 (1974) [hereinafter cited as *OSHA Hearing Notice*].

5. There have been several other studies of the regulation of VC: Krause, *Environmental Carcinogenesis: Regulation on the Frontiers of Science*, 7 ENVT'L. L. 83 (1976); N. Ashford, E. Zolt, D. Hattis, & J. Katz, The Impact of Governmental Restrictions on the Production and Use of Chemicals: Draft Final Report (appendices concerning regulation of VC in the workplace and as a food additive) (Dec. 1976) (report prepared for the Council on Environmental Quality); G. Adams,

Toxic Substance Control: Vinyl Chloride (unpublished master's thesis, Washington University, St. Louis, Mo., Dec. 1976).

6. For a more thorough description of the uses of VC and PVC, see text accompanying notes 84–87 and Figure 1 *infra*. [*Text and notes omitted.*]

7. For a more complete description of the sources of exposure, see text accompanying notes 148–167 *infra*. [Text and notes omitted.]

8. See text accompanying notes 98, 125–135 *infra*. [*Text and notes omitted.*]

9. See text accompanying notes 22–80, 148–167 *infra*. [*Text and notes omitted.*]

10. See text accompanying note 138 *infra*. [*Text and notes omitted.*]

11. On the vast number of hazardous substances needing regulatory attention, see Slesin & Sandler, *Categorization of Chemicals Under the Toxic Substances Control Act*, 7 ECOLOGY L.Q. 359 (1978); Page, *A Generic View of Toxic Chemicals and Similar Risks*, 7 ECOLOGY L.Q. 207 (1978). As an example of the numbers problem, see NATIONAL INSTITUTE FOR OCCUPATIONAL SAFETY & HEALTH, SUSPECTED CARCINOGENS (2d ed. 1976), which identifies 1,500–2,000 chemicals that animal experiments have implicated as possible carcinogens.

12. Maugh, *Chemicals: How Many Are There?* 199 SCIENCE 162 (1978).

13. Between 60 and 90 percent of human cancers are estimated to be caused, wholly or in part, by chemicals in food, water, workplaces, cigarette smoke, and the general environment. See COUNCIL ON ENVIRONMENTAL QUALITY, SIXTH ANNUAL REPORT 32–33 (1975). *See also* text accompanying note 33 *infra*.

14. Two possible exceptions are the components of cosmetics and of substances harmful to the natural environment which are components of food and drugs. *See generally* Page & Blackburn, *Behind the Looking Glass: Administrative, Legislative, and Private Approaches to Cosmetic Safety Substantiation*, 24 U.C.L.A. L. REV. 795 (1977); EPA, *Fully Halogenated Chlorofluoroalkanes, Proposed Rule*, 42 Fed. Reg. 24,544, 24,545 (1977).

15. *See* Interagency Regulatory Liaison Group, Joint Regulatory Developments, March 1, 1978, *reprinted in* 1 BNA CHEM. REG. REP.—CURR. REP. 1916–21 (1978) [hereinafter cited as IRLG List of Substances of Common Concern]. The list includes VC. For some of these substances, such as VC, some regulations are already in effect and more are under consideration.

16. The problem may be avoided for new chemicals, which under the Toxic Substances Control Act (TSCA) must be tested by manufacturers and evaluated by the Environmental Protection Agency prior to their entry into commerce. TSCA §4, 15 U.S.C. §2063 (Supp. V. 1975).

17. See text accompanying notes 672–674, 753–771, 793–795 *infra*. [*Text and notes omitted.*]

18. See text accompanying notes 557–561, 608 *infra*. [*Text and notes omitted.*]

19. See text accompanying notes 347–348, 470–472, 803–804 *infra*. [*Text and notes omitted.*]

20. See text accompanying notes 836–868 *infra*. [*Text and notes omitted.*]

21. 15 U.S.C. §§2601–2629 (West Supp. 1978).

22. The quoted phrase is taken from the title of a study of water project planning and, more particularly, from an article on similar issues in cost-benefit analysis in that context. *See* Bradford & Feiveson, *Benefits and Costs, Winners and Losers* in BOUNDARIES OF ANALYSIS: AN INQUIRY INTO THE TOCKS ISLAND DAM CONTROVERSY 125, 144 (H. Feiveson, F. Sinden, & R. Socolow eds. 1976).

23. *See* COUNCIL ON ENVIRONMENTAL QUALITY, SIXTH ANNUAL REPORT 13 (1975) (ch. 1, *Carcinogens in the Environment*) [hereinafter cited as CEQ SIXTH ANNUAL REPORT]. For explanations of the essentials of cancer directed to the lay reader, see M. SHIMKIN, SCIENCE AND CANCER, 1–6, 45–54, 87–98 (1973) [hereinafter cited as SCIENCE AND CANCER]; Cairns, *The Cancer Problem*, SCIENTIFIC AMERICAN, Nov. 1975, at 64 [hereinafter cited as *The Cancer Problem*].

24. CEQ SIXTH ANNUAL REPORT, *supra* note 23, at 9, table 2.

25. *Id.* at 12.

26. *The Cancer Problem*, *supra* note 23, at 66.

27. CANCER PATIENT SURVIVAL, REP. NO. 5, U.S. DEP'T HEALTH, EDUC., & WELF. PUB. NO. (NIH) 77–992, at 3 (1976).

28. *The Cancer Problem*, *supra* note 23, at 72.

29. See Hammond, *Tobacco* in PERSONS AT HIGH RISK OF CANCER: AN APPROACH TO CANCER ETIOLOGY AND CONTROL 131 (J. Fraumeni ed.1975) [hereinafter cited as PERSONS AT HIGH RISK OF CANCER].

30. CEQ SIXTH ANNUAL REPORT, *supra* note 23, at 23–26; Cole & Goldman, *Occupation* in PERSONS AT HIGH RISK OF CANCER, *supra* note 29, at 167.

31. EPA, *Interim Drinking Water Regulations: Control of Organic Chemical Contaminants in Drinking Water*, 43 Fed. Reg. 5756, 5758 (1978), *citing* NATIONAL ACADEMY OF SCIENCES, DRINKING WATER AND HEALTH (June 1977); Pike, *Air Pollution* in PERSONS AT HIGH RISK OF CANCER, *supra* note 29, at 225.

32. CEQ SIXTH ANNUAL REPORT, *supra* note 23, at 19; Hoover, Mason, McKay, & Fraumeni, *Geographic Patterns of Cancer Mortality in the United States* in PERSONS AT HIGH RISK OF CANCER, *supra* note 29, at 343–44 & table 1, at 345.

33. CEQ SIXTH ANNUAL REPORT, *supra* note 23, at 17; Higginson, *Importance of Environmental Factors in Cancer* in ENVIRONMENTAL POLLUTION AND CARCINOGENIC RISKS 15, 17 (C. Rosenfeld & W. Davis, eds. 1975) [hereinafter cited as ENVIRONMENTAL POLLUTION]; Boyland, *The Correlation of Experimental Carcinogenesis and Cancer in Man,* 11 PROGRESS IN EXPERIMENTAL TUMOR RESEARCH 222, 223 (1969); Epstein, *Environmental Determinants of Human Cancer,* 34 CANCER RESEARCH 2425 (1974). *See also* R. DOLL, PREVENTION OF CANCER: POINTERS FROM EPIDEMIOLOGY (1967) [hereinafter cited as PREVENTION OF CANCER].

34. CEQ SIXTH ANNUAL REPORT, *supra* note 23, at 30–32. The apparent exception is arsenic.

35. Occupational Safety and Health Administration, *Identification, Classification and Regulation of Toxic Substances Posing a Potential Occupational Carcinogenic Risk,* 42 Fed. Reg. 54,148 (1977).

36. Schneiderman, *Sources, Resources, and Tsouris* in PERSONS AT HIGH RISK OF CANCER, *supra* note 29, at 451, 452, 459.

37. *See generally* Schneiderman, Mantel, & Brown, *From Mouse to Man—Or How to Get from the Laboratory to Park Avenue and 59th Street,* 246 ANNALS N.Y. ACAD. SCI. 237, 243 (1975) [hereinafter cited as *From Mouse to Man*].

38. SCIENCE AND CANCER, *supra* note 23, at 45–54, 87–92.

39. *See generally* Mantel & Schneiderman, *Estimating "Safe" Levels, a Hazardous Undertaking,* 35 CANCER RESEARCH 1379 (1975) [hereinafter cited as *Estimating "Safe" Levels*].

40. *See* Cornfield, *Carcinogenic Risk Assessment,* 198 SCIENCE 693 (1977) [hereinafter cited as *Carcinogenic Risk Assessment*].

41. *See, e.g.,* Watanabe & Gehring. *Dose-Dependent Fate of Vinyl Chloride and Its Possible Relationship to Oncogenicity in Rats,* 17 ENVT'L. HEALTH PERSPECTIVES 145 (1976).

42. Some assumptions lead to the conclusion that threshold doses exist and that the risk at doses approaching the threshold declines to zero. *See* Kotin, *Dose-Response Relationship and Threshold Concepts,* 271 ANNALS N.Y. ACAD. SCI. 22, 25–27 [1976). *See also Carcinogenic Risk Assessment, supra* note 40; *DNA Repair: New Clues to Carcinogenesis,* 200 SCIENCES 518 (1978). Other models decline to decide whether there are thresholds. One major model has dose and response in a logarithmic relationship, with risk declining more rapidly than dose at low doses. This model yields higher risks for given doses than those which posit thresholds. *See Estimating "Safe" Levels, supra* note 39.

Other researchers argue that the dose-response relationship at low doses is likely to be linear, *i.e.,* that decreases in risk are probably proportional to reduc-

tions of dose. This approach yields a risk for a given dose higher than the risks estimated by the other two approaches at least at low doses. *See* Crump, Hoel, Langley, & Peto, *Fundamental Carcinogenic Processes and Their Implications for Low Dose Risk Assessment,* 36 CANCER RESEARCH 2973 (1976) [hereinafter cited as *Fundamental Carcinogenic Processes*].

The issues are summarized briefly in NATIONAL ACADEMY OF SCIENCES, PRINCIPLES FOR EVALUATION CHEMICALS IN THE ENVIRONMENT 86–88 (1975) [hereinafter cited as PRINCIPLES FOR EVALUATING CHEMICALS].

43. CEQ SIXTH ANNUAL REPORT, *supra* note 23, at 23–26.

44. *Id.* at 26–28.

45. *Id.* If the effect is mutation rather than cancer, the effect will not manifest itself for one or more generations.

For a general description of the nature of epidemiological evidence and of the uses and limitations of such research, see PREVENTION OF CANCER, *supra* note 33, at 15–29.

46. CEQ SIXTH ANNUAL REPORT, *supra* note 23, at 28–32; In re Shell Chem. Co., 6 ERC 2047, 2052 (EPA, FIFRA Docket, 1977); PRINCIPLES FOR EVALUATING CHEMICALS, *supra* note 42, at 135–39; T LOOMIS, ESSENTIALS OF TOXICOLOGY 206 (2d ed. 1974) [hereinafter cited as ESSENTIALS OF TOXICOLOGY].

47. CEQ SIXTH ANNUAL REPORT, *supra* note 23, at 30–32; *Estimating Safe Levels, supra* note 39, at 1381.

48. *See From Mouse to Man, supra* note 37. On the trade-off between the sensitivity and cost of tests, see Bates, *Laboratory Approaches to the Identification of Carcinogens,* 271 ANN. N.Y. ACAD. SCI. 29, 30–32 (1976).

49. For an explanation for laymen of the statistical issues, see W. LOWRANCE, OF ACCEPTABLE RISK 60–64 (1976) [hereinafter cited as OF ACCEPTABLE RISK].

50. This is not always the case, however. Some carcinogens are potent enough to cause cancers in experimental animals when administered at the dose levels to which people have been exposed. See text accompanying notes 133–146 *infra.* [*Text and notes omitted.*]

51. Three examples illustrate the point. In a test involving 100 animals each in an experimental and a control group, if no tumors are detected in either group, there is a 1.0% chance that the real rate of cancer is as high as 4.5%. With 1,000 animals in each group and no tumors, there remains a 1.0% chance that the real rate is as high as 0.46%, or 4.6 animals out of each 1,000. If only ten animals are used in each group and the results show no tumors, the potential error increases drastically; there is a 1.0% chance that the real rate is as high as 37.0%. *See* OF ACCEPTABLE RISK, *supra* note 49, at 62.

52. For a clear discussion of these points, see Saffiotti, *Comments on the Scientific Basis for the "Delaney Clause,"* 2 PREVENTIVE MEDICINE 125 (1973) [hereinafter cited as *Comments on the Scientific Basis for the "Delaney Clause"*]. *See also* World Health Organization, Assessment of the Carcinogenicity and Mutagenicity of Chemicals, Technical Report Series, No. 546, at 9–11 (1974); *Estimating "Safe" Levels*, *supra* note 42, at 1382–83.

53. *Estimating "Safe" Levels, supra* note 42, at 1383. *See also From Mouse to Man, supra* note 37, at 241.

54. *Carcinogenic Risk Assessment, supra* note 42, at 694.

55. For example, Schneiderman and his colleagues estimated on the basis of the animal experiments on VC completed by May 1974 "that a dose as low as 1 ppm [part per million] is almost certain to have a risk of less than 1 in 10,000" for animals. *From Mouse to Man, supra* note 37, at 241–42.

56. *See* Rall, *Problems of Low Doses of Carcinogens,* 64 J. WASH. ACAD. SCI. 63 (1974).

57. McCann & Ames, *A Simple Method for Detecting Environmental Carcinogens as Mutagens,* 271 ANNALS N.Y. ACAD. SCI. 5 (1976). *See also* Note, *From Microbes to Men: The New Toxic Substances Control Act and Bacterial Mutagenicity/Carcinogenicity Tests,* 6 ENVT'L. L. REP. 10,248 (1976).

58. *See* NATIONAL RESEARCH COUNCIL, DECISION MAKING IN THE ENVIRONMENTAL PROTECTION AGENCY 54–57 (1977) [hereinafter cited as DECISION MAKING IN EPA].

59. As an example of standard protocols for cancer testing, see Sontag, Page, & Saffiotti, Guidelines for Carcinogen Bioassay in Small Rodents, National Cancer Institute, Carcinogenesis Technical Report Series No. 1 (1976), *summarized in* Shubik & Clayson, *Application of the Results of Carcinogen Bioassays to Man* in ENVIRONMENTAL POLLUTION, *supra* note 33, at 241, 242. *See also* PRINCIPLES FOR EVALUATING CHEMICALS, *supra* note 42, at 134–55.

One other means for controlling the quality of data is to certify laboratories that meet minimum standards for their performance. *See* DECISION MAKING IN EPA, *supra* note 58, at 54–57. In addition, there are penalties in certain of the regulatory statutes for a company's misrepresenting or withholding toxicological data. Currently, the Food and Drug Administration is developing such certification procedures as part of "Good Laboratory Practice" regulations, and the agency has referred at least one case involving misrepresentation of data to the Justice Department with a recommendation for criminal prosecution. *See Creative Penmanship in Animal Testing Prompts FDA Controls,* 198 SCIENCE 1227 (1977). In addition, Velsicol Chemical Corporation has been indicted for withholding data from EPA regarding animal cancer tests on heptachlor/chlordane. *See Indictment*

Charges Velsicol, Six Persons, Withheld Chlordane, Heptachlordane Data, 1 BNA CHEM. REG. REP.— CURR. REP. 1413–14 (1977).

60. See text accompanying notes 67–71 *infra*.

61. *See generally* NATIONAL ACADEMY OF SCIENCES, DECISION MAKING FOR REGULATING CHEMICALS IN THE ENVIRONMENT 150–62 (1975) [hereinafter cited as DECISION MAKING FOR REGULATING CHEMICALS]. This study points out a fourth category of costs, effects of a regulation on market structure. A single decision or set of decisions may have the consequence of increasing concentration in an industry or of establishing barriers to entry, or may change the rate of innovation. *Id.* at 156. This topic is not addressed in this section. It is possible to argue, however, that other governmental mechanisms exist (*e.g.*, anti-trust regulation and research and development spending) to deal adequately with any such impacts. *See generally* R. NOLL, REFORMING REGULATION 29 (1971) [hereinafter cited as REFORMING REGULATION].

62. The general rule is illustrated in A. FREEMAN, R. HAVEMAN, & A. KNEESE, THE ECONOMICS OF ENVIRONMENTAL POLICY 86–87 (1973).

63. The increasing uncertainty is illustrated in W. ROWE, AN ANATOMY OF RISK 234 (1977) [hereinafter cited as AN ANATOMY OF RISK].

64. The economic term for this relationship is elasticity of demand.

65. The prime example of this problem is the continuing debate over whether the nearly complete ban on the use of DDT in the United States was a sensible or foolhardy decision. Much of the controversy concerns differences over the safety of the substance and differences between the parties on the acceptability of risks. In large part, however, the controversy concerns differences over the magnitude of the economic effects of the ban. *See* OF ACCEPTABLE RISK, *supra* note 49, at 155–73.

66. The recent history of aerosol products provides an example of the secondary adverse health consequences of a health-motivated regulation. Before 1974, VC was used in combination with fluorocarbons in some aerosols. When this use of VC was banned in 1974, no consideration was given to the possible adverse consequences of using a greater quantity of fluorocarbons. Subsequently, fluorocarbons were discovered to threaten the ozone layer in the upper atmosphere, and the use of this chemical in aerosol products will soon be ended. Thus the effect of regulating this use of VC was to aggravate the fluorocarbons problem, albeit for only a short period. On the regulation of VC in aerosols, see text accompanying notes 551–611 *infra*. [*Text and notes omitted.*]

67. *See, e.g.,* DECISION MAKING IN EPA, *supra* note 58, at 52–54, 57–58. The industries are also better organized to participate in regulatory decisions than is the generally affected public. The general public's in-

terest in a particular decision may be more weighty than in industry's, but there is a considerable cost to organizing. *See generally* M.OLSON, THE LOGIC OF COLLECTIVE ACTION 9–16 (1965). This organizational imbalance has been overcome only partly by the participation of environmental and consumer groups and labor unions in legislative and administrative proceedings.

68. *See generally* DECISION MAKING FOR REGULATING CHEMICALS, *supra* note 61, at 134–36.

69. See especially the misrepresentations of the VC and PVC industries regarding the impact of the OSHA standard, discussed at text accompanying notes 272–274, 325–338 *infra*. [*Text and notes omitted.*]

70. *See* DECISION MAKING IN EPA, *supra* note 58, at 51–54, 57–63. For example, OSHA and its companion research agency, the National Institute for Occupational Safety and Health, have been improving their capabilities to assess control possibilities and costs. *See* Hickey & Kearney, Engineering Control Research and Development Plan for Carcinogenic Materials, Research Triangle Institute, Research Triangle Park, North Carolina (Sept. 1977) (draft of study on contract from NIOSH).

71. Much of the necessary information is withheld from the government or the public on the grounds of trade secrecy claims. There is a great deal of controversy over how trade secrets will be treated in toxic substances regulation.

72. The rule penalizes an industry which presents data without exaggeration, because the data will be discounted rather than taken at face value.

73. *See* Schelling, *The Life You Save May Be Your Own* in PROBLEMS IN PUBLIC EXPENDITURE ANALYSIS 127, 129–33 (S. Chase ed. 1968) [hereinafter cited as *The Life You Save May Be Your Own*].

74. This discussion is derived mainly from *id.* and from Mishan, *Evaluation of Life and Limb: A Theoretical Approach*, 79 J. POLITICAL ECON. 687, 687–90 (1971) [hereinafter cited as *Evaluation of Life and Limb*]. The issues are summarized in DECISION MAKING IN EPA, *supra* note 58, at 219–34.

75. *The Life You Save May Be Your Own*, *supra* note 73, at 129–33, 142–44; *Evaluation of Life and Limb*, *supra* note 74, at 693–95. *See* DECISION MAKING IN EPA, *supra* note 58, at 232–34. *See also* Thaler & Rosen, Value of Saving a Life: Evidence from the Labor Market (unpublished 1975), cited in Kneese & Schulze, *Environment, Health, and Economics—The Case of Cancer*, 67 AM. ECON. REV. 326, 331 (1977) [hereinafter cited as *Environment, Health, and Economics*]. Thaler and Rosen estimate the value of an additional 0.001 risk of death at $260 per year, and consequently put the value of a life at $260,000.

76. *The Life You Save May Be Your Own*, *supra* note 73, at 158–62. *See generally* Starr, *Benefit-Cost Studies in Socio-technical Systems* in NATIONAL ACADEMY OF ENGINEERING, PERSPECTIVES ON ENVIRONMENTAL RISK DECISION MAKING 17 (1973).

77. *See* Coase, *The Problem of Social Cost*. 3 J.L. & ECON. 1 (1960).

78. See the chapter on equity considerations in DECISION MAKING FOR REGULATING CHEMICALS, *supra* note 61, at 121–29.

79. This is the thrust of most discussions of principles for judicial review of agency action regarding health and environmental hazards. *See, e.g.*, Ethyl Corp. v. EPA, 541 F.2d 1, 34, 8 ERC 1785, 1809–1811 (D.C. Cir. 1976). Judicial review is discussed in text accompanying notes 950–998 *infra*. [*Text and notes omitted.*]

80. *See, e.g.*, the Delaney Clause in the Food Additives Amendment to the Food, Drug, and Cosmetic Act, 21 U.S.C. §348(c)(3)(A) (1970), which prohibits the intentional addition to food of any amount of a substance determined to be carcinogenic in man or animal, and §112(a)(3)(B) of the Clean Air Act, 42 U.S.C. §7412(a)(3)(B) (West Supp. 1978), which states that a hazardous air pollutant standard must assure "an ample margin of safety" to protect health. See text accompanying notes 369–373, 492–494 *infra*. [*Text and notes omitted.*]

80a. *See, e.g.* §6(b)(5) of the Occupational Safety and Health Act, 29 U.S.C. §655(b)(5) (1970), which specifies that standards protect health "to the extent feasible." This provision, as well as certain others, has been held to be "technology-forcing," *i.e.*, to allow an agency to set standards whose requirements are somewhat beyond the conceded control capabilities of regulated industries, in order to stimulate the development of new devices and to counter the industries' underestimation of present capabilities. See text accompanying notes 213, 322–324 *infra*. [*Text and notes omitted.*] *See also* Portland Cement Ass'n v. Ruckelshaus, 486 F.2d 375, 384–85, 5 ERC 1593, 1599 (D.C. Cir. 1973) *cert. denied* 417 U.S. 921 (1974), 423 U.S. 1025 (1975), *reh. denied* 423 U.S. 1092 (1975) (interpreting the technology-forcing character of Clean Air Act §111, 42 U.S.C. §7411 (West Supp. 1978).

80b. Many value judgments are not so easily made as the distinction between food and food packaging. Typically, economists take the position that neutrality is required at all times in this regard, because of the difficulty of making so many of these value judgments. *See, e.g., Evaluation of Life and Limb, supra* note 74, at 695–96, 703. But the difficulty of making the hard decisions does not require us to avoid making the clearcut ones. And one need not accept the view that the values of a society must be regarded as inviolate. They change in a manner not fully understood, but certainly not free from the influences of groups, such as the business community, with strong financial interests in promoting the materialistic, consuming behavior of the public. As Professor Tribe puts it: "[W]e cannot simply assume that we must stand mute when confronting the ultimate question of whether we want our children, and their children's children, to live in—and *enjoy*—a plastic world." Tribe, *Ways Not to Think About Plastic Trees* in WHEN VALUES CONFLICT 61, 70 (L. Tribe, C. Schelling, & J. Voss eds.

1976) (emphasis in original). *See also* Dorfman, *An Afterword: Humane Values and Environmental Decisions,* in *id.* at 153–73.

* * *

3.4 A Philadelphia Story*

ANNETTE K. ALTSCHULER

Reprinted with permission of the Institute of Humane Studies, Inc., from 1 *Law & Liberty* 1, 11 and 12 (Winter 1975).

Just as chiropractors tend to believe that a great many of mankind's problems can be solved by manipulating the vertebrae, lawyers tend to put inordinate faith in manipulating the law. In the following tale, the Department of Housing and Urban Development, the City of Philadelphia, the United States Navy, assorted judges, poverty lawyers, and concerned citizens became involved in an elaborate legal imbroglio. It all started with a gift.

In the early 1960s, the United States Navy gave to the City of Philadelphia a huge quantity of surplus lead-based paint. The city fathers then passed on the paint to the citizens on a free, first-come-first-served basis. Since good lead paint is expensive, the program was a popular success. Everything in sight was painted.

There were a few problems. Lead was known to be toxic to humans, and there had been an outbreak of lead poisoning in children in Philadelphia in the 1950s. As time had passed, the public-health authorities had come to recognize the peril posed to young children who eat loose paint. Through the efforts of the Philadelphia Department of Public Health, that city took the initiative in eliminating this childhood health hazard by the adoption, in 1966, of an antilead-paint ordinance.

Since no one was in favor of poisoning children, it was assumed by the proponents of the measure that property owners would simply remove the newly recognized hazard. As so often seems to happen in our efforts to legislate a better world, cost was overlooked. Removal of lead-based paint and repainting could cost as much as $1,500 per unit. The owners of low-cost housing, most of which was tenant-occupied, could not pass on the cost to their tenants, for the tenants' rent-paying ability remained stationary. Serious economic difficulty was thus created in the area of low-income housing, which was, for the most part, composed of older houses with lead-based paint.

Changes in FHA mortgage insurance policies in 1968 brought about a large increase in the number of low-income owner-occupants. For a number of reasons beyond the scope of this article, the rental housing market had become untenable. Numerous problems arose for the new homeowners, many of whom had had no previous homeowner experience. Not the least of these problems was the responsibility for the removal of the leaded paint; the burden was now on him (the homeowner), whereas previously it had been on the landlord. Yet he was no better able to bear this cost as homeowner than he had been as renter.

The Department of Housing and Urban Development (HUD), apparently unaware of the

---

*I wish to express appreciation to CLS, HUD, the Department of Public Health, and the Research Section of the Oral Health Services of the University of Pennsylvania for their cooperation. The interpretations of information received are, of course, the author's.

lead-paint hazard, had insured the mortgages of this new group of homeowners. But then cases arose in which high-lead blood levels were discovered in children of these new homeowners. The parents were cited by the City of Philadelphia for lead-paint violations and were informed that it was their responsibility to remove the paint. When brought before the City's Common Pleas Court, the parents were threatened with large fines and criminal liability.

In August, 1972, the Community Legal Services (CLS), representing the City Wide Coalition Against Lead Paint Poisoning, and low-income purchasers of HUD-owned properties (acquired by HUD through foreclosure) instituted suit against the city and HUD. The suit was directed toward forcing HUD to remove lead-based paint from its properties prior to selling.

In January, 1973, U.S. District Court Judge Donald W. Van Artsdalen, in a preliminary hearing, enjoined HUD against selling, conveying, or transferring title or ownership to anyone for human habitation unless lead paint was removed from both interior and exterior surfaces. A HUD spokesman stated that a health problem had now become a housing nightmare, but the citizen groups and their public interest counsel considered it an important victory.

HUD then stopped selling its houses and the housing market drifted into confusion. Owners were confronted with three different legal standards defining a lead-paint hazard: the court's, the city ordinance, and HUD's. HUD's insurance standards require removal of cracked, peeled, or chipped paint, or that it be made tight. The city ordinance defines the problem in terms of a diagnosed health hazard. Judge Van Artsdalen demanded lead paint removal.

The impasse has serious implications for a city already in the throes of massive housing abandonment. Boarded-up vacant houses strongly affect property values. Elimination of this depressing environmental factor is critical for neighborhood preservation. HUD's boarded-up houses further depress and exacerbate a problem to monumental proportions. In January, 1973, when HUD stopped selling its units in Philadelphia, HUD owned about 1,650 houses; by January of 1974, the number had risen to 3,700. The cost to HUD for each vacant unit is approximately $1,440 a year. The time period before reoccupancy previously had been six months. It is now assumed the time span will be one year. Lead paint removal averages $600 for a three-bedroom house. While on a nationwide average HUD formerly had lost $5,800 without overhead on each house it acquired through foreclosure, repaired, and sold, the cost is now $6,500.

In the fall of 1973, HUD decided to comply with the court order and contracted with the city to identify what had to be done on each house—at $15 a unit. To date 1,500 have been inspected; 97 per cent have leaded paint.

A further complication involved *Page v. Romney* and *Davis v. Romney*. Both were individual cases represented by CLS and heard by U.S. District Court Judge Davis. HUD was ordered to remove the lead paint from the Page house, which had been in its inventory. The *Davis* case involved other repairs and HUD appealed. The Appellate Court sent it back to Judge Davis. HUD is now considering appealing both the original class-action suit and the *Page* case on the basis of the *Davis* case.

In September, 1973, HUD Assistant Secretary Sheldon B. Lubar issued a directive stating that commitments for mortgage insurance on existing properties within the city limits shall contain the condition that a certificate of inspection be secured, showing that the property is acceptable to the City of Philadelphia, pursuant to the terms of the local, lead-paint ordinance. A city ordinance was duly passed authorizing the Department of Public Health to inspect, on request, and state whether or not a house was in compliance with the Lead Poisoning Ordinance of 1966. Conditional mortgage commitments were issued as were Department of Public Health inspection certificates. HUD clarified its position: No HUD-insured mortgages would be granted unless the houses complied with Van Artsdalen's rulings; these units could, through foreclosure, become part of HUD's inventory.

Enormous areas of the city are almost totally dependent on HUD-insured mortgages for financing, so the market now is effectively frozen. Sellers cannot sell; buyers cannot buy. This development compounds the chaos existing in the low- and moderate-income rental market. The city has stated it cannot comply since its ordinance provides for the control of a health hazard to children resulting from lead-based paint. The child is the major focus rather than the house. In addition, portable testing equipment currently available cannot test as low a lead content as that required by new federal definition. Chemical methods are costly and deface the houses tested. The city also claims it has no authority to issue the types of certification requested by HUD. HUD stands fast with its projection of Van Artsdalen's ruling. Philadelphia is the only city in the nation that has no HUD-insured mortgages available to it. As usual, the ultimate victim is the low- and moderate-income purchaser of housing who has no other recourse open to him.

What started out as a sincere effort to remove a serious health hazard has resulted in the creation of a multiheaded monster primarily affecting those it was originally designed to help. Perhaps the present situation was best summed up by Mr. Robb, regional HUD chief, who said, "It is a horrible, heart-breaking, hell of a mess."

It is hard to disagree with that.

3.5 Dunson v. Friedlander Realty
369 So. 2d 792 (Ala. 1979)

SHORES, Justice.

The two cases involved in this appeal were consolidated by stipulation because they involve identical injuries and parties. The cases were filed by Frederick W. Dunson, individually and as father and next friend of his two minor daughters, against Friedlander Realty, a corporation, fictitious individuals designated John Doe I through John Doe V and fictitious parties designated X Company and Y Company.

Each complaint contains five separate claims for relief against the various defendants. In all counts, plaintiffs, while tenants of rental property located at 815 South Broad Street, Mobile, Alabama, sustained injuries when they consumed lead-based paint chips.

Count One alleges a landlord-tenant relationship between plaintiffs and defendants, Friedlander Realty, John Doe I–III, and alleges that these defendants were liable to the plaintiffs for injuries resulting to them from a hazardous, unsafe and dangerous defect in the premises, namely lead-based paint, which defect was known to these defendants at the time of the leasing and which they concealed from the plaintiffs.

Count Two alleges that the same defendants were aware of the defect; and they entered into a covenant to repair and remedy this condition but breached the agreement causing injuries to the minor children.

Count Three alleges that the same defendants knew of the presence of the lead-based paint and voluntarily undertook, through their agents or servants, to repair or correct the defect by employing John Doe IV and V ". . . to scrape and paint said dwelling . . . and they negligently failed to remove the scrapings containing lead paint from the premises."

Count Four attempts to state a claim against fictitious parties, X and Y Companies, for breach of warranties, express and implied. Such parties are alleged to be ". . . in the business of manufacturing, testing and/or selling paint. . . ." and that they warranted the paint purchase by defendants, John Doe IV and V, for painting the dwelling to be fit for ordinary purposes; that this warranty was breached because ". . . it failed to keep contact with certain paint on said dwelling that contained lead and further, that said paint failed to seal properly the paint on said dwelling that contained lead. . . ." and "Plaintiff and his minor daughter[s] relied upon the skill and judgment of the said Defendants to select and furnish a suitable paint to seal the lead paint on said dwelling and to stop the chipping or peeling of the lead paint from said dwelling . . ."

Count Five simply incorporates the other four and seeks damages for medical expenses and loss of services of his minor children.

Both children are alleged to have lived in the house involved since their respective births, which means that the premises were rented by their father before the birth of either child.

Defendant Friedlander Realty filed a motion under ARCP 12(b)(6) to dismiss each of the complaints on the ground that it failed to state a claim against this defendant upon which relief can be granted. The trial court entered judgment in compliance with ARCP 54(b) and plaintiff appealed.

The only issue presented is whether the complaint states a claim upon which relief may be granted as to Friedlander Realty inasmuch as the judgment appealed from adjudicates only the claims asserted against it. Because that is so, we do not address the validity of the breach of warranty claim against the manufacturer or seller of the paint used to paint the dwelling.

[1, 2] We hold that Count One was properly dismissed. The general rule is that a landlord is not liable in tort for injuries suffered by a tenant, whether there be a covenant to repair or not unless the defect existed at the time of the letting and was known to him and which he concealed from the tenant. *Bevis v. L. & L Services*, 360 So.2d 296 (Ala. 1978); *James & Sons, Inc. v. Breedlove*, 347 So.2d 1330 (Ala. 1977); *Chambers v. Buettner*, 295 Ala. 8, 321 So.2d 650 (1975); *Hallock v. Smith*, 207 Ala. 567, 93 So. 588 (1922). The allegations of Count One are that the existence of lead paint on the premises constituted a defect under the general rule; and that the defendant is liable because it concealed the defect. Restatement of the Law, Torts 2d, §358 (1965), states the rule as follows:

"Undisclosed Dangerous Conditions Known to Lessor
"(1) A lessor of land who conceals or fails to disclose to his lessee any condition, whether natural or artificial, which involves unreasonable risk of physical harm to persons on the land, is subject to liability to the lessee and others upon the land with the consent of the lessee or his sublessee for physical harm caused by the condition after the lessee has taken possession, if
  "(a) the lessee does not know or have reason to know of the condition or the risk involved, and
  "(b) the lessor knows or has reason to know of the condition, and realizes or should realize the risk involved, and has reason to expect that the lessee will not discover the condition or realize the risk."

Under the allegations of this count, should the landlord (even if it knew the lead-based paint was on the walls) have realized the risk involved or, to state the question in traditional tort language, was it reasonably foreseeable that the dangerous paint would chip and fall from the walls and be ingested by children? A landlord is expected to foresee only those dangers as would be foreseen by a reasonably prudent man under the same or similar circumstances. See *W. Prosser, The Law of Torts*, §63, page 401 (4th ed. 1971); *F. Harper & James, The Law of Torts*, §27.16, pages 1508–9 (1956).

[3] Lead-based paint was commonly used in buildings constructed prior to World War II. Only in recent years has the danger connected with chipping lead-based paint been appreciated. See: Legislative History of the Lead-Based Paint Poisoning Prevention Act, Pub.L. No. 91–695, 91st Congress, 2d Sess. (1970), 3 U.S. Code, Cong. & Admin. News, p. 6130, et seq. That act was passed by the Congress to provide federal assistance to aid cities and communities to carry out programs to eliminate the cause of the disease.

We think it unreasonable to expect a landlord to foresee that children would eat and be injured by this substance. According to testimony presented to the Congress during its deliberation of the act mentioned above, a condition known as Pica (defined as a craving for and eating of unnatural substances such as chalk, ashes, bones, etc. generally occurring in instances of nutritional deficiency) generally accounts for lead poisoning. Under the allegations of this count, we hold that it was not reasonably foreseeable that these children would be injured by the paint on the premises rented to their father.

[4] Under the law, a landlord is not an insurer of the safety of the premises. The law does not impose such a high duty. However, one can undertake a duty higher than that which the law imposes. By Counts Two and Three, the plaintiff alleges that Friedlander did just that. Count Two alleges that it covenanted and agreed to eliminate the hazardous condition and breached the agreement; Count Three alleges that, with knowledge of the hazardous condition, Friedlander voluntarily undertook to remedy the defect.

[5] These are claims upon which relief may be granted if the plaintiff can prove the allegations. The burden of proof, of course, is upon the plaintiff to prove the existence of a contract and he must establish, by the evidence, the terms of the agreement. *Madison Highlands Develop-*

ment Co. v. Hall, 283 Ala. 333, 216 So.2d 724 (1968). If he can show that the defendant agreed to eliminate the offending substance from the premises and breached that agreement, he can recover damages for breach of that agreement.

[6–8] Friedlander says this count states no claim upon which relief can be granted because it fails to aver that the alleged contract was supported by consideration. It is alleged that the premises were rented on a month-to-month basis. It is also alleged that the tenant threatened to terminate the rental contract because of the hazardous condition; and that Friedlander then promised and agreed to remedy the dangerous defect or condition. In *Adler v. Miller,* 218 Ala. 674, 677, 120 So. 153, 154 (1928), this court said:

"As applied to the relation of landlord and tenant and liability for injury to the latter from defects in the premises, where there was an express agreement to repair, the case of *Hart v. Coleman,* 201 Ala. 345, 78 So. 201, L.R.A. 1918E, 213, declares the rule of this court. In that case the holding was that, where the promise of a landlord to a tenant by the month to repair the porch was under the latter's threat to move unless such repairs were made, such promise was founded on a sufficient consideration; and the landlord, being notified or observing that the floor of considerable height was rotten in front of the door, failed after such promise to repair, and the tenant receiving injury by a fall through such insufficient and unsafe flooring was permitted to recover damages in an action ex contractu. . . ."

It is equally well-settled that:

". . . where the lessor, under no duty to repair, voluntarily undertakes so to do, he is liable for injuries proximately caused by negligence in so making repairs as to render the premises dangerous to life or limb of those rightfully occupying the premises. . . ." *Faucett v. Provident Mut. Life Ins. Co. of Philadelphia,* 244 Ala. 308, 312, 13 So.2d 182, 186 (1943).

This is the theory of the plaintiff's claim under Count Three.

We hold that the trial court erred in granting Friedlander's motion to dismiss Counts Two, Three and Five where applicable. Count One was properly dismissed. We express no opinion as to Count Four, it not being before us on this appeal from an ARCP 54(b) judgment. In so holding, we restate that, as against a motion to dismiss under ARCP 12(b)(6), the complaint must be construed in the light most favorable to the plaintiff and its allegations taken as true. Wright & Miller, Federal Practice and Procedure: Civil §1357.

[9] It is never proper to dismiss a complaint if it contains even a generalized statement of facts which will support a claim for relief under ARCP 8.

[10] The Supreme Court of the United States in *Conley v. Gibson,* 355 U.S. 41, 45, 46, 78 S.Ct. 99, 102, 2 L.Ed.2d 80 (1957), stated the rule which we follow:

". . . In appraising the sufficiency of the complaint we follow, of course, the accepted rule that a complaint should not be dismissed for failure to state a claim unless it appears beyond doubt that the plaintiff can prove no set of facts in support of his claim which would entitle him to relief. . . ."

AFFIRMED IN PART; REVERSED IN PART AND REMANDED.

TORBERT, C.J., and MADDOX and JONES, J.J., concur.

BEATTY, J., concurs in result.

ISSUES FOR CONSIDERATION AND SUGGESTIONS FOR FURTHER READING

The subject of environmental law is beyond the compass of the brief introduction given here. The Doniger article in its entirety is lengthy but well worth a student's time and serious attention. Students with specific interests could begin with William H. Rodgers, Jr., *Rodgers' Hornbook on Environmental Law* (1977) or one of several law school casebooks on environmental law.

Altshuler's article on the lead paint controversy in Philadelphia compresses the following cases: City of Philadelphia v. Page, 373 F.Supp. 453 (E.D. Pa. 1974); City of Philadelphia v. Page, 363 F.Supp. 148 (E.D. Pa. 1973); City-Wide Coalition against Childhood Lead Paint Poisoning v. Philadelphia Housing Authority, 356 F.Supp. 123 (E.D. Pa. 1973); Davis v. Romney, 490 F.2d 1360 (3d Cir. 1974); Davis v. Romney, 355 F.Supp. 29 (E.D. Pa. 1973); Davis v. Romney, 55 F.R.D. 337 (E.D. Pa. 1972); and Davis v. Romney, 53 F.R.D. 247 (E.D. Pa. 1971). See also, Davis v. Romney, 530 F.2d 963 (3d Cir. 1976) (unpublished opinion).

Children in cities are at risk not only from the lead they eat, but also from the lead they breathe, Ethyl Corp. v. EPA, 541 F.2d 1, 12 (D.C. Cir. 1976) (lead particulate emissions from automobiles a "significant risk" to urban children).

For a good analysis of the interactive problems of law and environmental concerns at the local level, see Passman, "Composting Municipal Sludge: Public Health and Legal Implications," 3 *Harvard Environmental L. Rev.* 381 (1979).

An interesting product liability case on the duty of a drug manufacturer to warn parents of vaccine danger is Reyes v. Wyeth Laboratories, 498 F.2d 1264 (5th Cir. 1974).

CHAPTER 4

THE ROLE OF LAW IN DEFINING AND REGULATING BEHAVIOR

OVERVIEW

The two articles and case in this chapter deal with the role of law in defining and regulating behavior. In a very provocative treatment, the Morse article invites critical examination of the scientific framework that underlies mental health law, particularly in relation to the regulation of behavior. Beauchamp's article examines whether an alcohol policy focused on individual responsibility can properly vindicate the public interest in discouraging alcoholism.

Both articles should be considered as vehicles for examining the limits of law as a restraint on human freedom and the proper role of law in promoting health-related concerns—an issue raised in the case of *People v. Carmichael*, which treats the requirement of helmets for motorcyclists.

4.1 Crazy Behavior, Morals, and Science: An Analysis of Mental Health Law*

STEPHEN J. MORSE

Reprinted with permission of Stephen J. Morse, from 51 *Southern California Law Review* 528–542, 553, 554–564, 603–604, 612–613, 625–626 (1978). Copyright © 1978 by Stephen J. Morse. All rights reserved.

People . . . talk about "traumatic experiences" all the time. I wish they would quit it.

When they use that rubbery, nerveless expression, they cheat us out of what our language should make us feel about gruesome events. They should talk about wounding experiences and painful experiences and shocking experiences and crippling experiences and murderous experiences and so on, instead.

I have looked up the meaning of the word "traumatic" in a dictionary, and its origins and meanings. I still think it was invented by a manufacturer of self-sealing gas tanks. If a bullet traumatizes such a gas tank, no harm is done.

> Kurt Vonnegut, Jr.,
> Letter to the Editor,
> *New York Times*
> (April 27, 1975)

Thou shalt not sit with statisticians nor commit a social science.

> W.H. Auden,
> *Under Which Lyre—A reactionary tract for the times* (1946)

*This Article was first presented to a Faculty Workshop at the University of Southern California Law Center. The author gratefully acknowledges the assistance of the commentators, Martin Levine and Alan Schwartz, and his other colleagues at the Workshop and thereafter. Alan Schwartz deserves special thanks for his continual help. Richard J. Bonnie of the University of Virginia Law School also made many helpful suggestions. The author further thanks the reference staff of the Law Center Library for their unflagging and good-natured assistance.

An abbreviated version of the paper was presented at a symposium on "Legal Issues in Psychology" at the 1977 Annual Convention of the American Psychological Association and at a symposium on "Social Science Information and the Legal Process" at the 1978 Annual Convention of the Public Choice Society. The abbreviated version will appear during the summer of 1978 in *Professional Psychology*.

For hundreds of years, the Anglo-American legal system has been developing special rules for dealing with problems caused by the inherently perplexing phenomenon of mentally disordered behavior.[1] In almost every area of civil and criminal law, from rules concerning preventive detention to rules concerning criminal responsibility, mentally disordered persons are treated differently from non-mentally disordered persons.

The purpose of this Article is to analyze in detail the social, moral, logical, and scientific bases of mental health law. The goals are to clarify the issues raised by mental health laws and to suggest how they ought to be understood and resolved. The first section introduces mental health law by exploring generally and briefly its nature and assumptions. The second section is the theoretical core of the Article. It examines in detail the three basic questions adjudicated by mental health law: Is the person normal?; Could the person have behaved otherwise?; and How will the person behave in the future? The first and second questions are demonstrated to be primarily social and moral. In addition, the discussion of the second question shows that craziness is only one cause of behavior among many and that it is a much less powerful cause of legally relevant behavior than other factors, such as poverty, which are not usually considered legally relevant. The discussion of the third question, which concerns the prediction of future behavior, points out that data does not itself decide legal and moral questions and that, in any case, there is very little data or expertise with which to predict accurately future behavior.

The third section applies the theoretical and empirical arguments of the second section to an analysis of the proper role of expertise in mental health law decisionmaking and substantive mental health laws. It argues first that if the law continues to treat disordered persons specially, the role of experts should be limited. The present use of expertise obfuscates moral issues and promotes the mistaken view that the issues that concern the law are primarily scientific in nature. These issues in fact are primarily social and moral, and mental health professionals have little expertise in resolving social and moral questions. The third section then suggests that the law should not treat mentally disordered persons significantly differently from nondisordered ones because there is little persuasive scientific evidence that the former have significantly less control over their legally relevant behavior or are more predictable than the latter.

I. THE NATURE OF MENTAL HEALTH LAW

The legal system and mental health science are both concerned with understanding and controlling human behavior. In polar terms, the legal system approaches human behavior in terms of moral evaluation and the imposition of values, whereas mental health science approaches human behavior in terms of scientific, value-neutral, empirical investigation. Further, the legal model of behavior holds that persons have free will: persons choose their behavior and are thus morally and legally responsible for it. By contrast, the scientific model is deterministic: behavior, like all phenomena, is caused by its antecedents, and questions of moral and legal responsibility are irrelevant.[2]

In most instances, the differing approaches of the legal system and mental health science cause few difficulties. It is generally believed that the fundamental assumptions of the legal system adequately interpret and deal with the problems of normal behavior. The problems associated with mental disorder, however, cause a very different reaction. Society and the legal system have always been confused and often frightened by mental disorder.[3]

Special legal rules seem compelled in response to problems created by disordered behavior because it intuitively seems that disordered persons are significantly different from most persons in fundamental ways. Most persons assume that almost everybody in their culture plays by the same behavioral and social rules they do, but that mentally ill persons do not. When the behavior of a normal individual causes a legal problem, it is believed that the same legal rules applicable to everyone else can be fairly applied to that person. Because the rules of disordered persons are not understood, however, society assumes that they must be different.[4] While society assumes that most persons have free choice concerning their behavior, disordered persons are viewed as having little or no choice.[5] Observers believe that persons who are normal would not freely choose to behave in a mentally disordered fashion. Consequently, when a disordered person engages in legally relevant behavior, the legal system must decide if it can properly apply the same generally applicable legal rules to persons who appear to be fundamentally different and to lack normal ability to control their behavior. The explanations of disordered behavior have changed over the centuries, but special legal treatment of disordered persons always has been bottomed upon the assumption of their fundamental difference from normal persons.

Applying special rules to the problems created by mental disorder raises fundamental moral and political issues. The special treatment authorized by mental health laws is usually based on the premises that the mentally disordered person is abnormal and less responsible causally, and thus legally, for his behavior than other persons. Application of mental health laws to a person, therefore, tends to deprive the actor of some form of liberty, autonomy, or dignity by confining him or by negating the usual legal significance of his actions. For example, mental health laws authorize preventive detention by civil commitment even though the person is not suspected of criminal behavior.[6] Mental health laws also authorize a defense, in some instances, to the enforcement of contracts.[7] The law's decision to treat a mentally disordered person specially, on the basis that there is something uncontrollably wrong with the actor's mind, is thus a decision fraught with social and moral implications.

The law recognizes these implications and generally presumes first, that persons are not mentally disordered and have control over their behavior and second, that persons should not be treated specially unless disorder and lack of control can be affirmatively shown.[8] On the one hand, to treat disordered persons like everyone else seems counterintuitive and morally improper. On the other hand, to treat disordered persons differently, usually to their disadvantage in terms of freedom and autonomy, is equally morally improper unless there is a powerful justification for doing so.

Proponents of mental health laws claim that such laws are humane and that they enhance both the dignity of disordered persons and the moral climate of the society. They argue that it is unjust to treat persons who are incapable[9] of behaving like everyone else as if they were so capable.[10] Critics of these laws, however, believe that they diminish the dignity of disordered persons.[11] Although disordered persons may indeed behave differently from most persons, critics claim that in many and perhaps most cases there is good reason to believe that mentally disordered persons are sufficiently like most people to be treated like all other persons and held responsible for their behavior. Thus, it erodes the moral climate of society and infringes on the rights of mentally disordered persons to subject them to special laws that deny their responsibility and consequently reduce their dignity. The choice between these two alternative views of the relevance of mental disorder to law clearly presents a difficult moral, social, political, and legal dilemma.

The difficulty in part explains the readiness of the legal system to turn to mental health experts—the professionals charged in our culture with the task of understanding, treating, and controlling mentally disordered behavior.[12] Confronted with problems caused by mystifying be-

havior, the legal system naturally turned to scientific experts for explanations and understanding. Much of the moral difficulty engendered by the issue of special treatment seems to be rendered moot if the question of how to treat disordered persons can be redefined from a legal question to essentially a medical or scientific question.[13]

The legal system, then, has come to rely primarily on the medical model of mental disorder that teaches, in part, that disordered behavior is a symptom of an underlying illness, a state that is not under the person's control.[14] This assumption implies that the actor is not causally responsible for his disordered behavior. The situation is analogized to that of a person with an infection who is not held responsible for a consequent fever. If legally relevant behavior is the product of illness or disease rather than of free choice, a special legal response seems justified. Then, rather than having to rely on a discomforting, intuitive justification for the different legal treatment of disordered persons, the legal system is comforted by the allegedly scientific justification offered by mental health science.

It is therefore not surprising that mental health science has had an enormous influence on mental health law. Much of the legal doctrine and operation of the mental health legal system depends on the assumptions and learning of mental health science. Most lawyers regard mental disorders as arcane and disturbing phenomena that are beyond their comprehension and are understood by only a few highly trained experts.[15] They view the response to problems created by mental disorder as primarily the concern of mental health professionals. Lawyers therefore tend to defer to mental health experts, and mental health law decisions at all levels, especially if the proceedings are not truly adversary, are often based more on psychiatric reasoning and conclusions than on legal reasoning.[16]

In addition to claiming that there is scientific justification for treating the mentally ill differently, some advocates of this strong influence also argue that decisions about the competence, freedom, and responsibility of the allegedly disordered person should be made primarily by experts.[17] Mentally disordered persons are allegedly so abnormal that legal decision-making about them is largely irrelevant. The legal factfinders and law-appliers must, of course, "make" the final decision; but, it is argued, the major influence on these decisions should be the experts who understand the behavior. The essential moral and legal nature of questions of freedom, competence, and responsibility then come to be seen as proper questions for largely expert determination. Some proponents of this view believe that these issues are resolved by the legal system only because of an historical precedent based on America's perhaps overzealous guarding of liberty.[18]

To explore the tension between legal and scientific decisionmaking further, Section II analyzes the social, moral, logical, and scientific bases of mental health law.

II. MORALS AND SCIENCE IN MENTAL HEALTH LAW

A. Introduction

The structure of all mental health laws is fundamentally the same: all require findings of (1) a *mental disorder;* (2) a *behavioral component;* and (3) a *causal connection* between the mental disorder and the behavioral component (at least in principle).[19] For instance, civil commitment is usually based on findings that the person is: (1) mentally ill; (2) dangerous to self or to others, or gravely disabled; and (3) that the dangerousness or grave disablement is a product or result of the mental disorder or defect.[20] A person is incompetent to stand trial if he is mentally ill and therefore unable to understand the charges against him or to assist counsel.[21] Guardianship or conservatorship may be imposed upon an individual if he is mentally ill and therefore unable to care for himself or his property.[22]

Two points concerning the behavioral component of mental health laws must be noted. First, in all cases the behavioral component of the law is the primary impetus for *legal* regulation.[23] What disturbs society, for example, is an individual's dangerousness, grave disablement, inability to assist counsel, or inability to manage his financial affairs. In other words, society believes that it must protect itself from dangerous persons, that it must protect disabled persons from themselves, that a criminal trial is unfair unless certain conditions are met, and that it is inhumane to let an incompetent person mismanage his property. Second, the behavioral standards alone, such as dangerousness or various incompetencies, also appear in the conduct of normal persons. The behavior is neither necessarily related to mental health problems nor is it exclusively or especially within the province of mental health science.

Mental illness alone does not warrant special legal intervention: a person who is simply mentally ill is left alone unless he behaves in one of the legally relevant ways described by the behavioral components. But when mentally disordered persons behave in legally relevant ways, such as dangerously or incompetently, special rules apply to these individuals that do not apply to "normal" dangerous or incompetent persons. For example, extremely dangerous but nonmentally disordered persons, even those who might be "reformed," are not preventively confinable by civil commitment upon the basis of dangerousness alone.

It is noteworthy that the special legal treatment of disordered persons is authorized even though the vast majority of mentally disordered persons do not meet the behavioral components of the mental health law standards and many normal persons do meet these behavioral standards. In other words, the mentally ill, as a class, are not especially dangerous or incompetent.[24] But, despite the over- and under-inclusive nature of mental disorder as grounds for furthering the social goals that are explicitly or implicitly identified by the behavioral component of mental health laws, the law is clearly instilled with the idea that mental disorder should authorize special treatment.

Mental health law standards are therefore legal rules that have been created to further the social goals identified above. As discussed in Part I, mentally disordered persons have been singled out for special legal treatment because it is believed that it is morally and socially inappropriate to treat them like everyone else. The moral and legal basis for this special treatment depends on three factual assumptions concerning mentally disordered persons: (1) They are significantly different from most persons because they are ill; (2) their legally relevant behavior is the product of their illness and not of their free, rational choice; and (3) their future behavior is predictable. The validity of these assumptions, especially the first two, is the foundation of mental health law. Only if a person is abnormal, non-responsible, and in some cases predictable should he or she be accorded special legal treatment.

Flowing from the structure and assumptions of mental health law, three general questions must be decided:

1. Is the person normal? That is, is the actor suffering from a mental disease, illness, or disorder?
2. Could the person have behaved otherwise? Is the legally relevant behavior the product of free choice, or is it the product of a disordered mind over which the person has no control? That is, is the person causally responsible for the behavior?
3. How will the person behave in the future? For instance, will the person be a danger to self or to others?

This section analyzes in detail the social, moral, logical, and scientific bases of mental health law by examining the three questions.[25]

The thesis of this Article is that these questions are fundamentally social, moral, and legal questions, not scientific ones. Although they appear to call for scientific answers, in fact they can be answered best on the basis of commonsense observations and social, moral, and commonsense evaluations of behavior. Further, many commonly believed assumptions about mentally disordered persons that are used to answer these questions are not scientifically proven. Experts may be useful in providing certain factual information, but the primary issues are not scientific. Hard moral issues raised by mental disorder should not be avoided by relying upon experts and allowing the questions to be "medicalized."

In summary, to define mental disorder for the purposes of mental health law, the best one can do is to state definitionally and tautologically that abnormal persons in the mental health sense are those who behave inordinately crazily. These are the people for whom special legal rules seem appropriate. If the definition of mental disorder as crazy behavior seems ambiguous, this is quite proper because there is no scientifically agreed on definition of mental disorder.[43] Attempts at more specific definitions are only theoretical. Experts agree only on the observation that in (probably) every society there are persons who behave in ways that society labels mentally ill, mentally disordered, crazy, or some equivalent term.

Of course, in our society crazy behavior is usually considered medically abnormal rather than, for example, morally abnormal. But the medical analogy is presently little more than an analogy; all that is known is that some people behave very crazily, and it is these people who are considered to be mentally disordered. Hereafter, the terms mental disorder, mental illness, and crazy behavior will be used interchangeably to ensure that the essential nature of the phenomenon in question is not lost.[44]

2. Who Is Crazy?

The previous section examined in some detail the nature of the question, "Is the person normal in the mental health sense?" It should now be recognized that for mental health law this question really should mean, in operational terms, "Does this person behave sufficiently crazily to warrant special legal treatment on moral and social grounds?" Once the nature of the question is clear, one can analyze how it should properly be answered. The major thesis of this section is that the question, "Who is sufficiently crazy?" is a social question, and that *for legal purposes* it can and should be answered by laypersons.

The number of persons who may be labeled "mentally disordered" according to current diagnostic categories is much larger than the number of persons who are clearly crazy[45] and thus arguably warrant special legal treatment on both moral and social grounds. Because there is no underlying, independently verifiable criterion other than behavior with which to determine if an actor is mentally disordered, it is especially hard to determine if the actor is "normal" in those cases where most observers would *not* agree that the actor is crazy. Mental health professionals can make such determinations by fiat, but these are not scientific decisions.[46] At the farthest extremes, it is relatively easy for anyone to differentiate a very crazy individual from a normal person, and we are not made uncomfortable by terming the person "crazy" although the conclusion of craziness in even the clearest cases is culturally relative to some degree. But the dividing line, near which most cases fall, is elusive.[47]

Let us consider some examples to analyze further the question of "who is crazy?" and how it should be answered. Suppose an adult walks down the street, accosting passersby and loudly uttering strange epithets. Asked why he is engaging in this behavior, he sincerely replies that electrochemical rays shot at him by supernatural beings are forcing him to behave in this way. This person clearly has a mental disorder according to the American Psychiatric Association,[48] but do we need an expert to tell us that he is crazy? Clearly not. Nor can an expert or anyone else tell us with any degree of certainty why this person behaves this way. All that is known, and this is clear to anyone in our culture—experts and laypersons alike—is that the actor is very crazy.

Let us now consider a much harder example: a man who is extremely neat, punctual, and precise. Indeed, he spends so much time ensuring that he is neat, punctual, and precise that he often accomplishes considerably less in his love life and work life than he might like, a fact that makes him unhappy. Despite his discontent, he finds that for some reason he feels that he just has to be that way, and in any case, he gets along all right with his family and his job. This person suffers from a mental disorder according to the currently dominant diagnostic scheme.[49] Indeed, excessive concern with neatness, punctuality, or anything else is a little crazy in the loosest colloquial sense. On the other hand, many persons would probably be inclined to say about this person, "Oh, so and so has some quirks like all of us, but that's just the way he is." Most persons would probably agree that his "quirks" are somewhat maladaptive, though others might admire an unusually neat, punctual, and precise person. Is this person normal? Again, does the ability to answer this question require medical expertise or merely common sense based on social rules and expectations?

Mental health experts are a bit more inclined than the average person to declare that particular behaviors are abnormal and evidence mental disorder.[50] Even so, most experts and laypersons would agree in their assessment of our second example. He is a person with some personality quirks (or in "psychiatrese," characterological symptoms) that interfere to some extent with his successful functioning. Thus, the final question of normality in this borderline case is simply, "How quirky must a person be before he or she will be labeled *abnormal?*" There is no scientific answer to this question. There exists no objectively identifiable underlying abnormal condition that distinguishes this person from those with fewer, different, or no quirks. Even if there were an identifiable underlying condition, for legal purposes the answer depends on social tolerance for quirkiness or on social value preferences concerning how much a person can "normally" hinder his own functioning by quirkiness before we consider him crazy.

A final example is a person whose sexual orientation is exclusively homosexual but who maintains adequate interpersonal relations, whose work life is generally unimpaired, and who has no significantly maladaptive personality quirks. This case illustrates the difficulty in answering the question "who is crazy?" and exemplifies the processes by which professionals sometimes decide such questions.

Our example is a person who would be regarded as quite normal by both experts and laypersons except for his homosexuality. But is this person normal in the mental health sense? If jargon is deleted from scientific definitions, experts and laypersons define homosexuality similarly: the occurrence of a (more or less) persistent sexual preference for members of the same sex. There is no test other than homosexual behavior itself with which to "diagnose" homosexuality. Until 1973, the American Psychiatric Association, the organization responsible for the promulgation of the currently dominant diagnostic scheme of mental disorders, considered homosexuality per se a mental disorder.[51] In that year, by a vote of its membership, the Association decided that homosexuality was not a mental disorder.[52] The nature of homosexuality did not change, nor were there any startling breakthroughs in the scientific understanding of homosexual behavior. No one is sure why the sexual orientation of some persons is homosexual; all that was known to a certainty prior to and after the 1973 vote was that some persons behave homosexually.

What changed were the *values* of a professional group empowered to affix labels of deviancy. Historically, many societies considered homosexuality sinful. The ascendancy of the medical model of deviant behavior led to a redefinition of this deviant behavior as sick. The majority of mental health experts, although by no means all, now view homosexuality per se as neither sick nor bad; rather, it is viewed as one possible form of human sexual orientation. A homosexual may still be considered mentally disordered, but not on the basis of the homosexuality per se.

For many reasons, homosexual behavior raises particularly difficult questions of defining behavioral normality. Homosexuals are not necessarily dysfunctional in ways important to them or, except for sexual orientation, to the rest of society. Nor is homosexual behavior particularly irrational, weird, or inexplicable; that is, it does not seem crazy. Yet, the unproven notion remains deeply rooted among professionals and laypersons that homosexuality is somewhat per se biologically and/or socially abnormal and/or maladaptive. Homosexuals are no longer officially considered sick not because of a scientific finding, but because a majority of professionals with the power to affix the "sick" label changed their minds. If the decision of whether homosexual behavior is abnormal really reduces to a statement of value preferences, however, the assistance professionals can give to laypersons to discern such abnormalities is negligible.

Mental health experts are neither moral experts nor social value experts, nor even experts on any mental health issue about which there is little scientific data or agreement; and mental health is a field of little agreement.[53] For the most part, the experts do not have tests or instruments that reliably and validly demonstrate the presence or absence of abnormal conditions. Certainly, no responsible expert would diagnose mental disorder on the basis of a test result if the person otherwise behaved normally. Any data that experts might use to determine whether a subject meets the *legal* test of craziness is perfectly accessible to lay observers as well.[54]

In sum, laypersons and experts both form judgments based largely on their observations of behavior. In commonsense language, their observations are likely to be remarkably similar. In cases where mental health experts readily agree that an actor suffers from a severe mental disorder,[55] laypersons would agree that the actor is crazy. Where persons are less crazy but still arguably irrationally quirky (as in our earlier case of the extremely neat, precise, and punctual man), laypersons and experts would agree on the description although experts would be more likely to diagnose mental disorder than laypersons would be likely to "diagnose" craziness.[56] Yet there would be no scientific reason to call our second person "mentally disordered" as

opposed to "quirky" or even normal. "Mental disorder" and "quirky" are both labels affixed to the same behavior. Any extra meaning connoted by "mental disorder," such as neurological dysfunction or underlying psychological forces, is currently unverified.

The best measuring instrument for determining if a person is crazy is to find out as much as possible about the actor from those persons who have had an opportunity to observe him directly in a wide variety of circumstances. When much is learned about how the actor has behaved at many different times and in many different circumstances, or at a particular time and in particular circumstances, then all members of society will be competent to judge if the person is crazy in general or if he was crazy at the particular time in question.[57] The current deference the law accords mental health experts is misplaced. For legal purposes, the question of who is crazy must be recognized as a social and moral judgment that must be decided as such.

3. Summary

Mental disorder fundamentally refers to crazy behavior. Theories about abnormal underlying causes of the behavior are yet unproven. Further, what behavior is considered crazy depends largely on social and cultural norms and expectations and on the particular situational context in which the behavior occurs. Except in the clearest cases, determinations of who is crazy are difficult to make because the criteria of craziness are very imprecise. Because determinations of craziness depend on observations of behavior and social norms, such determinations can be made by laypersons and experts alike.

When the legal system must decide if a person is crazy enough to warrant special legal treatment, it should recognize the social and moral nature and significance of the decision. Consequently, the question of who is crazy should be decided by society's representatives—judges and juries of laypersons.

C. Could the Person Have Behaved Otherwise?

Once an initial determination is made that a person has behaved sufficiently crazily to justify labeling him "mentally disordered," *i.e.*, a crazy person, the next important question for the legal system is whether the person could have behaved otherwise. In other words, were the crazy behavior and related legally relevant behavior products of free choice or were they the product of a disordered mind? Was the person a free agent and causally responsible for the behavior? Being different enough to be clearly crazy seems to be a necessary but not sufficient reason for special legal treatment. A further factual assumption appears morally and legally compelled—that the legally relevant behavior was the result of uncontrollable illness.[58] In such instances, the crazy actor, unlike most persons, is not regarded as a free agent and special legal treatment does not seem to infringe unduly the actor's dignity and autonomy.

This section first briefly explores the differing views of personal responsibility held by the law and mental health scientists. It then examines in general the degree to which crazy persons have less control over their behavior than normal persons. Finally, the section considers the two crucial questions for the law: whether crazy persons are responsible for their legally relevant behavior and how this question can be determined. These questions are analyzed by first examining the threshold issue of the relationship between craziness and other legally relevant behavior. It is concluded that whether a relationship exists is a commonsense determination. Then, on the assumption that there is a clear relationship between craziness and legally relevant behavior, the section explores whether and when the legally relevant behavior was a product of the actor's free choice. It is argued that crazy persons do have a good deal of choice about the consequences of their craziness, and again, the question of responsibility is to be answered on moral and commonsense grounds.

1. Scientific and Legal Models of Personal Responsibility

The concepts of free will or personal responsibility have little meaning to mental health scientists, as scientists. Simplistically put, the sci-

entific model is deterministic: all phenomena, including behavior, are allegedly the effects of their multiple interacting antecedent causes. According to this model, human thoughts, feelings, and actions are not the products of free will directed by the actor; rather, human behavior is the probabilistic outcome of the many biological, psychological, and social antecedent variables that have operated on the person.[59] Responsibility is thus a moral term that is allegedly scientifically irrelevant.[60] The various models of behavior assume that different causes are crucial for explaining behavior and that causality is extremely complex. All deterministic scientific models, however, view *all* behavior as phenomena subject to the same probabilistic laws as the rest of the phenomena of the universe.

Scientists who are strict determinists are aware that at present they are not able to specify all the antecedent causes that would allow them to state perfectly the probabilities that particular behavior will occur, but they believe that this is a result of lack of knowledge, not a flaw in principle in the scientific model. They believe that when behavior can be perfectly predicted and controlled, notions of responsibility will then wither away.[61]

The legal system takes a quite different view of personal responsibility. Law is a normative enterprise that treats nearly all persons in all situations as responsible for their acts and often for the natural and probable consequences of those acts.[62] In most cases, the law adheres to the commonsense and subjectively experienced view that behavior is a matter of choice: it is the actor's act.[63] Nevertheless, the law acknowledges that all persons are subjected to various biological, psychological, and sociocultural factors or pressures that affect their choices of action. All such factors affect choices, making some choices easy and some hard. As a result, the law recognizes that some behavioral choices may be too hard to serve as the basis for the imposition of legal responsibility.[64] For instance, in cases of duress the law excuses otherwise criminally culpable behavior not because the actor absolutely lacked choice in a causal sense, but because society feels the actor's choice to obey the law was too difficult to consider him culpable. In other instances, such as cases of automatism, the law reflects the view that the actor was not causally responsible for his behavior; the act was not his and, therefore, the actor cannot be morally and legally responsible for his behavior.[65]

While acknowledging that some choices are so hard that it is inappropriate for society to ascribe responsibility for them to the actor, the legal system allows few exceptions to the rule that persons are causally and legally responsible for their behavior. But which choices are too hard? In another article, the author has analyzed this question as follows:

> There is no bright line between free and unfree choices. Harder and easier choices are arranged along a continuum of choice: there is no scientifically dictated cutting point where legal and moral responsibility begins or ends. Nor is there a higher moral authority which can tell society where to draw the line. All society can do is to determine the cutting point that comports with our collective sense of morality. The real issue is where society ought to draw the line of responsibility—and by whom it should be drawn.[66]

The central question for our inquiry, then, is whether the choice to behave in legally relevant ways is too hard a choice for society fairly to ascribe moral and legal responsibility to actors whose legally relevant behavior seems caused by craziness. Throughout the analysis, this Article will adopt this commonsense model of harder and easier choices.[67] Scientific data will be relied on, but its relevance to legal determinations will be assessed in the light of this model.

Although the legal system does not generally adopt a deterministic model of behavior, if an actor's behavior is apparently and inexplicably irrational and crazy, the law and also persons in general assume that because of mental disorder the actor was not in control of his behavior—that it was not chosen.[68] After all, the generally rational model of behavior held by most persons and the law is unable to explain how and why an actor would choose to behave inexplicably crazily. When the law adopts the intuitive and perhaps correct view that the crazy person has great difficulty controlling his behavior, the law comports with and is reinforced in its view by mental health science, even if the correspondence in view only extends to the class of persons considered crazy.[69] Where there is such a correspondence of views, the legal system

calls upon mental health experts to help resolve and legitimize the decision as to whether a crazy actor's legally relevant behavior was caused by his mental disorder rather than by his free choice.

It must be remembered, however, that although determinations of legal causation and responsibility rest in part on factual scientific notions of causation and responsibility, legal and scientific determinations are separable and serve different purposes. Scientists may provide information about pressures and probabilities, but the legal system must determine for its own purposes when those pressures and probabilities are too great to hold the actor legally responsible for his behavior.[70] Although crazy behavior should perhaps be considered an illness for some purposes, doing so when the actor's moral and legal responsibility is in issue begs the question and prematurely ends the analysis. Are legally relevant behaviors simply uncontrollable symptoms? As noted, mental health laws assume that mental illness is such a powerful cause in fact that it robs actors of their free choice and thus renders them legally nonresponsible. Rather than accepting the validity of this assumption, this Article will examine in the succeeding sections the degree to which the law's assumption is founded in scientific fact and the extent to which mental health science provides assistance in deciding questions of both factual and legal responsibility.

* * *

Responsibility for deciding legal questions concerning crazy behavior must be accepted by legal decisionmakers. If crazy persons are to be deprived of liberty, "fixed" against their wills, or are to have the usual legal significance of their actions negated, such decisions should be made with the full realization that they are extremely difficult social and moral decisions and not simply legal ratifications of scientific judgments. This Article contends that laypersons are perfectly competent both to provide most of the observational data necessary for mental health decisions and to make such decisions. Despite the general competence of laypersons and the dangers of reliance on experts, it is also argued that for limited purposes experts will be able to furnish helpful data. They should not, however, be allowed to draw conclusions or to state their data in other than commonsense and observational terms. There are no scientific answers to legal questions such as whether the actor's behavior is normal or whether he could have behaved otherwise. Moreover, the categories and theories of mental health science are at present too imprecise and speculative to help clarify legal questions.[157] When scientific expertise is used, it should be based on direct observations or other hard data. The legal decisionmaker should not be offered unscientific theories or conclusions that are supported mostly by the Aesculapian authority of unproven expertise.[158]

* * *

For example, experts should not testify that an actor is "hallucinatory and probably schizophrenic." Instead, the expert should testify that the actor told the expert that on some (specified) occasions, the actor heard or hears voices despite the fact that no one was or is talking to him and the voices told or tell him the following (specified) things. For another example, experts should not testify that an actor "suffers from loose associations when questioned on an ego-threatening topic and is therefore probably schizophrenic." Rather, the expert should testify that when the expert asked the actor certain (specified) questions about topics that seem to mean a lot to the actor, the actor responded in the following way (specified by examples).[179] Of course, if laypersons such as family, friends, coworkers, or neighbors are aware of such behavior, they too can testify about it.

Using lay as well as expert testimony about the actor's behavior, the decisionmaker can then decide if the person is sufficiently crazy to be an appropriate candidate for the application of mental health laws. If the factfinder's response to the behavioral data it hears is "so what," then the actor probably does not meet the legal criterion of mental disorder; if the response is "that's crazy" or "he's crazy," then the criterion of mental abnormality may be met.

* * *

5. Summary and Conclusions

Mental health experts should be limited to testifying about those matters in which they are more skilled than laypersons. This Article has suggested that experts may be useful in two specific ways: (1) as acute and efficient first-hand observers of crazy behavior; and (2) as sources of scientifically rigorous data. Further, descriptions and data should be presented in a commonsense and ordinary language fashion. If experts are so limited, their testimony will tend to be far more useful than it is at present. They should not, however, be allowed to draw conclusions about any issue to be decided by mental health law. These are moral and legal issues that should be decided by legal decisionmakers.

In addition to suggesting the type of expert testimony that ought to be considered and the form in which it should be offered, some further suggestions flow from the analysis of expertise. First, psychiatric experts cannot be value-neutral scientists and should properly function as advocates. In proceedings such as civil commitment where liberty is at stake, defendants should be entitled as a matter of due process to an advocate expert of their choice paid for by the state.[209] It is almost impossible to defend oneself against or to prove mental health allegations without the assistance of an advocate expert. Even though the battles of the experts may be confusing, it is submitted that if expert testimony is limited in the manner proposed in this Article, confusion will be reduced enormously because legal factfinders will not be led to believe that there are scientific "answers" to the questions being presented. Moreover, disputes over the precision of observational data or over the soundness of probability statistics reflect the uncertainties and ambiguities in the field, and there is no reason for juries and judges not to be aware of the level of uncertainty of mental health science.

Second, in those cases where an advocate expert is not required by due process or is not available for any other reason, the court should attempt to ensure that the jury recognize that the sole expert is not impartial. The court should also ensure that the expert is fully cross-examined. Judges should know and juries should be instructed first, that unopposed testimony should be assessed cautiously, and second, that unopposed testimony may be disregarded. Finally, it is suggested that an appellate or trial court should never overturn as a matter of law a judge or jury's decision, even if the decision clearly disregards unanimous psychiatric expertise to the contrary. Mental health law decisions involve too little science and too much social and moral judgment to allow a factfinder's decision to be overriden because it opposes the weight of "expert" testimony.

* * *

NOTES

1. Throughout this Article, the term "behavior" will refer to *thoughts, feelings,* and *actions* and will not be limited to externally perceivable actions. The preference for the generic term behavior should not be interpreted to mean that the writer is an adherent exclusively of behavioral psychology.

As explored in greater detail below, mentally disordered behavior refers to thoughts, feelings, and actions that would be described by the word "crazy" or some similar term. The word "crazy" is used because in the author's opinion it is, for legal purposes, the least question-begging and most accurate word to describe the behavior regulated by mental health laws. No disrespect or flippancy towards disordered persons or those individuals trying to help them is implied. *See* text accompanying notes 26–57 *infra.*

Legal problems created by mental retardation are related to those created by mental illness, but they are distinct and will not be considered in this Article.

2. *See* notes 58–70 and accompanying text *infra.*

3. Rabkin, *Opinions About Mental Illness: A Review of the Literature,* 77 PSYCHOLOGICAL BULL. 153 (1972) and sources cited therein; Sarbin & Mancuso, *Failure of a Moral Enterprise: Attitudes of the Public Toward Mental Illness,* 35 J. CONSULTING & CLINICAL PSYCHOLOGY 159 (1970); *see* Kirk, *The Psychiatric Sick Role and Rejection,* 161 J. NERVOUS & MENTAL DISEASE 318, 318, 324 (1975) (ascribing of psychiatric sickness to deviant behavior increases social rejection).

For various historical approaches from differing points of view, see F. ALEXANDER & S. SELESNICK, THE HISTORY OF PSYCHIATRY (1968); M. FOUCAULT, MADNESS & CIVILIZATION (1971); G. ROSEN, MADNESS IN SOCIETY (1969); D. ROTHMAN, THE DISCOVERY OF THE ASYLUM (1971); T. SZASZ, THE MANUFACTURE OF MADNESS (1970); White, *The Forms of Wildness: Archaeology of an Idea,* in THE WILD MAN WITHIN: AN IMAGE IN WESTERN THOUGHT FROM THE RENAISSANCE TO ROMANTICISM 3–38 (E. Dudley & M. Novak eds. 1972); Kenny, *Mental Health in Plato's* Republic, 55 PROC. BRIT. ACAD. 229 (1969); Scull, *From Madness to Mental Illness,* 16 EUROPEAN J. SOC. 218 (1975). *See generally* Mora, *Historiography of Psychiatry and Its Development: A Re-evaluation,* 1 J. HIST. BEHAVIORAL SCI. 43 (1965).

4. *See, e.g.,* Edgerton, *On the "Recognition" of Mental Illness,* in CHANGING PERSPECTIVES IN MENTAL ILLNESS 49–72 (S. Plog & R. Edgerton eds. 1969); Mechanic, *Some Factors in Identifying and Defining Mental Illness,* in THE MAKING OF A MENTAL PATIENT 19 (R. Price & B. Denner eds. 1973).

5. Gross, *Mental Abnormality as a Criminal Excuse,* in PHILOSOPHY OF LAW 466–76 (J. Feinberg & H. Gross eds. 1975). For a recent psychiatric opinion to this effect, see Chodoff, *The Case for Involuntary Hospitalization of the Mentally Ill,* 133 AM. J. PSYCHIATRY 496 (1976). After describing the crazy behavior of some persons, Chodoff notes that "they are *incapable* by an effort of will of stopping or changing their destructive behavior. . . . [I]t must also be acknowledged that these severely ill people are *not capable* at a conscious level of deciding what is best for themselves. . . ." *Id.* at 498 (emphasis added). *But see* text accompanying notes 58–112 *infra* (analysis of the assumption that crazy persons have no free choice).

6. *See, e.g.,* CAL. WELF. & INST. CODE §§ 5150, 5250 (West 1972 & Supp. 1978). *See generally Developments in the Law—Civil Commitment of the Mentally Ill,* 87 HARV. L. REV. 1190 (1974) [hereinafter cited as *Developments*]; Note, *"Who Says I'm Crazy?"—A Proposal for Mandatory Judicial Review of Emergency Detention in California,* 51 S. CAL. L. REV. 695 (1978).

7. Ortelere v. Teachers' Retirement Bd., 25 N.Y.2d 196, 250 N.E.2d 460, 303 N.Y.S.2d 362 (1969); J. MURRAY, MURRAY ON CONTRACTS §14 (2d rev. ed. 1974). Of course, mentally disordered persons are not the only group protected from the enforcement of their contracts. Minors too, for example, enjoy special treatment. It is interesting to note that the justification is similar in both cases—members of the protected groups are considered incapable of protecting their rights.

8. 31A C.J.S. *Evidence* §147 (1964) ("It is to be presumed that a person is mentally sound . . . ."). For example, the criminal law presumes that all defendants are sane. People v. Silver, 33 N.Y.2d 475, 310 N.E.2d 520, 354 N.Y.S.2d 915 (1974). Modern case law has recognized the social and moral implications of mental health laws; when actors may be legally disabled on the basis of alleged insanity, the burden of persuasion

for proving mental health law criteria has been raised in areas such as civil commitment and quasi-criminal confinement from a "preponderance" to "clear and convincing" or "beyond a reasonable doubt." Stachulak v. Coughlin, 520 F.2d 931, 937 (7th Cir. 1975), *cert. denied,* 424 U.S. 947 (1976); *In re* Ballay, 482 F.2d 648, 667 (D.C. Cir. 1973); Lynch v. Baxley, 386 F. Supp. 378, 393–94 (M.D. Ala. 1974).

9. *See* note 5 and accompanying text *supra.*

10. Chodoff, *supra* note 5; *see* A. GOLDSTEIN, THE INSANITY DEFENSE 9–22, 211–26 (1967); A. STONE, MENTAL HEALTH AND LAW: A SYSTEM IN TRANSITION 43–82 (1972); American Psychiatric Association, *Position Statement on Involuntary Hospitalization of the Mentally Ill* (revised), 130 AM. J. PSYCHIATRY 392 (1973); Slovenko, *Civil Commitment in Perspective,* 20 J. PUB. L. 3 (1971); Treffert, *The Practical Limits of Patients' Rights,* 5 PSYCHIATRIC ANN. 158 (1975); Note, *Testamentary Capacity in a Nutshell: A Psychiatric Reevaluation,* 18 STAN. L. REV. 1119, 1125–26 (1966). *See generally* A. STONE, *supra.*

It should be noted that the vast majority of commentary on mental health laws, both pro and con, deals with the insanity defense and civil commitment. Therefore, most examples in this Article will be drawn from or refer to these aspects of mental health law.

11. R. LEIFER, IN THE NAME OF MENTAL HEALTH (1969); K. MILLER, MANAGING MADNESS: THE CASE AGAINST CIVIL COMMITMENT (1976); T. SZASZ, LAW, LIBERTY & PSYCHIATRY (1963); Alexander & Szasz, *From Contract to Status via Psychiatry,* 13 SANTA CLARA LAW. 537 (1973); Alexander & Szasz, *Mental Illness as an Excuse for Civil Wrongs,* 43 NOTRE DAME LAW. 24 (1967); Dershowitz, *Psychiatry in the Legal Process: A Knife that Cuts Both Ways,* TRIAL, Feb./Mar. 1968, at 29. *See generally* N. KITTRIE, THE RIGHT TO BE DIFFERENT (1971).

12. The professionals who have the most contact with and influence on the mental health legal system are psychiatrists, psychoanalysts, and psychologists. These professionals are believed to have special expertise concerning the description, causes, and treatment of disordered behavior. Because they play such a crucial role in the mental health legal system, it will be useful to have a brief description of their training.

The *psychiatrist* is a physician who specializes in the treatment of mental and emotional disorders. Although any physician may call himself a psychiatrist, the usual course of psychiatric training is for a new physician to enter postgraduate training, termed a psychiatric "residency." Residencies are three- or four-year programs in psychiatric settings approved by the Council on Medical Education of the American Medical Association. A psychiatric residency is similar to other medical residences; residents are trained largely by being responsible for much of the day-to-day patient care in the institution. Psychiatric residency training varies widely in quality, but usually includes experience with patients in various types of treatment settings, supervised training in methods of treatment, and some academic training in the theory and practice of psychiatry. Psychiatric training rarely involves much emphasis on normal psychology, other behavioral sciences, or behavioral science methodology; it is usually more clinical in orientation. After finishing the residency the psychiatrist may receive certification by passing an examination in psychiatry given by the American Board of Psychiatry and Neurology. If he or she is eligible to take the examination but has not passed, the psychiatrist is said to be "Board eligible." If he or she passes, the psychiatrist is said to be "Board certified."

A *psychoanalyst* is a person trained in the theory and practice of psychoanalysis. Psychoanalysis is one theory of human behavior and one form of psychotherapy, first developed by Sigmund Freud and then modified by later writers and practitioners. Psychoanalytic training and certification is usually conducted by private associations of analysts. There is nothing to prevent any psychotherapist from terming himself a psychoanalyst, but the appellation is usually reserved for graduates of psychoanalytic institutes. Although psychoanalysis is only one theory and method, trained psychoanalysts deserve separate attention because in the United States psychoanalysis and psychoanalysts have enjoyed singular influence compared to the other schools and practitioners of mental health science. In this country the psychoanalytic institutes have largely reserved their training for physicians, especially psychiatrists. Recently, increasing numbers of nonphysicians are being trained, and such psychoanalysts are called "lay analysts." Psychoanalytic training usually involves three phases: First, the candidate undergoes a personal psychoanalysis; second, he engages in academic coursework concerned with the theory and practice of psychoanalysis; and third, he psychoanalyzes a small number of patients under the close supervision of senior members of his institute. Psychoanalytic training does not require the candidate's full time (at most it requires a few hours a day), but because of the lengthy nature of psychoanalytic treatments (the candidate's own analysis and those he conducts under supervision), the training usually takes over five years before the candidate is "graduated" as a psychoanalyst.

The *psychologist* has earned the Ph.D. degree in psychology. (Persons with bachelor's or master's degrees in psychology are called psychologists in some contexts, but the psychologists involved with the legal system nearly always have doctorates.) There are many specialty areas of psychology, but most psychologists who work in the mental health field are clinical psychologists, and, therefore, this discussion shall focus on these psychologists. Training in psychology usually begins with two years of postgraduate coursework that emphasizes the specialty branch for which the student is training. Clinical psychologists take courses dealing with normal and abnormal psychology, human development, treatment methods, psychodiagnostics (including psychological testing), research methodology, and statistics. After completion of coursework, clinical psychology training requires the student to complete a year-long clinical internship in a program approved by the American Psychological Association. These programs are usually based in psychiatric hospitals (including community mental health centers) and offer the trainee supervised clinical experience in diagnosis, especially psychological diagnostic testing, and psychological treatment methods. Like psychiatric residencies, psychology internships vary widely in their quality. They usually offer the trainee supervised experience with a wide variety of patients, treatment settings, and treatment methods. After completing the internship, the psychologist must write a doctoral dissertation that is typically a major, empirical research effort. After finishing their dissertations and earning their doctorates, many clinical psychologists, especially those who wish to practice as well as to teach and do research, then enter postdoctoral programs of one to two years where they receive further clinical training. The vast majority of states now require that psychologists who practice with patients or consult in the community (as opposed to those who mainly teach and do research) be licensed. Although the licensing requirements vary from state to state, most states require the candidate to have completed one or two years of approved postdoctoral experience, and to pass an examination. In addition to licensing by the various states, psychologists with considerably more experience may qualify for a certification in clinical psychology given by the American Board of Professional Psychology. If the psychologist meets the requirements of the ABPP, he is then said to be a "Diplomate in Clinical Psychology."

In addition to psychiatrists, psychoanalysts, and psychologists, there are other professionals such as psychiatric social workers and psychiatric nurses whose primary responsibility is working with mentally disordered persons. Only the first three groups, however, have significant contact with the mental health legal system.

13. Bazelon, *Can Psychiatry Humanize the Law?*, 7 PSYCHIATRIC ANN. 292, 295 (1977); Hardisty, *Mental Illness: A Legal Fiction*, 48 WASH. L. REV. 735 (1973); Horstman, *Protective Services for the Elderly: The Limits of Parens Patriae*, 40 MO. L. REV. 215, 225–29 (1975); Suarez, *A Critique of the Psychiatrist's Role as Expert Witness*, 12 J. FORENSIC SCI. 172 (1967); Szasz, *Psychiatric Expert Testimony—Its Covert Meaning and Social Function*, 20 PSYCHIATRY 313, 315–16 (1957).

14. *See* Kety, *From Rationalization to Reason*, 131 AM. J. PSYCHIATRY 957, 959 (1974). Although the "medical model" is a complex construct that is often oversimplified and misunderstood, the statement in the text is one fundamental tenet of the model. Generally, the "sick" role in our society includes the assumption that the person's illness or consequent incapacity is not his voluntary act and he is therefore not responsible for it. T. PARSONS, *Definitions of Health and Illness in the Light of American Values and Social Structure*, in SOCIAL STRUCTURE AND PERSONALITY 257, 274 (1970); Kirk, *supra* note 3, at 318–19, 323–24; Siegler & Osmond, *The 'Sick Role' Revisited*, HASTINGS CENTER STUD. 41, 46 (1973).

There is currently enormous debate concerning the propriety of applying the medical model to psychiatric disorders, a debate that has also generated other competing models. *See* T. SCHEFF, BEING MENTALLY ILL (1966); M. SIEGLER & H. OSMOND, MODELS OF MADNESS, MODELS OF MEDICINE (1974); T. SZASZ, THE MYTH OF MENTAL ILLNESS (1961); T. SZASZ, SCHIZOPHRENIA (1976); E. TORREY, THE DEATH OF PSYCHIATRY (1974); Ullmann & Krasner, *Introduction*, in CASE STUDIES IN BEHAVIOR MODIFICATION 2–15 (L. Ullmann & L. Krasner eds. 1965); Blaney, *Implications of the Medical Model and Its Alternatives*, 132 AM. J. PSYCHIATRY 911 (1975); Lazare, *Hidden Conceptual Models in Clinical Psychiatry*, 288 NEW ENG. J. MED. 345 (1973); Roth, *Schizophrenia and the Theories of Thomas Szasz*, 129 BRIT. J. PSYCHIATRY 317 (1976); Sarasen & Ganzer, *Concerning the Medical Model*, 23 AM. PSYCHOLOGIST 507 (1968); Sarbin, *On the Futility of the Proposition that Some People Be Labeled "Mentally Ill,"* 31 J. CONSULTING PSYCHOLOGY 447 (1967); Taylor, *The Medical Model of the Disease Concept*, 128 BRIT. J. PSYCHIATRY 588 (1976). *See generally* LABELING MADNESS (T. Sheff ed. 1975); R. LEIFER, IN THE NAME OF MENTAL HEALTH (1969); Gove, *Labelling and Mental Illness: A Critique*, in THE LABELLING OF DEVIANCE 38–81 (W. Gove ed. 1975); Eisenberg, *Psychiatry and Society*, 296 NEW ENG. J. MED. 903 (1977); Engel, *The Need for a New Medical Model: A Challenge for Biomedicine*, 196 SCI. 129 (1977); Imershein & Simons, *Rules and Examples in Lay and Professional Psychiatry: An Ethnomethodological Comment on the Scheff-Gove Controversy*, 41 AM. SOC. REV. 559 (1976); Sarbin & Mancuso, *supra* note 3, at 159; Scheff, *Reply to Chauncey and Gove*, 40 AM. SOC. REV. 252 (1975). The most forceful and well-reasoned critique of the "myth of mental illness" position is set forth in Moore, *Some Myths of "Mental Illness,"* 32 ARCHIVES OF GENERAL PSYCHIATRY 1483 (1975). *See* note 25 *infra*.

For an account of the medical model of psychiatry in law (the following of which is confined largely to the U.S. Court of Appeals for the District of Columbia), see Wales, *The Rise, The Fall, and the Resurrection of the Medical Model,* 63 GEO. L.J. 87 (1974).

This Article will not attempt to resolve the dispute about whether a medical or illness model of disordered behavior is useful. The position taken here is that the illness model may or may not be useful depending on the context in which one is considering the behavior that might be labeled as ill. Thus, whereas an illness model might be useful for clinical or research purposes, it might not be for legal purposes. It will be argued that uncritical acceptance of all possible implications of a medical or illness model of disordered behavior is mistaken when legal decisionmaking is involved. *See* note 43 *infra.*

15. *See* Cohen, *The Function of the Attorney and the Commitment of the Mentally Ill,* 44 TEX. L. REV. 449–50 (1966). *See generally* A. BROOKS, LAW, PSYCHIATRY AND THE MENTAL HEALTH SYSTEM 801–02 (1974).

16. Hall, *Science, Common Sense, and Criminal Law Reform,* 49 IOWA L. REV. 1044, 1066 (1964). The most noteworthy discussion of expert dominance in legal proceedings was provided by Chief Judge Bazelon in Washington v. United States, 390 F.2d 444, 446–47, 451–57 (D.C. Cir. 1967).

This point has been demonstrated empirically in numerous studies of civil commitment (proceedings that are rarely truly adversary) in which the legal decisionmaking is almost completely perfunctory and in which the concordance rate between psychiatric opinion and ultimate legal disposition is extraordinarily high. Cohen, *supra* note 15, at 427–31 (in a sample of 40 commitment cases observed, all defendants were committed in accordance with psychiatric recommendation at perfunctory hearings); Fein & Miller, *Legal Processes and Adjudication in Mental Incompetency Proceedings,* 20 SOC. PROB. 57, 58, 60 n.2 (1972) (in a sample of 756 commitment cases, there was perfunctory adjudication in concordance with expert recommendation of examining committee composed of two physicians and one layman in all but two cases; in the two cases of court disagreement with the committee recommendation, there were unusual circumstances that indicated that the judge did not necessarily disagree with the experts); Maisel, *Decision-Making in Commitment Court,* 33 PSYCHIATRY 352 (1970) (in a sample of approximately 50 commitment hearings, no exact figures given, but by implication it seems clear that expert recommendations were perfunctorily followed in all cases, including those in which there was no tangible evidence of mental illness); Miller & Schwartz, *County Lunacy Commission Hearings: Some Observations of Commitments to a State Mental Hospital,* 14 SOC. PROB. 26, 27–28, 34 (1966) (in a sample of 58 commitment hearings, medical recommendation followed 75% of time by judge; demeanor of patient played crucial role in commitment decision); Scheff, *Social Conditions for Rationality:*

How Urban and Rural Courts Deal with the Mentally Ill, AM. BEHAVIORAL SCIENTIST, Mar., 1964, at 21 (in a sample of 43 commitment hearings, psychiatrists recommended commitment in all cases, and all defendants were committed after a perfunctory hearing even though there was no evidence of craziness in some); Scheff, *The Societal Reaction to Deviance: Ascriptive Elements in the Psychiatric Screening of Mental Patients in a Midwestern State,* 11 SOC. PROB. 401, 405 (1964) (in a sample of 116 judicial commitment hearings, psychiatrists recommended commitment in all cases despite lack of evidence in many; in informal discussions, judges and other court officials noted that they would rarely release a person against the advice of the experts); Wenger & Fletcher, *The Effect of Legal Counsel on Admissions to a State Mental Hospital, A Confrontation of Professions,* 10 J. HEALTH & HUMAN BEHAVIOR 66 (1969) (in a sample of 81 commitment cases, 80% of defendants were committed and 20% released, *all* in accordance with expert recommendation; legal decisionmaking was largely perfunctory; extremely high statistical association [Q=.942] was noted between representation by attorney and decision not to hospitalize); Wexler, Special Project, *The Administration of Psychiatric Justice: Theory and Practice in Arizona,* 13 ARIZ. L. REV. 1, 60 & n.195 (1971) (in samples of 196 commitment cases in one county and 367 in another, physicians' recommendations perfunctorily followed in 97.9% and 96.1% of cases, respectively; where physician's recommendation not followed, the judge was usually precluded from doing so because the recommendation was not provided for by statute).

Even under "reformed" procedures in which defendant-patients have greater due process protections, the concordance rate is still extremely high. Hiday, *Reformed Commitment Procedures: An Empirical Study in the Courtroom,* 11 LAW & SOC'Y REV. 651, 660–64 (1977) (77% concordance; in 15.6% of contested cases, judge committed patient in concordance with psychiatric recommendation despite lack of evidence of statutorily required danger; but hearings were longer than those reported in previous studies and decisionmaking was considerably less perfunctory). A recent, fascinating study examined the differential nature of commitment hearings in two counties in Wisconsin, one of which followed the stringent due process requirements of Lessard v. Schmidt, 349 F.Supp. 1078 (E.D. Wis. 1972), and one of which did not. In the latter, trials averaged 13 minutes, decisionmaking was perfunctory, and the court followed psychiatric advice in most cases. In the former, trials averaged 2 1/2 hours, there was true adjudication of the issues, and the court made an independent determination of whether the statutory criteria were met. Zander, *Civil Commitment in Wisconsin: The Impact of Lessard v. Schmidt,* 1976 WIS. L. REV. 503, 552.

Numerous appellate decisions, both old and new, also confirm the truth of the statement in the text. *E.g., In re* Oakes, in 8 THE LAW REPORTER 122 (P. Chandler ed. 1846). "Dr. Fox [the expert witness] testifies that he has no doubt that Mr. Oakes is insane. His opinion must have great weight in this case, from his skill and experience in the treatment of insanity. . . . If we cannot rely upon the opinion of those who have charge of the institution, and there is no law to restrain the persons confined, we must set all the insane at large who are confined in the McLean Asylum." *Id.; see* Sas v. Maryland, 334 F.2d 506, 511 (4th Cir. 1964) (expert findings and conclusions are to be given serious consideration and must be relied on to a considerable degree in defective delinquent proceedings); Logan v. Arafeh, 346 F. Supp. 1265, 1267–70 (D. Conn. 1972) (denied due process challenge to length of pretrial hearing on civil commitment; decision based on testimony of expert witnesses), *aff'd sub. nom.* Briggs v. Arafeh, 411 U.S. 911 (1973); Commonwealth v. Mutina, 366 Mass. 810, 323 N.E.2d 294, 298 (1975) (defendant convicted by jury of first degree murder; prosecution relied on presumption of sanity and defense introduced psychiatric testimony about defendant's insanity; held, verdict against the weight of the evidence); People *ex rel.* Rogers v. Stanley, 17 N.Y.2d 256, 260–61, 262–64, 217 N.E.2d 636, 637–39, 270 N.Y.S.2d 573, 574–75, 576–78 (1966) (Bergan, J., dissenting) (right to counsel in civil commitment should be denied because it will interfere with proper medical treatment).

Numerous commentators have also noted the legal abdication to psychiatric experts. *See* sources in note 13 *supra;* LAW REFORM COMMISSION OF CANADA, FITNESS TO STAND TRIAL 7 (1973); Bazelon, *Institutional Psychiatry—"The Self Inflicted Wound,"* 23 CATH. U.L. REV. 643 (1974); Dershowitz, *supra* note 11; Halleck, *The Psychiatrist and the Legal Process,* PSYCHOLOGY TODAY, Feb., 1969, at 25.

In recent years, there has been increasing judicial recognition of the fact that the issues involved in mental health cases are fundamentally legal and that overreliance on experts is a danger. *See* Humphrey v. Cady, 405 U.S. 504, 509–10 (1972); United States v. Brawner, 471 F.2d 969, 1006 (D.C. Cir. 1972); Washington v. United States, 390 F.2d at 446; Lessard v. Schmidt, 349 F.Supp. 1078 (E.D. Wis. 1972), *vacated and remanded on procedural grounds,* 414 U.S. 473, *new judgment entered,* 379 F. Supp. 1376, 1378 (E.D. Wis. 1974), *vacated and remanded,* 421 U.S. 957 (1975) (for reconsideration in light of Huffman v. Pursue, Ltd., 420 U.S. 592 (1975)), *reaff'd,* 413 F. Supp. 1318 (E.D. Wis. 1976). For an interesting case that upheld allowing a criminal prosecution to go to the jury although expert testimony that the defendant was insane was unanimous and rebutted only by cross-examination and lay evidence, see United States v. Dube, 520 F.2d 250, 251 (1st Cir. 1975).

Of course, where proceedings are truly adversary and each side has psychiatric as well as legal representation, there cannot be simple judicial concordance with one expert. Still, as *Washington* and *Brawner* discuss, experts often dominate the proceedings and the issues are defined as scientific. *See* notes 12–16 and accompanying text *supra.*

17. *See* H. DAVIDSON, FORENSIC PSYCHIATRY 237, 271–74 (1965). *See generally* S. BRAKEL & R. ROCK, THE MENTALLY DISABLED AND THE LAW 59–61 (rev. ed. 1971); L. KOLB, MODERN CLINICAL PSYCHIATRY 656–59 (8th ed. 1973); T. SZASZ, *supra* note 11, at 41–45; Wexler, *supra* note 16, at 69–73.

More recently, medically oriented writers have taken note of the changing legal climate exemplified by *Lessard,* and have argued that significant due process rights must be granted to civilly committed. American Psychiatric Association, *supra* note 10. A fair reading of many current writers is that the decision still ought to be largely medical even if much due process is granted. Chodoff, *supra* note 5; Treffert, *supra* note 10; Psychiatric News, Aug. 5, 1977, at 5, col. 1 (a code of ethical guidelines to be considered for adoption by the World Psychiatric Association).

> Whenever there is compulsory treatment or detention of a person on psychiatric grounds, that person must have available on appeal, with legal aid, to a *panel of psychiatrists* . . . .

Id. at 5 (emphasis added). The draft of ethical guidelines finally adopted in principle by the entire World Psychiatric Association provided:

> Whenever there is compulsory treatment or detention there must be an independent and neutral body of appeal for regular inquiry into these cases.

Psychiatric News, Oct. 7, 1977, at 23, col. 1. The American Psychiatric Association criticized the W.P.A. draft because it was "vague" and "subject to broad interpretation," and because it "did not mandate a psychiatrically knowledgeable panel." The A.P.A. continues to prefer appeal, with legal aid, to a panel of psychiatrists. *Id.* at 22. *See generally* Blomquist, *From the Oath of Hippocrates to the Declaration of Hawaii,* 4 ETHICS SCI. & MED. 139 (1977).

18. A. DEUTSCH, THE MENTALLY ILL IN AMERICA 418–41 (2d ed. 1949); J. KATZ, J. GOLDSTEIN, & A. DERSHOWITZ, PSYCHOANALYSIS, PSYCHIATRY AND LAW 462–63 (1967) (statement of W. Overholser, Sup't of St. Elizabeth's Hospital); T. Szasz, *supra* note 11, at 57–62. *See generally* Dershowitz, *The Origins of Preventive Confinement in Anglo-American Law—Part II: The American Experience,* 43 U. CIN. L. REV. 781 (1974).

19. *E.g.,* CAL. WELF. & INST. CODE § 5250 (West 1972) ("[T]he person is, as a result of mental disorder . . ."); Weihofen, *The Definition of Mental Illness,* 21 OHIO ST. L.J. 1 (1960). The causal connection criterion is often not recognized or stated explicitly by

commentators (including Weihofen) and mental health statutes. The causal criterion is always implicit, however, and in probably the substantial majority of statutes it is included by terms such as, "as a result of" or "because of." The causal connection criterion is a reflection of the critical rationale of mental health law—that the legally relevant behavior of mentally disordered persons is a product of their mental disorder and not of their free choice. *See* texts accompanying notes 58–112 *infra*.

20. *E.g.*, CAL. WELF. & INST. CODE §§5150, 5250 (West 1972 & Supp. 1978); *Developments*, *supra* note 6, at 1201–07.

21. Drope v. Missouri, 420 U.S. 162 (1975); Dusky v. United States, 362 U.S. 402 (1960) (per curiam); CAL. PENAL CODE §1367 (West Supp. 1977). Although some statutes and cases do not make specific reference to mental disorder as the cause of the incompetence, it is nearly always the case that incompetence will be found only if a mental disorder or defect is present. Stilten & Tullis, *Mental Competency in Criminal Proceedings*, 28 HASTINGS L.J. 1053, 1053–54 (1977); *see* HOME OFFICE, DEPARTMENT OF HEALTH AND SOCIAL SECURITY, REPORT OF THE COMMITTEE ON MENTALLY ABNORMAL OFFENDERS 143 (1975).

22. CAL. PROB. CODE §1460 (West Supp. 1977); CAL. WELF. & INST. CODE §5350 (West Supp. 1978). *See generally* Horstman, *Protective Services for the Elderly: The Limits of* Parens Patriac, 40 MO. L. REV. 215, 217–22, 225–30 (1975). On the distinction between involuntary civil commitment and guardianship or conservatorship, see *id*. at 224–25.

23. This Article will refer to the various behavioral components of the standards as "legally relevant behavior."

24. *See* Diamond, *The Psychiatric Prediction of Dangerousness*, 123 U. PA. L. REV. 439, 447–50 (1974); Greenberg, *Involuntary Psychiatric Commitments to Prevent Suicide*, 49 N.Y.U. L. REV. 227, 233–36, 259–63 (1974); Steadman, Cocozza, & Melick, *Explaining the Increased Arrest Rate Among Mental Patients: The Changing Clientele of State Hospitals*, 135 AM. J. PSYCHIATRY 816, 819–20 (1978); Psychiatric News, Nov. 18, 1977, at 42, col. 1. *See also* Zitrin, Hardesty, Burdock, & Drossman, *Crime and Violence Among Mental Patients*, 133 AM. J. PSYCHIATRY 147 (1976) (arrest rates for mentally ill persons are quite low, albeit somewhat higher than for normals). Many studies seem to show the mental patients are less dangerous than the population at large. *But see* Sosowsky, *Crime and Violence Among Mental Patients Reconsidered in View of the New Legal Relationship Between the State and the Mentally Ill*, 135 AM. J. PSYCHIATRY 33, 40–42 (1978) (higher arrest rates for patients; conviction rates not given and no control for prior arrests and social class). *See generally* THE CLINICAL EVALUATION OF THE DAN-

GEROUSNESS OF THE MENTALLY ILL (J. Rappeport ed. 1967). Indeed, even persons who are considered criminally insane and highly dangerous often exhibit low rates of violence if, for some reason, they are released prior to being considered cured. R. STEADMAN & J. COCOZZA, CAREERS OF THE CRIMINALLY INSANE 137–39, 183–89 (1974); Monahan, *The Prediction of Violence*, in VIOLENCE AND CRIMINAL JUSTICE 15, 19–20 (D. Chappell & J. Monahan eds. 1975).

On the issue of incompetence, see, *e.g.*, Vecchione v. Wohlgemuth, 377 F. Supp. 1361, 1367–69 (E.D. Pa. 1974); R. ALLEN, E. FERSTER, & H. WEIHOFEN, MENTAL IMPAIRMENT AND LEGAL INCOMPETENCY 46–68 (1968); Buttiglieri, Woodson, Guenette, & Thompson, *Driver Accidents and the Neuropsychiatric Patient*, 33 J. CONSULTING & CLINICAL PSYCHOLOGY 381 (1969) (neuropsychiatric patients had more traffic violations than normals but a comparable accident rate; psychiatric variables accounted for only a small percentage of difference in accident involvement; diagnosis of schizophrenic reaction seemed associated with a lower accident rate than rates associated with other, less serious diagnoses); Howard, *The Ex-Mental Patient as an Employee: An On-the-Job Evaluation*, 45 AM. J. ORTHOPSYCHIATRY 497 (1975); Tolor, Kelly, & Stebbins, *Altruism in Psychiatric Patients: How Socially Concerned Are the Emotionally Disturbed?*, 44 J. CONSULTING & CLINICAL PSYCHOLOGY 503 (1976) (psychiatric patients compared to normals on a paper and pencil test and in a devised "real world" situation that both measured altruism; no differences found on paper and pencil test; patients demonstrated significantly more altruism in the devised situation). *See generally* L.A. Times, Oct. 30, 1975, pt. 1, at 1, col. 1 ("1 in 5 Adults Lack Basic Living Skills, Study Finds").

25. A substantial portion of the argument in this section and the remainder of the Article depends heavily on the findings of mental health science and the writer's assessment of those findings. It is, of course, impossible to know or to cite every study that may be relevant to the broad statements that are made herein about mental disorder. Broad statements will therefore be supported either by reference to authorities who agree or to representative studies that support the position taken. At present, there can be few correct answers—the mental health field is too vast and is beset by too many methodological and substantive ambiguities and uncertainties. Before beginning the analysis, therefore, it will be helpful to set forth a brief statement of why knowledge is so hard to achieve in mental health science.

Research on mental disorder, which involves primarily research on human behavior, is at best difficult to perform—few certain conclusions can be reached. Although there are many reasons for the lack of certainty, two deserve special notice here: the imprecision in defining and categorizing mental disorder, and the difficulty in devising adequate tools for measuring human behavior. Chapman, *Schizomimetic Conditions and Schizophrenia*, 33 J. CONSULTING & CLINICAL PSYCHOLOGY 646, 648 (1969); *see* Spitzer, Endicott, & Robins, *Clinical Criteria for Psychiatric Diagnosis and DSM-III*, 132 AM. J. PSYCHIATRY 1187 (1975). It is indeed difficult to reach firm conclusions about any aspect of mental disorder when there is little agreement about the boundaries of the condition being studied and when there are few reliable and valid tools with which to perform the studies. Progress is being made in these regards, but the essential problems remain. *See, e.g.*, Helzer, Robins, Taibleson, Woodruff, Reich, & Wish, *Reliability of Psychiatric Diagnosis: I. A Methodological Review*, 34 ARCHIVES OF GENERAL PSYCHIATRY 129 (1977); text accompanying notes 26, 29–30, 54, 161–77 *infra*.

For discussions of these definitional difficulties in the context of the conditions most relevant to legal issues, see Kendell, *The Classification of Depressions: A Review of Contemporary Confusion*, 129 BRIT. J. PSYCHIATRY 15 (1976); van Praag, *About the Impossible Concept of Schizophrenia*, 17 COMPREHENSIVE PSYCHIATRY 481 (1976); Treves-Brown, *Who is the Psychopath?*, 17 MED. SCI. & L. 56 (1977); Letter from J.E. Cooper to editors, 127 BRIT. J. PSYCHIATRY 191 (1975).

On the difficulties of psychiatric and behavioral classification and measurement, see generally T. BARBER, PITFALLS IN HUMAN RESEARCH (1976); G. FRANK, PSYCHIATRIC DIAGNOSIS: A REVIEW OF RESEARCH (1975); R. KENDELL, THE ROLE OF DIAGNOSIS IN PSYCHIATRY (1975); Berman & Kenny, *Correlational Bias in Observer Ratings*, 34 J. PERSONALITY & SOC. PSYCHOLOGY 263 (1976); Blashfield & Draguns, *Evaluative Criteria for Psychiatric Classification*, 85 J. ABNORMAL PSYCHOLOGY 140 (1976) [hereinafter cited as *Evaluative Criteria*]; Blashfield & Draguns, *Toward A Taxonomy of Psychopathology: The Purpose of Psychiatric Classification*, 129 BRIT. J. PSYCHIATRY 574 (1976); Kazdin, *Artifact, Bias, and Complexity of Assessment: The ABCs of Reliability*, 10 J. APPLIED BEHAVIOR ANALYSIS 141 (1977); note 54 *infra*. For a penetrating methodological guide to the analysis of behavioral science for purposes of applying it to legal problems, see Meehl, *Law and the Fireside Inductions: Reflections of a Clinical Psychologist*, 27 J. SOC. ISSUES 65 (1971).

As we have seen, moreover, note 14 *supra*, there is enormous debate about the entire enterprise of considering abnormal behaviors as illness. Many writers feel that studying abnormal behavior on this basis is theoretically and morally misconceived and that knowledge about disordered behavior will inevitably be flawed.

The two most complete, albeit highly critical, reviews of mental health science literature pertaining to legal questions are J. ZISKIN, COPING WITH PSYCHIATRIC AND PSYCHOLOGICAL TESTIMONY (2d ed. 1975) and Ennis & Litwack, *Psychiatry and the Presumption of Expertise: Flipping Coins in the Courtroom*, 62 CALIF. L. REV. 693 (1974).

Finally, nearly all references are to the literature of adult mental health science. It should be noted, however, that the conclusions of this Article apply to child and adolescent mental health science as well. Morse, *Psychological and Psychiatric Issues*, in J. WILSON, THE RIGHTS OF ADOLESCENTS IN THE MENTAL HEALTH SYSTEM 81–122 (1978).

43. Spitzer & Wilson, *supra* note 26, at 827. *See also* note 14 *supra* (sources concerning the medical model in psychiatry).

Unlike Szasz and others, this author has no major theoretical objections to the use of illness language in general in discussion of crazy behavior. If it is useful for clinicians, researchers, and others, there is no harm in employing it. Whatever conceptual models are useful for different purposes should be employed. The major difficulty, however, is that illness language carries with it many unproven assumptions about crazy behavior that may have profound implications in non-mental health contexts such as legal decisionmaking. *See* note 14 *supra*. For instance, it is assumed that mentally ill persons lack control over their crazy behavior and its consequences much in the same way that physically ill persons are assumed to lack control over their illnesses and symptoms. As is shown at text accompanying notes 58 to 112 *infra*, however, this assumption about mentally ill persons is not proven. Unfortunately, when illness language is used to characterize behavior in the legal context, it reinforces the unproven assumption that the crazy person is not responsible for his behavior. *Cf.* Farina, Fisher, Getler, & Fischer, *Some Consequences of Changing People's Views Regarding the Nature of Mental Illness*, 87 J. ABNORMAL PSYCHOLOGY 272, 277–79 (1978) (subjects who were told that a behavioral problem was a product of social learning were compared to subjects who were told that the behavioral problem was a disease; the latter were more likely to feel helpless and less likely to believe they had control over the problem). This point is recognized by sophisticated lawyers and mental health professionals. Until nearly all people who work in the area of mental health law recognize this, the use of illness language may have the undesirable effect of begging the question of legal responsibility.

44. Jargon terms have question-begging connotations about the causes or nature of the phenomenon. Thus, this Article uses a nonjargon term interchangeably with the dominant jargon terms. It is difficult, however, to find a nonjargon term that both describes the behavior considered mental disorder and avoids unwanted connotations. No term is perfect, but "crazy" seems to avoid both legal and mental health science connotations while preserving a sense of serious abnormality. The author owes his preference for the term

"crazy" to his former teacher, Professor Alan Stone of Harvard Law School. In Professor Stone's courses on mental health law, it was a term often used and this writer has had an affection for it ever since. It is also widely used by mental health professionals, in discussion both among themselves and with patients. For a similar attempt to find a proper word, see Rosenhan, *The Contextual Nature of Psychiatric Diagnosis*, 84 J. ABNORMAL PSYCHOLOGY 462, 465 n.2 (1975).

45. . . . . *See generally* DSM-II, *supra* note 26.

46. Of course, mental health professionals can define for their own purposes whatever behavior they wish as abnormal, but unless the behavior so categorized is crazy or arguably so, society and the legal system would not accept special treatment of the persons so categorized—they would not seem sufficiently abnormal and different.

47. Edgerton, *supra* note 4, at 51. When mental health professionals attempt to break crazy behavior into "disease" categories or clusters, agreement that the person fits into a category is not high, even for those categories that map the craziest behavior. *See* Helzer, Clayton, Pambakian, Reich, Woodruff, & Reveley, *Reliability of Psychiatric Diagnosis: II. The Test/Retest Reliability of Diagnostic Classification*, 34 ARCHIVES OF GENERAL PSYCHIATRY 136 (1977); Spitzer & Fleiss, *A Re-analysis of the Reliability of Psychiatric Diagnosis*, 125 BRIT. J. PSYCHIATRY 341 (1974). In the seven studies reported by these two articles, the interrater reliability for schizophrenia was .57. For the reasons why diagnostic agreement is difficult to achieve, see notes 25 *supra* and 161–71 and accompanying text *infra*.

48. The diagnosis would probably be "Schizophrenia, Paranoid Type," according to DSM-II, *supra* note 26, at 34, or DSM-III, *supra* note 26, at C:10.

49. The diagnosis would probably be "Obsessive compulsive personality" according to DSM-II, *supra* note 26, at 43, or "Compulsive personality disorder" according to DSM-III, *supra* note 26, at K:15.

50. G. NEWMAN, COMPARATIVE DEVIANCE: PERCEPTION AND LAW IN SIX CULTURES 39–40 (1976); D'Arcy & Brockman, *Changing Public Recognition of Psychiatric Symptoms? Blackfoot Revisited*, 17 J. HEALTH & SOC. BEHAVIOR 303 (1976); Sarbin & Mancuso, *supra* note 3. *See generally* Scheff, *Decision Rules, Types of Error, and their Consequences in Medical Diagnosis*, 8 BEHAVIORAL SCI. 97 (1963); note 38 *supra; see also* Coie, Costanzo & Cox, *Behavioral Determinants of Mental Illness Concerns: A Comparison of "Gatekeeper" Professions*, 43 J. CONSULTING & CLINICAL PSYCHOLOGY 626, 635 (1975). On occasion, this tendency can assume outrageous proportions. *See* Cleary, *The Writ Writer*, 130 AM. J. PSYCHIATRY 319 (1973) (behavior of patient-prisoners in forensic psychiatry units who petitioned in order to secure their release interpreted as possibly "the expression of om-

nipotent fantasies, the idea that oppressive external forces can be routed by a stroke of the pen. The magic is not only in the written communication itself but also in the arcane, stylized phraseology so peculiar to legal documents." *Id*. at 320); Rosenhan, *On Being Sane in Insane Places*, 179 SCI. 250, 253 (1973) (pseudopatients who were admitted to mental hospitals as part of an experiment took notes of their experiences while on the ward; the note-taking was seen as evidence of psychopathology according to nursing records in three cases).

There is also evidence that, compared to laypersons, psychiatrists consistently place lower social value on behaviors labeled psychiatric symptoms. B.P. DOHRENWEND & B.S. DOHRENWEND, SOCIAL STATUS AND PSYCHOLOGICAL DISORDER: A CAUSAL INQUIRY 81–88 (1969).

51. DSM-II, *supra* note 26, at 44.

52. American Psychiatric Association, *Position Statement on Homosexuality and Civil Rights*, 131 AM. J. PSYCHIATRY 497 (1974). *See also A Symposium: Should Homosexuality Be in the APA Nomenclature?*, 130 AM. J. PSYCHIATRY 1207 (1973).

53. *Cf.* Rippere, *Commonsense Beliefs About Depression and Antidepressive Behavior: A Study of Social Consensus*, 15 BEHAVIOUR RESEARCH & THERAPY 465, 466–67, 471–73 (1977) (subjects who were psychologists were tested on their degree of consensus about beliefs concerning depression and antidepressive behavior; subjects agreed on commonsense propositions verifiable by first hand experience or observation, but disagreed on abstract matters debated by experts; support for validity of lay beliefs about psychopathology). For an interesting series of articles by mental health professionals that deal with the appropriate ethical and professional responses that professionals should make when they are consulted by gay persons, see Bieber, *A Discussion of "Homosexuality: The Ethical Challenge,"* 44 J. CONSULTING & CLINICAL PSYCHOLOGY 163 (1976); Davison, *Homosexuality: The Ethical Challenge*, 44 J. CONSULTING & CLINICAL PSYCHOLOGY 157 (1976); Halleck, *Another Response to "Homosexuality: The Ethical Challenge,"* 44 J. CONSULTING & CLINICAL PSYCHOLOGY 167 (1976). These articles evidence substantial disagreement among professionals.

54. A possible exception to the statement in the text would occur if experts used psychological test results. There are, of course, numerous tests that measure the supposed presence or absence of mental disorders. *See generally* M. MALONEY & M. WARD, PSYCHOLOGICAL ASSESSMENT, A CONCEPTUAL APPROACH 311–408 (1976); CLINICAL METHODS IN PSYCHOLOGY 61–279 (I. Weiner ed. 1976). For legal purposes, however, there are two major difficulties with these tests. First, there is considerable reason to doubt their usefulness in general; tests may not produce reliable and valid information about the person

tested. Second, in addition to possible general reliability and validity problems, present psychological tests do not define those persons who are crazy enough to meet the legal standard of mental illness. For the law, it is not the person's behavior on a test that is at issue, but *his behavior in the real world.* If the tests accurately predicted who behaved sufficiently crazily in the real world, then they might help determine whether the legal standard of mental illness is met. To date, however, there is no indication that tests can do this. *See, e.g.,* M. MALONEY & M. WARD, *supra* at 336–43, 363–70; W. MISCHEL, PERSONALITY AND ASSESSMENT 59–70, 110–13 (1968); J. ZISKIN, COPING WITH PSYCHIATRIC AND PSYCHOLOGICAL TESTIMONY 144–80 (2d ed. 1975); Blatt, *The Validity of Projective Techniques and Their Research and Clinical Contribution,* 39 J. PERSONALITY ASSESSMENT 327 (1975); Cleveland, *Reflections on the Rise and Fall of Psychodiagnosis,* 7 PROFESSIONAL PSYCHOLOGY 309 (1976); Lewandowski & Saccuzzo, *The Decline of Psychological Testing,* 7 PROFESSIONAL PSYCHOLOGY 177 (1976).

It is not suggested here that critics of testing in general are correct about the uselessness of the enterprise. *Cf.* Wade & Baker, *Opinions and Uses of Psychological Tests: A Survey of Clinical Psychologists,* 32 AM. PSYCHOLOGIST 874, 879–881 (1977) (despite criticism of tests, they are still widely used by clinicians of all therapeutic orientations; clinicians recognize the psychometric flaws of tests, but question the reliability and validity of the negative studies; clinicians are probably unaffected by negative results concerning tests because of the need to assess, the lack of weight given to experimental evidence, and the lack of practical alternatives). This writer believes that testing is worthwhile and that some tests are very useful for some purposes. It is claimed here, however, that present tests do not offer data that answer legal questions about normality. By and large, tests of psychopathology track present psychiatric categories that themselves are of little value in legal decisionmaking. *See* notes 161–77 and accompanying text *infra.*

55. *See* note 47 and accompanying text *supra.*

56. *See* note 50 and accompanying text *supra.*

57. Hall, *supra* note 16, at 1049; *see* note 47 and accompanying text *supra. See also* Vestre & Zimmermann, *Validity of Informants' Ratings of the Behavior and Symptoms of Psychiatric Patients,* 33 J. CONSULTING & CLINICAL /PSYCHOLOGY 175 (1969). It is sometimes suggested that psychiatric categories help *limit* the number of cases of deviant behavior where mental health law intervention would be justified. Shapiro, *Therapeutic Justifications for Intervention into Mentation and Behavior,* 13 DUQ. L. REV. 673, 772–73 (1975). Perhaps so, but why should mental health professionals be delegated the power to decide for society and the law the social and moral question of

which persons ought to be subject to special legal treatment?

58. *See, e.g., Developments, supra* note 6, at 1212–19, 1228–35 (analysis of the relevance to civil commitment decisions of various forms of legally relevant incapacity caused by mental illness; contention that the policies behind special treatment and due process are both satisfied only if the person treated specially is incapacitated as a result of mental illness).

59. J. MACKIE, ETHICS 216 (1977); . . . Wender, *On Necessary and Sufficient Conditions in Psychiatric Explanation,* 16 ARCHIVES OF GENERAL PSYCHIATRY 41 (1967). The modern view of the determinism thesis recognizes that there are no certain laws and that events are best understood in terms of probabilities and contingencies. E. NAGEL, PRINCIPLES OF THE THEORY OF PROBABILITY 1–4 (1939); E. NAGEL, THE STRUCTURE OF SCIENCE 73–78 (1961). Determinism in modern science also serves as a regulative methodological principle that holds that it is useful to look for lawful relations between events. A. KAPLAN, THE CONDUCT OF INQUIRY 124–25 (1964); E. NAGEL, *supra,* at 605–06. *See generally* A. KAPLAN, *supra,* at 121–24; Edel, *Psychiatry and Philosophy,* in 1 AMERICAN HANDBOOK OF PSYCHIATRY 961, 964–66 (2d ed. S. Arieti ed. 1974).

On the difficulty of formulating an adequate general theory of behavior, see Alexander, *The Search for a General Theory of Behavior,* 20 BEHAVIORAL SCI. 77 ‹1975).

60. M. FELDMAN, CRIMINAL BEHAVIOUR: A PSYCHOLOGICAL ANALYSIS 271 (1977); B.F. SKINNER, BEYOND FREEDOM AND DIGNITY (1971); Katz, *Law, Psychiatry, and Free Will,* 22 U. CHI. L. REV. 397, 398 (1955). *But see* Meehl, *Psychology and the Criminal Law,* 5 U. RICH L. REV. 1, 3 (1970) (critique of those who argue for the scientific irrelevance of responsibility).

61. For the most strikingly optimistic and perhaps frightening example of this view, see B.F.SKINNER, *supra* note 60. Some determinists react to the present incomplete state of knowledge by believing that the orderly functioning of society requires that persons be treated *as if* they were responsible for their behavior, even if such treatment is based on an allegedly incorrect view of reality. . . . Katz, *supra* note 60, at 398–99. *See generally* Waelder, *Psychiatry and the Problem of Criminal Responsibility,* 101 U. PA. L. REV. 378 (1952). In any case, the determinist does not believe that lack of knowledge or a rejection of the behaviorist approach means behavior is free: behavior is still determined, but by unplanned and unknown determinants. M. FELDMAN, *supra* note 60, at 272.

62. United States v. Ceccolini, 98 S. Ct. 1054, 1063 (1978) (Burger, C.J., concurring); *see, e.g.,* State v. Sikora, 44 N.J. 453, 476–79, 210 A.2d 193, 205–07 (1965) (Weintraub, C.J., concurring); J. HALL,

GENERAL PRINCIPLES OF CRIMINAL LAW 455–58 (2d ed. 1960) (discussion of conflict of perspectives between law and mental health science). *See generally* Katz, *supra* note 60; Waelder, *supra* note 60. Most legal discussion of responsibility occurs in the criminal law context, but the assumption of responsibility holds generally.

63. Morse, *The Twilight of Welfare Criminology: A Reply to Judge Bazelon*, 49 S. CAL. L. REV. 1247, 1251–54 (1976). *See generally* W. LaFave & A. Scott, CRIMINAL LAW 179–81 (1972).

64. Morse, *supra* note 63, at 1251–54. *See also* H.L.A. HART, PUNISHMENT AND RESPONSIBILITY 15 (1968).

> The special features of Mitigation are that a good reason for administering a less severe penalty is made out if the situation or mental state of the convicted criminal is such that he was exposed to an unusual or specially great temptation, or his ability to control his actions is thought to have been impaired or weakened otherwise than by his own actions, so that conformity to the law which he has broken was a matter of special difficulty for him as compared with normal persons normally placed.

Id. Presumably, if the actor's ability to conform to law is weakened sufficiently, the law would consider the actor completely nonresponsible. *Id.* at 14.

It is recognized that philosophers consider substantive determinism to be an all-or-none proposition. Determinism and indeterminism, however, are both unprovable. J. MACKIE, *supra* note 59, at 216. The law cannot proceed on the assumption of either. The law is a moral-evaluative institution that must make decisions concerning real world problems of human interaction. Thus, the law cannot afford to be philosophically pure, but must adopt a commonsense cosmology, congruent with ordinary experience and useful for making decisions. That various factors or pressures make some choices harder and others easier and that such factors bear on the moral and legal responsibility of actors is certainly a commonsense view of the world that accords with ordinary experience. *See generally* Katz, *supra* note 60.

65. W. LaFave & A. Scott, *supra* note 63, at 337–41; N. MORRIS & C. HOWARD, STUDIES IN CRIMINAL LAW 61–73 (1964).

66. Morse, *supra* note 63, at 1253.

67. This Article will not attempt to resolve either the philosophical dispute about free will and determinism or the philosophical and scientific quagmire of causation. Interested readers are referred to the following works, which have furnished the general background for much of the argument in this section. H. BLALOCK, CAUSAL INFERENCES IN NONEXPERIMENTAL RESEARCH (1964); H.L.A. HART, *supra* note 64; A. KAPLAN, *supra* note 59; E. NAGEL, *supra* note 59; D. O'CONNOR, FREE WILL (1971); K. POPPER, *Of Clouds and Clocks,* in OBJECTIVE KNOWLEDGE 206 (1972); A. ROSS, ON GUILT, RESPONSIBILITY AND PUNISHMENT (1975); M. SUSSER, CAUSAL THINKING IN THE HEALTH SCIENCES (1973); DETERMINISM AND FREEDOM (S. Hook ed. 1958); DETERMINISM, FREE WILL, AND MORAL RESPONSIBILITY (G. Dworkin ed. 1970); ESSAYS ON FREEDOM OF ACTION (T. Honderich ed. 1973); FREEDOM & RESPONSIBILITY 1–51, 282–342 (H. Morris ed. 1961); FREE WILL AND DETERMINISM (B. Berofsky ed. 1966).

68. The causal hypothesis is expressed by locutions such as "result of," "because of," "due to," "incapacity," "unable," and the like. *See, e.g.,* CAL. WELF. & INST. CODE § 5150 (West Supp. 1978).

69. *See* M. FELDMAN, *supra* note 60, at 270.

70. *See generally* Waelder, *supra* note 60; notes 62–67 and accompanying text *supra.*

* * *

157. Livermore, Malmquist, & Meehl, *On the Justifications for Civil Commitment,* 117 U. Pa. L. Rev. 75, 80 (1968).

158. Some commentators have suggested that physicians possess a unique kind of authority that is based on a combination of knowledge and expertness, moral authority, and charisma. This authority is strengthened by the facts that medicine deals with death and was once unified with religion. Siegler & Osmond, *Aesculapian Authority,* 1 HASTINGS CENTER STUD. 41–43 (1973). This unique authority may be extended, however, to spheres where it is not applicable. Many commentators believe that crazy conduct is not a medical matter and that the psychiatrist's authority in judicial proceedings is improper and derives solely from the magico-religious background of much of medicine. *See generally* authorities cited in notes 13–14 *supra.* Of course, Siegler and Osmond believe that crazy behavior is a sphere where the authority of physicians is appropriate. In either case, the concept is useful for understanding the power of medical experts in the mental health legal system. *See generally* Bazelon, *The Perils of Wizardry,* 131 AM. J. PSYCHIATRY 1317 (1974); Starr, *Medicine and the Waning of Professional Sovereignty,* 107 DAEDALUS 175, 175–76 (1978).

* * *

179. Descriptions and conclusions may be difficult to distinguish in some instances. Ennis & Litwak, *supra* note 25, at 743–45. Terms such as "depressed" have both commonsense, descriptive connotations and technical connotations. Experts should carefully avoid using technical terms and should put their observations in commonsense language. Because psychiatric terms generally describe behavior, nearly always there will be ordinary language equivalents for jargon. Also, since conclusion terms, whether or not technical, are based on observable referents, the referents should be described. If possible, it would be most useful if the factfinder could hear a tape recording of the interview or see a videotape of it.

It is assumed, too, that the adversary model would ensure, through the use of adversary experts or effective cross-examination, that the person's *normal* as well as crazy behavior would be described by the experts. Otherwise, it is far too easy to make a person appear crazy by selective testimony. Ennis & Litwak, *supra* note 25, at 745. The problem of selective testimony would be reduced if the factfinder has access to a tape of the interview.

One difficulty that will arise from the suggested mode of testifying concerns the presentation of psychological test results. The results of such tests are unlike the data of ordinary experience—lay observers have no baseline to measure them against. If there were tests that validly answered legally relevant questions (which at present there are not), the expert would have to describe the validity studies, specifying the probability that a person who achieved a certain test result also behaves sufficiently crazy for legal purposes in real life.

* * *

209. *See* Farrell, *The Right of an Indigent Civil Commitment Defendant to Psychiatric Assistance of His Own Choice at State Expense,* 11 Idaho L. Rev. 141 (1975).

* * *

4.2 Exploring New Ethics for Public Health: Developing a Fair Alcohol Policy

DAN E. BEAUCHAMP

Reprinted with permission of the Department of Health Administration, Duke University, from 1 *Journal of Health Politics, Policy and Law* 338–354 (1976). Copyright © 1976 by the Department of Health Administration, Duke University. All rights reserved.

Public policies for a society are based on prevailing visions of justice and the common good. In the United States we have extolled a theory of justice under which individuals are entitled only to material ends such as status, income or employment that have been acquired by fair rules of entitlement, e.g., by individual efforts or abilities. Ideally this market theory of justice emphasizes individual responsibility, the pursuit of self-interest, minimal collective action and, except for the prohibition against causing direct harm to others or interfering with other persons' fundamental rights, freedom from collective obligations.

We have compromised these market-justice[1] principles to protect the public's health, usually when it has been in the interest of the entire community, and especially the most powerful or the most numerous elements, to do so. We have been willing to undertake collective action when the well-being of the whole populace has been threatened (infectious disease campaigns) or for the sake of collective amenities which can be secured only through organized community effort (chlorination, sanitary codes, immunization, fluoridation or social insurance for the aged), most often when such measures did not severely impinge upon majorities or powerful interests.

We have been less willing to undertake collective action to protect minorities or the least powerful, especially when such action would deprive key groups—this despite the evidence that most of our vexing public health problems (controlling the hazards of our workplaces, modes of transportation, the commodities we use or consume, and the air we breathe) are problems of social justice and equality[2] in that they affect a minority of the population and cannot be reduced significantly without the majority in society accepting painful new burdens. We have acquiesced in collective action to provide treatment and rehabilitation services for disadvantaged minorities such as the handicapped and the poor, though such action often has been taken grudgingly and minimally; but we are still far from accepting the egalitarian principle that the numbers of that minority who suffer preventable disability and premature death ought to be minimized, and that all persons and groups—including the most powerful and the most numerous—ought to bear their fair share of the burdens of prevention.

This is not to deny that we have adopted sometimes stringent public health measures to combat specific threats to the public's health. Yet public policy in health has leaned more heavily toward support for research and education of professionals, limited areawide planning, and public subsidization of the costs of medical care for the poor and aged. These governmental policies often serve to protect powerful medical interests and to perpetuate essentially private mechanisms for the delivery of health services. More seriously, these policies often leave manufacturing groups free to operate with minimal regard for the public's health while spreading the costs of treating casualties throughout the population.

Often when we have undertaken collective action to protect the health of a minority we have yet managed to explain the problem in a way that subtly reaffirms the norms of market-justice and individual responsibility, and carefully protects powerful groups and majorities from the burdens and responsibilities of prevention. One particularly interesting form of this (William Ryan[3] has called it "victim-blaming") involves admitting that for certain health problems such as mental illness, addictions, suicide, and accidental injury, the rule of individual responsibility is not operable—*for a minority of individuals*. Since the majority of individuals do not fall into the problem category, it is mistakenly assumed that they have some saving attribute or capacity—e.g., they are "capable" of behaving responsibly—which the minority who experience the problem must lack. The problem is defined (falsely) as occurring because the minority "fails" where the majority "succeeds," and the majority (and more importantly powerful interests) are automatically absolved of any responsibility for serious collective action to prevent death and disability.

ALCOHOL POLICY AND THE ALCOHOLIC MINORITY

This process of explaining public problems in a way that protects powerful interests from the burdens of collective action is nowhere more conspicuous than in the case of alcohol and alcohol problems. The concept of alcoholism is based on the seemingly straightforward observation that the vast *majority* of drinkers do not experience alcohol problems. This has led to acceptance of the idea (in reality the myth) that the minority with problems lack an ability possessed by the majority. Many experts see the inability to control one's use of alcohol as a disease condition predisposed by hereditary, social, cultural or psychological factors.[4] Obviously, then, there would be little point—and what is more, little justice—in more stringent controls on alcohol in order to reduce problems.

Our public policy for alcohol problems reflects this thinking. Despite the fact that alcohol problems cost the nation $25 billion annually in disease, death and loss of productivity,[5] and despite the alarming evidence that per capita consumption of alcohol has increased by one-third over the past fifteen years,[6] the Department of Health, Education and Welfare agency responsible for developing policy for alcohol problems—the National Institute on Alcohol Abuse and Alcoholism (NIAAA)—has no alcohol control policy. Instead, the NIAAA concentrates on developing treatment resources for the suffering alcoholic; searching for the causes of the "disease" of alcoholism; and mounting a national campaign to teach people "how to drink responsibly."[7] All of these policies are based squarely on the view that the nation's alcohol problems occur mainly because a minority of persons lack the ability to control their use of alcohol. Clearly, the policies of the NIAAA do not require the liquor industry or the majority of the drinking public to share any significant burdens of preventing problems.

NEW EVIDENCE FOR ALCOHOL CONTROL

There is impressive new empirical evidence, however, that offers a direct challenge to the alcoholism paradigm[8] and its implications—rooted in market-justice—that producer groups and all persons who drink need not, or should not, share the cost of minimizing the numbers of the minority who suffer alcohol problems.

This evidence demonstrates that it is the low overall or per capita consumption of alcohol in society (and by implication the factors that influence this low consumption, such as rules governing the use of alcohol—that produces low rates of such major alcohol related problems as cirrhosis.[9]

The evidence is clear: in countries where the average consumption of alcohol is high, alcohol-related cirrhosis rates are high; in countries where the average consumption of alcohol is lower, the rates of alcohol-related cirrhosis are lower. Further, as the average rates of consumption go up so do the rates of cirrhosis and other afflictions.

Later I will discuss these findings and their implications for alcohol policy in more detail. For now, suffice it to say they indicate that protection of the community from rising alcohol problems is not to be achieved primarily by strengthening individual abilities or capacities to use alcohol correctly, but by imposing community and societal rules that are designed to limit and control everyone's use of alcohol and thus to minimize the number of the minority who suffer problems. (Indeed, I shall argue that the entire question of "why" some people are unable to control their drinking—the attempt to define alcohol problems in an idiom of individual powers, abilities and capacities—is fundamentally misconceived.)[10]

These findings imply that to minimize alcohol problems burdens must be placed on the most powerful or the most numerous in order to benefit the least powerful or the least numerous. In this view, alcohol problems are not different from other serious social problems of inequality—unemployment, racial inequality, poverty, the abandonment of the aged—all problems of minorities which can only be solved by redistributing the burdens and benefits of society.

This perspective suggests that the primary obstacle to minimizing alcohol problems is not in the realm of biomedical research or technology but is a social ethic—market-justice—which unfairly protects the alcohol industry and the majority who drink from the burdens of more stringent controls. What is needed is a new public health ethic—an ethic based on justice and equality—that subjects alcohol, and other hazards of this world, to fair limitation, in order to minimize the number of persons who suffer damage. Such an ethic would necessitate that all who participate in the manufacture, distribution, sale and consumption of alcohol have, unequal (but still fair) responsibility to bear the burdens of these controls. The balance of this article is devoted to outlining the broad principles of an egalitarian public health ethic and to specifying what this new ethic would imply for alcohol policy.

PUBLIC HEALTH AS SOCIAL JUSTICE[11]

The ideal of market-justice has been challenged in Western liberal thought by a tradition of equality and social justice.[12] This tradition—in contrast to market-justice[13]—argues that some harms are so inimical to the interests of all human beings that collective measures should be taken to ensure that all persons are protected from them equally and to the greatest extent possible. A list of these harms might include: threats to security and survival; lack of minimal education; poverty; deprivation of basic human liberties; and, especially significant for our purposes, serious disability and premature death.

John Rawls has recently given the most exhaustive treatment of the dream of social justice in his *A Theory of Justice*.[14] Rawls argues that persons placed in a position of radical impartiality (what he terms the original position) and ignorant of their respective positions, talents, or attributes would agree to adopt mutually binding rules protecting each other against serious harms—harms which would thwart any person in securing his particular ends in life. These protections (which Rawls calls *primary goods*[15]) would be necessary to assure protection and redress against the lottery of heredity and the powerful inequalities generated by the environment or social structure.

Regardless of whether one starts with the Rawlsian position or draws upon the visions of other social philosophers, the essentials of social justice remain fairly constant: equality, impartiality, autonomy, and the protection of all persons against serious harms to the greatest extent possible.[16]

The historic ideal of public health—to minimize preventable death and disability—can be treated as an objective of equality and social justice; however, this egalitarian interpretation has not emerged for several reasons. First, despite the fact that one can find social justice influences in the classics of public health literature,[17] public health—at least in England—was more directly influenced by mercantilist and utilitarian streams of thought.[18] Second, the great emphasis on individual liberty and markets in England and the U.S. tended to restrict the scope of public health to problems of market failures or externalities. Third, public health measures were then (as they are now) public goods[19] offering protection against threats to the entire community (e.g., the campaigns for sanitary reform and against infectious disease). For these public goods the rule of individual responsibility seemed inapplicable, but the issue of a more equal distribution of benefits and burdens was not very crucial; as everyone seemed threatened and everyone benefitted equally, roughly speaking. Finally, new discoveries in medical science (such as immunization) afforded "technological shortcuts"[20] to avoid the pain of social change.

However, the current situation does not permit the treatment of public health as an acceptable deviation from the norms of market-justice. In the case of current problems of disability and premature death, it is clearly a minority who are affected (although that minority may number in the millions). Further, there seem to be no easy technological short-cuts to eliminating disability or early death; indeed the evidence indicates that technology is a major source of hazard.[21] Moreover, reducing the numbers of the affected minority in most cases requires painful reallocations of the burdens of collective action. Thus, there is a central need for a more adequate public health ethic, with the social justice and egalitarian goals of minimizing the numbers of the minority who suffer preventable disability and premature death. Such an ethic would ensure that no group or person was arbitrarily excluded from protection and that the burdens of collective action were fairly shouldered by all.

Linking public health to the tradition of social justice and equality and seeing public health from the standpoint of ethics has several key logical implications for public health policy which are referred to here as "principles." These principles are not new to public health. To the contrary, making these egalitarian influences visible only serves to add ethical coherence and order to pre-existing public health principles. These principles of an egalitarian public health ethic are: (1) controlling the hazards of this world (2) to prevent death and disability (3) through organized collective action (4) shared equally by all except where unequal burdens result in increased protection for everyone and especially for potential victims of death and disability.[22]

Controlling the Hazards

A key principle of an egalitarian public health ethic would be to identify and control the hazards of this world rather than focus on the behavioral defects of individuals damaged by those hazards. Against this principle it is usually argued that today the causes of death and disability are multiple and frequently are behavioral in origin. Further, since it is usually only a minority of the public that suffer death and disability from most known hazards, additional controls on those hazards would not seem effective or just.[23] Instead we should ask why some people expose themselves to known hazards or perils, or act in an unsafe or careless manner.

A public health ethic rooted in equality would be suspicious of behavioral explanations for public health problems, since such explanations tend to "blame the victim" and unfairly protect powerful groups from the burdens of prevention. Whether the issue is alcohol, other drugs, large dogs, noxious chemicals, infectious diseases, exploding bombs, crashing automobiles, damaging levels of noise, avalanches, earthquakes, polluted air, radiation, contaminated water, starvation, the unjust distribution of medical care, or the "escape of tigers,"[24] the focus of a health ethic seeking to minimize disability and premature death would not be on explaining "why" some individuals fall victim to perils. Rather, its point would be to ensure that all hazards, and all essential goods were controlled by fair and equitable rules to minimize the risks of death and disability.

Public health, ideally, should not be concerned with explaining the successes and failures of differing individuals (dispositional explanations)[25] in dealing with the hazards of this world. These failures instead should be seen as signs of weak and ineffective limits or controls over those conditions, practices, commodities, products, or services which are either hazardous to the safety of members of the public, or which are vital to protect the public's health.

Prevention

The second principle of a new public health ethic—prevention—is based directly on an egalitarian commitment to minimizing the numbers of persons who suffer disability and premature death. The only way known to minimize death and disability rates is to prevent damaging exposures in the first place or to seek to minimize damage when exposures cannot be controlled. Thus the familiar public health options are creating rules to[26]:

1. minimize the exposure of groups of individuals to hazards and thereby to reduce the rates of hazardous exchanges
2. provide safeguards against damage in the event that hazardous exchanges occur anyway, where such techniques (e.g., fluoridation, seat-belts or immunization) are feasible
3. organize treatment resources in the community so as to minimize damage that does

occur, since it can rarely be prevented totally.

Compulsory Measures

The third principle of an egalitarian public health ethic is that the control of hazards must be achieved, not through voluntary or market mechanisms, but by governmental or non-governmental agencies through planned, organized, and obligatory collective action. This is for two reasons. The first is that market, or voluntary, action is characteristically inadequate for providing what are called public goods. Again, public goods are those public policies (as for reducing the rates of crime, disease, injury, or alcohol problems) that are universal or general in impact, affecting everyone equally, and hence not easily withheld from those individuals in the community who choose not to pay for them. Individuals acting out of self-interest as is typical in market situations, might choose not to share in the cost of reducing the rate of alcohol problems since they will realize the benefits of the policy in any event. Many individuals also might calculate that they need not bear the costs and inconveniences for clean air and water, fluoridation, safe neighborhoods, or low rates of alcohol problems, since in large groups such as communities or societies their contribution, or lack of it, would be negligible.[27]

A second reason why it is often not in the interest of self-regarding individuals to pay the costs of public goods is that policies to provide them and improve protection for everyone impose burdens that are greater than every individual will voluntarily accept. With these temptations for individual noncompliance, justice demands assurance that all persons share equally the costs of collective action through obligatory or sanctioned policies. These arguments for compulsory measures are essentially the same as those behind Hardin's parable of the "tragedy of the commons."[28] If the public good (protecting the commons) is to be assured, society must accept mutual obligations—mutually agreed upon—that are binding and compulsory.

Fair-Sharing

The final principle of a new public health ethic is that all persons are equally responsible for sharing the burdens—as well as the benefits—of

protection against death and disability, except where unequal burdens result in greater protection for every person, and especially for those most threatened. In practice this means that policies to control the hazards of a given substance, service or commodity fall unequally (but still fairly) on those involved in the production, provision or consumption of the service, commodity or substance.

LIMITS TO PUBLIC HEALTH

A public health ethic rooted in the tradition of equality and social justice places a very high priority on the protection and preservation of human life. At the same time, equality and justice give rise to other values and protections which constitute important limits to public health and collective action. I will list, without elaboration, the most crucial of these limits to demonstrate that the egalitarian ethic being advocated here rejects collectivist or paternalistic remedies. Its emphasis is always upon the creation of mutually agreed upon obligations, in order to minimize rates and number of persons who suffer serious disability and early death.[29] Very tentatively the limits to collective action for public health would seem to be as follows:

1. the broad injunction against public health measures that unreasonably and coercively interfere with the *fundamental* rights of privacy of individual citizens
2. the injunction against pursuing the goals of public health at the expense of other primary goods such as basic education, elimination of poverty and, especially, basic political liberties
3. the injunction against the undue emphasis on controlling some public health hazards to the exclusion of others, especially where the control of others might achieve more dramatic results in terms of minimizing disability or early death
4. the injunction against measures that increase over the long run the risks of death and disability
5. the injunction to consider the problems of "redistributive justice," or the special problems of achieving a transition from one model of justice to another; a corollary of this injunction would seem to be that

where two or more policy options promise roughly equivalent results, that option should be chosen that is least disruptive of other social or economic values.

FOUNDATIONS FOR A FAIR ALCOHOL CONTROL POLICY

The final portion of this article is devoted to outlining a policy for alcohol that is consistent with an ethic stressing the minimization of serious disability or early death. I will not attempt to provide detailed specifics but will only sketch out the most salient characteristics of a just alcohol control policy.[30]

The most important feature of this new policy of course, would be a shift in public attention away from the "failure" of the alcoholic and toward controlling the overall use of alcohol. Under an ethic stressing the *minimization*[31] of alcohol-related damage, the chief focus becomes the creation of adequate control structures for alcohol at all levels of government and in the private sector. This control structure would seek to reduce or restrict the per capita consumption of alcohol through more adequate public and private limits over the manufacture, import, distribution, advertising, sale and consumption of alcohol.

Controlling Per Capita Consumption

The thrust of a fair alcohol policy—both official and private—would need to be conservative and should discourage the use of alcohol. As a start, the goal could be zero growth in total alcohol consumption. The strategy should be to make alcohol a little more expensive, a little harder to come by, and its use a little less approved.

This new alcohol policy cannot be solely federal, but the federal government must take the lead. Fair and adequate control structures can never be established unless the power of the federal government is exercised to urge uniform and appropriately high levels of taxation, stringent regulation of advertising, and controls over marketing practices. Below the federal level the federal government should encourage the states and localities to exert more control over the industry and to enact stricter measures regarding the availability of alcohol. The alternative is the current situation, with a "balkanized" alcohol con-

trol structure that merely reflects the checkered distribution of influence between the industry and temperance forces across the fifty states.

Haddon[32] has called attention to the fact that for many kinds of public health hazards we can reduce losses even if we do not control per capita or overall exposure to hazards; we can use techniques (sometimes called "technological shortcuts")[33] that are socially and politically less disruptive. Seatbelts, as a strategy against highway injuries, may be unpopular, but the opposition to an overall planned reduction of exposure of groups to the private automobile might be significantly more unpopular. If such techniques were available for alcohol problems, we would be justified in using them if for no other reason than that such techniques usually disrupt other values less than direct controls over exposure to hazards.

But in the case of drugs, and perhaps many other chemical hazards of man's environment, there seem to be few known techniques to protect individuals without controlling per capita exposure to the substance. As Terris has pointed ed out, there seems to be no presently available technology for "immunizing" individuals against hazardous chemical exposures.[34] Even if such techniques were available, it is clear that there would be problems in implementing them as collective policies.

For all hazardous drugs then, including alcohol, it seems that much of the focus of preventive strategy must be aimed at controlling exposure in the first place.

The Myth of "Safe Drinking"

In response to the perennial question of how much an individual should drink, a fair and just alcohol policy would seek to restrict (not forbid) the use of alcohol, and would encourage people to use alcohol either not at all or minimally, giving it a relatively minor place in their lives. *The overall goal of alcohol control policy will be to encourage high rates of minimal or non-use of alcohol so as to promote low rates of excessive use of alcohol.*[35]

A fair alcohol policy would avoid confusing the issue of what is "safe" for an individual to drink and what all individuals ought to drink. This is in sharp contrast to recent federal policy. When asked to define the level of "safe" drinking, the past Director of the NIAAA, Morris

Chafetz, responded by endorsing a nineteenth-century actuarial study which found that persons who drank no more than the equivalent of three ounces of whiskey a day did not seem to suffer an increase in health problems or mortality.[36] The interesting thing about this response is that less than ten percent of the persons in the United States drink as much as the equivalent of three ounces of whiskey daily.[37] In fact, the NIAAA's *Second Special Report to Congress on Alcohol and Health* classifies a daily intake of three ounces of alcohol as heavy drinking![38]

The entire notion of "safe drinking" ignores the fact that the rules governing what is "safe" for a given individual to drink are far different from the rules governing what individuals "should" drink in order to minimize alcohol problems in the community. This is essentially the difference between prudential, or self-regarding, rules and ethical rules governing conduct which are designed to achieve fair and just protection for everyone from known hazards. The latter, ethical norms are much more conservative, allowing for a factor of failure, and require that individuals drink at rates that are far lower than might be safe for them individually. (The empirical evidence from the work of deLint and Schmidt and others[39] tends to suggest that cultural and social norms are rooted not in prudence but rather in the common good. In most countries the modal group of drinkers drink at rates far lower than would be safe for them as individuals.)

Abandoning Voluntary Campaigns

The NIAAA's answer to primary prevention has been a campaign labelled "responsible drinking." Its argument is that alcohol is here to stay and instead of stricter compulsory controls over the availability of alcohol, Americans need to learn (voluntarily) to drink responsibly where responsibility suggests avoiding intoxication.

The responsible-drinking campaign is yet another variant of a familiar tenet of American social policy; if people can be sufficiently apprised of the facts bearing on their own and society's welfare, they will voluntarily follow that standard—especially if the government devotes enough resources to training and education.

A fair alcohol control policy, however, would be rooted in an ethic that is not so sentimental and optimistic about human capabilities; it would stand opposed to the naive—if not cynical—practice of advocating that the majority or the most powerful voluntarily accept the burdens of painful collective action. Rather, such a policy would recognize that an effective control structure that justly distributes the burdens of prevention would meet with powerful opposition. Not the least of this resistance could be expected from the alcohol interests—a $27 billion industry with advertising expenditures exceeding $250 million.[40] Thus, it should go without saying that measures to achieve fairer controls over alcohol—public and private—would be compulsory and nonvoluntary.

While the policy outlined here will place great emphasis on primary prevention, treatment resources would not be neglected. We can never prevent all, or even most, alcohol problems. Despite the efforts of the NIAAA, treatment resources still are sadly underdeveloped. While the fears of the alcoholism-treatment industrial complex—that primary prevention would challenge their base of support—are understandable, the policy outlined here should make the social costs of alcohol more visible and therefore should help, not hinder, attempts to build public support for treatment programs.

Fair Shares: A New Approach to Alcohol Education

Although "a fair alcohol" policy would reject educational campaigns aiming to teach individuals "how to drink"—as if avoiding alcohol problems were a skill analogous to driving, education would play a vital role in such a policy.

Education is needed for two key purposes: first, to increase the visibility of alcohol problems and, especially, the collective or structural basis of these problems; and second, to promote public acceptance of the fairness of more effective control structures and a more equitable distribution of responsibility for prevention among all those who manufacture, import, distribute, advertise, market or consume alcoholic beverages.

Alcohol problems will be made automatically more visible and manifest to the entire society by focusing on the control of the substance itself rather than on the failures and hidden attributes of the minority who suffer problems. The frank focus on alcohol dictated by a fair alcohol policy, and the stress upon the need for controlling per capita or overall consumption, would in themselves begin to communicate the collective aspects of alcohol problems.

Problem visibility has been sorely lacking in the past, mainly because of the ideological biases of the "alcoholism paradigm." As it defines the situation, alcohol, drinking, the neighborhood bar, the cocktail hour, the dry martini—all of these are seen only as aspects of a widespread and legitimate social custom. But under the new policy outlined here—with its emphasis on controlling overall consumption—these aspects and instances of drinking are no longer taken as safe and innocent practices; they also refer to strong forces found everywhere in our society and contributing to ever-increasing levels of per capita consumption.

In fact, the prevailing definition of the problem of alcoholism has the explicit *political* function of restricting public attention and concern to the problem group. This helps in part to explain why alcohol problems—our most serious drug problems—have never reached the national agenda. This is in sharp contrast to other, lesser drug problems such as heroin and marijuana that receive massive political attention. Redefining alcoholism in terms of the availability of alcohol and the need for all persons to bear the burden of its restriction expands the issue. Such expansion would occur through the redirection of public attention from an exclusive focus on those suffering an illness, to the much broader and more general issue of equality and more just controls. This issue expansion is a precondition for moving alcohol problems to the public agenda, and necessary for the adoption and implementation of a new alcohol policy.[41]

This redefinition of alcohol problems will help achieve the second goal of education for alcohol, public acceptance of the principle of fair shares in the task of preventing alcohol problems. As long as the myth persists that alcohol problems result from the "failure" of a minority, public acceptance of the fairness of alcohol control policies that affect all drinkers and the industry will be frustrated.[42]

By placing alcohol at the center of policy, and by refusing to resort to "victim-blaming," we also will help remove some of the stigma implied in the current approach, which still locates the problem within the skin of the alcoholic. Although we label alcoholism a disease, we at the same time tacitly acknowledge that the vast majority of drinkers are able to use alcohol without problems. Thus, under the current paradigm the alcoholic is still stigmatized: the disease label indicates that the alcoholic cannot successfully perform a widely legitimate social practice.

Broad acceptance of the fairness of the alcohol control approach cannot be achieved without destroying the myth of alcoholism, and without greater public awareness of the connection between alcohol restriction and the possibility of enlarging the circle of those who are saved from alcohol damage, serious disability or early death. The [basis for] alcohol education would not be self-regard but regard for others and the necessity and justice of control mechanisms on all hazards of this world—including alcohol.

These control measures are likely to be represented, especially by the alcohol industry, as another instance of gross governmental interference with the private decisions of individual citizens. But the burdens imposed by these controls can just as easily be seen as acts of sharing, gifts of life, and as the distinguishing signs of a just community.

If public acceptance of these measures is to be won, the *limits* to a fair alcohol policy also must be clearly communicated. For example, the public must be reassured that an egalitarian public health ethic is strictly opposed to prohibitionism. Prohibitionism not only entails the risk of jeopardizing other primary goods, such as protection of basic political liberties; it also encourages the false supposition that the "alcohol issue" is our leading or only health or social problem.

If these measures are to be accepted, the public must be reassured that control mechanisms will stop short of coercive interference in the private and purely voluntary choices of citizens, since respect for the autonomy and dignity of individual persons is a cardinal tenet of equality and social justice.

As a brief aside, the control policy outlined here offers hope of bringing order and coherence to the present chaos surrounding our national drug policy. We have, on the one hand, harsh and punitive approaches to the control of some substances such as heroin and marijuana. On the other hand, we have relatively ineffective control mechanisms for alcohol and prescription drugs. Current policy seems to vacillate between complete laissez-faire—an enlightened liberal approach that mainly stresses humane treatment and ignores prevention—and harsh and coercive policies for the so-called "hard drugs."

The ethic outlined here suggests a more balanced approach. It maintains the need for control mechanisms and primary prevention, but it rejects labelling or stigmatizing those who suffer drug damage, not so much because they are "sick," as because drug-damaged people are the predictable consequence of the widespread availability of drugs. The policy here would also reject primary reliance on punitive or coercive mechanisms, although realism dictates the participation of law enforcement officials and the courts to restrict illicit drug traffic. Finally, a coherent drug policy stressing fairness and justice would offer a new and promising avenue for all of drug education—one that stresses the collective nature of these problems and the fairness and justice of reasonable collective burdens.

CONCLUSION

The purpose of this article has been to sketch the basis of an egalitarian public health ethic for the control of alcohol and to demonstrate that this policy would differ sharply from the current alcoholism policy paradigm.

The health ethic outlined here is the logical and ethical consequence of accepting the premise that society ought to accept reasonable and just rules to minimize the numbers of persons who suffer the harm of serious disability or premature death. Thus alcohol problems are not different from health problems such as injury or the distribution of medical care services. In the broadest sense, alcohol controls are simply part of the larger question of whether society will accept and implement fair policies to protect the public against *all* threats of disability and death, and whether the burdens of these policies will be fairly shared. How to move the American public to accept a strikingly different ethic for health and a new perspective on alcohol problems remains an important issue. This task, in a democratic society, must be educational and informational.

Initiating this redefinition process, including mobilizing support for the creation of public health strategies to reduce the rates of alcohol problems, can be seen as the primary task of all agencies—public and private—concerned with alcohol problems. I am not unaware of the tremendous resistance and skepticism that will greet any new attempt to restore controls as a cornerstone of our social policy concerning alcohol. Nonetheless, I see the most important challenge facing alcoholism authorities and the agencies involved as being that of convincing the public that this redefinition process is in order.

NOTES

1. My joining of the terms "market" and "justice" is not without controversy. One theory of the market holds that it is a blind hand that rewards without regard to merit or individual effort. For this point of view, see Milton Friedman, *Capitalism and Freedom: Constitution of Liberty* (Chicago: University of Chicago Press, 1962) and F. Hayek, *The Constitution of Liberty* (Chicago: University of Chicago Press, 1960). But Irving Kristol in "When Virtue Loses All Her Loveliness," *The Public Interest* 21 (Fall, 1970): 3–15, argues that this is a minority view, that most persons accept the marriage of the market ideal and the merits of individual effort and performance. I agree with Kristol; the dominant model of justice in America seems a merger of the notions of meritarian and market norms. See my "Public Health As Social Justice," *Inquiry* 13 (March 1976): 3–14.

2. J. Rawls, *A Theory of Justice* (Cambridge: Harvard University Press, 1971).

3. W. Ryan, *Blaming the Victim* (New York: Vintage Books, 1971).

4. M. Keller, "Alcoholism." *The Annals of the American Academy of Political and Social Science* 315 (January 1958): 1–11; S. Bacon, "Alcoholics Do Not Drink," *The Annals* 315 (January 1958): 55–64; T.F.A. Plaut, *Alcohol Problems: A Report to the Nation* (New York: Oxford University Press, 1967). For an interesting critique of the circularity involved in these explanations, see W.P. Rohan, "Drinking Behavior and 'Alcoholism'," *Journal of Studies on Alcohol* 36 (July 1975): 908–917.

5. United States Department of Health, Education, and Welfare, Alcohol, Drug Abuse and Mental Health Administration, *Second Special Report of the U.S. Congress on Alcohol and Health* (Washington, D.C.: Government Printing Office, 1974).

6. Ibid.

7. For an elaboration of the concept of "responsible drinking" see M. Chafetz, "The Prevention of Alcoholism," *International Journal of Psychiatry* 9 (1970–1971): 329–348. Chafetz was the first director of the National Institute on Alcohol Abuse and Alcoholism. He left that post in September 1975.

8. See my "Alcoholism as Blaming the Alcoholic," *International Journal of the Addictions* 11 (1976): 41–52, for a discussion of the alcoholism "paradigm" or "myth."

9. For some of the most pertinent evidence of the relationship between overall consumption and alcoholic cirrhosis—as well as evidence for the efficacy of alcohol controls—see: W. Schmidt and J. deLint, "Estimating the Prevalence of Alcoholism from Alcohol Consumption and Mortality Data," *Quarterly Journal of Studies on Alcohol* 31 (September 1970) 957–964; M. Terris, "Epidemiology of Cirrhosis of the Liver," *American Journal of Public Health* 58 (January 1958) 5–12; P.C. Whitehead, and C. Harvey, "Explaining Alcoholisms," *Journal of Health and Social Behavior 15 (March 1974) 57–65;* J. deLint, and W. Schmidt, "Consumption Averages and Alcoholism Prevalence," *British Journal of Addictions* 66 (September 1971) 97–107; K. Makela, "The Case of the Personnel Strike in the Stores of the Finnish Alcohol Monopoly." Paper presented at the 20th International Institute on the Prevention and Treatment of Alcoholism, Manchester, England, June 1974; and S. Ledermann, "Can One Reduce Alcoholism Without Changing Total Alcohol Consumption . . . ?" Proceedings of the 27th International Congress on Alcohol and Alcoholism, Frankfort-am Main, September 6–12, 1964.

10. See Beauchamp, "Alcoholism As Blaming the Alcoholic," and "The Alcohol Alibi: Blaming Alcoholics," *Society* 12 (Sept./Oct. 1975) 12–17.

11. The argument in this next section follows closely my earlier article "Public Health As Social Justice."

12. See R. Tawney, *Equality* (London: G. Allen and Unwin, 1964) and L.T. Hobhouse. *Liberalism* (New York: Oxford University Press, 1964). For the latest and most elegant statement, see Rawls.

13. The classic statement of utilitarianism is J.S. Mill. See M. Cohen, ed. *The Philosophy of John Stuart Mill* (New York: Modern Library, 1961).

14. Rawls.

15. *Ibid.*

16. For two good discussions relating the notion of social justice to health policy see: A.R. Jonsen, and A.E. Hellegers, "Conceptual Foundations for an Ethics of Medical Care," in *Ethics of Health Care,* ed: L.R. Tancredi (Washington, D.C.: National Academy of Sciences, 1974); and G. Outka, "Social Justice and Equal Access to Health Care," *The Journal of Religious Ethics* 2 (Spring, 1974) 11–32.

17. For example, see S. Smith, *The City That Was* (Metuchen, N.J.: Scarecrow Reprint Corporation, 1973); and C.-E.A. Winslow, *The Life of Hermann Biggs, Physician and Statesman of the Public Health* (Philadelphia: Lea and Febiger, 1929).

18. George Robsen in his *A History of Public Health* (New York: MD Publications, Inc., 1948) traces the mercantilist influences on public health. Audrey Robinson has traced the utilitarian influences on public health, "Government and Public Health," in *The*

Libertarian Alternative, ed: T.R. Machan (Chicago: Nelson Hall, 1974), pp. 275–288.

19. See M. Olson, *The Logic of Collective Action* (Cambridge: Harvard University Press, 1965) for an excellent discussion of the notion of public or collective goods.

20. A. Etzioni and R. Remp, "Technological 'Shortcuts' to Social Change," *Science* 175 (Jan. 7, 1972) 31–38.

21. V. Fuchs, *Who Shall Live?* (New York: Basic Books, 1974).

22. This fourth principle of public health is similar to John Rawl's "difference principle."

23. R. Brotman, and F. Suffet, "The Concept of Prevention and Its Limitations," *Annals* 417 (January 1975) 53–65.

24. The "escape of tigers" is the famous example used in Haddon's excellent discussion of the options for control of public health hazards. See W. Haddon, Jr., "Energy Damage and the Ten Countermeasure Strategies," *The Journal of Trauma* 13 (April 1973) 321–331; W. Haddon, Jr., "The Changing Approach to the Epidemiology, Prevention and Amelioration of Trauma," *American Journal of Public Health* 58 (August 1968) 1431–4138; and W. Haddon, Jr., "Exploring the Options," in *Research Directions Toward the Reduction of Injury,* U.S. Department of Health, Education and Welfare (Washington, D.C.: Government Printing Office, 1973), pp. 73–124, 38–59.

25. See R. Brown, *Explanations in Social Science* (Chicago: Aldine, 1963) for an excellent discussion of the limitations of dispositional explanations in social science.

26. M. Terris Haddon, "Breaking the Barriers to Prevention," Paper presented to the Annual Health Conference, New York Academy of Medicine, April 26, 1974.

27. Olson.

28. G. Hardin, "The Tragedy of the Commons," *Science* 162 (Dec. 13, 1968) 1243–1248.

29. R. Room, "Governing Images and the Prevention of Alcohol Problems," *Preventive Medicine* 3 (March 1974) 11–23. Room seems to see minimization in a cost-benefit or utilitarian context.

30. Some of these broad principles were first traced in my "Federal Alcohol Policy: Captive to an Industry and a Myth," *Christian Century* 92 (Sept. 13, 1975) 788–791.

31. For a different use of the term "minimization," see Room.

32. "Breaking the Barriers."

33. Etzioni and Remp.

34. Terris.

35. Again, the logic of this strategy is borne out by a growing body of scientific evidence suggesting that

control measures (both public and private) that limit the availability of alcohol and that encourage all people to use it minimally are the best guarantees against rising alcohol problems (see note nine).

Canadian researchers have found that in nearly every society where alcohol is widely used, the largest groups of drinkers use alcohol infrequently. Another and much smaller group uses it fairly frequently but still not heavily. Finally, there is a much smaller group that is exposed to damaging levels of alcohol. As the overall level of consumption of alcohol in a society goes up, the number of persons who drink infrequently decreases and the number of those who drink at moderate and "alcoholic" rates tends to increase. The overall pattern of alcohol in society suggests a gradual and smooth shift from the infrequent categories to moderate categories and finally to the heavier, damaging category (see J. deLint and S. Lederman).

The most plausible interpretation of these findings is that the general or per capita consumption of alcohol is an index of the adequacy of existing public and private controls over alcohol. These controls on the substance of alcohol, especially as they encourage high rates of minimal or infrequent exposure to alcohol, are the crucial policy variables that promote low rates of damaging exposure to alcohol.

36. "Anstie's limit: not more than 1½ ounces of absolute alcohol (approximately 3 oz. of whiskey, ½ bottle of wine, or 4 glasses of beer) taken only with meals or food, and with all hard liquor in well diluted form. This is the amount calculated by Francis Anstie (1862) that an adult man could drink daily without being adversely affected in general health," statement by Morris E. Chafetz, M.D., Seminar for Health Writers, The White House, Washington, D.C., July 10, 1974, cited in E. Edelstein, "Dr. Anstie's Magic Formula," *Addictions* 3 (September 1974): 10.

37. D. Cahalan, I.H. Cisin and H.M. Crossley, *American Drinking Practices* (New Brunswick, N.J.: Rutgers Center of Alcohol Studies, 1969).

38. *Second Special Report.*

39. See note nine.

40. These data are for 1973 and are taken from standard and Poor's *Industry Survey (Liquor)*, October 18, 1973 and *Leading National Advertisers' National Advertising Investments.*

41. For an excellent discussion of the notion of agenda-setting, see Roger W. Cobb, and Charles D. Elder, *Participation in American Politics: The Dynamics of Agenda Building* (Baltimore: The Johns Hopkins University Press, 1972).

42. Many will insist that limiting alcohol to reduce alcohol problems is either unfair because the majority has "succeeded" in using alcohol without problems, or is ineffective because there is not yet sufficient evidence that we can indeed reduce alcoholism by controlling the substance of alcohol. These two arguments usually are related, albeit in a subtle way. Many experts doubt the effectiveness of alcohol control measures because they still see alcoholism as a condition located primarily inside the skin of the alcoholic (usually expressed as an incapacity or inability to control the use of alcohol). However, there is a serious logical reason to question the whole notion of dividing the drinking population into two groups—those who have problems and those who do not—and then inferring that these two populations differ in terms of behavioral abilities and capacities. This amounts to *explaining* (rather than describing) the problem by the subtle process of converting structural data (rates of problems) into individual attributes that carry etiological significance. As I have argued elsewhere ("The Alcoholism Alibi" and "Alcoholism") what we are doing is committing a "category mistake" by discussing a class of phenomena (in this case alcohol problems) in the wrong idiom. Saying that all individuals who do not fall into a certain category have the ability to avoid falling into that category often leads to logical confusion. This would be like holding a marksmanship contest in which the winners all are those who do not hit the target. There is no criterion for establishing that all those who do not hit the target had to overcome some difficulty or hazard in order to perform this action. Abilities and skills are attributes assigned to tasks that are "hard" or "easy." For the most part, drinking relates to categories classified as "safe" and "unsafe." When we mix these two categories and start treating members of the safe group ("social drinkers") as if they had done something difficult the confusion is compounded.

4.3 PEOPLE V. CARMICHAEL
53 MISC. 2D 584, 279 N.Y.S. 2D
272 (CT. SPEC. SESS. 1967)

DECISION

RICHARD D. YUNKER, Justice of Peace

The defendant was charged with violation of Section 381 subd. 6 of the Vehicle and Traffic Law in that he operated a motorcycle without a protective helmet on February 15, 1967 in the Town of Oakfield, Genesee County, New York. The defendant appeared in court to answer the charge and raised the issue that the Subdivision of the Statute under which he was charged is unconstitutional.

Subdivision 6 of the Vehicle and Traffic Law Section 381, designated "Motorcycle Equipment" reads as follows:

"It shall be unlawful . . . for any person to operate or ride upon a motorcycle unless he wears a protective helmet of a type approved by the commissioner. . . ."

It is apparent that the purpose of this statute is the protection of the person who is required to wear the helmet.

* * *

Many requirements concerning equipment for vehicles that are used upon the highway are imposed by law. For instance, it is common knowledge that vehicles operated in the hours of darkness are required, not only by common sense, but also by law to have suitable head lights and tail lights. However, the requirement of the statute now challenged is unique in that so far as use of highways is involved it affects only the safety of the person who is required to wear the protective helmet. It is obvious that the requirement for head lights and tail lights will make the highways safer for other users of the highway. However, it cannot be argued that the motorcyclist who does not wear a protective helmet has any different effect upon the safety of other users of the highway than a motorcyclist who does wear a helmet.

The question then is whether the state can by such a statute require a motorcyclist to wear a protective helmet for the purpose of protecting himself from injury. Two issues can be distinguished. One issue is whether this particular statute . . . is definite enough to sustain a criminal conviction. The other issue is whether the government has power to require a motorcycle operator or any other person to wear a protective helmet to protect himself. . . . This other issue would be presented by any statute requiring all persons to wear protective helmets and seatbelts while operating a motor vehicle or by a statute requiring all persons to refrain from smoking.

* * *

It is the opinion of this court that [the statute at issue] as applied to operator of a motorcycle, is too indefinite to sustain a criminal conviction.

The second issue must now be considered, that is, whether the state has the authority even by a statute definite in its terms to require a motorcycle operator to wear a protective helmet.

Our government is a government of limited powers. Our Federal Government has all the powers given to it in the Federal Constitution. All the other powers are reserved to the states and to the people. Our state government has all the power commonly referred to as police power, which can be defined as the power to make the necessary laws to maintain public order, public health, public safety, public morals and public welfare. There are many reported cases illustrating the extent of the police power. To the knowledge of this court there is no reported case which will fit closely the facts of the case at bar.

There are many definitions of the police power. All of the definitions, when properly understood, involve the principle of regulating the conduct of one person so that another person will not be unreasonably endangered or restricted in the use and enjoyment of public and private property; the regulation of the conduct of one person is justified because of the effect of that conduct on other persons. In the case of the Vehicle and Traffic Laws, the police power authorizes statutes that tend to make the highways safer or more useful to the general public. It can be argued that the statute here questioned affects public welfare because if a person suffers injury that could have been avoided by wearing a protective helmet, that person will perhaps become a public charge because of a disabling injury and that those who have been dependent upon that person for support may also become a public charge. The possibility and even likelihood of this happening cannot be denied. If a statute required every person to refrain from smoking there could be no serious argument that many persons would be spared crippling illnesses that cause premature disability and death. If a statute required every person to retire to bed by 10:00 p.m. every evening, it would probably benefit the general health of many citizens. A court cannot say as a matter of law that there is no public benefit from a statute requiring motorcyclists to wear a protective helmet, or a statute requiring all persons to refrain from smoking, or a statute requiring all persons to retire to bed by 10:00 p.m. every evening.

To state this argument and concede that it has weight does not decide the issue. If the fact that this argument has validity were taken to decide a question such as presented by this case, then it would justify almost any rule imposed by the legislature, for our society is so complex today that there are very few things that cannot be said to affect some other person or the public treasury. If this argument were to decide questions such as presented by this case, then the hypothetical statute requiring people to go to bed early would be valid. But such an argument does not decide the question but merely poses one factor to be considered with other factors.

The statute challenged in this case has the direct effect of protecting the physical well being of the person who is subject to the mandate of the statute, and the indirect effect of protecting other persons from the burdens that might result from the death or disability of the person subject to the mandate; the direct effect is to safeguard the motorcyclist and the indirect effect the prevention of the motorcyclist and his dependents from becoming public charges.

As the police power is understood by the court, it justifies the regulation of the conduct of one person because of the effect of that conduct upon other persons. Therefore, the police power does not justify the statute on the basis of the direct effect alone. Is the indirect effect such that the police power authorizes the statute?

In the opinion of the court it is not. The police power traditionally has not included the power to make a citizen protect his own physical well being. To hold that a citizen may be required to protect his health alone would be an enlargement of the police power beyond traditional limits; it would introduce a novel basis for government power, a new principle upon which to authorize the regulation of the lives of the citizens in a manner and to an extent hitherto unknown. As our society has grown more complex, governmental regulation has necessarily become more complex and complete. Yet for all the extent to which the conduct of citizens has been subject to regulation, there has been no regulation for the sole purpose of making the citizen protect his own physical well being so that others may benefit from it. There are statutes that regulate a citizen in matters that affect his own health. For example, the citizen is restricted in the use of alcohol and narcotics. However it must be noted such restriction is not the exercise of the police power to make a citizen maintain himself in a state of physical and mental well being so that other persons may not be deprived of sharing in the fruits of his good health; it is the exercise of the police power to protect other persons from the harmful conduct of citizens whose behavior toward others is affected by the use of alcohol or narcotics.

It is the holding of this court that [the statute at issue], which requires the operator of a motorcycle to wear a protective helmet, is unconstitutional as applied to this defendant because it is not sufficiently definite to sustain a criminal conviction, and because the police power does not authorize statutes requiring a citizen to protect his own physical well-being.

The charge is dismissed.

The decision in the *Carmichael* case was reversed on appeal, 56 Misc. 2d 388, 288 N.Y.S. 2d 931 (Genesee County Ct. 1968). See also Penny v. City of North Little Rock, 248 Ark. 1158, 1160, 455 S.W.2d 132, 133 (1970). In upholding a similar Arkansas helmet requirement statute the court had this to say:

The appellant [party bringing the appeal] contends that the Act involved is unconstitutional "in that it is beyond the police power of the legislature. The Act was passed for protection of the rider himself and not the general public." The appellant insists that the Act is unconstitutional and urges us in so holding, to adopt the view of the Michigan, Ohio, New York and Louisiana courts as announced in the following cases: By Michigan in American Motorcycle Association v. Davids, 11 Mich. App. 351, 158 N.W.2d 72; by Ohio in State v. Betts, Ohio Mun. Ct., 252 N.E.2d 866; by New York in People v. Carmichael, 53 Misc. 2d 584, 279 N.Y.S.2d 272; and by the Court of Appeals of Louisiana as announced in Everhardt v. City of New Orleans, 208 So. 2d 423.

We are of the opinion that the better reasoning favors the courts who have held similar statutes constitutional and we feel more comfortable aligned with the final decision of the New York court in People v. Carmichael, as announced in 56 Misc. 2d 388, 288 N.Y.S.2d 931, and the final Louisiana Supreme Court decision in Everhardt v. City of New Orleans, as announced in 253 La. 285, 217 So.2d 400. In reversing the Special Sessions Court in Carmichael, the Genessee County Court in 288 N.Y.S. 2d 931, said:

". . . While concededly the instant legislation may infringe on the rights of the individual, it is equally apparent that such is incidental to a valid exercise of the police power and is not unreasonable. . . . The use of protective helmets is an accepted and widely used safety device in our society. A standard by its nature may be a general one and nonetheless valid if it is capable of reasonable application under the circumstances."

ISSUES FOR CONSIDERATION AND SUGGESTIONS FOR FURTHER READING

Contrast the concept of an "egalitarian public health ethic for the control of alcohol" postulated by Beauchamp with the attitude toward protective legislation reflected by the trial court judge who, in People v. Carmichael, dismissed a criminal charge against a person accused of operating a motorcycle without a helmet because he found the statute upon which the charge was based to be unconstitutional.

You may wish to compare the motorcycle helmet regulations considered in the foregoing cases with a Puerto Rican law requiring automobile safety belts, P.R. Laws Ann. tit. 9 §§1211–1214. §1212 requires "[a]ny person who drives or rides [on a public street in a car equipped with seat belts] to fasten [the] belt around his body." Violations are punishable by a fine. Is a criminal sanction an appropriate enforcement mechanism for laws designed to protect individual's health and safety? For a more extensive discussion of helmet laws, you should consult "Validity of Traffic Regulations Requiring Motorcyclists to Wear Protective Headgear," Annot., 32 A.L.R.3d 1270 (1970).

The question of therapeutic intervention on a large scale is raised by the fluoridation of public water supplies. See Annot., 43 *A.L.R.* 2d 453 (1955).

For an example of regulations on smoking you may wish to examine the rules of the Civil Aeronautics Board (CAB) on the provision of designated No Smoking areas aboard aircraft, operated by certificated air carriers, 44 *Fed. Reg.* 5071 (1979) (14 C.F.R. §252). The conclusions of the CAB with respect to health considerations supporting the rules should be of particular interest.

There are a variety of conditions that, like the crazy behavior of which Morse writes, are affected by the definitions that the law affixes to them and the technique of accommodation that is frequently prescribed by the law. You may wish to read portions of the symposium on Mentally Retarded People and the Law in 31 *Stanford Law Review* 541 (1979), which discusses an area of emerging legal significance.

For a historically oriented introduction to mental health, you may wish to consult H. Foley, *Community Mental Health Legislation: The Formative Process* (1975).

CHAPTER 5

THE ROLE OF LAW IN SHAPING AND REFLECTING ETHICAL CONCERNS: EUTHANASIA

OVERVIEW

This chapter takes up the way in which law and ethics interact in an area of high significance, the question of life and death. Two leading cases presented here, *In re Quinlan* and *Saikewicz,* consider the question of the propriety of withholding life-sustaining procedures from seriously ill patients who are unable to participate in the medical decisions affecting them.

The article by Kaplan presents a statutory approach to the matter of euthanasia. Mueller and Phoenix treat the euthanasia problem in relation to defective newborns.

5.1 *In re* Quinlan
70 N.J. 10, 355 A. 2d 647 (1976)

C. J. HUGHES

THE LITIGATION

The central figure in this tragic case is Karen Ann Quinlan, a New Jersey resident. At the age of 22, she lies in a debilitated and allegedly moribund state at Saint Clare's Hospital in Denville, New Jersey. The litigation has to do, in final analysis, with her life,—its continuance or cessation,—and the responsibilities, rights and duties, with regard to any fateful decision concerning it, of her family, her guardian, her doctors, the hospital, the State through its law enforcement authorities, and finally the courts of justice.

The issues are before this Court following its direct certification of the action under the rule, R. 2:12–1, prior to hearing in the Superior Court, Appellate Division, to which the appellant (hereafter "plaintiff") Joseph Quinlan, Karen's father, had appealed the adverse judgment of the Chancery Division.

Due to extensive physical damage fully described in the able opinion of the trial judge, Judge Muir, supporting that judgment, Karen allegedly was incompetent. Joseph Quinlan sought the adjudication of that incompetency. He wished to be appointed guardian of the person and property of his daughter. It was proposed by him that such letters of guardianship, if granted, should contain an express power to him as guardian to authorize the discontinuance of all extraordinary medical procedures now allegedly sustaining Karen's vital processes and hence her life, since these measures, he asserted, present no hope of her eventual recovery. A guardian *ad litem* was appointed by Judge Muir to represent the interest of the alleged incompetent.

By a supplemental complaint, in view of the extraordinary nature of the relief sought by plaintiff and the involvement therein of their several rights and responsibilities, other parties were added. These included the treating physicians and the hospital, the relief sought being that they be restrained from interfering with the carrying out of any such extraordinary authorization in the event it were to be granted by the court. Joined, as well, was the Prosecutor of Morris County (he being charged with responsibility for enforcement of the criminal law), to enjoin him from interfering with, or projecting a criminal prosecution which otherwise might ensue in the event of, cessation of life in Karen resulting from the exercise of such extraordinary authorization were it to be granted to the guardian.

The Attorney General of New Jersey intervened as of right pursuant to R. 4:33–1 on behalf of the State of New Jersey, such intervention being recognized by the court in the pretrial conference order (R. 4:25–1 *et seq.*) of September 22, 1975. Its basis, of course, was the interest of the State in the preservation of life, which has an undoubted constitutional foundation.[1]

The matter is of transcendent importance, involving questions related to the definition and existence of death, the prolongation of life through artificial means developed by medical technology undreamed of in past generations of the practice of the healing arts;[2] the impact of such durationally indeterminate and artificial life prolongation on the rights of the incompetent, her family and society in general; the bearing of constitutional right and the scope of judicial responsibility, as to the appropriate response of an equity court of justice to the extraordinary prayer for relief of the plaintiff. Involved as well is the right of the plaintiff, Joseph Quinlan, to guardianship of the person of his daughter.

Among his "factual and legal contentions" under such Pretrial Order was the following:

I. Legal and Medical Death
   (a) Under the existing legal and medical definitions of death recognized by the State of New Jersey, Karen Ann Quinlan is dead.

This contention, made in the context of Karen's profound and allegedly irreversible coma and physical debility, was discarded during trial by the following stipulated amendment to the Pretrial Order:

Under any legal standard recognized by the State of New Jersey and also under standard medical practice, Karen Ann Quinlan is presently alive.

Other amendments to the Pretrial Order made at the time of trial expanded the issues before the court. The Prosecutor of Morris County sought a declaratory judgment as to the effect any affirmation by the court of a right in a guardian to terminate life-sustaining procedures would have with regard to enforcement of the criminal laws of New Jersey with reference to homicide. Saint Clare's Hospital, in the face of trial testimony on the subject of "brain death," sought declaratory judgment as to:

Whether the use of the criteria developed and enunciated by the Ad Hoc Committee of the Harvard Medical School on or about August 5, 1968, as well as similar criteria, by a physician to assist in determination of the death of a patient whose cardiopulmonary functions are being artificially sustained, is in accordance with ordinary and standard medical practice.[3]

It was further stipulated during trial that Karen was indeed incompetent and guardianship was necessary, although there exists a dispute as to the determination later reached by the court that such guardianship should be bifurcated, and that Mr. Quinlan should be appointed as guardian of the trivial property but not the person of his daughter.

After certification the Attorney General filed as of right (R. 2:3–4) a cross-appeal[3.1] challenging the action of the trial court in admitting evidence of prior statements made by Karen while competent as to her distaste for continuance of life by extraordinary medical procedures, under circumstances not unlike those of the present case. These quoted statements were made in the context of several conversations with regard to others terminally ill and being subjected to like heroic measures. The statements were advanced as evidence of what she would want done in such a contingency as now exists. She was said to have firmly evinced her wish, in like circumstances, not to have her life prolonged by the otherwise futile use of extraordinary means. Because we agree with the conception of the trial court that such statements, since they were remote and impersonal, lacked significant probative weight, it is not of consequence to our opinion that we decide whether or not they were admissible hearsay. Again, after certification, the guardian of the person of the incompetent (who had been appointed as a part of the judgment appealed from) resigned and was succeeded by another, but that too seems irrelevant to decision. It is, however, of interest to note the trial court's delineation (in its supplemental opinion of November 12, 1975) of the extent of the personal guardian's authority with respect to medical care of his ward:

Mr. Coburn's appointment is designed to deal with those instances wherein Dr. Morse,[4] in the process of administering care and treatment to Karen Quinlan, feels there should be concurrence on the extent or nature of the care or treatment. If Mr. and Mrs. Quinlan are unable to give concurrence, then Mr. Coburn will be consulted for his concurrence.

Essentially then, appealing to the power of equity, and relying on claimed constitutional rights of free exercise of religion, of privacy and of protection against cruel and unusual punishment, Karen Quinlan's father sought judicial authority to withdraw the life-sustaining mechanisms temporarily preserving his daughter's life, and his appointment as guardian of her person to that end. His request was opposed by her doctors, the hospital, the Morris County Prosecutor, the State of New Jersey, and her guardian *ad litem*.

THE FACTUAL BASE

An understanding of the issues in their basic perspective suggests a brief review of the factual base developed in the testimony and documented in greater detail in the opinion of the trial judge. *In re Quinlan*, 137 N.J.Super. 227, 348 A.2d 801 (Ch.Div.1975).

On the night of April 15, 1975, for reasons still unclear, Karen Quinlan ceased breathing for at least two 15 minute periods. She received some ineffectual mouth-to-mouth resuscitation from friends. She was taken by ambulance to Newton Memorial Hospital. There she had a temperature of 100 degrees, her pupils were unreactive and she was unresponsive even to deep pain. The history at the time of her admission to that hospital was essentially incomplete and uninformative.

Three days later, Dr. Morse examined Karen at the request of the Newton admitting physician, Dr. McGee. He found her comatose with evidence of decortication, a condition relating to derangement of the cortex of the brain causing a physical posture in which the upper extremities are flexed and the lower extremities are extended. She required a respirator to assist her breathing. Dr. Morse was unable to obtain an adequate account of the circumstances and events leading up to Karen's admission to the Newton Hospital. Such initial history or etiology is crucial in neurological diagnosis. Relying as he did upon the Newton Memorial records and his own examination, he concluded that prolonged lack of oxygen in the bloodstream, anoxia, was identified with her condition as he saw it upon first observation. When she was later transferred to Saint Clare's Hospital she was still unconscious, still on a respirator and a tracheotomy had been performed. On her arrival Dr. Morse conducted extensive and detailed examinations. An electroencephalogram (EEG) measuring electrical rhythm of the brain was performed and Dr. Morse characterized the result as "abnormal

but it showed some activity and was consistent with her clinical state." Other significant neurological tests, including a brain scan, an angiogram, and a lumbar puncture were normal in result. Dr. Morse testified that Karen has been in a state of coma, lack of consciousness, since he began treating her. He explained that there are basically two types of coma, sleep-like unresponsiveness and awake unresponsiveness. Karen was originally in a sleep-like unresponsive condition but soon developed "sleep-wake" cycles, apparently a normal improvement for comatose patients occurring within three to four weeks. In the awake cycle she blinks, cries out and does things of that sort but is still totally unaware of anyone or anything around her.

Dr. Morse and other expert physicians who examined her characterized Karen as being in a "chronic persistent vegetative state." Dr. Fred Plum, one of such expert witnesses, defined this as a "subject who remains with the capacity to maintain the vegetative parts of neurological function but who * * * no longer has any cognitive function."

Dr. Morse, as well as the several other medical and neurological experts who testified in this case, believed with certainty that Karen Quinlan is not "brain dead." They identified the Ad Hoc Committee of Harvard Medical School report (*infra*) as the ordinary medical standard for determining brain death, and all of them were satisfied that Karen met none of the criteria specified in that report and was therefore not "brain dead" within its contemplation.

In this respect it was indicated by Dr. Plum that the brain works in essentially two ways, the vegetative and the sapient. He testified:

We have an internal vegetative regulation which controls body temperature, which controls breathing, which controls to a considerable degree blood pressure, which controls to some degree heart rate, which controls chewing, swallowing, and which controls sleeping and waking. We have a more highly developed brain which is uniquely human which controls our relation to the outside world, our capacity to talk, to see, to feel, to sing, to think. Brain death necessarily must mean the death of both of these functions of the brain, vegetative and the sapient. Therefore, the presence of any function which is regulated or governed or controlled by the deeper parts of the brain which in laymen's terms might be considered purely vegetative would mean that the brain is not biologically dead.

Because Karen's neurological condition affects her respiratory ability (the respiratory system being a brain stem function) she requires a respirator to assist her breathing. From the time of her admission to Saint Clare's Hospital Karen has been assisted by an MA–1 respirator, a sophisticated machine which delivers a given volume of air at a certain rate and periodically provides a "sigh" volume, a relatively large measured volume of air designed to purge the lungs of excretions. Attempts to "wean" her from the respirator were unsuccessful and have been abandoned.

The experts believe that Karen cannot now survive without the assistance of the respirator; that exactly how long she would live without it is unknown; that the strong likelihood is that death would follow soon after its removal, and that removal would also risk further brain damage and would curtail the assistance the respirator presently provides in warding off infection.

It seemed to be the consensus not only of the treating physicians but also of the several qualified experts who testified in the case, that removal from the respirator would not conform to medical practices, standards and traditions.

The further medical consensus was that Karen in addition to being comatose is in a chronic and persistent "vegetative" state, having no awareness of anything or anyone around her and existing at a primitive reflex level. Although she does have some brain stem function (ineffective for respiration) and has other reactions one normally associates with being alive, such as moving, reacting to light, sound and noxious stimuli, blinking her eyes, and the like, the quality of her feeling impulses is unknown. She grimaces, makes stereotyped cries and sounds and has chewing motions. Her blood pressure is normal.

Karen remains in the intensive care unit at Saint Clare's Hospital, receiving 24-hour care by a team of four nurses characterized, as was the medical attention, as "excellent." She is nourished by feeding by way of a nasal-gastro tube and is routinely examined for infection, which under these circumstances is a serious life threat. The result is that her condition is considered remarkable under the unhappy circumstances involved.

Karen is described as emaciated, having suffered a weight loss of at least 40 pounds, and undergoing a continuing deteriorative process. Her posture is described as fetal-like and grotesque; there is extreme flexion-rigidity of the arms, legs and related muscles and her joints are severely rigid and deformed.

From all of this evidence, and including the whole testimonial record, several basic findings in the physical area are mandated. Severe brain and associated damage, albeit of uncertain etiology, has left Karen in a chronic and persistent vegetative state. No form of treatment which can cure or improve that condition is known or available. As nearly as may be determined, considering the guarded area of remote uncertainties characteristic of most medical science predictions, she can *never* be restored to cognitive or sapient life. Even with regard to the vegetative level and improvement therein (if such it may be called) the prognosis is extremely poor and the extent unknown if it should in fact occur.

She is debilitated and moribund and although fairly stable at the time of argument before us (no new information having been filed in the meanwhile in expansion of the record), no physician risked the opinion that she could live more than a year and indeed she may die much earlier. Excellent medical and nursing care so far has been able to ward off the constant threat of infection, to which she is peculiarly susceptible because of the respirator, the tracheal tube and other incidents of care in her vulnerable condition. Her life accordingly is sustained by the respirator and tubal feeding, and removal from the respirator would cause her death soon, although the time cannot be stated with more precision.

The determination of the fact and time of death in past years of medical science was keyed to the action of the heart and blood circulation, in turn dependent upon pulmonary activity, and hence cessation of these functions spelled out the reality of death.[5]

Developments in medical technology have obfuscated the use of the traditional definition of death. Efforts have been made to define irreversible coma as a new criterion for death, such as by the 1968 report of the Ad Hoc Committee of the Harvard Medical School (the Committee comprising ten physicians, an historian, a lawyer and a theologian), which asserted that:

From ancient times down to the recent past it was clear that, when the respiration and heart stopped, the brain would die in a few minutes; so the obvious criterion of no heart beat as synonymous with death was sufficiently accurate. In those times the heart was considered to be the central organ of the body; it is not surprising that its failure marked the onset of death. This is no longer valid when modern resuscitative and supportive measures are used. These improved activities can now restore "life" as judged by the ancient standards of persistent respiration and continuing heart beat. This can be the case even when there is not the remotest possibility of an individual recovering consciousness following massive brain damage. ["A Definition of Irreversible Coma," 205 J.A. M.A. 337, 339 (1968)].

The Ad Hoc standards, carefully delineated, included absence of response to pain or other stimuli, pupilary reflexes, corneal, pharyngeal and other reflexes, blood pressure, spontaneous respiration, as well as "flat" or isoelectric electroencephalograms and the like, with all tests repeated "at least 24 hours later with no change." In such circumstances, where all of such criteria have been met as showing "brain death," the Committee recommends with regard to the respirator:

The patient's condition can be determined only by a physician. When the patient is hopelessly damaged as defined above, the family and all colleagues who have participated in major decisions concerning the patient, and all nurses involved, should be so informed. Death is to be declared and *then* the respirator turned off. The decision to do this and the responsibility for it are to be taken by the physician-in-charge, in consultation with one or more physicians who have been directly involved in the case. It is unsound and undesirable to force the family to make the decision. [205 J.A. M.A., *supra* at 338 (emphasis in original)].

But, as indicated, it was the consensus of medical testimony in the instant case that Karen, for all her disability, met none of these criteria, nor indeed any comparable criteria extant in the medical world and representing, as does the Ad Hoc Committee report, according to the testimony in this case, prevailing and accepted medical standards.

We have adverted to the "brain death" concept and Karen's disassociation with any of its criteria, to emphasize the basis of the medical decision made by Dr. Morse. When plaintiff and his family, finally reconciled to the certainty of Karen's impending death, requested the withdrawal of life support mechanisms, he demurred. His refusal was based upon his conception of medical standards, practice and ethics described in the medical testimony, such as in the evidence given by another neurologist, Dr. Sidney Diamond, a witness for the State. Dr. Diamond asserted that no physician would have failed to provide respirator support at the outset, and none would interrupt its life-saving course thereafter, except in the case of cerebral death. In the latter case, he thought the respirator would in effect be disconnected from one already dead, entitling the physician under medical standards and, he thought, legal concepts, to terminate the supportive measures. We note Dr. Diamond's distinction of major surgical or transfusion procedures in a terminal case not involving cerebral death, such as here:

The subject has lost human qualities. It would be incredible, and I think unlikely, that any physician would respond to a sudden hemorrhage, massive hemorrhage or a loss of all her defensive blood cells, by giving her large quantities of blood. I think that * * * major surgical procedures would be out of the question even if they were known to be essential for continued physical existence.

This distinction is adverted to also in the testimony of Dr. Julius Korein, a neurologist called by plaintiff. Dr. Korein described a medical practice concept of "judicious neglect" under which the physician will say:

Don't treat this patient anymore, * * * it does not serve either the patient, the family, or society in any meaningful way to continue treatment with this patient.

Dr. Korein also told of the unwritten and unspoken standard of medical practice implied in the foreboding initials DNR (do not resuscitate), as applied to the extraordinary terminal case:

> Cancer, metastatic cancer, involving the lungs, the liver, the brain, multiple involvements, the physician may or may not write: Do not resuscitate. * * * [I]t could be said to the nurse: if this man stops breathing don't resuscitate him. * * * No physician that I know personally is going to try and resuscitate a man riddled with cancer and in agony and he stops breathing. They are not going to put him on a respirator. * * * I think that would be the height of misuse of technology.

While the thread of logic in such distinctions may be elusive to the non-medical lay mind, in relation to the supposed imperative to sustain life at all costs, they nevertheless relate to medical decisions, such as the decision of Dr. Morse in the present case. We agree with the trial court that that decision was in accord with Dr. Morse's conception of medical standards and practice.

We turn to that branch of the factual case pertaining to the application for guardianship, as distinguished from the nature of the authorization sought by the applicant. The character and general suitability of Joseph Quinlan as guardian for his daughter, in ordinary circumstances, could not be doubted. The record bespeaks the high degree of familial love which pervaded the home of Joseph Quinlan and reached out fully to embrace Karen, although she was living elsewhere at the time of her collapse. The proofs showed him to be deeply religious, imbued with a morality so sensitive that months of tortured indecision preceded his belated conclusion (despite earlier moral judgments reached by the other family members, but unexpressed to him in order not to influence him) to seek the termination of life-supportive measures sustaining Karen. A communicant of the Roman Catholic Church, as were other family members, he first sought solace in private prayer looking with confidence, as he says, to the Creator, first for the recovery of Karen and then, if that were not possible, for guidance with respect to the awesome decision confronting him.

[1] To confirm the moral rightness of the decision he was about to make he consulted with his parish priest and later with the Catholic chaplain of Saint Clare's Hospital. He would not, he testified, have sought termination if that act were to be morally wrong or in conflict with the tenets of the religion he so profoundly respects. He was disabused of doubt, however, when the position of the Roman Catholic Church was made known to him as it is reflected in the record in this case. While it is not usual for matters of religious dogma or concepts to enter a civil litigation (except as they may bear upon constitutional right, or sometimes, familial matters; cf. In re Adoption of E, 59 N.J. 36, 279 A.2d 785 (1971)), they were rightly admitted in evidence here. The judge was bound to measure the character and motivations in all respects of Joseph Quinlan as prospective guardian; and insofar as these religious matters bore upon them, they were properly scrutinized and considered by the court.

Thus germane, we note the position of that Church as illuminated by the record before us. We have no reason to believe that it would be at all discordant with the whole of Judeo-Christian tradition, considering its central respect and reverence for the sanctity of human life. It was in this sense of relevance that we admitted as amicus curiae the New Jersey Catholic Conference, essentially the spokesman for the various Catholic bishops of New Jersey, organized to give witness to spiritual values in public affairs in the statewide community. The position statement of Bishop Lawrence B. Casey, reproduced in the amicus brief, projects these views:

(a) The verification of the fact of death in a particular case cannot be deduced from any religious or moral principle and, under this aspect, does not fall within the competence of the church;—that dependence must be had upon traditional and medical standards, and by these standards Karen Ann Quinlan is assumed to be alive.

(b) The request of plaintiff for authority to terminate a medical procedure characterized as "an extraordinary means of treatment" would not involve euthanasia. This upon the reasoning expressed by Pope Pius XII in his "allocutio" (address) to anesthesiologists on November 24, 1957, when he dealt with the question:

Does the anesthesiologist have the right or is he bound, in all cases of deep unconsciousness, even in those that are completely hopeless in the opinion of the competent doctor, to use modern artificial respiration apparatus, even against the will of the family?

His answer made the following points:

1. In ordinary cases the doctor has the right to act in this manner, but is not bound to do so unless this is the only way of fulfilling another certain moral duty.
2. The doctor, however, has no right independent of the patient. He can act only if the patient explicitly or implicitly, directly or indirectly gives him the permission.
3. The treatment as described in the question constitutes extraordinary means of preserving life and so there is no obligation to use them nor to give the doctor permission to use them.
4. The rights and the duties of the family depend on the presumed will of the unconscious patient if he or she is of legal age, and the family, too, is bound to use only ordinary means.
5. This case is not to be considered euthanasia in any way; that would never be licit. The interruption of attempts at resuscitation, even when it causes the arrest of circulation, is not more than an indirect cause of the cessation of life, and we must apply in this case the principle of double effect.

So it was that the Bishop Casey statement validated the decision of Joseph Quinlan:

Competent medical testimony has established that Karen Ann Quinlan has no reasonable hope of recovery from her comatose state by the use of any available medical procedures. The continuance of mechanical (cardiorespiratory) supportive measures to sustain continuation of her body functions and her life constitute extraordinary means of treatment. *Therefore,*

*the decision of Joseph * * * Quinlan to request the discontinuance of this treatment is, according to the teachings of the Catholic Church, a morally correct decision.* (emphasis in original)

And the mind and purpose of the intending guardian were undoubtedly influenced by factors included in the following reference to the interrelationship of the three disciplines of theology, law and medicine as exposed in the Casey statement:

The right to a natural death is one outstanding area in which the disciplines of theology, medicine and law overlap; or, to put it another way, it is an area in which these three disciplines convene.

Medicine with its combination of advanced technology and professional ethics is both able and inclined to prolong biological life. Law with its felt obligation to protect the life and freedom of the individual seeks to assure each person's right to live out his human life until its natural and inevitable conclusion. Theology with its acknowledgment of man's dissatisfaction with biological life as the ultimate source of joy * * * defends the sacredness of human life and defends it from all direct attacks.

These disciplines do not conflict with one another, but are necessarily conjoined in the application of their principles in a particular instance such as that of Karen Ann Quinlan. Each must in some way acknowledge the other without denying its own competence. The civil law is not expected to assert a belief in eternal life; nor, on the other hand, is it expected to ignore the right of the individual to profess it, and to form and pursue his conscience in accord with that belief. Medical science is not authorized to directly cause natural death; nor, however, is it expected to prevent it when it is inevitable and all hope of a return to an even partial exercise of human life is irreparably lost. Religion is not expected to define biological death; nor, on its part, is it expected to relinquish its responsibility to assist man in the formation and pursuit of a correct conscience as to the acceptance of natural death when science has confirmed its inevitability beyond any hope other than that of preserving biological life in a merely vegetative state.

And the gap in the law is aptly described in the Bishop Casey statement:

In the present public discussion of the case of Karen Ann Quinlan it has been brought out that responsible people involved in medical care, patients and families have exercised the freedom to terminate or withhold certain treatments as extraordinary means in cases judged to be terminal, i. e., cases which hold no realistic hope for some recovery, in accord with the expressed or implied intentions of the patients themselves. To whatever extent this has been happening it has been without sanction in civil law. Those involved in such actions, however, have ethical and theological literature to guide them in their judgments and actions. Furthermore, such actions have not in themselves undermined society's reverence for the lives of sick and dying people.

It is both possible and necessary for society to have laws and ethical standards which provide freedom for decisions, in accord with the expressed or implied intentions of the patient, to terminate or withhold extraordinary treatment in cases which are judged to be hopeless by competent medical authorities, without at the same time leaving an opening for euthanasia. Indeed, to accomplish this, it may simply be required that courts and legislative bodies recognize the present standards and practices of many people engaged in medical care who have been doing what the parents of Karen Ann Quinlan are requesting authorization to have done for their beloved daughter.

Before turning to the legal and constitutional issues involved, we feel it essential to reiterate that the "Catholic view" of religious neutrality in the circumstances of this case is considered by the Court only in the aspect of its impact upon the conscience, motivation and purpose of the intending guardian, Joseph Quinlan, and not as a precedent in terms of the civil law. If Joseph Quinlan, for instance, were a follower and strongly influenced by the teachings of Buddha, or if, as an agnostic or atheist, his moral judgments were formed without reference to religious feelings, but were nevertheless formed and viable, we would with equal attention and high respect consider these elements, as bearing upon his character, motivations and purposes as relevant to his qualification and suitability as guardian.

It is from this factual base that the Court confronts and responds to three basic issues:

1. Was the trial court correct in denying the specific relief requested by plaintiff, i. e., authorization for termination of the life-supporting apparatus, on the case presented to him? Our determination on that question is in the affirmative.
2. Was the court correct in withholding letters of guardianship from the plaintiff and appointing in his stead a stranger? On that issue our determination is in the negative.
3. Should this Court, in the light of the foregoing conclusions, grant declaratory relief to the plaintiff? On that question our Court's determination is in the affirmative.

This brings us to a consideration of the constitutional and legal issues underlying the foregoing determinations.

CONSTITUTIONAL AND LEGAL ISSUES

At the outset we note the dual role in which plaintiff comes before the Court. He not only raises, derivatively, what he perceives to be the constitutional and legal rights of his daughter Karen, but he also claims certain rights independently as parent.

[2, 3] Although generally litigant may assert only his own constitutional rights, we have no doubt that plaintiff has sufficient standing to advance both positions.

[4, 5] While no express constitutional language limits judicial activity to cases and controversies, New Jersey courts will not render advisory opinions or entertain proceedings by plaintiffs who do not have sufficient legal standing to maintain their actions. *Walker v. Stanhope*, 23 N.J. 657, 660, 130 A.2d 372 (1957). However, as in this case, New Jersey courts commonly grant declaratory relief. Declaratory Judgments Act, N.J.S.A. 2A:16–50 *et seq.* And

our courts hold that where the plaintiff is not simply an interloper and the proceeding serves the public interest, standing will be found. *Walker v. Stanhope, supra,* 23 N.J. at 661–66, 130 A.2d 372; *Koons v. Atlantic City Bd. of Comm'rs,* 134 N.J.L. 329, 338–39, 47 A.2d 589 (Sup.Ct.1946), *aff'd,* 135 N.J.L. 204, 50 A.2d 869 (E. & A. 1947). In *Crescent Park Tenants Ass'n v. Realty Equities Corp.,* 58 N.J. 98, 275 A.2d 433 (1971), Justice Jacobs said:

> * * * [W]e have appropriately confined litigation to those situations where the litigant's concern with the subject matter evidenced a sufficient stake and real adverseness. In the overall we have given due weight to the interests of individual justice, along with the public interest, always bearing in mind that throughout our law we have been sweepingly rejecting procedural frustrations in favor of "just and expeditious determinations on the ultimate merits." [58 N.J. at 107–08, 275 A.2d at 438 (quoting from *Tumarkin v. Friedman,* 17 N.J.Super. 20, 21, 85, A.2d 304 (App.Div.1951), certif. den, 9 N.J. 287, 88 A.2d 39 (1952))].

The father of Karen Quinlan is certainly no stranger to the present controversy. His interests are real and adverse and he raises questions of surpassing importance. Manifestly, he has standing to assert his daughter's constitutional rights, she being incompetent to do so.

I. The Free Exercise of Religion

We think the contention as to interference with religious beliefs or rights may be considered and dealt with without extended discussion, given the acceptance of distinctions so clear and simple in their precedential definition as to be dispositive on their face.

[6] Simply stated, the right to religious beliefs is absolute but conduct in pursuance thereof is not wholly immune from governmental restraint. *John F. Kennedy Memorial Hosp. v. Heston,* 58 N.J. 576, 580–81, 279 A.2d 670 (1971). So it is that, for the sake of life, courts sometimes (but not always) order blood transfusions for Jehovah's Witnesses (whose religious beliefs

abhor such procedure), *Application of President & Directors of Georgetown College, Inc.,* 118 U.S.App.D.C. 80, 331 F.2d 1000 (D.C.Cir.), *cert.* den., 377 U.S. 978, 84 S.Ct. 1883, 12 L.Ed.2d 746 (1964); *United States v. George,* 239 F.Supp. 752 (D.Conn.1965); *John F. Kennedy Memorial Hosp. v. Heston, supra; Powell v. Columbian Presbyterian Medical Center,* 49 Misc.2d 215, 267 N.Y.S.2d 450 (Sup.Ct.1965); *but see In re Osborne,* 294 A.2d 372 (D.C.Ct.App.1972); *In re Estate of Brooks,* 32 Ill.2d 361, 205 N.E.2d 435 (Sup.Ct.1965); *Erickson v. Dilgard,* 44 Misc.2d 27, 252 N.Y.S.2d 705 (Sup.Ct.1962); *see generally* Annot., "Power Of Courts Or Other Public Agencies, In The Absence Of Statutory Authority, To Order Compulsory Medical Care for Adult," 9 A.L.R.3d 1391 (1966); forbid exposure to death from handling virulent snakes or ingesting poison (interfering with deeply held religious sentiments in such regard), *e. g., Hill v. State,* 38 Aa.App. 404, 88 So.2d 880 (Ct.App.), *cert.* den., 264 Ala. 697, 88 So.2d 887 (Sup.Ct. 1956); *State v. Massey,* 229 N.C. 734, 51 S.E.2d 179 (Sup.Ct.), appeal dismissed *sub nom., Bunn v. North Carolina,* 336 U.S. 942, 69 S.Ct. 813, 93 L.Ed. 1099 (1949); *State ex rel. Swann v. Pack,* Tenn., 527 S.W.2d 99 (Sup.Ct.1975), *cert.* den., — U.S. —, 96 S.Ct. 1429, 46 L.Ed.2d 360, 44 U.S.L.W. 3498, No. 75–956 (March 8, 1976); and protect the public health as in the case of compulsory vaccination (over the strongest of religious objections), *e. g., Wright v. DeWitt School Dist. 1,* 238 Ark. 906, 385 S.W.2d 644 (Sup.Ct.1965); *Mountain Lakes Bd. of Educ. v. Maas,* 56 N.J.Super. 245, 152 A.2d 394 (App.Div.1959), *aff'd o. b.,* 31 N.J. 537, 158 A.2d 330 (1960), *cert.* den., 363 U.S. 843, 80 S.Ct. 1613, 4 L.Ed.2d 1727 (1960); *McCartney v. Austin,* 57 Misc.2d 525, 293 N.Y.S.2d 188 (Sup.Ct.1968). The public interest is thus considered paramount, without essential dissolution of respect for religious beliefs.

[7, 8] We think, without further examples, that, ranged against the State's interest in the preservation of life, the impingement of religious belief, much less religious "neutrality" as here, does not reflect a constitutional question, in the circumstances at least of the case presently before the Court. Moreover, like the trial court, we do not recognize an independent parental right of religious freedom to support the relief requested. 137 N.J.Super. at 267–68, 348 A.2d 801.

II. Cruel and Unusual Punishment

[9] Similarly inapplicable to the case before us is the Constitution's Eighth Amendment protection against cruel and unusual punishment which, as held by the trial court, is not relevant to situations other than the imposition of penal sanctions. Historic in nature, it stemmed from punitive excesses in the infliction of criminal penalties.[6] We find no precedent in law which would justify its extension to the correction of social injustice or hardship, such as, for instance, in the case of poverty. The latter often condemns the poor and deprived to horrendous living conditions which could certainly be described in the abstract as "cruel and unusual punishment." Yet the constitutional base of protection from "cruel and unusual punishment" is plainly irrelevant to such societal ills which must be remedied, if at all, under other concepts of constitutional and civil right.

[10] So it is in the case of the unfortunate Karen Quinlan. Neither the State, nor the law, but the accident of fate and nature, has inflicted upon her conditions which though in essence cruel and most unusual, yet do not amount to "punishment" in any constitutional sense.

Neither the judgment of the court below, nor the medical decision which confronted it, nor the law and equity perceptions which impelled its action, nor the whole factual base upon which it was predicated, inflicted "cruel and unusual punishment" in the constitutional sense.

III. The Right of Privacy[7]

It is the issue of the constitutional right of privacy that has given us most concern, in the exceptional circumstances of this case. Here a loving parent, *qua* parent and raising the rights of his incompetent and profoundly damaged daughter, probably irreversibly doomed to no more than a biologically vegetative remnant of life, is before the court. He seeks authorization to abandon specialized technological procedures which can only maintain for a time a body having no potential for resumption or continuance of other than a "vegetative" existence.

We have no doubt, in these unhappy circumstances, that if Karen were herself miraculously lucid for an interval (not altering the existing prognosis of the condition to which she would soon return) and perceptive of her irreversible

condition, she could effectively decide upon discontinuance of the life-support apparatus, even if it meant the prospect of natural death. To this extent we may distinguish *Heston, supra,* which concerned a severely injured young woman (Delores Heston), whose life depended on surgery and blood transfusion; and who was in such extreme shock that she was unable to express an informed choice (although the Court apparently considered the case as if the patient's own religious decision to resist transfusion were at stake), but most importantly a patient apparently salvable to long life and vibrant health;—a situation not at all like the present case.

We have no hesitancy in deciding, in the instant diametrically opposite case, that no external compelling interest of the State could compel Karen to endure the unendurable, only to vegetate a few measurable months with no realistic possibility of returning to any semblance of cognitive or sapient life. We perceive no thread of logic distinguishing between such a choice on Karen's part and a similar choice which, under the evidence in this case, could be made by a competent patient terminally ill, riddled by cancer and suffering great pain; such a patient would not be resuscitated or put on a respirator in the example described by Dr. Korein, and *a fortiori* would not be kept *against his will* on a respirator.

Although the Constitution does not explicitly mention a right of privacy, Supreme Court decisions have recognized that a right of personal privacy exists and that certain areas of privacy are guaranteed under the Constitution. *Eisenstadt v. Baird,* 405 U.S. 438, 92 S.Ct. 1029, 31 L.Ed.2d 349 (1972); *Stanley v. Georgia,* 394 U.S. 557, 89 S.Ct. 1243, 22 L.Ed.2d 542 (1969). The Court has interdicted judicial intrusion into many aspects of personal decision, sometimes basing this restraint upon the conception of a limitation of judicial interest and responsibility, such as with regard to contraception and its relationship to family life and decision. *Griswold v. Connecticut,* 381 U.S. 479, 85 S.Ct. 1678, 14 L.Ed.2d 510 (1965).

[11] The Court in *Griswold* found the unwritten constitutional right of privacy to exist in the penumbra of specific guarantees of the Bill of Rights "formed by emanations from those guarantees that help give them life and substance." 381 U.S. at 484, 85 S.Ct. at 1681, 14 L.Ed.2d at 514. Presumably this right is broad

enough to encompass a patient's decision to decline medical treatment under certain circumstances, in much the same way as it is broad enough to encompass a woman's decision to terminate pregnancy under certain conditions. *Roe v. Wade,* 410 U.S. 113, 153, 93 S.Ct. 705, 727, 35 L.Ed.2d 147, 177 (1973).

Nor is such right of privacy forgotten in the New Jersey Constitution. N.J.Const. (1947), Art. I, par. 1.

[12] The claimed interests of the State in this case are essentially the preservation and sanctity of human life and defense of the right of the physician to administer medical treatment according to his best judgment. In this case the doctors say that removing Karen from the respirator will conflict with their professional judgment. The plaintiff answers that Karen's present treatment serves only a maintenance function; that the respirator cannot cure or improve her condition but at best can only prolong her inevitable slow deterioration and death; and that the interests of the patient, as seen by her surrogate, the guardian, must be evaluated by the court as predominant, even in the face of an opinion *contra* by the present attending physicians. Plaintiff's distinction is significant. The nature of Karen's care and the realistic chances of her recovery are quite unlike those of the patients discussed in many of the cases where treatments were ordered. In many of those cases the medical procedure required (usually a transfusion) constituted a minimal bodily invasion and the chances of recovery and return to functioning life were very good. We think that the State's interest *contra* weakens and the individual's right to privacy grows as the degree of bodily invasion increases and the prognosis dims. Ultimately there comes a point at which the individual's rights overcome the State interest. It is for that reason that we believe Karen's choice, if she were competent to make it, would be vindicated by the law. Her prognosis is extremely poor,—she will never resume cognitive life. And the bodily invasion is very great,—she requires 24 hour intensive nursing care, antibiotics, the assistance of a respirator, a catheter and feeding tube.

[13] Our affirmation of Karen's independent right of choice, however, would ordinarily be based upon her competency to assert it. The sad truth, however, is that she is grossly incompetent and we cannot discern her supposed choice

based on the testimony of her previous conversations with friends, where such testimony is without sufficient probative weight. 137 N.J.Super. at 260, 348 A.2d 801. Nevertheless we have concluded that Karen's right of privacy may be asserted on her behalf by her guardian under the peculiar circumstances here present.

If a putative decision by Karen to permit this non-cognitive, vegetative existence to terminate by natural forces is regarded as a valuable incident of her right of privacy, as we believe it to be, then it should not be discarded solely on the basis that her condition prevents her conscious exercise of the choice. The only practical way to prevent destruction of the right is to permit the guardian and family of Karen to render their best judgment, subject to the qualifications hereinafter stated, as to whether she would exercise it in these circumstances. If their conclusion is in the affirmative this decision should be accepted by a society the overwhelming majority of whose members would, we think, in similar circumstances, exercise such a choice in the same way for themselves or for those closest to them. It is for this reason that we determine that Karen's right of privacy may be asserted in her behalf, in this respect, by her guardian and family under the particular circumstances presented by this record.

[14] Regarding Mr. Quinlan's right of privacy, we agree with Judge Muir's conclusion that there is no parental constitutional right that would entitle him to a grant of relief *in propria persona. Id.* at 266, 348 A.2d 801. Insofar as a parental right of privacy has been recognized, it has been in the context of determining the rearing of infants and, as Judge Muir put it, involved "continuing life styles." *See Wisconsin v. Yoder,* 406 U.S. 205, 92 S.Ct. 1526, 32 L.Ed.2d 15 (1972); *Pierce v. Society of Sisters,* 268 U.S. 510, 45 S.Ct. 571, 69 L.Ed. 1070 (1925); *Meyer v. Nebraska,* 262 U.S. 390, 43 S.Ct. 625, 67 L.Ed. 1042 (1923). Karen Quinlan is a 22 year old adult. Her right of privacy in respect of the matter before the Court is to be vindicated by Mr. Quinlan as guardian, as hereinabove determined.

IV. The Medical Factor

Having declared the substantive legal basis upon which plaintiff's rights as representative of Karen must be deemed predicated, we face and respond to the assertion on behalf of defendants that our premise unwarrantably offends prevailing medical standards. We thus turn to consideration of the medical decision supporting the determination made below, conscious of the paucity of pre-existing legislative and judicial guidance as to the rights and liabilities therein involved.

A significant problem in any discussion of sensitive medical-legal issues is the marked, perhaps unconscious, tendency of many to distort what the law is, in pursuit of an exposition of what they would like the law to be. Nowhere is this barrier to the intelligent resolution of legal controversies more obstructive than in the debate over patient rights at the end of life. Judicial refusals to order lifesaving treatment in the face of contrary claims of bodily self-determination or free religious exercise are too often cited in support of a preconceived "right to die," even though the patients, wanting to live, have claimed no such right. Conversely, the assertion of a religious or other objection to lifesaving treatment is at times condemned as attempted suicide, even though suicide means something quite different in the law. [Byrn, "Compulsory Lifesaving Treatment For The Competent Adult," 44 Fordham L. Rev. 1 (1975)].

Perhaps the confusion there adverted to stems from mention by some courts of statutory or common law condemnation of suicide as demonstrating the state's interest in the preservation of life. We would see, however, a real distinction between the self-infliction of deadly harm and a self-determination against artificial life support or radical surgery, for instance, in the face of irreversible, painful and certain imminent death. The contrasting situations mentioned are analogous to those continually faced by the medical profession. When does the institution of life-sustaining procedures, ordinarily mandatory, become the subject of medical discretion in the context of administration to persons *in extremis?* And when does the withdrawal of such procedures, from such persons already supported by them, come within the orbit of medical discretion? When does a determination as to either of the foregoing contingencies court the

hazard of civil or criminal liability on the part of the physician or institution involved?

The existence and nature of the medical dilemma need hardly be discussed at length, portrayed as it is in the present case and complicated as it has recently come to be in view of the dramatic advance of medical technology. The dilemma is there, it is real, it is constantly resolved in accepted medical practice without attention in the courts, it pervades the issues in the very case we here examine. The branch of the dilemma involving the doctor's responsibility and the relationship of the court's duty was thus conceived by Judge Muir:

Doctors * * * to treat a patient, must deal with medical tradition and past case histories. They must be guided by what they do know. The extent of their training, their experience, consultation with other physicians, must guide their decision-making processes in providing care to their patient. The nature, extent and duration of care by societal standards is the responsibility of a physician. The morality and conscience of our society places this responsibility in the hands of the physician. What justification is there to remove it from the control of the medical profession and place it in the hands of the courts? [137 N.J.Super. at 259, 348 A.2d at 818].

[15] Such notions as to the distribution of responsibility, heretofore generally entertained, should however neither impede this Court in deciding matters clearly justiciable nor preclude a re-examination by the Court as to underlying human values and rights. Determinations as to these must, in the ultimate, be responsive not only to the concepts of medicine but also to the common moral judgment of the community at large. In the latter respect the Court has a nondelegable judicial responsibility.

Put in another way, the law, equity and justice must not themselves quail and be helpless in the face of modern technological marvels presenting questions hitherto unthought of. Where a Karen Quinlan, or a parent, or a doctor, or a hospital, or a State seeks the process and response of a court, it must answer with its most informed conception of justice in the previously unexplored circumstances presented to it. That is its obligation and we are here fulfilling it, for the actors and those having an interest in the matter should not go without remedy.

Courts in the exercise of their *parens patriae* responsibility to protect those under disability have sometimes implemented medical decisions and authorized their carrying out under the doctrine of "substituted judgment." *Hart v. Brown,* 29 Conn.Sup. 368, 289 A.2d 386, 387–88 (Super.Ct.1972); *Strunk v. Strunk,* 445 S.W.2d 145, 147–48 (Ky.1969). For as Judge Muir pointed out:

"As part of the inherent power of equity, a Court of Equity has full and complete jurisdiction over the persons of those who labor under any legal disability. * * * The Court's action in such a case is not limited by any narrow bounds, but it is empowered to stretch forth its arm in whatever direction its aid and protection may be needed. While this is indeed a special exercise of equity jurisdiction, it is beyond question that by virtue thereof the Court may pass upon purely personal rights." [137 N.J. Super. at 254, 348 A.2d at 816 (quoting from *Am.Jur.*2d, Equity §69 (1966))].

But insofar as a court, having no inherent medical expertise, is called upon to overrule a professional decision made according to prevailing medical practice and standards, a different question is presented. As mentioned below, a doctor is required

"to exercise in the treatment of his patient the degree of care, knowledge and skill ordinarily possessed and exercised in similar situations by the average member of the profession practicing in his field." *Schueler v. Strelinger,* 43 N.J. 330, 344, 204 A.2d 577, 584 (1964). If he is a specialist he "must employ not merely the skill of a general practitioner, but also that special degree of skill normally possessed by the average physician who devotes special study and attention to the particular organ or disease or injury involved, having regard to the present state of scientific knowledge". *Clark v. Wichman,* 72 N.J.Super. 486, 493, 179 A.2d 38, 42 (App.Div.1962). This is the duty that establishes his legal obligations to his patients. [137 N.J.Super. at 257–58, 348 A.2d at 818].

The medical obligation is related to standards and practice prevailing in the profession. The physicians in charge of the case, as noted above, declined to withdraw the respirator.

That decision was consistent with the proofs below as to the then existing medical standards and practices.

Under the law as it then stood, Judge Muir was correct in declining to authorize withdrawal of the respirator.

However, in relation to the matter of the declaratory relief sought by plaintiff as representative of Karen's interests, we are required to reevaluate the applicability of the medical standards projected in the court below. The question is whether there is such internal consistency and rationality in the application of such standards as should warrant their constituting an ineluctable bar to the effectuation of substantive relief for plaintiff at the hands of the court. We have concluded not.

In regard to the foregoing it is pertinent that we consider the impact on the standards both of the civil and criminal law as to medical liability and the new technological means of sustaining life irreversibly damaged.

The modern proliferation of substantial malpractice litigation and the less frequent but even more unnerving possibility of criminal sanctions would seem, for it is beyond human nature to suppose otherwise, to have bearing on the practice and standards as they exist. The brooding presence of such possible liability, it was testified here, had no part in the decision of the treating physicians. As did Judge Muir, we afford this testimony full credence. But we cannot believe that the stated factor has not had a strong influence on the standards, as the literature on the subject plainly reveals. (See footnote 8, *infra*). Moreover our attention is drawn not so much to the recognition by Drs. Morse and Javed of the extant practice and standards but to the widening ambiguity of those standards themselves in their application to the medical problems we are discussing.

The agitation of the medical community in the face of modern life prolongation technology and its search for definitive policy are demonstrated in the large volume of relevant professional commentary.[8]

The wide debate thus reflected contrasts with the relative paucity of legislative and judicial guides and standards in the same field. The medical profession has sought to devise guidelines such as the "brain death" concept of the Harvard Ad Hoc Committee mentioned above. But it is perfectly apparent from the testimony we have quoted of Dr. Korein, and indeed so clear as almost to be judicially noticeable, that humane decisions against resuscitative or maintenance therapy are frequently a recognized *de facto* response in the medical world to the irreversible, terminal, pain-ridden patient, especially with familial consent. And these cases, of course, are far short of "brain death."

We glean from the record here that physicians distinguish between curing the ill and comforting and easing the dying; that they refuse to treat the curable as if they were dying or sought to die, and that they have sometimes refused to treat the hopeless and dying as if they were curable. In this sense, as we were reminded by the testimony of Drs. Korein and Diamond, many of them have refused to inflict an undesired prolongation of the process of dying on a patient in irreversible condition when it is clear that such "therapy" offers neither human nor humane benefit. We think these attitudes represent a balanced implementation of a profoundly realistic perspective on the meaning of life and death and that they respect the whole Judeo-Christian tradition of regard for human life. No less would they seem consistent with the moral matrix of medicine, "to heal," very much in the sense of the endless mission of the law, "to do justice."

Yet this balance, we feel, is particularly difficult to perceive and apply in the context of the development by advanced technology of sophisticated and artificial life-sustaining devices. For those possibly curable, such devices are of great value, and, as ordinary medical procedures, are essential. Consequently, as pointed out by Dr. Diamond, they are necessary because of the ethic of medical practice. But in light of the situation in the present case (while the record here is somewhat hazy in distinguishing between "ordinary" and "extraordinary" measures), one would have to think that the use of the same respirator or like support could be considered "ordinary" in the context of the possibly curable patient but "extraordinary" in the context of the forced sustaining by cardio-respiratory processes of an irreversibly doomed patient. And this dilemma is sharpened in the face of the malpractice and criminal action threat which we have mentioned.

We would hesitate, in this imperfect world, to propose as to physicians that type of immunity which from the early common law has surrounded judges and grand jurors, *see e.g.,* *Grove v. Van Duyn,* 44 N.J.L. 654, 656–57 (E & A.1882); *O'Regan v. Schermerhorn,* 25 N.J.Misc. 1, 19–20, 50 A.2d 10 (Sup.Ct.1940), so that they might without fear of personal retaliation perform their judicial duties with independent objectivity. In *Bradley v Fisher,* 80 U.S. (13 WALL.)335, 347, 20 L.Ed. 646, 649 (1872), the Supreme Court held:

> [I]t is a general principle of the highest importance to the proper administration of justice that a judicial officer, in exercising the authority vested in him, shall be free to act upon his own convictions, without apprehension of personal consequences to himself.

Lord Coke said of judges that "they are only to make an account to God and the King [the State]." 12 Coke Rep. 23, 25, 77 Eng.Rep. 1305, 1307 (S.C.1608).

Nevertheless, there must be a way to free physicians, in the pursuit of their healing vocation, from possible contamination by self-interest or self-protection concerns which would inhibit their independent medical judgments for the well-being of their dying patients. We would hope that this opinion might be serviceable to some degree in ameliorating the professional problems under discussion.

A technique aimed at the underlying difficulty (though in a somewhat broader context) is described by Dr. Karen Teel, a pediatrician and a director of Pediatric Education, who writes in the *Baylor Law Review* under the title "The Physician's Dilemma: A Doctor's View: What The Law Should Be." Dr. Teel recalls:

> Physicians, by virtue of their responsibility for medical judgments are, partly by choice and partly by default, charged with the responsibility of making ethical judgments which we are sometimes ill-equipped to make. We are not always morally and legally authorized to make them. The physician is thereby assuming a civil and criminal liability that, as often as not, he does not even realize as a factor in his decision. There is little or no dialogue in this

whole process. The physician assumes that his judgment is called for and, in good faith, he acts. Someone must and it has been the physician who has assumed the responsibility and the risk.

I suggest that it would be more appropriate to provide a regular forum for more input and dialogue in individual situations and to allow the responsibility of these judgments to be shared. Many hospitals have established an Ethics Committee composed of physicians, social workers, attorneys, and theologians, * * * which serves to review the individual circumstances of ethical dilemma and which has provided much in the way of assistance and safeguards for patients and their medical caretakers. Generally, the authority of these committees is primarily restricted to the hospital setting and their official status is more that of an advisory body than of an enforcing body.

The concept of an Ethics Committee which has this kind of organization and is readily accessible to those persons rendering medical care to patients, would be, I think, the most promising direction for further study at this point. * * * [This would allow] some much needed dialogue regarding these issues and [force] the point of exploring all of the options for a particular patient. It diffuses the responsibility for making these judgments. Many physicians, in many circumstances, would welcome this sharing of responsibility. I believe that such an entity could lend itself well to an assumption of a legal status which would allow courses of action not now undertaken because of the concern for liability. [27 Baylor L.Rev. 6, 8–9 (1975)].

The most appealing factor in the technique suggested by Dr. Teel seems to us to be the diffusion of professional responsibility for decision, comparable in a way to the value of multi-judge courts in finally resolving on appeal difficult questions of law. Moreover, such a system would be protective to the hospital as well as the doctor in screening out, so to speak, a case which might be contaminated by less than worthy motivations of family or physician. In the real world and in relationship to the momentous decision contemplated, the value of additional views and diverse knowledge is apparent.

[16] We consider that a practice of applying to a court to confirm such decisions would generally be inappropriate, not only because that would be a gratuitous encroachment upon the medical profession's field of competence, but because it would be impossibly cumbersome. Such a requirement is distinguishable from the judicial overview traditionally required in other matters such as the adjudication and commitment of mental incompetents. This is not to say that in the case of an otherwise justiciable controversy access to the courts would be foreclosed; we speak rather of a general practice and procedure.

And although the deliberations and decisions which we describe would be professional in nature they should obviously include at some stage the feelings of the family of an incompetent relative. Decision-making within health care if it is considered as an expression of a primary obligation of the physician, *primum non nocere*, should be controlled primarily within the patient-doctor-family relationship, as indeed was recognized by Judge Muir in his supplemental opinion of November 12, 1975.

If there could be created not necessarily this particular system but some reasonable counterpart, we would have no doubt that such decisions, thus determined to be in accordance with medical practice and prevailing standards, would be accepted by society and by the courts, at least in cases comparable to that of Karen Quinlan.

The evidence in this case convinces us that the focal point of decision should be the prognosis as to the reasonable possibility of return to cognitive and sapient life, as distinguished from the forced continuance of that biological vegetative existence to which Karen seems to be doomed.

[17] In summary of the present Point of this opinion, we conclude that the state of the pertinent medical standards and practices which guided the attending physicians in this matter is not such as would justify this Court in deeming itself bound or controlled thereby in responding to the case for declaratory relief established by the parties on the record before us.

V. Alleged Criminal Liability

[18] Having concluded that there is a right of privacy that might permit termination of treat-

ment in the circumstances of this case, we turn to consider the relationship of the exercise of that right to the criminal law. We are aware that such termination of treatment would accelerate Karen's death. The County Prosecutor and the Attorney General maintain that there would be criminal liability for such acceleration. Under the statutes of this State, the unlawful killing of another human being is criminal homicide. N.J.S.A. 2A:113-1, 2, 5. We conclude that there would be no criminal homicide in the circumstances of this case. We believe, first, that the ensuing death would not be homicide but rather expiration from existing natural causes. Secondly, even if it were to be regarded as homicide, it would not be unlawful.

These conclusions rest upon definitional and constitutional bases. The termination of treatment pursuant to the right of privacy is, within the limitations of this case, *ipso facto* lawful. Thus, a death resulting from such an act would not come within the scope of the homicide statutes proscribing only the unlawful killing of another. There is a real and in this case determinative distinction between the unlawful taking of the life of another and the ending of artificial life-support systems as a matter of self-determination.

[19–21] Furthermore, the exercise of a constitutional right such as we have here found is protected from criminal prosecution. *See Stanley v. Georgia, supra,* 394 U.S. at 559, 89 S.Ct. at 1245, 22 L.Ed.2d at 546. We do not question the State's undoubted power to punish the taking of human life, but that power does not encompass individuals terminating medical treatment pursuant to their right of privacy. *See id.* at 568, 89 S.Ct. at 1250, 22 L.Ed.2d at 551. The constitutional protection extends to third parties whose action is necessary to effectuate the exercise of that right where the individuals themselves would not be subject to prosecution or the third parties are charged as accessories to an act which could not be a crime. *Eisenstadt v. Baird, supra,* 405 U.S. at 445–46, 92 S.Ct. at 1034–35, 31 L.Ed.2d at 357–58; *Griswold v. Connecticut, supra,* 381 U.S. at 481, 85 S.Ct. at 1679–80, 14 L.Ed.2d at 512–13. And, under the circumstances of this case, these same principles would apply to and negate a valid prosecution for attempted suicide were there still such a crime in this State.[9]

VI. The Guardianship of the Person

[22] The trial judge bifurcated the guardianship, as we have noted, refusing to appoint Joseph Quinlan to be guardian of the person and limiting his guardianship to that of the property of his daughter. Such occasional division of guardianship, as between responsibility for the person and the property of an incompetent person, has roots deep in the common law and was well within the jurisdictional capacity of the trial judge. *In re Rollins,* 65 A.2d 667, 679–82 (N.J.Cty.Ct.1949).

The statute creates an initial presumption of entitlement to guardianship in the next of kin, for it provides:

In any case where a guardian is to be appointed, letters of guardianship shall be granted * * * to the next of kin, or if * * * it is proven to the court that no appointment from among them will be to the best interest of the incompetent or his estate, then to such other proper person as will accept the same. [N.J.S.A. 3A:6–36. *See In re Roll,* 117 N.J.Super. 122, 124, 283 A.2d 764, 765 (App.Div.1971)].

[23] The trial court was apparently convinced of the high character of Joseph Quinlan and his general suitability as guardian under other circumstances, describing him as "very sincere, moral, ethical and religious." The court felt, however, that the obligation to concur in the medical care and treatment of his daughter would be a source of anguish to him and would distort his "decision-making processes." We disagree, for we sense from the whole record before us that while Mr. Quinlan feels a natural grief, and understandably sorrows because of the tragedy which has befallen his daughter, his strength of purpose and character far outweighs these sentiments and qualifies him eminently for guardianship of the person as well as the property of his daughter. Hence we discern no valid reason to overrule the statutory intendment of perference to the next of kin.

DECLARATORY RELIEF

[24] We thus arrive at the formulation of the declaratory relief which we have concluded is

appropriate to this case. Some time has passed since Karen's physical and mental condition was described to the Court. At that time her continuing deterioration was plainly projected. Since the record has not been expanded we assume that she is now even more fragile and nearer to death than she was then. Since her present treating physicians may give reconsideration to her present posture in the light of this opinion, and since we are transferring to the plaintiff as guardian the choice of the attending physician and therefore other physicians may be in charge of the case who may take a different view from that of the present attending physicians, we herewith declare the following affirmative relief on behalf of the plaintiff. Upon the concurrence of the guardian and family of Karen, should the responsible attending physicians conclude that there is no reasonable possibility of Karen's ever emerging from her present comatose condition to a cognitive, sapient state and that the life-support apparatus now being administered to Karen should be discontinued, they shall consult with the hospital "Ethics Committee" or like body of the institution in which Karen is then hospitalized. If that consultative body agrees that there is no reasonable possibility of Karen's ever emerging from her present comatose condition to a cognitive, sapient state, the present life-support system may be withdrawn and said action shall be without any civil or criminal liability therefor on the part of any participant, whether guardian, physician, hospital or others.[10] We herewith specifically so hold.

CONCLUSION

We therefore remand this record to the trial court to implement (without further testimonial hearing) the following decisions:

1. To discharge, with the thanks of the Court for his service, the present guardian of the person of Karen Quinlan, Thomas R. Curtin, Esquire, a member of the Bar and an officer of the court.
2. To appoint Joseph Quinlan as guardian of the person of Karen Quinlan with full power to make decisions with regard to the identity of her treating physicians.

We repeat for the sake of emphasis and clarity that upon the concurrence of the guardian and family of Karen, should the responsible attending physicians conclude that there is no reasonable possibility of Karen's ever emerging from her present comatose condition to a cognitive, sapient state and that the life-support apparatus now being administered to Karen should be discontinued, they shall consult with the hospital "Ethics Committee" or like body of the institution in which Karen is then hospitalized. If that consultative body agrees that there is no reasonable possibility of Karen's ever emerging from her present comatose condition to a cognitive, sapient state, the present life-support system may be withdrawn and said action shall be without any civil or criminal liability therefor on the part of any participant, whether guardian, physician, hospital or others.

By the above ruling we do not intend to be understood as implying that a proceeding for judicial declaratory relief is necessarily required for the implementation of comparable decisions in the field of medical practice.

Modified and remanded.

For modification and remandment: Chief Justice HUGHES, Justices MOUNTAIN, SULLIVAN, PASHMAN, CLIFFORD and SCHREIBER and Judge CONFORD—7.

Opposed: None.

NOTES

1. The importance of the preservation of life is memorialized in various organic documents. The Declaration of Independence states as self-evident truths "that all men * * * are endowed by their Creator with certain unalienable Rights, that among these are Life, Liberty and the pursuit of Happiness." This ideal is inherent in the Constitution of the United States. It is explicitly recognized in our Constitution of 1947 which provides for "certain natural and unalienable rights, among which are those of enjoying and defending life * * *." N.J.Const. (1947), Art. I, par. 1. Our State government is established to protect such rights, N.J.Const. (1947), Art. I, par. 2, and, acting through the Attorney General (N.J.S.A. 52:17A–4(h)), it enforces them.

2. Dr. Julius Korein, a neurologist, testified:

A. * * * [Y]ou've got a set of possible lesions that prior to the era of advanced technology and advances in medicine were no problem inasmuch as the patient would expire. They could do nothing for themselves and even external care was limited. It was—I don't know how many years ago they couldn't keep a person alive with intravenous feedings because they couldn't give enough calories. Now they have these high caloric tube feedings that can keep people in excellent nutrition for years so what's happened is these things have occurred all along but the technology has now reached a point where you can in fact start to replace anything outside of the brain to maintain something that is irreversibly damaged.

Q. Doctor, can the art of medicine repair the cerebral damage that was sustained by Karen?

A. In my opinion, no. * * *

Q. Doctor, in your opinion is there any course of treatment that will lead to the improvement of Karen's condition?

A. No.

3. The Harvard Ad Hoc standards, with reference to "brain death," will be discussed *infra*.

3.1. This cross-appeal was later informally withdrawn but in view of the importance of the matter we nevertheless deal with it.

4. Dr. Robert J. Morse, a neurologist, and Karen's treating physician from the time of her admission to Saint Clare's Hospital on April 24, 1975 (reference was made *supra* to "treating physicians" named as defendants; this term included Dr. Arshad Javed, a highly qualified pulmonary internist, who considers that he manages that phase of Karen's care with primary responsibility to the "attending physician," Dr. Morse).

5. Death. The cessation of life; the ceasing to exist; defined by physicians as a total stoppage of the circulation of the blood, and a cessation of the animal and vital functions consequent thereon, such as respiration, pulsation, etc. *Black's Law Dictionary* 488 (rev. 4th ed. 1968).

6. It is generally agreed that the Eighth Amendment's provision of "[n]or cruel and unusual punishments inflicted" is drawn verbatim from the English Declaration of Rights. *See* 1 Wm. & M., sess. 2, c. 2 (1689). The prohibition arose in the context of excessive punishments for crimes, punishments that were barbarous and savage as well as disproportionate to the offense committed. *See generally* Granucci " 'Nor Cruel and Unusual Punishments Inflicted:' The Original Meaning," 57 Calif.L.Rev. 839, 844–60 (1969); Note, "The Cruel and Unusual Punishment Clause and the Substantive Criminal Law," 79 Harv.L.Rev. 635, 636–39 (1966). The principle against excessiveness in criminal punishments can be traced back to Chapters 20–22 of the *Magna Carta* (1215). The historical background of the Eighth Amendment was examined at some length in various opinions in *Furman v. Georgia*, 408 U.S. 238, 92 S.Ct. 2726, 33 L.Ed.2d 346 (1972).

The Constitution itself is silent as to the meaning of the word "punishment." Whether it refers to the variety of legal and non-legal penalties that human beings endure or whether it must be in connection with a criminal rather than a civil proceeding is not stated in the document. But the origins of the clause are clear. And the cases construing it have consistently held that the "punishment" contemplated by the Eighth Amendment is the penalty inflicted by a court for the commission of a crime in the enforcement of what is a criminal law. *See, e. g., Trop v. Dulles*, 356 U.S. 86, 94–99, 78 S.Ct. 590, 594–97, 2 L.Ed.2d 630, 638–41 (1957). *See generally* Note, "The Effectiveness of the Eighth Amendment: An Appraisal of Cruel and Unusual Punishment," 36 N.Y.U.L.Rev. 846, 854–57 (1961). A deprivation, forfeiture or penalty arising out of a civil proceeding or otherwise cannot be "cruel and unusual punishment" within the meaning of the constitutional clause.

7. The right we here discuss is included within the class of what have been called rights of "personality." *See* Pound, "Equitable Relief against Defamation and Injuries to Personality," 29 Harv.L.Rev. 640, 668–76 (1916). Equitable jurisdiction with respect to the recognition and enforcement of such rights has long been recognized in New Jersey. *See, e. g., Vanderbilt v. Mitchell*, 72 N.J.Eq. 910, 919–20, 67 A. 97 (E. & A. 1907).

8. *See, e. g., Downing, Euthanasia and the Right to Death* (1969); *St. John-Stevas, Life, Death and the Law* (1961); *Williams, The Sanctity of Human Life and the Criminal Law* (1957); Appel, "Ethical and Legal Questions Posed by Recent Advances in Medicine," 205 J.A.M.A. 513 (1968); Cantor, "A Patient's Decision To Decline Life-Saving Medical Treatment: Bodily Integrity Versus The Preservation Of Life," 26 Rutgers L.Rev. 228 (1973); Claypool, "The Family Deals with Death," 27 Baylor L.Rev. 34 (1975); Elkington, "The Dying Patient, The Doctor and The Law," 13 Vill.L.Rev. 740 (1968); Fletcher, "Legal Aspects of the Decision Not to Prolong Life," 203 J.A.M.A. 65 (1968); Foreman, "The Physician's Criminal Liability for the Practice of Euthanasia," 27 Baylor L.Rev. 54 (1975); Gurney, "Is There A Right To Die?—A Study of the Law of Euthanasia," 3 Cumb.-Sam.L.Rev. 235 (1972): Mannes, "Euthanasia vs. The Right to Life," 27 Baylor L.Rev. 68 (1975); Sharp & Crofts, "Death with Dignity and The Physician's Civil Liability," 27 Baylor L.Rev. 86 (1975); Sharpe & Hargest, "Lifesaving Treatment for Unwilling Patients," 36 Fordham L.Rev. 695 (1968); Skegg, "Irreversibly Comatose Individuals: 'Alive' or 'Dead'?," 33 Camb.L.J. 130 (1974); Comment, "The Right to Die," 7 Houston L.Rev. 654 (1970); Note, "The Time Of Death—A Legal, Ethical and Medical Dilemma," 18 Catholic Law. 243 (1972); Note, "Compulsory Medical Treatment: The State's Interest Reevaluated," 51 Minn.L.Rev. 293 (1966).

9. An attempt to commit suicide was an indictable offense at common law and as such was indictable in this State as a common law misdemeanor. 1 *Schlosser, Criminal Laws of New Jersey* §12.5 (3d ed. 1970); *see*

N.J.S.A. 2A:85–1. The legislature downgraded the offense in 1957 to the status of a disorderly persons offense, which is not a "crime" under our law. N.J.S.A. 2A:170–25.6. And in 1971, the legislature repealed all criminal sanctions for attempted suicide. N.J.S.A. 2A:85–5.1. Provision is now made for temporary hospitalization of persons making such an attempt. N.J.S.A. 30:4–26.3a. We note that under the proposed New Jersey Penal Code (Oct. 1971) there is no provision for criminal punishment of attempted suicide. *See*

Commentary, §2C:11–6. There is, however, an independent offense of "aiding suicide." §2C:11–6b. This provision, if enacted, would not be incriminatory in circumstances similar to those presented in this case.
10. The declaratory relief we here award is not intended to imply that the principles enunciated in this case might not be applicable in divers other types of terminal medical situations such as those described by Drs. Korein and Diamond, *supra*, not necessarily involving the hopeless loss of cognitive or sapient life.

5.2 Superintendent of Belchertown v. Saikewicz

1977 Mass. Ad. Sh. 2461, 370 N.E. 2d 417 (1977)

Before HENNESSEY, C. J., and BRAUCHER, KAPLAN, WILKINS and LIACOS, JJ.

LIACOS, Justice.

On April 26, 1976, William E. Jones, superintendent of the Belchertown State School (a facility of the Massachusetts Department of Mental Health), and Paul R. Rogers, a staff attorney at the school, petitioned the Probate Court for Hampshire County for the appointment of a guardian of Joseph Saikewicz, a resident of the State school. Simultaneously they filed a motion for the immediate appointment of a guardian ad litem, with authority to make the necessary decisions concerning the care and treatment of Saikewicz, who was suffering with acute myeloblastic monocytic leukemia. The petition alleged that Saikewicz was a mentally retarded person in urgent need of medical treatment and that he was a person with disability incapable of giving informed consent for such treatment.

On May 5, 1976, the probate judge appointed a guardian ad litem. On May 6, 1976, the guardian ad litem filed a report with the court. The guardian ad litem's report indicated that Saikewicz's illness was an incurable one, and that although chemotherapy was the medically indicated course of treatment it would cause Saikewicz significant adverse side effects and discomfort. The guardian ad litem concluded that these factors, as well as the inability of the ward to understand the treatment to which he would be subjected and the fear and pain he would suffer as a result, outweighed the limited prospect of any benefit from such treatment, namely, the possibility of some uncertain but limited extension of life. He therefore recommended "that not treating Mr. Saikewicz would be in his best interests."

A hearing on the report was held on May 13, 1976. Present were the petitioners and the guardian ad litem.[1] The record before us does not indicate whether a guardian for Saikewicz was ever appointed. After hearing the evidence, the judge entered findings of fact and an order that in essence agreed with the recommendation of the guardian ad litem. The decision of the judge appears to be based in part on the testimony of Saikewicz's two attending physicians who recommended against chemotherapy. The judge then reported to the Appeals Court the two questions set forth in the margin.[2] An application for direct appellate review was allowed by this court. On July 9, 1976, this court issued an order answering the questions reported in the affirmative with the notation "rescript and opinion . . . will follow."[3] We now issue that opinion.

I.

The judge below found that Joseph Saikewicz, at the time the matter arose, was sixty-seven years old, with an I.Q. of ten and a mental age of approximately two years and eight months. He was profoundly mentally retarded. The record discloses that, apart from his leukemic condition, Saikewicz enjoyed generally good health. He was physically strong and well built, nutritionally nourished, and ambulatory. He was not, however, able to communicate verbally— resorting to gestures and grunts to make his wishes known to others and responding only to gestures or physical contacts. In the course of treatment for various medical conditions arising during Saikewicz's residency at the school, he had been unable to respond intelligibly to inquiries such as whether he was experiencing pain. It was the opinion of a consulting psychologist, not contested by the other experts relied on by the judge below, that Saikewicz was not aware of dangers and was disoriented outside his immediate environment. As a result of his condition, Saikewicz had lived in State institutions since 1923 and had resided at the Belchertown State School since 1928. Two of his sisters, the only members of his family who could be located, were notified of his condition and of the hearing, but they preferred not to attend or otherwise become involved.

On April 19, 1976, Saikewicz was diagnosed as suffering from acute myeloblastic monocytic leukemia. Leukemia is a disease of the blood. It arises when organs of the body produce an excessive number of white blood cells as well as other abnormal cellular structures, in particular undeveloped and immature white cells. Along with these symptoms in the composition of the blood the disease is accompanied by enlargement of the organs which produce the cells, e.g., the spleen, lymph glands, and bone marrow. The disease tends to cause internal bleeding and weakness, and, in the acute form, severe anemia and high susceptibility to infection. Attorneys' Dictionary of Medicine L–37–38 (1977). The particular form of the disease present in this case, acute myeloblastic monocytic leukemia is so defined because the particular cells which increase are the myeloblasts, the youngest form of a cell which at maturity is known as the granulocytes. *Id.* at M–138. The disease is invariably fatal.

Chemotherapy, as was testified to at the hearing in the Probate Court, involves the administration of drugs over several weeks, the purpose of which is to kill the leukemia cells. This treatment unfortunately affects normal cells as well. One expert testified that the end result, in effect, is to destroy the living vitality of the bone marrow. Because of this effect, the patient becomes very anemic and may bleed or suffer

infections—a condition which requires a number of blood transfusions. In this sense, the patient immediately becomes much "sicker" with the commencement of chemotherapy, and there is a possibility that infections during the initial period of severe anemia will prove fatal. Moreover, while most patients survive chemotherapy, remission of the leukemia is achieved in only thirty to fifty per cent of the cases. Remission is meant here as a temporary return to normal as measured by clinical and laboratory means. If remission does occur, it typically lasts for between two and thirteen months although longer periods of remission are possible. Estimates of the effectiveness of chemotherapy are complicated in cases, such as the one presented here, in which the patient's age becomes a factor. According to the medical testimony before the court below, persons over age sixty have more difficulty tolerating chemotherapy and the treatment is likely to be less successful than in younger patients.[4] This prognosis may be compared with the doctors' estimates that, left untreated, a patient in Saikewicz's condition would live for a matter of weeks or, perhaps, several months. According to the testimony, a decision to allow the disease to run its natural course would not result in pain for the patient, and death would probably come without discomfort.

An important facet of the chemotherapy process, to which the judge below directed careful attention, is the problem of serious adverse side effects caused by the treating drugs. Among these side effects are severe nausea, bladder irritation, numbness and tingling of the extremities, and loss of hair. The bladder irritation can be avoided, however, if the patient drinks fluids, and the nausea can be treated by drugs. It was the opinion of the guardian ad litem, as well as the doctors who testified before the probate judge, that most people elect to suffer the side effects of chemotherapy rather than to allow their leukemia to run its natural course.

Drawing on the evidence before him including the testimony of the medical experts, and the report of the guardian ad litem, the probate judge issued detailed findings with regard to the costs and benefits of allowing Saikewicz to undergo chemotherapy. The judge's findings are reproduced in part here because of the importance of clearly delimiting the issues presented in this case. The judge below found:

"5. That the majority of persons suffering from leukemia who are faced with a choice of receiving or foregoing such chemotherapy, and who are able to make an informed judgment thereon, choose to receive treatment in spite of its toxic side effects and risks of failure.

"6. That such toxic side effects of chemotherapy include pain and discomfort, depressed bone marrow, pronounced anemia, increased chance of infection, possible bladder irritation, and possible loss of hair.

"7. That administration of such chemotherapy requires cooperation from the patient over several weeks of time, which cooperation said JOSEPH SAIKEWICZ is unable to give due to his profound retardation.[5]

"8. That, considering the age and general state of health of said JOSEPH SAIKEWICZ, there is only a 30–40 percent chance that chemotherapy will produce a remission of said leukemia, which remission would probably be for a period of time of from 2 to 13 months, but that said chemotherapy will certainly not completely cure such leukemia.

"9. That if such chemotherapy is to be administered at all it should be administered immediately, inasmuch as the risks involved will increase and the chances of successfully bringing about remission will decrease as time goes by.

"10. That, at present, said JOSEPH SAIKEWICZ's leukemia condition is stable and is not deteriorating.

"11. That said JOSEPH SAIKEWICZ is not now in pain and will probably die within a matter of weeks or months a relatively painless death due to the leukemia unless other factors should intervene to themselves cause death.

"12. That it is impossible to predict how long said JOSEPH SAIKEWICZ will probably live without chemotherapy or how long he will probably live with chemotherapy, but it is to a very high degree medically likely that he will die sooner, without treatment than with it."

[Balancing these various factors, the judge] concluded that the following considerations weighed *against* administering chemotherapy to Saikewicz: "(1) his age, (2) his inability to cooperate with the treatment, (3) probable adverse side effects of treatment, (4) low chance of producing remission, (5) the certainty that treatment will cause immediate suffering, and (6) the quality of life possible for him even if the treatment does bring about remission."

The following considerations were determined to weigh in *favor* of chemotherapy: "(1) the chance that his life may be lengthened thereby, and (2) the fact that most people in his situation when given a chance to do so elect to take the gamble of treatment."

Concluding that, in this case, the negative factors of treatment exceeded the benefits, the probate judge ordered on May 13, 1976, that no treatment be administered to Saikewicz for his condition of acute myeloblastic monocytic leukemia except by further order of the court. The judge further ordered that all reasonable and necessary supportive measures be taken, medical or otherwise, to safeguard the well-being of Saikewicz in all other respects and to reduce as far as possible any suffering or discomfort which he might experience.

It is within this factual context that we issued our order of July 9, 1976.

Saikewicz died on September 4, 1976, at the Belchertown State School hospital. Death was due to bronchial pneumonia, a complication of the leukemia. Saikewicz died without pain or discomfort.[6]

II.

We recognize at the outset that this case presents novel issues of fundamental importance that should not be resolved by mechanical reliance on legal doctrine. Our task of establishing a framework in the law on which the activities of health care personnel and other persons can find support is furthered by seeking the collective guidance of those in health care, moral ethics, philosophy, and other disciplines. Our attempt to bring such insights to bear in the legal context has been advanced by the diligent efforts of the guardian ad litem and the probate judge, as well as the excellent briefs of the parties and amici curiae.[7] As thus illuminated, the principal areas of determination are:

A. The nature of the right of any person, competent or incompetent, to decline potentially life-prolonging treatment.

B. The legal standards that control the course of decision whether or not potentially life-prolonging, but not life-saving, treatment should be administered to a person who is not competent to make the choice.

C. The procedures that must be followed in arriving at that decision.

For reasons we develop in the body of this opinion, it becomes apparent that the questions to be discussed in the first two areas are closely interrelated. We take the view that the substantive rights of the competent and the incompetent person are the same in regard to the right to decline potentially life-prolonging treatment. The factors which distinguish the two types of persons are found only in the area of how the State should approach the preservation and implementation of the rights of an incompetent person and in the procedures necessary to that process of preservation and implementation. We treat the matter in the sequence above stated because we think it helpful to set forth our views on (A) what the rights of all persons in this area are and (B) the issue of how an incompetent person is to be afforded the status in law of a competent person with respect to such rights. Only then can we proceed to (C) the particular procedures to be followed to ensure the rights of the incompetent person.

A.

1. It has been said that "[t]he law always lags behind the most advanced thinking in every area. It must wait until the theologians and the moral leaders and events have created some common ground, some consensus." Burger, The Law and Medical Advances, 67 Annals Internal Med. Supp. 7, 15, 17 (1967), quoted in Elkinton, The Dying Patient, the Doctor, and the Law, 13 Vill.L.Rev. 740 (1968). We therefore think it advisable to consider the framework of medical ethics which influences a doctor's decision as to how to deal with the terminally ill patient. While these considerations are not controlling, they ought to be considered for the insights they give us.

Advances in medical science have given doctors greater control over the time and nature of death. Chemotherapy is, as evident from our previous discussion, one of these advances. Prior to the development of such new techniques the physician perceived his duty as that of making every conceivable effort to prolong life. On the other hand, the context in which such an ethos prevailed did not provide the range of options available to the physician today in terms of taking steps to postpone death irrespective of the effect on the patient. With the development of the new techniques, serious questions as to what may constitute acting in the best interests of the patient have arisen.

The nature of the choice has become more difficult because physicians have begun to realize that in many cases the effect of using extraordinary measures to prolong life is to "only prolong suffering, isolate the family from their loved one at a time when they may be close at hand or result in economic ruin for the family." Lewis, Machine Medicine and Its Relation to the Fatally Ill, 206 J.A.M.A. 387 (1968).

Recognition of these factors led the Supreme Court of New Jersey to observe "that physicians distinguish between curing the ill and comforting and easing the dying; that they refuse to treat the curable as if they were dying or ought to die, and that they have sometimes refused to treat the hopeless and dying as if they were curable." *In re Quinlan,* 70 N.J. 10, 47, 355 A.2d 647, 667 (1976).

The essence of this distinction in defining the medical role is to draw the sometimes subtle distinction between those situations in which the withholding of extraordinary measures may be viewed as allowing the disease to take its natural course and those in which the same actions may be deemed to have been the cause of death. See Elkinton, *supra* at 743. Recent literature suggests that health care institutions are drawing such a distinction, at least with regard to respecting the decision of competent patients to refuse such measures. Rabkin, Gillerman & Rice, Orders Not to Resuscitate, 293 N.E.J. of Med. 364 (1976). Cf. Beecher, Ethical Problems Created by the Hopelessly Unconscious Patient, 278 N.E.J. of Med. 1425 (1968).

The current state of medical ethics in this area is expressed by one commentator who states that: "we should not use *extraordinary* means of prolonging life or its semblance when, after careful consideration, consultation and the application of the most well conceived therapy it becomes apparent that there is no hope for the recovery of the patient. Recovery should not be defined simply as the ability to remain alive; it should mean life without intolerable suffering.'' *Lewis, supra*. See Collins, Limits of Medical Responsibility in Prolonging Life, 206 J.A.M.A. 389 (1968); Williamson, Life or Death—Whose Decision? 197 J.A.M.A. 793 (1966).

Our decision in this case is consistent with the current medical ethos in this area.

[1] 2. There is implicit recognition in the law of the Commonwealth, as elsewhere, that a person has a strong interest in being free from nonconsensual invasion of his bodily integrity. *Thibault v. Lalumiere*, 318 Mass. 72, 60 N.E.2d 349 (1945). *Commonwealth v. Clark*, 2 Metc. 23 (1840). *Union Pac. Ry. v. Botsford*, 141 U.S. 250, 251, 11 S.Ct. 1000, 35 L.Ed. 734 (1891). In short, the law recognizes the individual interest in preserving "the inviolability of his person." *Pratt v. Davis*, 118 Ill.App. 161, 166 (1905), aff'd, 224 Ill. 300, 79 N.E. 562 (1906). One means by which the law has developed in a manner consistent with the protection of this interest is through the development of the doctrine of informed consent. While the doctrine to the extent it may justify recovery in tort for the breach of a physician's duty has not been formally recognized by this court, *Schroeder v. Lawrence*, —— Mass. ——[a], 359 N.E.2d 1301 (1977); see *Baird v. Attorney Gen.*, — Mass. —[b], 360 N.E.2d 288 (1977); *Reddington v. Clayman*, 334 Mass. 244, 134 N.E.2d 920 (1956); G.L. c. 112, §12F, it is one of widespread recognition. Capron, Informed Consent in Catastrophic Disease Research and Treatment, 123 U.Pa.L.Rev. 340, 365 (1975); Cantor, A Patient's Decision to Decline Life-Saving Medical Treatment: Bodily Integrity Versus the Preservation of Life, 26 Rutgers L.Rev. 228, 236–238 (1973). W. Prosser, Torts §18 (4th ed. 1971). As previously suggested, one of the foundations of the doctrine is that it protects the patient's status as a human being. Capron, *supra* at 366–367.

[2] Of even broader import, but arising from the same regard for human dignity and self-determination, is the unwritten constitutional right of privacy found in the penumbra of specific guaranties of the Bill of Rights. *Griswold v. Connecticut*, 381 U.S. 479, 484, 85 S.Ct. 328, 13 L.Ed.2d 339 (1965). As this constitutional guaranty reaches out to protect the freedom of a woman to terminate pregnancy under certain conditions, *Roe v. Wade*, 410 U.S. 113, 153, 93 S.Ct. 705, 35 L.Ed.2d 147 (1973), so it encompasses the right of a patient to preserve his or her right to privacy against unwanted infringements of bodily integrity in appropriate circumstances. *In re Quinlan, supra* 70 N.J. at 38–39, 355 A.2d 647. In the case of a person incompetent to assert this constitutional right of privacy, it may be asserted by that person's guardian in conformance with the standards and procedures set forth in sections II(B) and II(C) of this opinion. See *Quinlan* at 39, 355 A.2d 647.

3. The question when the circumstances are appropriate for the exercise of this privacy right depends on the proper identification of State interests. It is not surprising that courts have, in the course of investigating State interests in various medical contexts and under various formulations of the individual rights involved, reached differing views on the nature and the extent of State interests. We have undertaken a survey of some of the leading cases to help in identifying the range of State interests potentially applicable to cases of medical intervention.

In a number of cases, no applicable State interest, or combination of such interests, was found sufficient to outweigh the individual's interests in exercising the choice of refusing medical treatment. To this effect are *Erickson v. Dilgard*, 44 Misc.2d 27, 252 N.Y.S.2d 705 (N.Y.Sup.Ct.1962) (scheme of liberty puts highest priority on free individual choice); *In re Estate of Brooks*, 32 Ill.2d 361, 205 N.E.2d 435 (1965) (patient may elect to pursue religious beliefs by refusing life-saving blood transfusion provided the decision did not endanger public health, safety or morals); see *In re Osborne*, 294 A.2d 372 (D.C.App.1972); *Holmes v. Silver Cross Hosp. of Joliet, Ill.*, 340 F.Supp. 125 (D.Ill.1972); Byrn, Compulsory Lifesaving Treatment for the Competent Adult, 44 Fordham L.Rev. 1 (1975). See also *In re Guardianship of Pescinski*, 67 Wis.2d 4, 226 N.W.2d 180 (1975).

Subordination of State interests to individual interests has not been universal, however. In a leading case, *Application of the President & Directors of Georgetown College, Inc.*, 118 U.S.App.D.C. 80, 331 F.2d 1000, cert. denied,

---

a. Mass.Adv.Sh. (1977) 286.

b. Mass.Adv.Sh. (1977) 96.

377 U.S. 978, 84 S.Ct. 1883, 12 L.Ed.2d 746 (1964), a hospital sought permission to perform a blood transfusion necessary to save the patient's life where the person was unwilling to consent due to religious beliefs. The court held that it had the power to allow the action to be taken despite the previously expressed contrary sentiments of the patient. The court justified its decision by reasoning that its purpose was to protect three State interests, the protection of which was viewed as having greater import than the individual right: (1) the State interest in preventing suicide, (2) a parens patriae interest in protecting the patient's minor children from "abandonment" by their parent, and (3) the protection of the medical profession's desire to act affirmatively to safe life without fear of civil liability. In *John F. Kennedy Memorial Hosp. v. Heston,* 58 N.J. 576, 279 A.2d 670 (1971), a case involving a fact situation similar to *Georgetown,* the New Jersey Supreme Court also allowed a transfusion. It based its decision on *Georgetown,* as well as its prior decisions. See *Raleigh Fitkin-Paul Morgan Memorial Hosp. v. Anderson,* 42 N.J. 421, 201 A.2d 537, cert. denied, 377 U.S. 985, 84 S.Ct. 1894, 12 L.Ed.2d 1032 (1964);[8] *State v. Perricone,* 37 N.J. 463, 181 A.2d 751, cert. denied, 371 U.S. 890, 83 S.Ct. 189, 9 L.Ed.2d 124 (1962). The New Jersey court held that the State's paramount interest in preserving life and the hospital's interest in fully caring for a patient under its custody and control outweighed the individual decision to decline the necessary measures. See *United States v. George,* 239 F. Supp. 752 (D.Conn.1965); *Long Island Jewish-Hillside Medical Center v. Levitt,* 73 Misc. 2d 395, 342 N.Y.S.2d 356 (N.Y. Sup.Ct. 1973); *In re Sampson,* 65 Misc.2d 658, 317 N.Y.S.2d 641 (Fam.Ct.1970), aff'd 37 App. Div.2d 668, 323 N.Y.S.2d 253 (1971), aff'd per curiam, 29 N.Y.2d 900, 328 N.Y.S.2d 686, 278 N.E.2d 915 (1972); *In re Weberlist,* 79 Misc.2d 753, 360 N.Y.S.2d 783 (N.Y. Sup. Ct.1974); *In re Karwath,* 199 N.W.2d 147 (Iowa 1972).

This survey of recent decisions involving the difficult question of the right of an individual to refuse medical intervention or treatment indicates that a relatively concise statement of countervailing State interests may be made. As distilled from the cases, the State has claimed interest in: (1) the preservation of life; (2) the protection of the interests of innocent third parties; (3) the prevention of suicide; and (4) maintaining the ethical integrity of the medical profession.

[3, 4] It is clear that the most significant of the asserted Stated interests is that of the preservation of human life. Recognition of such an interest, however, does not necessarily resolve the problem where the affliction or disease clearly indicates that life will soon, and inevitably, be extinguished. The interest of the State in prolonging a life must be reconciled with the interest of an individual to reject the traumatic cost of that prolongation. There is a substantial distinction in the State's insistence that human life be saved where the affliction is curable, as opposed to the State interest where, as here, the issue is not whether but when, for how long, and at what cost to the individual that life may be briefly extended. Even if we assume that the State has an additional interest in seeing to it that individual decisions on the prolongation of life do not in any way tend to "cheapen" the value which is placed in the concept of living, see *Roe v. Wade, supra,* we believe it is not inconsistent to recognize a right to decline medical treatment in a situation of incurable illness. The constitutional right to privacy, as we conceive it, is an expression of the sanctity of individual free choice and self-determination as fundamental constituents of life. The value of life as so perceived is lessened not by a decision to refuse treatment, but by the failure to allow a competent human being the right of choice.[9]

A second interest of considerable magnitude, which the State may have some interest in asserting, is that of protecting third parties, particularly minor children, from the emotional and financial damage which may occur as a result of the decision of a competent adult to refuse lifesaving or life-prolonging treatment. Thus, in *Holmes v. Silver Cross Hosp. of Joliet, Ill.,* 340 F.Supp. 125 (D.Ill.1972), the court held that, while the State's interest in preserving an individual's life was not sufficient, by itself, to outweigh the individual's interest in the exercise of free choice, the possible impact on minor children would be a factor which might have a critical effect on the outcome of the balancing process. Similarly, in the *Georgetown* case the court held that one of the interests requiring protection was that of the minor child in order to avoid the effect of "abandonment" on that child as a result of the parent's decision to refuse the necessary medical measures. See Byrn, *supra* at 33; *United States v. George, supra.*[10] We need not reach this aspect of claimed State interest as it is not in issue on the facts of this case.

The last State interest requiring discussion[11] is that of the maintenance of the ethical integrity of the medical profession as well as allowing hospitals the full opportunity to care for people under their control. See *Georgetown, supra; United States v. George, supra; John F. Kennedy Memorial Hosp. v. Heston, supra.* The force and impact of this interest is lessened by the prevailing medical ethical standards, see Byrn, *supra* at 31. Prevailing medical ethical practice does not, without exception, demand that all efforts toward life prolongation be made in all circumstances. Rather, as indicated in *Quinlan,* the prevailing ethical practice seems to be to recognize that the dying are more often in need of comfort than treatment. Recognition of the right to refuse necessary treatment in appropriate circumstances is consistent with existing medical mores; such a doctrine does not threaten either the integrity of the medical profession, the proper role of hospitals in caring for such patients or the State's interest in protecting the same. It is not necessary to deny a right of self-determination to a patient in order to recognize the interests of doctors, hospitals, and medical personnel in attendance on the patient. Also, if the doctrines of informed consent and right of privacy have as their foundations the right to bodily integrity, see *Union Pac. Ry. v. Botsford,* 141 U.S. 250, 11 S.Ct. 1000, 35 L.Ed. 734 (1891), and control of one's own fate, then those rights are superior to the institutional considerations.[12]

Applying the considerations discussed in this subsection to the decision made by the probate judge in the circumstances of the case before us, we are satisfied that his decision was consistent with a proper balancing of applicable State and individual interests. Two of the four categories of State interests that we have identified, the protection of third parties and the prevention of suicide, are inapplicable to this case. The third, involving the protection of the ethical integrity of the medical profession was satisfied on two grounds. The probate judge's decision was in accord with the testimony of the attending physicians of the patient. The decision is in accord with the generally accepted views of the medical profession, as set forth in this opinion. The fourth State interest—the preservation of

life—has been viewed with proper regard for the heavy physical and emotional burdens on the patient if a vigorous regimen of drug therapy were to be imposed to effect a brief and uncertain delay in the natural process of death. To be balanced against these State interests was the individual's interest in the freedom to choose to reject, or refuse to consent to, intrusions of his bodily integrity and privacy. We cannot say that the facts of this case required a result contrary to that reached by the probate judge with regard to the right of any person, competent or incompetent, to be spared the deleterious consequences of life-prolonging treatment. We therefore turn to consider the unique considerations arising in this case by virtue of the patient's inability to appreciate his predicament and articulate his desires.

B.

[5] The question what legal standards govern the decision whether to administer potentially life-prolonging treatment to an incompetent person encompasses two distinct and important subissues. First, does a choice exist? That is, is it the unvarying responsibility of the State to order medical treatment in all circumstances involving the care of an incompetent person? Second, if a choice does exist under certain conditions, what considerations enter into the decision-making process?

We think that principles of equality and respect for all individuals require the conclusion that a choice exists. For reasons discussed at some length in subsection A, *supra,* we recognize a general right in all persons to refuse medical treatment in appropriate circumstances. The recognition of that right must extend to the case of an incompetent, as well as a competent, patient because the value of human dignity extends to both.

This is not to deny that the State has a traditional power and responsibility, under the doctrine of parens patriae, to care for and protect the "best interests" of the incompetent person. Indeed, the existence of this power and responsibility has impelled a number of courts to hold that the "best interests" of such a person mandate an unvarying responsibility by the courts to order necessary medical treatment for an incompetent person facing an immediate and severe danger to life. *Application of the President*

& *Directors of Georgetown College, Inc.*, 118
U.S.App.D.C. 80, 331 F.2d 1000, cert. denied,
377 U.S. 978, 84 S.Ct. 1883, 12 L.Ed.2d 746
(1964). *Long Island Jewish-Hillside Medical
Center v. Levitt*, 73 Misc.2d 395, 342 N.Y.S.2d
356 (N.Y.Sup.Ct.1973). Cf. *In re Weberlist*, 79
Misc.2d 753, 360 N.Y.S.2d 783 (N.Y.Sup.
Ct.1974). Whatever the merits of such a policy
where lifesaving treatment is available—a situation unfortunately not presented by this case—a
more flexible view of the "best interests" of the
incompetent patient is not precluded under other
conditions. For example, other courts have refused to take it on themselves to order certain
forms of treatment or therapy which are not immediately required although concededly beneficial to the innocent person. *In re CFB*, 497
S.W.2d 831 (Mo.App.1973). *Green's Appeal*,
448 Pa. 338, 292 A.2d 387 (1972). *In re Frank*, 41
Wash.2d 294, 248 P.2d 553 (1952). Cf. *In re Rot-
kowitz*, 175 Misc. 948, 25 N.Y.S.2d 624 (N.Y.
Dom.Rel.Ct.1941); *Mitchell v. Davis*, 205 S.W.
2d 812 (Tex.App.1947). While some of these
cases involved children who might eventually be competent to make the necessary decisions without judicial interference, it is also clear
that the additional period of waiting might make
the task of correction more difficult. See, e.g., *In
re Frank, supra*. These cases stand for the proposition that, even in the exercise of the parens
patriae power, there must be respect for the bodily integrity of the child or respect for the rational decision of those parties, usually the parents, who for one reason or another are seeking
to protect the bodily integrity or other personal
interest of the child. See *In re Hudson*, 13
Wash.2d 673, 126 P.2d 765 (1942).

[6] The "best interests" of an incompetent
person are not necessarily served by imposing
on such persons results not mandated as to competent persons similarly situated. It does not advance the interest of the State or the ward to
treat the ward as a person of lesser status or
dignity than others. To protect the incompetent
person within its power, the State must recognize the dignity and worth of such a person and
afford to that person the same panoply of rights
and choices it recognizes in competent persons.
If a competent person faced with death may
choose to decline treatment which not only will
not cure the person but which substantially may
increase suffering in exchange for a possible yet
brief prolongation of life, then it cannot be said

that it is always in the "best interests" of the
ward to require submission to such treatment.
Nor do statistical factors indicating that a majority of competent persons similarly situated
choose treatment resolve the issue. The significant decisions of life are more complex than
statistical determinations. Individual choice is
determined not by the vote of the majority but
by the complexities of the singular situation
viewed from the unique perspective of the person called on to make the decision. To presume
that the incompetent person must always be subjected to what many rational and intelligent persons may decline is to downgrade the status of
the incompetent person by placing a lesser value
on his intrinsic human worth and vitality.

The trend in the law has been to give incompetent persons the same rights as other individuals.
Boyd v. Registrars of Voters of Belchertown, 368
Mass. ——[c], 334 N.E.2d 629 (1975). Recognition
of this principle of equality requires understanding that in certain circumstances it may be
appropriate for a court to consent to the withholding of treatment from an incompetent individual. This leads us to the question of how the
right of an incompetent person to decline treatment might best be exercised so as to give the
fullest possible expression to the character and
circumstances of that individual.

The problem of decision-making presented in
this case is one of first impression before this
court, and we know of no decision in other jurisdictions squarely on point. The well publicized
decision of the New Jersey Supreme Court in *In
re Quinlan*, 70 N.J. 10, 355 A.2d 647 (1976), provides a helpful starting point for analysis, however.

Karen Ann Quinlan, then age twenty-one,
stopped breathing for reasons not clearly identified for at least two fifteen-minute periods on
the night of April 15, 1975. As a result, this formerly healthy individual suffered severe brain
damage to the extent that medical experts
characterized her as being in a "chronic persistent vegetative state." *Id.* at 24, 355 A.2d 647.
Although her brain was capable of a certain degree of primitive reflex-level functioning, she
had no cognitive function or awareness of her
surroundings. Karen Quinlan did not, however,
exhibit any of the signs of "brain death" as iden-

---

c. Mass.Adv.Sh. (1975) 2853.

tified by the Ad Hoc Committee of the Harvard Medical School.[13] She was thus "alive" under controlling legal and medical standards. *Id.* at 25, 355 A.2d 647. Nonetheless, it was the opinion of the experts and conclusion of the court that there was no reasonable possibility that she would ever be restored to cognitive or sapient life. *Id.* at 26, 355 A.2d 647. Her breathing was assisted by a respirator, without which the experts believed she could not survive. It was for the purpose of getting authority to order the disconnection of the respirator that Quinlan's father petitioned the lower New Jersey court.

The Supreme Court of New Jersey, in a unanimous opinion authored by Chief Justice Hughes, held that the father, as guardian, could, subject to certain qualifications,[14] exercise his daughter's right to privacy by authorizing removal of the artificial life-support systems. *Id.* at 55, 355 A.2d 647. The court thus recognized that the preservation of the personal right to privacy against bodily intrusions, not exercisable directly due to the incompetence of the rightholder, depended on its indirect exercise by one acting on behalf of the incompetent person. The exposition by the New Jersey court of the principle of substituted judgment, and of the legal standards that were to be applied by the guardian in making this decision, bears repetition here.

"If a putative decision by Karen to permit this non-cognitive, vegetative existence to terminate by natural forces is regarded as a valuable incident of her right of privacy, as we believe it to be, then it should not be discarded solely on the basis that her condition prevents her conscious exercise of the choice. The only practical way to prevent destruction of the right is to *permit the guardian and family of Karen to render their best judgment,* subject to the qualifications [regarding consultation with attending physicians and hospital 'Ethics Committee'] hereinafter stated, *as to whether she would exercise it in these circumstances.* If their conclusion is in the affirmative this decision should be accepted by a society the overwhelming majority of whose members would, we think, in similar circumstances, exercise such a choice in the same way for themselves or for those closest to them. It is for this reason that we determine that Karen's right of privacy may be asserted in her behalf, in this respect, by her guardian and family under the particular circumstances presented by this

record" (emphasis supplied). *Id.* at 41–42, 355 A.2d 647.

The court's observation that most people in like circumstances would choose a natural death does not, we believe, detract from or modify the central concern that the guardian's decision conform, to the extent possible, to the decision that would have been made by Karen Quinlan herself. Evidence that most people would or would not act in a certain way is certainly an important consideration in attempting to ascertain the predilections of any individual, but care must be taken, as in any analogy, to ensure that operative factors are similar or at least to take notice of the dissimilarities. With this in mind, it is profitable to compare the situations presented in the *Quinlan* case and the case presently before us. Karen Quinlan, subsequent to her accident, was totally incapable of knowing or appreciating life, was physically debilitated, and was pathetically reliant on sophisticated machinery to nourish and clean her body. Any other person suffering from similar massive brain damage would be in a similar state of total incapacity, and thus it is not unreasonable to give weight to a supposed general, and widespread, response to the situation.

Karen Quinlan's situation, however, must be distinguished from that of Joseph Saikewicz. Saikewicz was profoundly mentally retarded. His mental state was a cognitive one but limited in his capacity to comprehend and communicate. Evidence that most people choose to accept the rigors of chemotherapy has no direct bearing on the likely choice that Joseph Saikewicz would have made. Unlike most people, Saikewicz had no capacity to understand his present situation or his prognosis. The guardian ad litem gave expression to this important distinction in coming to grips with this "most troubling aspect" of withholding treatment from Saikewicz: "If he is treated with toxic drugs he will be involuntarily immersed in a state of painful suffering, the reason for which he will never understand. Patients who request treatment know the risks involved and can appreciate the painful side-effects when they arrive. They know the reason for the pain and their hope makes it tolerable." To make a worthwhile comparison, one would have to ask whether a majority of people would choose chemotherapy if they were told merely that something outside of their previous experience was going to be done to them, that this something would cause them pain and discomfort, that they would be removed to strange surroundings and possibly restrained for extended periods of time, and that the advantages of this course of action were measured by concepts of time and mortality beyond their ability to comprehend.

[7] To put the above discussion in proper perspective, we realize that an inquiry into what a majority of people would do in circumstances that truly were similar assumes an objective viewpoint not far removed from a "reasonable person" inquiry. While we recognize the value of this kind of indirect evidence, we should make it plain that the primary test is subjective in nature—that is, the goal is to determine with as much accuracy as possible the wants and needs of the individual involved.[15] This may or may not conform to what is thought wise or prudent by most people. The problems of arriving at an accurate substituted judgment in matters of life and death vary greatly in degree, if not in kind, in different circumstances. For example, the responsibility of Karen Quinlan's father to act as she would have wanted could be discharged by drawing on many years of what was apparently an affectionate and close relationship. In contrast, Joseph Saikewicz was profoundly retarded and noncommunicative his entire life, which was spent largely in the highly restrictive atmosphere of an institution. While it may thus be necessary to rely to a greater degree on objective criteria, such as the supposed inability of profoundly retarded persons to conceptualize or fear death, the effort to bring the substituted judgment into step with the values and desires of the affected individual must not, and need not, be abandoned.

The "substituted judgment" standard which we have described commends itself simply because of its straightforward respect for the integrity and autonomy of the individual. We need not, however, ignore the substantial pedigree that accompanies this phrase. The doctrine of substituted judgment had its origin over 150 years ago in the area of the administration of the estate of an incompetent person. *Ex parte Whitbread in re Hinde, a Lunatic,* 35 Eng.Rep. 878 (1816). The doctrine was utilized to authorize a gift from the estate of an incompetent person to an individual when the incompetent owed no duty of support. The English court accomplished this purpose by substituting itself as nearly as possible for the incompetent, and acting on the

same motives and considerations as would have moved him. *City Bank Farmers Trust Co. v. McGowan,* 323 U.S. 594, 599, 65 S.Ct. 496, 89 L.Ed. 483 (1945). In essence, the doctrine in its original inception called on the court to "don the mental mantle of the incompetent." *In re Carson,* 39 Misc.2d 544, 545, 241 N.Y.S.2d 288, 289 (N.Y.Sup.Ct.1962). Cf. *Strange v. Powers,* 358 Mass. 126, 260 N.E.2d 704 (1970).

In modern times the doctrine of substituted judgment has been applied as a vehicle of decision in cases more analogous to the situation presented in this case. In a leading decision on this point, *Strunk v. Strunk,* 445 S.W.2d 145 (Ky.Ct.App.1969), the court held that a court of equity had the power to permit removal of a kidney from an incompetent donor for purposes of effectuating a transplant. The court concluded that, due to the nature of their relationship, both parties would benefit from the completion of the procedure, and hence the court could presume that the prospective donor would, if competent, assent to the procedure. Accord, *Hart v. Brown,* 29 Conn.Supp. 368, 289 A.2d 386 (1972). But see *In re Guardianship of Pescinski,* 67 Wis.2d 4, 226 N.W.2d 180 (1975). See generally Baron and others, Life Organ and Tissue Transplants from Minor Donors in Massachusetts, 55 B.U.L.Rev. 159 (1975).[16]

[8, 9] With this historical perspective, we now reiterate the substituted judgment doctrine as we apply it in the instant case. We believe that both the guardian ad litem in his recommendation and the judge in his decision should have attempted (as they did) to ascertain the incompetent person's actual interests and preferences. In short, the decision in cases such as this should be that which would be made by the incompetent person, if that person were competent, but taking into account the present and future incompetency of the individual as one of the factors which would necessarily enter into the decision-making process of the competent person. Having recognized the right of a competent person to make for himself the same decision as the court made in this case, the question is, do the facts on the record support the proposition that Saikewicz himself would have made the decision under the standard set forth. We believe they do.

The two factors considered by the probate judge to weigh in favor of administering chemotherapy were: (1) the fact that most people elect chemotherapy and (2) the chance of a longer life. Both are appropriate indicators of what Saikewicz himself would have wanted, provided that due allowance is taken for this individual's present and future incompetency. We have already discussed the perspective this brings to the fact that most people choose to undergo chemotherapy. With regard to the second factor, the chance of a longer life carries the same weight for Saikewicz as for any other person, the value of life under the law having no relation to intelligence or social position. Intertwined with this consideration is the hope that a cure, temporary or permanent, will be discovered during the period of extra weeks or months potentially made available by chemotherapy. The guardian ad litem investigated this possibility and found no reason to hope for a dramatic breakthrough in the time frame relevant to the decision.

[10] The probate judge identified six factors weighing against administration of chemotherapy. Four of these—Saikewicz's age,[17] the probable side effects of treatment, the low chance of producing remission, and the certainty that treatment will cause immediate suffering—were clearly established by the medical testimony to be considerations that any individual would weigh carefully. A fifth factor—Saikewicz's inability to cooperate with the treatment—introduces those considerations that are unique to this individual and which therefore are essential to the proper exercise of substituted judgment. The judge heard testimony that Saikewicz would have no comprehension of the reasons for the severe disruption of his formerly secure and stable environment occasioned by the chemotherapy. He therefore would experience fear without the understanding from which other patients draw strength. The inability to anticipate and prepare for the severe side effects of the drugs leaves room only for confusion and disorientation. The possibility that such a naturally uncooperative patient would have to be physically restrained to allow the slow intravenous administration of drugs could only compound his pain and fear, as well as possibly jeopardize the ability of his body to withstand the toxic effects of the drugs.

[11] The sixth factor identified by the judge as weighing against chemotherapy was "the quality of life possible for him even if the treatment does bring about remission." To the extent that this formulation equates the value of life with any measure of the quality of life, we firmly reject it. A reading of the entire record clearly reveals, however, the judge's concern that special care be taken to respect the dignity and worth of Saikewicz's life precisely because of his vulnerable position. The judge, as well as all the parties, were keenly aware that the supposed ability of Saikewicz, by virtue of his mental retardation, to appreciate or experience life had no place in the decision before them. Rather than reading the judge's formulation in a manner that demeans the value of the life of one who is mentally retarded, the vague, and perhaps ill-chosen, term "quality of life" should be understood as a reference to the continuing state of pain and disorientation precipitated by the chemotherapy treatment. Viewing the term in this manner, together with the other factors properly considered by the judge, we are satisfied that the decision to withhold treatment from Saikewicz was based on a regard for his actual interests and preferences and that the facts supported this decision.

C.

We turn now to a consideration of the procedures appropriate for reaching a decision where a person allegedly incompetent is in a position in which a decision as to the giving or withholding of life-prolonging treatment must be made.[18] As a preliminary matter, we briefly inquire into the powers of the Probate Court in this context.

[12] The Probate Court is a court of superior and general jurisdiction. G.L. c. 215, §2. *Wilder v. Orcutt,* 257 Mass. 100, 153 N.E. 332 (1926). The Probate Court is given equity jurisdiction by statute. G.L. c. 215, §6. It has been given the specific grant of equitable powers to act in all matters relating to guardianship. G.L. c. 215, §6. *Buckingham v. Alden,* 315 Mass. 383, 387, 53 N.E.2d 101 (1944). The Probate Court has the power to appoint a guardian for a retarded person. G.L. c. 201, §6A. It may also appoint a temporary guardian of such a person where immediate action is required. G.L. c. 201, §14. Additionally, the Probate Court may appoint a guardian ad litem whenever the court believes it necessary to protect the interests of a person in a proceeding before it. *Buckingham v. Alden, supra.* This power is inherent in the court even apart from statutory authorization, and its exercise at times becomes necessary for the proper

function of the court. *Lynde v. Vose*, 326 Mass. 621, 96 N.E.2d 172 (1951). *Buckingham v. Alden, supra.*

[13] In dealing with matters concerning a person properly under the court's protective jurisdiction, "[t]he court's action . . . is not limited by any narrow bounds, but it is empowered to stretch forth its arm in whatever direction its aid and protection may be needed. . . ." *In re Quinlan,* 70 N.J. 10, 45, 355 A.2d 647, 666 (1976), quoting from 27 Am.Jur.2d Equity §69 (1966). In essence the powers of the court to act in the best interests of a person under its jurisdiction, *Petition of the Dep't of Pub. Welfare to Dispense with Consent to Adoption,* —— Mass. ——d, 358 N.E.2d 794 (1976); must be broad and flexible enough "to afford whatever relief may be necessary to protect his interests." *Strunk v. Strunk,* 445 S.W.2d 145, 147 (Ky.Ct.App.1969), quoting from 27 Am.Jur.2d Equity §69, at 592 (1966). The Probate Court is the proper forum in which to determine the need for the appointment of a guardian or a guardian ad litem. It is also the proper tribunal to determine the best interests of a ward.

In this case, a ward of a State institution was discovered to have an invariably fatal illness, the only effective—in the sense of life-prolonging—treatment for which involved serious and painful intrusions on the patient's body. While an emergency existed with regard to taking action to begin treatment, it was not a case in which immediate action was required. Nor was this a case in which life-saving, as distinguished from life-prolonging, procedures were available. Because the individual involved was thought to be incompetent to make the necessary decisions, the officials of the State institutions properly initiated proceedings in the Probate Court.

The course of proceedings in such a case is readily determined by reference to the applicable statutes. The first step is to petition the court for the appointment of a guardian. (G.L. c. 201, §6A) or a temporary guardian (G.L. c. 201, §14). The decision under which of these two provisions to proceed will be determined by the circumstances of the case, that is, whether the exigencies of the situation allow time to comply with the seven-day notice requirement prior to the hearing on the appointment of a guardian. G.L. c. 201, §§6A, 7. If appointment of a temporary guardian is sought, the probate judge will make such orders regarding notice as he deems appropriate. G.L. c. 201, §14. At the hearing on the appointment of a guardian or temporary guardian, the issues before the court are (1) whether the person involved is mentally retarded within the meaning of the statute (G.L. c. 201, §6A) and (2), if the person is mentally retarded, who shall be appointed guardian. *Id.* As an aid to the judge in reaching these two decisions, it will often be desirable to appoint a guardian ad litem, sua sponte or on motion, to represent the interests of the person. Moreover, we think it appropriate, and highly desirable, in cases such as the one before us to charge the guardian ad litem with an additional responsibility to be discharged if there is a finding of incompetency. This will be the responsibility of presenting to the judge, after as thorough an investigation as time will permit, all reasonable arguments in favor of administering treatment to prolong the life of the individual involved. This will ensure that all viewpoints and alternatives will be aggressively pursued and examined at the subsequent hearing where it will be determined whether treatment should or should not be allowed. The report of the guardian or temporary guardian will, of course, also be available to the judge at this hearing on the ultimate issue of treatment.[19] Should the probate judge then be satisfied that the incompetent individual would, as determined by the standards previously set forth, have chosen to forego potentially life-prolonging treatment, the judge shall issue the appropriate order. If the judge is not so persuaded, or finds that the interests of the State require it, then treatment shall be ordered.

[14] Commensurate with the powers of the Probate Court already described, the probate judge may, at any step in these proceedings, avail himself or herself of the additional advice or knowledge of any person or group. We note here that many health care institutions have developed medical ethics committees or panels to consider many of the issues touched on here. Consideration of the findings and advice of such groups as well as the testimony of the attending physicians and other medical experts ordinarily would be of great assistance to a probate judge faced with such a difficult decision. We believe it desirable for a judge to consider such views wherever available and useful to the court. We do not believe, however, that this option should

---

d. Mass.Adv.Sh. (1976) 2981.

be transformed by us into a required procedure. We take a dim view of any attempt to shift the ultimate decision-making responsibility away from the duly established courts of proper jurisdiction to any committee, panel or group, ad hoc or permanent. Thus, we reject the approach adopted by the New Jersey Supreme Court in the *Quinlan* case of entrusting the decision whether to continue artificial life support to the patient's guardian, family, attending doctors, and hospital "ethics committee."[20] 70 N.J. at 55, 355 A.2d 647, 671. One rationale for such a delegation was expressed by the lower court judge in the *Quinlan* case, and quoted by the New Jersey Supreme Court: "The nature, extent and duration of care by societal standards is the responsibility of a physician. The morality and conscience of our society places this responsibility in the hands of the physician. What justification is there to remove it from the control of the medical profession and place it in the hands of the courts?" *Id.* at 44, 355 A.2d at 665. For its part, the New Jersey Supreme Court concluded that "a practice of applying to a court to confirm such decisions would generally be inappropriate, not only because that would be a gratuitous encroachment upon the medical profession's field of competence, but because it would be impossibly cumbersome. Such a requirement is distinguishable from the judicial overview traditionally required in other matters such as the adjudication and commitment of mental incompetents. This is not to say that in the case of an otherwise justiciable controversy access to the courts would be foreclosed; we speak rather of a general practice and procedure." *Id.* at 50, 355 A.2d at 669.

We do not view the judicial resolution of this most difficult and awesome question—whether potentially life-prolonging treatment should be withheld from a person incapable of making his own decision—as constituting a "gratuitous encroachment" on the domain of medical expertise. Rather, such questions of life and death seem to us to require the process of detached but passionate investigation and decision that forms the ideal on which the judicial branch of government was created. Achieving this ideal is our responsibility and that of the lower court, and is not to be entrusted to any other group purporting to represent the "morality and conscience of our society," no matter how highly motivated or impressively constituted.

III.

Finding no State interest sufficient to counterbalance a patient's decision to decline life-prolonging medical treatment in the circumstances of this case, we conclude that the patient's right to privacy and self-determination is entitled to enforcement. Because of this conclusion, and in view of the position of equality of an incompetent person in Joseph Saikewicz's position, we conclude that the probate judge acted appropriately in this case. For these reasons we issued our order of July 9, 1976, and responded as we did to the questions of the probate judge.

NOTES

1. In addition to the report of the guardian ad litem, the probate judge had before him the clinical team reports of a physician, a psychologist, and a social worker, as required by G.L. c. 201, §6A. Expert testimony was taken from a staff physician of the Belchertown State School and two consulting physicians from the Baystate Medical Center, formerly Springfield Hospital.

2."1. Does the Probate Court under its general or any special jurisdiction have the authority to order, in circumstances it deems appropriate, the withholding of medical treatment from a person even though such withholding of treatment might contribute to a shortening of the life of such person?

"2. On the facts reported in this case, is the Court correct in ordering that no treatment be administered to said JOSEPH SAIKEWICZ now or at any time for his condition of acute myeloblastic monocetic leukemia except by further order of the Court?"

3. After briefly reviewing the facts of the case, we stated in that order: "Upon consideration, based upon the findings of the probate judge, we answer the first question in the affirmative, and a majority of the Court answer the second question in the affirmative. However, we emphasize that upon receiving evidence of a significant change either in the medical condition of Saikewicz or in the medical treatment available to him for successful treatment of his condition, the probate judge may issue a further order."

4. On appeal, the petitioners have collected in their brief a number of recent empirical studies which cast doubt on the view that patients over sixty are less successfully treated by chemotherapy. E. g., Bloomfield & Theologides, Acute Granulocytic Leukemia in Elderly Patients, 226 J.A.M.A. 1190, 1192 (1973); Grann and others, The Therapy of Acute Granulocytic Leukemia in Patients More Than Fifty Years Old, 80 Annals Internal Med. 15, 16 (1974). (Acute myeloblastic monocytic leukemia is a subcategory of acute

granulocytic leukemia.) Other experts maintain that older patients have lower remission rates and are more vulnerable to the toxic effects of the administered drugs. E. g., Crosby, Grounds for Optimism in Treating Acute Granulocytic Leukemia, 134 Archives Internal Med. 177 (1974). None of these authorities was brought to the consideration of the probate judge. We accept the judge's conclusion, based on the expert testimony before him and in accordance with substantial medical evidence, that the patient's age weighed against the successful administration of chemotherapy. See note 17 *infra*.

5. There was testimony as to the importance of having the full cooperation of the patient during the initial weeks of the chemotherapy process as well as during follow-up visits. For example, the evidence was that it would be necessary to administer drugs intravenously for extended periods of time—twelve or twenty-four hours a day for up to five days. The inability of Saikewicz to comprehend the purpose of the treatment, combined with his physical strength, led the doctors to testify that Saikewicz would probably have to be restrained to prevent him from tampering with the intravenous devices. Such forcible restraint could, in addition to increasing the patient's discomfort, lead to complications such as pneumonia.

6. This information comes to us from the supplemental briefs of the parties.

7. Submitting the brief for the defendant was the guardian ad litem, Patrick J. Melnik. The Attorney General submitted the brief for the plaintiffs. The Civil Rights and Liberties Division of the Department of the Attorney General prepared a brief amicus curiae on behalf of the defendant. Briefs amicus curiae were also submitted by the Mental Health Legal Advisors Committee, the Massachusetts Association for Retarded Citizens, Inc., and the Developmental Disabilities Law Project of the University of Maryland Law School.

8. While *Quinlan* would seem to limit the effect of these decisions, the opinion therein does not make clear the extent to which this is so.

9. *Commonwealth v. O'Neal,* 367 Mass. 440, 327 N.E.2d 662 (1975), does not compel a different result. That case considered the magnitude of the State interest in preserving life in the context of an intentional State deprivation. It does not apply to a situation where an individual, without State involvement, may make a decision resulting in the shortening of life by natural causes.

10. The nature of the third party interest discussed here is not one where the decision has clear, immediate, and adverse effects on the third party such as in *Raleigh Fitkin-Paul Morgan Memorial Hosp.*, *supra,* where a blood transfusion was necessary to preserve the life of a child in utero, as well as the mother. Clearly, different considerations are presented in such a case.

11. The interest in protecting against suicide seems to require little if any discussion. In the case of the competent adult's refusing medical treatment such an act does not necessarily constitute suicide since (1) in refusing treatment the patient may not have the specific intent to die, and (2) even if he did, to the extent that the cause of death was from natural causes the patient did not set the death producing agent in motion with the intent of causing his own death. Byrn, *supra* at 17–18. Cantor, *supra* at 255. Furthermore, the underlying State interest in this area lies in the prevention of irrational self-destruction. What we consider here is a competent, rational decision to refuse treatment when death is inevitable and the treatment offers no hope of cure or preservation of life. There is no connection between the conduct here in issue and any State concern to prevent suicide. Cantor, *supra* at 258.

12. Any threats of civil liability may be removed by a valid giving or withholding of consent by an informed patient. See generally Note, Statutory Recognition of the Right to Die: The California Natural Death Act, 57 B.U.L.Rev. 148 (1977), for a comprehensive discussion of the common law foundations of physicians' duties and patients' rights, one legislative attempt to modernize the law, and an analysis of the ramifications for doctors and patients of recognizing the option of withholding life-sustaining procedures from a patient incapable of indicating his or her wishes.

13. The brain death criteria developed by the Ad Hoc Committee was recently recognized by this court as a medically and legally acceptable definition of death. *Commonwealth v. Golston,* —— Mass. ——, —— – —— (Mass.Adv.Sh. [1977] 1778, 1779–1783), 336 N.E.2d 744 (1977).

14. The mandatory involvement of the family, attending doctors, and the hospital "ethics committee" was also provided for by the court. See note 20 *infra*.

15. In arriving at a philosophical rationale in support of a theory of substituted judgment in the context of organ transplants from incompetent persons, Professor Robertson of the University of Wisconsin Law School argued that "maintaining the integrity of the person means that we act toward him 'as we have reason to believe [he] would choose for [himself] if [he] were [capable] of reason and deciding rationally.' It does not provide a license to impute to him preferences he never had or to ignore previous preferences. . . . If preferences are unknown, we must act with respect to the preferences a reasonable, competent person in the incompetent's situation would have." Robertson, Organ Donations by Incompetents and the Substituted Judgment Doctrine, 76 Colum.L.Rev. 48, 63 (1976), quoting J. Rawls, A Theory of Justice 209 (1971). In this way, the "free choice and moral dignity" of the incompetent person would be recognized. "Even if we were mistaken in ascertaining his preferences, the person [if he somehow became competent] could still agree that he had been fairly

treated, if we had a good reason for thinking he would have made the choices imputed to him.'' Robertson, *supra* at 63.

16. In a similar matter before a single justice of this court, *Nathan v. Farinelli*, Suffolk Eq. 74–87, use of the doctrine was rejected, but primarily because the facts of the case involved potential conflicts of interest and made it inapplicable.

17. This factor is relevant because of the medical evidence in the record that people of Saikewicz's age do not tolerate the chemotherapy as well as younger people and that the chance of a remission is decreased. Age is irrelevant, of course, to the question of the value or quality of life.

18. We decline the invitation of several of the amicus and party briefs to formulate a comprehensive set of guidelines applicable generally to emergency medical situations involving incompetent persons. Such a wide-ranging effort is better left to the legislative branch after appropriate study.

19. We note that the probate judge in the instant case would more appropriately have appointed a temporary guardian under G.L. c. 201, §14, subsequent to an initial determination that Saikewicz was incompetent to make his own decision regarding treatment. Instead the judge appointed a guardian ad litem to discharge the duties of a general guardian. In view of the facts, however, we are of the view that nothing of substance turns on this distinction in this case. We also note the existence of some confusion and doubt concerning the power of a probate judge to appoint a temporary guardian for a mentally retarded person prior to the amendment in 1976 of G.L. c. 201, §14, by St.1976, c. 277.

20. Specifically, the court held that ''upon the concurrence of the guardian and family of Karen, should the responsible attending physicians conclude that there is no reasonable possibility of Karen's ever emerging from her present comatose condition to a cognitive, sapient state and that the life-support apparatus now being administered to Karen should be discontinued, they shall consult with the hospital 'Ethics Committee' or like body of the institution in which Karen is then hospitalized. If that consultative body agrees that there is no reasonable possibility of Karen's ever emerging from her present comatose condition to a cognitive, sapient state, the present life-support system may be withdrawn and said action shall be without any civil or criminal liability therefor on the part of any participant, whether guardian, physician, hospital or others.''

''By the above ruling we do not intend to be understood as implying that a proceeding for judicial declaratory relief is necessarily required for the implementation of comparable decisions in the field of medical practice—'' *In re Quinlan*, 70 N.J. at 55, 355 A.2d at 672.

5.3 Euthanasia Legislation: A Survey and a Model Act

RONALD P. KAPLAN, J.D.

With increasing frequency, state legislators have been proposing legislation which would permit euthanasia—the allowance of "death with dignity"—under certain circumstances. These proposals indicate varying degrees of awareness of the issues and problems involved in drafting euthanasia legislation. This Article focuses on such issues and problems, studies the methods proposed by legislators to deal with them, and offers a Model Euthanasia Act designed to achieve their optimal solution.

I. INTRODUCTION

The subject of euthanasia[1] has been given considerable attention in recent years.[2] Advances in medical technology have contributed to this increased attention, allowing growing numbers of people to live through serious illness to old age and increasing the chance of lingering death. Broad interpretation of the Constitution, as in the case of *Griswold v. Connecticut*,[3] has called attention to the individual's role in determining the time and manner of his own death.[4] Public opinion,[5] keeping pace with these medical and legal changes, also has played a role in stimulating free and open debate on euthanasia.

Consideration of euthanasia is no longer confined to the scholarly journal or the seminar in philosophy. Euthanasia is now recognized to be an issue which can affect every person. For this reason, the debate on euthanasia is taking tangible form through the filing of an increasing number of euthanasia bills in the various state legislatures. Although proposed euthanasia legislation existed as early as the 1930's,[6] only very recently have efforts at passing such legislation been made with frequency and vigor. At the time of this writing, none of the proposed euthanasia statutes have been enacted into law.

The purpose of this Article is to provide the legislator, the legislative draftsman, the individual testifying before legislative committees, and other interested parties with an analysis of the problems with which a euthanasia statute should deal, and with recommended provisions for solving those problems. The method chosen to accomplish this objective is to draw primarily upon the euthanasia bills already introduced in state legislatures and to analyze those bills for their strengths and weaknesses.

This Article begins with a discussion of some of the key terms and concepts relevant to euthanasia legislation (Part II). Next, the Article briefly reviews British and American proposals for euthanasia legislation, focusing on those proposals as examples of the variety of possible approaches (e.g., active versus passive euthanasia; voluntary versus involuntary euthanasia) to the task of drafting effective legislation (Part III). The Article then develops a series of issues with which effective legislation aimed at creating a system of *voluntary passive euthanasia* should deal and evaluates, in terms of their strengths and weaknesses, the manner in which American euthanasia bills have treated those issues (Part IV). Finally, the Article sets forth a Model Euthanasia Act which builds on the best of the earlier proposals and attempts to resolve the problems that those bills either generate or ignore (Part V).

The Model Act permits only voluntary, passive euthanasia. A detailed discussion of these terms will be found in Part II. Briefly, however, *voluntary* euthanasia as that term is used herein requires the consent of the patient to the acts or omissions constituting euthanasia. In the strictest sense this would mean, for example, that a wife could not give legally valid consent for her incompetent husband. As will be seen, however, the Model Act does not adopt this strict approach, but rather speaks of voluntary euthanasia in the sense that at some point the patient himself must have expressed competently his consent to euthanasia. Thus, the ultimate decision might well be made by a relative or physician, so long as the patient, at some time while he was competent to do so, had permitted the decision to be so made. The method used by the Model Act to accomplish this is the so-called "advance declaration."

There is no uniform view with respect to the meaning of *passive* euthanasia. It is often characterized as the omission of an act or acts, the result of the omission being an earlier death than would have occurred had the act been carried out. An example of such an omission would be the decision not to put a patient on a respirator. Such a definition, however, may be interpreted to classify activities such as turning off the respirator as active euthanasia, placing them in the same category as such obviously active measures as administering a lethal dose of some foreign substance. An alternative approach—defining euthanasia as "withholding or terminating treatment"—characterizes "pulling the plug" as passive euthanasia; this is the approach of the Model Act. The discussion of the passive-active distinction in Part II will demonstrate the importance to all legislators of fully considering their underlying approach before drafting euthanasia legislation.

Each state legislature must determine for itself which of these types of euthanasia, if any, a statute should permit. The author may not impose his judgment upon that of the legislators. His decision to restrict the Model Act to voluntary passive euthanasia is based largely on an admit-

tedly subjective desire to test the waters before diving in. In an area such as this, where neither legislators nor legislative committees can study the results of existing legislation, this author believes that the initial statutes should adopt an approach which may be narrow, but which can be studied and later expanded if found successful.

By trying to accomplish too much at first, draftsmen risk grave practical consequences such as euthanasia decisions being made by persons other than the patient who stand to profit or benefit from the patient's death. A broader statute authorizing active euthanasia also risks the loss of what may be a solid legal foundation for the statute. In the narrower (passive euthanasia) approach, it can be argued that withholding or terminating treatment of persons suffering from terminal illness or brain death is not "killing" at all. Arguably, in the case of terminal illness, the person is not killed but simply allowed to die of a pre-existing terminal condition; and, in the case of brain death, no killing exists because the person already is medically and legally dead. A statute permitting active euthanasia which allowed, for example, a lethal injection could be protested more easily than a statute permitting passive euthanasia on the ground that an active euthanasia statute legalizes killing because the injection would lead to an earlier death than would have occurred if nature had taken its course. (Query: Are the elements of man's technology now a part of "nature"? If so, does the withholding of such treatment lead to an "unnatural" death?)

In choosing to draft a voluntary passive euthanasia law, the author also was influenced by his belief that an involuntary or active euthanasia bill would have little chance of being enacted into law. Since those who introduce bills presumably do so with the intention that the bills become law, a Model Act which does not consider "passage-ability" is little more than an academic exercise. In addition, the vast majority of recent euthanasia proposals call for voluntary passive euthanasia, and the author feels that, at the present time, the most useful analysis is one which deals with the same type of legislation now confronting the legislators.

Finally, one may ask whether there is even any need for euthanasia legislation—that is, whether there may be alternatives to extensive legislation which would accomplish the same ends with less difficulty in both the implementing and operating stages. Changing the criminal laws dealing with homicide to exclude certain categories of "killings" has been suggested as one simple way to deal with euthanasia.[7] A similar but distinct approach is to make euthanasia a defense to a charge of homicide, rather than a complete exception, or, at least, to reduce sentences for euthanasia-related homicides. These approaches have been criticized, however, as not being in accord with the American system of criminal justice in which liability is founded on intent rather than on motive.[8]

Another alternative to special euthanasia legislation might be a judicial pronouncement of a state or federal constitutional "right to die." Until the recent *Karen Quinlan* case, no such pronouncement had been made; in *Quinlan,* however, the New Jersey Supreme Court found what may be at least a functional equivalent of a "right to die" in the right of a patient to decline medical treatment under certain circumstances.[9]

Even if the right enunciated in *Quinlan* survives future judicial tests, there would still be a need for legislation. First, the holding in *Quinlan* may only apply to patients whose conditions are as extreme as Karen Quinlan's. It might not apply to others whose conditions are nevertheless severe enough to warrant euthanasia.

Second, there would remain the problem of devising an appropriate mechanism for giving the constitutional pronouncement operative effect. An analogy could be drawn to the abortion cases, where, although the courts have found a constitutionally-rooted "right" to have an abortion,[10] there have been great difficulties in translating this "right" into practical terms.[11] The presence of such difficulties necessitates the creation of effective legislation to carry out any such constitutional mandate. Hence, the need for a skillfully drafted Model Act in any event.

Still another suggestion, and one which no doubt has many supporters, is simply to maintain the status quo—that is, keep the present criminal laws which make euthanasia a crime, but which at the same time allow prosecutors not to prosecute and allow sympathetic juries to acquit.[12] This alternative, while it works to a certain extent in practice, nevertheless lacks the certainty upon which physicians, among others, would like to rely. Carefully drafted legislation, on the other hand, could provide certainty in the form of fixed guidelines which constitute a "safe

harbor" for the complying physician or other person involved in the euthanasia process.

This Article is directed primarily toward those who have already determined that legislation is the most desirable vehicle for legalizing euthanasia. It focuses only peripherally on the relative merits of the above and other alternatives to legislation.[13] It is hoped, however, that even people who do not view legislation as the appropriate vehicle will profit from a consideration of the issues herein discussed.

II. SOME KEY TERMS AND CONCEPTS

This Part considers some of the basic conceptual issues involved in drafting a euthanasia statute. To some extent it overlaps with the discussion in Parts IV and V. However, it is important that the reader become acquainted at the outset with a number of key concepts which both illustrate problems of clarity of language and reflect distinctive approaches to euthanasia legislation.

A. Defining "Euthanasia"

An appropriate starting point is the term "euthanasia" itself. At least one commentator has said that ". . . euthanasia is the *taking* of human life, . . . *not* permitting death to occur or allowing the inevitable to come about."[14] A leading pro-legislation spokesman deliberately has refrained from using the term "euthanasia" in bills he has sponsored because of its connotation.[15] Significantly, these views emphasize the existence of negative connotations with respect to the term "euthanasia" as it is commonly understood;[16] equating the term "euthanasia" with "taking a life" reduces euthanasia legislation to little more than "legalized killing"—a difficult proposition to advocate.[17]

The question is whether euthanasia can be viewed as something other than "taking a life." If it can, much of the negative connotation possibly may be eliminated. It is the author's belief that in a situation where a person's illness or injury is terminal, the withholding or termination of treatment does not "kill" him by "causing" death, but simply does not prolong the inevitable. Nor does such withholding or termination of treatment "kill" a person if he has already suffered brain death, since it is, by definition, impossible to "kill" a cadaver. By drafting a euthanasia statute which permits only the termination or withholding of treatment ("passive" euthanasia), one may take a major step in combating the negative connotations which have accompanied euthanasia in the past.

Some commentators have followed the suggestions not to use the term "euthanasia."[18] The Model Act adopts this approach and also employs terminology which arguably removes euthanasia from the "killing" class and presents it instead as simply not taking steps to avoid certain death, or not continuing to treat a person whose brain has died. This distinction—"not avoiding" death, versus "killing"—is commonly phrased in terms of "passive" versus "active" euthanasia.

B. The "Active-Passive" Distinction

As previously noted in the Introduction, depending on how one defines "passive" and "active," a single statute may be interpreted as dealing differently with the same situation. The example in the Introduction involved pulling the plug on a respirator, which is passive if one supports the "withholding or terminating treatment" approach, but arguably is active under the "omission-commission" view. Another, the perhaps even more critical, example is the use of drugs administered to relieve pain[19] which, in some cases, may be known to hasten death. Is their administration passive or active euthanasia? Arguably, it is active under both definitions. Thus, a legislature enacting a passive euthanasia act might fail to protect individuals (such as the physician administering drugs to relieve pain) whom in all good faith it had intended to protect, because it had not given adequate thought to the meaning of "passive" euthanasia.

This "passive" versus "active" euthanasia controversy emphasizes the initial need to define the *substance* of these terms (i.e., situations included and excluded from the definition), and then to consider the substantive passive-active distinction as it affects the *procedure* (e.g., statutory definitions) by which the subject legislation will accomplish (or fail to accomplish) its goals. Only then can the statute expressly cover everything it was intended to cover and exclude everything else.

C. The "Voluntary-Involuntary" Distinction

The second major distinction noted in the Introduction was the "voluntary-involuntary" distinction. As previously noted, the crux of this distinction is not the extent to which the patient has participated in the euthanasia decision, but whether he has participated at all. Where the patient has not participated, ethical[20] and legal[21] arguments can be invoked to criticize the concept of euthanasia. Few informed persons would disagree with the proposition that the individual should have some say in the decision to allow his body to die.

However, there is a gray area between clear voluntariness and clear involuntariness which clouds the distinction and makes the procedure by which a voluntary euthanasia statute is structured somewhat difficult. One part of the problem is the very nature of the subject matter, for it should be clear that in many instances pain, or the effect of drugs, or perhaps simply acute depression will prevent the patient from expressing that consent which is the very manifestation of voluntariness.[22] In other words, the draftsmen of a voluntary euthanasia bill must consider the effect of the nature of the patient's condition on his ability to consent, lest persons who were intended to be covered by the act be deemed legally incompetent to consent.[23] The vehicle employed by the Model Act in an attempt to solve this problem is the so-called "advance declaration."

Even the advance declaration does not solve the problem raised by another facet of the gray area between voluntariness and involuntariness—the applicability of the statute to the minor child.[24] Unlike the incompetent patient who presumably could have expressed his consent while he was still competent, the minor never may have been able to do so because his young age may have prevented him from fully understanding the nature of the act to which he was consenting. Thus, it may be that, if a euthanasia statute is to apply to minors as well as to adults, a specific provision permitting a parent or guardian to consent on the minor's behalf will be necessary. The presence of such a provision, however, will take the statute out of the realm of truly voluntary euthanasia, and place it in the realm of legal fictions. The draftsmen must recognize this, however, if their goal is to keep their statute truly voluntary.

D. The "Withholding-Terminating" Distinction

Still another important distinction must be drawn between "withholding" and "terminating" treatment. Fortunately for the draftsmen, the line between the two is fairly clear-cut and the distinction creates few, if any, foreseeable problems. Only by permitting one without the other could a statute give rise to any great difficulties, for in that case treatment arguably could never legally be stopped once it was initiated. This is a rather obvious point which is difficult to ignore and, in fact, few legislative draftsmen have ignored it.

E. The "Mandatory-Permissive" Distinction

An additional distinction, noted here because of its importance, is that between "mandatory" legislation which *requires* that the patient's request for euthanasia be honored and "permissive" legislation which says euthanasia is *allowable* if requested. This dichotomy is considered in greater detail in subsequent parts of this Article.

F. The "Ordinary-Extraordinary" Distinction

Finally, there is the difficult distinction between "ordinary" and "extraordinary" treatment. As discussed hereinafter, a number of the recent bills fail even to raise this issue,[25] while those that do often handle this complex issue ineffectively. The importance of this distinction cannot be overstated. If a statute permits only voluntary euthanasia, then one who brings about involuntary euthanasia will be exposed to civil and criminal liability. Similarly, if only passive euthanasia is permitted, then the performance of active euthanasia will create the potential for such liability. The same logic dictates that if a statute permits only extraordinary treatment to be withheld or discontinued, then the withholding of ordinary treatment might give rise to such liability. Thus, precision in making the foregoing distinctions is essential to the adequate protection of physicians and others involved in the euthanasia process.

G. Summary

Central to this problem is the sheer difficulty in characterizing treatment as either voluntary or involuntary, active or passive, or ordinary or extraordinary in an age of rapid medical and technological advances. Correlative to this issue is the question of *who* makes the distinction and from whose perspective are the decision-making criteria viewed—that of the patient, his relatives, the physician in charge, or society as a whole. Is the line to be drawn in terms of certainty of results? Social acceptability? Longevity of use? Expense? Different frameworks produce different answers. Heart transplants, which almost certainly would have been considered extraordinary treatment by any standard several years ago, may now be considered ordinary treatment where, for example, there is a ready donor whose heart is compatible with a recipient who can afford the expense of the operation. Would failure to undertake such an operation implicitly expose a physician to liability where the euthanasia statute permits only extraordinary treatment to be withheld? If so, could this possibly have been the result intended by the legislature when it enacted the statute?

The foregoing discussion obviously has not set forth any hard and fast definitions. That task is undertaken in Parts IV and V. Part II was intended to point out that legislative draftsmen must know where they are going (i.e., the issues and situations to be covered) before they decide how to get there (the drafting of the statute). Part II hopefully has pointed out some of the key concepts and approaches which must be considered no matter what type of euthanasia statute is being drawn.

III. SURVEY OF PROPOSED EUTHANASIA LEGISLATION

A. Early Proposals

Legislative proposals dealing with euthanasia date back to the 1930's. It was in that decade that voluntary euthanasia bills were first introduced into legislatures in the United States and Great Britain. The best known early British proposal, introduced under the sponsorship of the English Euthanasia Society, was put before the House of Lords in 1936.[26] It was rather narrow in scope compared with some of its modern counterparts, but it failed to pass largely because its procedural safeguards (e.g., forms and certificates to be signed by the patient in the presence of witnesses, and interviews of the patient by a "referee") were felt by its opponents to "bring too much formality into the sickroom."[27] This British proposal was limited to voluntary euthanasia performed on mentally competent adults. It did not distinguish between passive and active means.[28] A major failing of this early proposal was its paradoxical treatment of the competency requirement: on the one hand, euthanasia could be performed only on a consenting adult who was competent; on the other hand, the patient was also required to be suffering from a terminal and incurable illness.[29] As noted in Part II, arguably the very nature of a terminal illness prevents the terminal patient from giving competent consent. As hereinafter discussed, subsequent American proposals have introduced the idea of an "advance declaration of intent" designed to eliminate this problem.

Following the British lead, the American Euthanasia Society was formed in 1938.[30] The Society immediately drafted a proposal that was submitted, in slightly different forms, in both the New York and Nebraska Assemblies;[31] both bills were defeated.[32] Although the American bills were similar to the British proposal, a greater role for the courts was added with respect to the approval of applications for euthanasia.[33] The Nebraska bill differed from both the New York and British proposals in two respects: it authorized a limited form of involuntary euthanasia, allowing certain competent adults to consent on behalf of minors and mentally incompetent adults; and it provided that euthanasia could be performed even where the illness was not terminal.[34] This latter feature of the Nebraska bill has not appeared in any subsequent legislative proposal, although some recent bills have included somewhat analogous provisions.[35]

B. Proposals Made During the Late Sixties and Early Seventies

After these early defeats, the legislative push waned for a lengthy period. Then, perhaps due to previously described circumstances, such as advances in medical technology, broader interpretation of Constitutional rights, and public opinion, the issue gathered renewed momentum in the late 1960's. In 1969 the proposed Voluntary Euthanasia Act in Great Britain became the first serious attempt at euthanasia legislation since the early failures.[36] This proposal included the use of the "advance certificate of intent" in order to circumvent partially the competency problem.[37] As did the 1936 proposal, it failed to distinguish clearly between active and passive forms of euthanasia; the definition of euthanasia that was used—"the painless inducement of death"[38]—was quite vague. The advance certificate of intent, in which the declarant requests that ". . . no active steps should be taken . . . to prolong my life . . . ,"[39] suggested that the Act permitted active euthanasia for it did not bar active steps taken to cause the declarant's death. Elaborate procedural safeguards, which had been criticized for their formality, were for the most part replaced by a thirty-day waiting period before the application for euthanasia became effective.[40] The 1969 proposal nevertheless failed to pass; once again, the reasons given were poor drafting, vague definition of terms, and procedural difficulties.[41]

In 1970, legislative effort related to euthanasia was reactivated in the United States, this time in Florida. Rep. Walter W. Sackett, Jr., himself a physician, had in 1969 introduced, as an amendment to the Florida Constitution, a proposal[42] dealing with the "right to death with dignity."[43] After the amendment failed, Rep. Sackett reintroduced his proposal in the Florida House of Representatives in the form of a proposed statute.[44] The bill, which passed the House, but died on the Senate Calendar, declared the existence of an inalienable right to die with dignity, the first legislative proposal to do so, although many subsequent bills have included a similar section. The bill also incorporated the advance declaration of intent.[45] But in stating that life ". . . shall not be prolonged beyond the point of meaningful existence . . ." the bill was unclear as to whether it permitted cessation of extraordinary treatment only, or of ordinary measures of prolonging life as well. Some subsequent proposals have been more explicit in this regard.

C. Recent Proposals

Since 1969, at least 35 bills[46] dealing with some form of euthanasia[47] have been introduced in some 22 state legislatures (including Florida). A number of these bills were introduced only recently and have not yet had a chance to progress. Of those bills that have been introduced, the great majority have died in committee. In fact, as of the time of this writing, only two bills have survived to the point of a House or Senate vote.[48] Not one has been enacted into law.

The bills encompass a variety of approaches to euthanasia legislation. They vary greatly as to precision of terms, procedural complexities, and control of potential abuses. Nevertheless, there exist a few generalizations about them that can be made fairly.

The great majority of the bills permit only passive euthanasia. These are usually characterized by language to the effect that medical treatment may be withheld or discontinued. Of the half-dozen or so bills which clearly are not passive in nature, only one is clear as to whether or not it permits active as well as passive euthanasia.[49] The uncertainty generally arises from having the patient consent to "the administration of euthanasia," with euthanasia defined as "the painless inducement of death." Such language reasonably might or might not be read to permit active as well as passive euthanasia.

The only bill which clearly permits active euthanasia is A.B. 1207 in Wisconsin. That bill provides that "any person may request any person 14 years of age or older to terminate the life of the requestor." The requestor may be as young as seven years of age, and the request may be oral. The possibilities for abuse of such a proposal are staggering.

The proportion of voluntary to involuntary bills is about equal to that of passive to active bills. The bills classified as involuntary are those which permit euthanasia in the case of one who has neither consented to it nor consented to let someone else make the decision. Some of the involuntary measures permit only relatives to consent on behalf of the patient.[50] Others permit the physician, the attorney, or even a mere friend to do so.[51] However, the latter type afford some protection against abuse in that they require court approval of any euthanasia decision in which the patient himself did not participate.

Oddly enough, the greatest common denominator among the legislative proposals appears to be the almost total absence of bills which *require* that the patient's request for euthanasia be honored. Considering that the de-

sire to create a *legally binding* document is one of the reasons commonly given in support of euthanasia legislation,[52] this absence is alarming. Only H.B. 1082, proposed in Missouri, and H.B. 618, proposed in Illinois, purport to give the patient's request some binding effect by punishing the physician who fails to honor it.[53] Several other bills announce the duty of a physician to transfer the patient to another physician if the transfering physician refuses to comply with the patient's request, but include no punishment if a transfer is not made.[54] The great majority of bills simply exempt from liability those physicians who perform authorized euthanasia, but say nothing about the physician who refuses to do so.[55]

Another common denominator among most of the recent proposals is their failure to define adequately the type of treatment which may be withheld or terminated. The problem typically lies in the difficulty of adequately drawing the line between ordinary and extraordinary treatment. A few bills, however, do not even make the effort and therefore arguably permit even ordinary treatment to be terminated or withheld.[56]

At first, the author had intended to place each bill into one of several broad categories and to select one representative bill from each category for detailed analysis in Part IV. However, because many of the bills are similar in some respects but very different in others and because some of the more unique bills nevertheless contain one or more provisions of particular interest, it seems preferable to draw from all the bills as illustrations of different approaches to some of the key issues involved in drafting euthanasia legislation. This Article now turns to that task.

IV. LEARNING FROM THE PAST: SOME GUIDELINES FOR A MODEL ACT

This Part enumerates the key issues with which the Model Act should deal and evaluates the strengths and weaknesses of provisions in post-1969 American euthanasia bills which have purported to deal with these issues. To a large extent, the material presented here records the author's thought processes in moving from those proposals to the actual drafting of the Model Euthanasia Act set forth in Part V of this Article. The discussion here, combined with the analysis of the Model Act in Part V, should help the reader to understand the intended function of the Act.

The ultimate goal is to draft a Model Act using language that evidences both a recognition of the potential problem areas and an unambiguous approach to resolving them. Many of the American proposals have failed to achieve one or both of these goals. This Part is organized to permit the reader to observe that the Model Act was drafted in a manner that recognized and dealt with potential problems.

A. The "Right to Die"

Some of the recent American euthanasia proposals include as an introductory provision the declaration of a "right to death with dignity."[57] Whether such a right actually exists under federal or state constitutions is a question too broad for extensive discussion in this Article.[58] The relevance of the question to the drafting of the Model Act lies in whether a declaration of a right to die—a right which arguably does not exist under such constitutions—has any effect on the validity of the Act and, if so, what that effect is.

The mere absence of such a right (either express or implied) under federal or state constitutions should not render invalid the Act if it declares the existence of such a right. The Act would be invalid only if shown to be unconstitutional. Being based upon something other than a constitutional right does not make a statute unconstitutional, for if it did, few statutes would be valid. Rather than focusing upon the existence or nonexistence of a right to die, the important question is whether euthanasia legislation in general, and the Model Act in particular, violates or abridges some other federal or state constitutional right that we know does exist. Because of the state to state variation in constitutional provisions, the following discussion will focus on those rights arising under the federal constitution only.

The logical right to consider is the right to ". . . *life,* liberty, and the pursuit of happiness. . . ." Would a euthanasia statute violate a federal constitutional "right to life?" It might if the "right to life" were absolute. But clearly it is not absolute.[59] Exceptions have been carved out in a number of areas, and, therefore, the existence of a "right to life" should not necessarily preclude the existence of a "right to die" as well.

In sum, if euthanasia legislation in general, and the Model Act in particular, is unconstitutional, it is not so because of the inclusion of a provision declaring the existence of a right to die. While such a provision adds little, if anything, to the substance of the Act (it is for this reason that it is omitted from the Model Act), a legislature desiring to include it in legislation for its own reasons would not be remiss in so doing.

B. Type of Euthanasia Permitted

The author's reasons for choosing to write a Model Act limited to voluntary passive euthanasia have already been given in Part I. The author further pointed out in Part III that most of the American bills have likewise been confined to this type of euthanasia.

Assuming, then, that the voluntary and passive decisions have been made, the next question is how to draft the Model Act so as to avoid ambiguity surrounding these issues. The bills that have had the most difficulty in this area are the ones that have permitted the physician to "administer euthanasia," where euthanasia is defined as "the painless inducement of death."[60] Such language arguably permits active as well as passive euthanasia, since a fatal injection, for example, might painlessly induce death. It is sufficiently vague, however, to raise the possibility that a passive bill was intended, but was poorly drafted.

The potentially disastrous results of such ambiguities perhaps can be prevented by the avoidance of general terms like "the painless inducement of death," and, in fact, by the avoidance of the word "euthanasia" altogether. The problem with the word "euthanasia" is that any verb preceding it (administer; perform; bring about; cause; etc.), tends to suggest the performance of an affirmative act—namely, *active* euthanasia. Such an interpretation is acceptable for purposes of general discussion but creates real problems in a statute.

Rather than using the word "euthanasia," the more explicit statutes simply delineate the permitted acts or omissions wherever explanation is needed. Thus, a qualified patient may be permitted to ". . . refuse the use of medical or surgical means or procedures calculated to prolong the person's life . . . ;"[61] or to ". . . execute a document directing that no maintenance medical treatment be utilized for the prolongation of his life . . . ;"[62] or to ". . . execute in writing a dated document directing that . . . medical treatment . . . not be effectuated or, if said medical treatment is being effectuated, that it be discontinued."[63] Both the awkward use of the term "euthanasia" and the resulting confusion concerning the permitting of active euthanasia are thus avoided.

The previous examples also illustrate different approaches to the question of whether a given passive statute permits both the withholding and the termination of treatment. Part II emphasized that there is little difficulty in drafting language that clearly carries out the legislature's intent in this respect; all that is required, therefore, is the recognition of the issue.[64] Each of the three examples given above arguably permits both the withholding and termination of treatment, but the third example is superior to the others in that it actually spells out the distinction between withholding ("not be effectuated") and terminating ("be discontinued") treatment.

Whether to permit the withholding and termination of ordinary or only of extraordinary treatment, and how to distinguish between them, are two of the most difficult problems facing would-be draftsmen. As noted in Part II, potential physician liability may result if the distinction never is made[65] or, if made, is done inadequately.[66] On the other hand, this distinction between ordinary and extraordinary treatment may be merely illusory since, arguably, in the case of a qualified patient (e.g., one with a terminal illness), even the most basic treatment may be "extraordinary" in the sense that it cannot cure a terminal illness.

This paradox is illustrated by a number of provisions which are typical of recent attempts to draw the ordinary-extraordinary distinction. A number of draftsmen have permitted refusal of "medical treatment designed solely to sustain the life processes."[67] Others have drafted such provisions in somewhat greater detail. An example of this kind of provision is contained in an Iowa bill which permits refusal of "medical treatment which induces or improves the vital signs of a patient without improving the chances for a reversal in the patient's condition."[68] The most detailed provisions are those proposed in three states to permit the refusal of:

> . . . medical treatment which, in accepted medical practice in the community[69] in

which the patient is being treated, is known as heroic or extraordinary measures designed not for the cure or recovery of the patient from the terminal condition from which the patient suffers but rather is supportive medical treatment designed solely to prevent the death of the patient . . . .[70]

One state's bill would permit the patient himself to designate the type of treatment he wishes to have terminated or withheld,[71] thereby eliminating the need for the ordinary-extraordinary determination.

Arguably, under most of these typical provisions, virtually *all* treatment could be withheld because even the most basic treatment could not cure or reverse the condition of a qualified patient. However, those definitions are drawn not in realistic terms of what the treatment *does* do or *can* do in a particular case, but rather in terms of what it generally was *designed* to do. Thus, even though a blood transfusion may do nothing to cure a given terminal patient, it is "ordinary" treatment because its purpose is to cure patients and in many instances it may do so. Sophisticated machines (e.g., dialysis) which were not designed to cure or reverse the patient's condition, on the other hand, might be deemed extraordinary and therefore their use might be withheld or terminated.

The definition quoted above is not perfect (query whether a heart transplant is ordinary or extraordinary under it). But, in a context in which all qualified patients are, by definition, terminal and incurable, it may be the best distinction that can be made.

Finally, as noted in Part II, the administration of drugs to relieve pain creates a special problem under a passive euthanasia statute because it arguably may be viewed as active euthanasia. A few bills indicate that their draftsmen have recognized this problem. One such proposal provides that:

> For the purpose of removing any doubt as to its legal effect, it is declared that a patient suffering from an irremediable condition medically thought in his case to be terminal shall be entitled to the administration of whatever quantity of drugs may be required to keep him free from pain, and such a patient in whose case severe distress cannot be otherwise relieved shall, if he so

requests, be entitled to drugs rendering him continuously unconscious.[72]

The Model Act includes a provision of this nature. If the Act did not contain such a provision, potential liability might be created in a situation where drugs are administered which hasten or cause death.

C. Who Qualifies for Euthanasia?

An effective Model Act must state precisely the state of physical condition, mental condition, or both,[73] at which the patient first qualifies for euthanasia. The most limited provisions permit euthanasia only where the patient's condition is terminal; a patient who will not, within medical certainty, *die* from whatever it is he is suffering does not qualify for euthanasia. A number of the proposals express this test with precision.[74]

Other proposals require a condition which, although severe, falls short of certain death. These bills vary, however, in their approach. One such bill requires an incurable physical illness or impairment before euthanasia is permitted.[75] Several similar bills expand on this by permitting euthanasia not only where there is incurable *physical* illness or impairment, but also where there is severe *mental* impairment.[76]

Severe mental impairment can be justified as a legitimate euthanasia-permitting condition on either of two grounds: because "brain death" is "death" in the legal sense, or because brain death is typically followed by death so that brain death is in effect a "terminal" condition. Because only a few states now have statutes defining "death" to include "brain death,"[77] the latter justification may be more persuasive at the present time. While it may therefore be true that "brain death" fits within the coverage of legislation permitting euthanasia where the patient has a disability which is diagnosed as incurable and terminal, many of the proposed statutes specify brain death as an alternative qualifying condition so that there will be no doubt as to whether or not the statute was intended to apply in cases where the brain is dead but the patient is otherwise technically "alive."

With one exception, however, the draftsmen who have included mental impairment in their bills have done so in an undesirable manner. They have declared that the patient qualifies for euthanasia when his mental disabilities have

rendered him "incapable of leading a rational existence" or have brought him "beyond the point of a meaningful existence."[78] The vagueness of such definitions stems from their highly subjective nature. The dangerous possibility exists (under the "wedge" theory[79]) that such a subjective standard for determining on whom euthanasia may be performed will be the first step on the road to indiscriminate "extinction" of the aged and others whose lives may, to some people, seem "beyond the point of a meaningful existence." Of the proposals which would permit euthanasia in cases of severe mental impairment, only the Idaho draftsmen have avoided the use of this type of subjective language.[80]

D. Advance Declaration of Intent

Having established appropriate standards for deciding who qualifies for euthanasia under the legislation, the recent proposed statutes then set up an operative provision which establishes a means for carrying out the statute's intent. In most bills, the crux of such a provision is the requirement of a declaration by the patient that he wishes euthanasia to be performed if he should qualify.[81] Some of the proposed statutes have included a form to be signed by the patient, which serves as his declaration; such statutes require that any declaration be made in substantially that form.[82] Other bills have required the execution of a document but have not specified any particular form to be followed.[83]

Specified declaration forms are important. If patients are allowed to use their own form of declaration, they might "authorize" a type of euthanasia (e.g., "active" euthanasia) which is not permitted by the statute. It is reasonably arguable that the *entire* declaration would thus be ruled invalid, even as to types of euthanasia which *are* permitted by the statute. The use of a uniform declaration form which all persons substantially must follow avoids this problem by enabling the draftsmen to include in the patient's declaration all types of euthanasia which are permitted under the statute and only those types.[84]

The use of the "advance declaration" is a mechanism for getting the patient's consent to euthanasia. The advance declaration requirement—or any requirement stipulating the need for consent—limits allowable euthanasia to the voluntary variety. Only with the patient's written consent would euthanasia be allowed. Few proposed bills, however, have provided specifically that the written declaration is conclusive (in the absence of fraud or coercion) evidence of the patient's consent. For the most part, the proposed bills simply have enumerated safeguards which tend to suggest that the patient has in fact consented to euthanasia. Such safeguards include (in addition to the almost universal requirement that the declaration be in writing) requirements that the declaration be witnessed,[85] that it be notarized,[86] that it include the patient's fingerprints,[87] and that it be filed with a court or other appropriate authority.[88] Some proposals simply require that the declaration be made with the same formalities required by that state for the execution of a will.[89]

As noted in Part II, the fact that valid consent cannot be given by one who is incompetent raises the possibility that a dying or severely injured patient, perhaps influenced by pain and drugs and not thinking clearly, will be legally incapable of giving or withdrawing his consent. This might create a paradox in which voluntary euthanasia could be carried out only if the patient were both rational (for consent purposes) and irrational (e.g., in great pain, for purposes of qualifying for euthanasia) at the same time.[90] This situation is avoided in the Model Act by the use of the advance declaration of intent, which permits an individual to consent to euthanasia while he is healthy. If he subsequently becomes incompetent, his prior consent will still be valid, although in such situations he would also be incapable of withdrawing his consent. In any event, euthanasia, of course, could not be performed until the qualifications discussed earlier had been met.

Of the many American proposals which have incorporated the concept of the advance declaration, some have done so by permitting "any person" to execute a declaration.[91] The language used in these bills makes it unmistakable that "any person" includes even those persons not suffering from a qualifying illness or injury at the time of such execution.[92]

The bills vary in the length of time the declaration remains effective. Almost all the bills put no limit on the effective period of the declaration, but only one bill does this by express language.[93] The other bills imply lifetime validity (absent express revocation) by saying nothing to the contrary. Only two bills limit the period during

which the declaration is effective. One such bill is S.B. 179, Oregon Legislature (1973), which provides that:

1. Subject to the provisions of this section, a declaration shall come into force 30 days after being made and shall remain in force, unless revoked, for three years.
2. A declaration re-executed after the lapse of one year from its execution date and prior to its expiration date shall remain in force, unless revoked, during the lifetime of the declarant.[94]

The danger with such a provision is that a declarant is too likely to make his declaration once and forget about re-executing it a year later, thinking his initial consent is good forever.

The absence from virtually all of the American bills of any provision *requiring* that the advance declaration be honored and euthanasia performed was considered in Part III. Instead, the majority of bills permit physicians to decline any involvement in the euthanasia process.[95] There is an obvious conflict between assuring a patient that his declaration will be honored and simply permitting the doctor not to take part. It is important for the legislature to be concerned with all persons involved in the performance of euthanasia—the doctor as well as the patient. Yet, by making euthanasia discretionary with the physician even though the patient has requested it, the majority of bills seem to be more concerned with the doctor than with the patient. One may question whether such emphasis undercuts the stated purpose of euthanasia legislation, which almost always focuses on the patient's right to death with dignity.

E. Vicarious Consent

Most of the American bills have provided for truly voluntary euthanasia by requiring the declaration to be signed by the person on whom euthanasia is to be performed.[96] Others, however, delve into the gray area described in the discussion of the voluntary-involuntary dichotomy in Part II by permitting euthanasia even though the patient himself never has consented to it. Each of the bills which permits "vicarious consent" allows such consent to be given on behalf of mental incompetents.[97] Two of these bills additionally allow vicarious consent to be given on behalf of minors.[98]

Unfortunately, the language used in a majority of the bills to describe those persons for whom vicarious consent may be given is so broad that it arguably includes more than just mental incompetents. For example, S.B. 670, Wisconsin Legislature (1971), allows vicarious consent on behalf of minors and on behalf of:

> . . . an adult who is physically or mentally unable to execute or is otherwise incapacitated from executing such document. . . .

This language covers not only mental incompetents, but *all* persons suffering from a terminal illness who have not signed a declaration.

The danger of such a provision is illustrated by the hypothetical case of a man who wants to be kept alive as long as possible; he does not want euthanasia, even though he may qualify for it, and refuses throughout his entire competent life to sign a declaration authorizing it. He becomes terminally ill and comatose. Under the type of provision quoted above, his spouse or some other person then might be allowed to authorize euthanasia, despite the fact that the patient never wanted it. The problem lies in the fact that although a person's declaration in favor of euthanasia will result in the performance of euthanasia,[99] his failure to sign a declaration does not set up a conclusive presumption that he does *not* want euthanasia. In some cases such a presumption indeed would be unwarranted; for example, failure to sign a declaration may be due to ignorance of one's statutory power to do so rather than opposition to euthanasia. In other cases, however, the individual's failure to sign a declaration will in fact be due to his affirmative desire that euthanasia not be performed.

At least one state legislature has recognized this problem and attempted to resolve it.[100] However, its requirement that the patient must have expressed affirmatively his preference against euthanasia puts the burden on the *patient* to make it clear that he *does not* want euthanasia. Such a burden would require each person, upon reaching the age of majority, to sign a document either authorizing euthanasia or rejecting it. This may be onerous; but the alternative—permitting involuntary euthanasia

—may be contrary to the intentions of the draftsmen.

The bills which do permit vicarious consent vary in several respects. Most such bills enumerate a number of the patient's relatives who may consent on the patient's behalf;[101] on the other hand, one bill allows only relatives of "first degree kinship" to give consent.[102] Some bills permit not only relatives, but friends, attorneys,[103] or physicians[104] to consent vicariously. Some bills list the priority by which the person who may make the decision is selected;[105] others, by not doing so, may result in confusion over who makes the decision in a given case.[106] None of the statutes permitting vicarious consent require that the person giving vicarious consent disclaim his right to any portion of the patient's estate so as to assure that self-interest will not affect the consenting individual's decision.

F. Revocation of Consent

Few of the proposed statutes lock the individual into his initial decision to consent to euthanasia. Some bills establish a short waiting period before the declaration becomes effective;[107] such a provision serves little apparent purpose, since the individual may change his mind after the waiting period. A better method (which is utilized in almost all the present bills) permits the individual to revoke his consent to euthanasia.[108] The bills vary with respect to when the revocation must be made, who may make it, and how it may be made.

The bills are virtually unanimous in permitting a declaration to be revoked "at any time." Some bills state this explicitly,[109] while others say nothing and thereby permit it by implication. Either approach exposes the statute to the potential problem of the patient who, having executed a declaration while healthy, has a change of heart after becoming terminally ill. For the same reasons (i.e., drugs, pain, depression) that consent may not be valid during terminal illness or injury, revocation of consent also may not be valid. Thus the situation may arise in which the patient revokes his consent, but his family, not wishing to see him suffer and perhaps also influenced by the financial burden of keeping him in a "semi-living" state, strenuously contends that he "did not know what he was doing," and argues that the physician is bound by statute to withhold treatment pursuant to the original declaration. Of the American proposals, only one expressly permits a revocation whether or not the patient is competent.[110]

It may be, however, that the failure to recognize this problem has no effect on the statutes. If a revocation made while one is a qualified patient is invalid as a matter of law, then the statutes permitting revocation "at any time" must be read as permitting revocation "at any time before becoming a qualified (and therefore presumably legally incompetent) patient," whether or not the statute contains such limiting language. Nevertheless, there may be some value in expressly stating in the statute those limitations the law would imply anyway, in order that the declarant be informed of the legal limitation on revocation. On the other hand, to do so would prevent revocation by terminal patients who, because of the nature of their particular case, were in fact competent to revoke even though terminally ill or injured. On balance, the simple "at any time" language used by the majority of the states, though imperfect, may be the best approach to the question of when a declaration may be revoked.

Most of the bills are also in agreement concerning *who* may revoke a declaration. In only a few bills is a person other than the declarant himself expressly permitted to revoke a declaration, and, even in such bills, revocation by another must be made at the declarant's order.[111] American draftsmen uniformly have been careful to avoid language which creates some ambiguity regarding whether a person other than the declarant may revoke a declaration.[112]

In addition, the bills vary with regard to *how* the revocation must be made. Virtually all proposals permit a revocation to be made in writing, and most permit it to be made orally as well, provided that such oral revocations are properly witnessed.[113] Some states permit revocation by physical destruction[114] or by cancellation on the face of the declaration.[115]

For example, H.B. 2997, Oregon Legislature (1973), provides as follows:

> Revocation may be accomplished by destroying such document [declaration of intent], or by contrary indication expressed in the presence of two witnesses 18 years of age or older.

This bill illustrates the defects found in most revocation provisions. It is too easy for the declaration document to be destroyed by someone other than the declarant, or for it to be destroyed accidentally; in the absence of specific proof by the declarant that he did not destroy the document, it might be presumed that the fact of destruction would be sufficient to constitute revocation. Although in situations in which the purpose of the destruction is unclear it might be better to err in favor of the patient's continued life rather than his death, a provision like H.B. 2997 is too broad and would establish a revocation even where clearly none was intended. In addition, since the declarant normally is instructed to give a copy of his declaration to his lawyer, his physician, his family, and his clergyman,[116] it might be difficult for him to destroy all these documents.

The other manner of revocation—revocation by "contrary indication"—is rather vague. Some bills attempted to avoid this problem by establishing a more formal procedure similar to that in H.B. 137, Montana Legislature (1973)[117] which requires a revocation request to be filed with a designated public official who, after having ascertained that the person requesting the revocation is the same person who made the declaration, will write "Revoked" across the filed copy of the declaration and refile the declaration together with the revocation request. This procedure is admirable in that it attempts to establish a central site so that revocations (and subsequent declarations) will not go unnoticed. However, the attempt fails because there is nothing in the bill designed to get the revocation from the county clerk to those persons who should know about it. As a practical matter, it is crucial that a revocation be communicated to those involved in the euthanasia process. Yet, few states have specific provisions to accomplish this.[118]

To avoid confusion where conflicting documents exist, some bills provide that the most recently dated document is controlling.[119] Few, however, clearly specify the events that will take place where an oral revocation is made. And surprisingly few require that the documents actually be dated, an important requirement if the most recently dated document is to be given effect.[120]

G. The Physician's Role

In the preceding sections issues such as the competency for consent and the point at which a patient will qualify for euthanasia have been considered. A question not heretofore discussed is: *Who decides* whether the patient is suffering from a qualifying illness or injury and whether he is competent to give consent to euthanasia? These decisions, as well as the responsibility for actually "performing" the euthanasia act or omission, typically are left to the physician.

With the exception of about a half dozen bills which do not consider the issue, all the American proposals require certification by one or more licensed physicians that the patient is suffering from one of the conditions which qualifies him for euthanasia under the state's statute. It seems appropriate that this decision be given to the physician because it falls within his area of expertise, but it cannot be overlooked that such delegation of authority also gives the physician great control over the euthanasia process.[121]

Although, as will be shown subsequently, nearly all bills provide immunity from liability for physicians who withdraw or terminate treatment pursuant to the statute, few of the bills provide immunity for physicians who certify that the patient has a qualifying illness or injury. One of the few bills that addresses the issue states that:

> Physicians who certify a terminal illness under this act are presumed to be acting in good faith. Unless it is alleged and proved that their actions violated standards of reasonable professional care and judgment under the circumstances, they are immune from civil or criminal liability for such actions.[122]

Such a provision, however, does no more than codify the common-law standard that probably would apply even in the absence of such a provision—that is, it provides little or no greater protection to the physician than would be available without it. Hence, under virtually every bill, the physician certifying the patient's qualifying condition is open to liability for negligence resulting in the death of the patient (if he has diagnosed a qualifying illness where none exists) or negligence resulting in the failure to comply with the patient's wishes (if he has failed to diagnose an existing qualifying illness).

Should a court or other delegated adjudicatory authority be utilized to certify the existence of a qualifying illness? One suggestion has been to appoint a special "euthanasia referee" to serve in such capacity.[123] If a court or referee were used, the physician's medical opinion presumably would be considered as persuasive, although not conclusive, evidence of a qualifying condition. Yet, it is hard to envision the type of evidence which might exist that could outweigh it.[124] An adjudicatory proceeding might be established for cases in which the physician's decision is disputed, but otherwise, unless there is some reason to feel that erroneous diagnoses are likely,[125] there seems to be no reason for the Model Act to depart from the practice used by the majority of the statutes, giving the ultimate authority to the physician to decide whether the patient qualifies for euthanasia.

The problem of physician participation in resolution of the question of whether the patient has the capacity to consent to or to revoke his declaration is more difficult. Pain, drugs, and mental anguish may affect the patient's ability to give valid consent; these are all within the province of the physician's expertise. But, unlike determination of the qualifying condition, which is essentially a medical issue under the proposed statutes, the determination of whether consent is valid is as much a legal issue as a medical one. The physician can provide the medical facts, but he is not qualified to determine whether the legal standard of consent has been met. Thus, proposals (such as that made in Alaska) which require the physician to ascertain whether the patient validly has authorized euthanasia probably are inadequate.[126] The better alternative is employed by a number of bills which permit the physician to presume, in the absence of some contrary knowledge, that the patient's consent was validly given, and which require the court to settle all disputes that might arise.[127]

Once it has been determined that a qualified patient validly has authorized the administration of euthanasia, the great majority of states permit treatment to be withheld or terminated only by the physician (or, in some cases, by a nurse or other medical personnel).[128] One state allows family members as well as the physician to perform euthanasia;[129] a number of others allow anyone to do so.[130] Regardless of which group is selected, the draftsmen must see to it that immunity from liability is given to all persons in that group. With one possible exception, this point has been addressed by every proposal.[131]

H. Immunity from Liability

Most American proposals include a provision removing liability for participation in euthanasia.[132] The inclusion of such a provision is crucial, since permitting physicians to become involved in the euthanasia process without fear of liability is one of the central purposes behind euthanasia legislation.

The extent to which immunity is granted varies from bill to bill. One proposal states merely that a physician performing euthanasia "shall be immune from liability."[133] Others state that such a person is "not guilty of any offense."[134] Such provisions are deficient in that they do not indicate whether the physician is protected against civil liability, criminal liability, or both. The former provision is simply vague; the latter suggests that there is no immunity from civil liability. It may be that a state employing the "not guilty of any offense" standard indeed intended to grant immunity from criminal liability only. Yet, it would be simple enough for such a state to have its statute speak in terms of "civil" and "criminal" liability so as to avoid such confusion.

A number of draftsmen have expressly avoided blanket immunity. Some of these draftsmen prescribe immunity "unless it is proved that such person [the physician] was negligent or acted in bad faith."[135] Most of these provisions are coupled with a presumption that a physician who relies on a declaration is presumed to be acting non-negligently and in good faith. In those situations where, in lieu of such presumption, the physician himself has the duty to ascertain the validity of the declaration, there is much greater chance of negligence on the physician's part.

But the majority of draftsmen who avoid blanket immunity do so by means of a good faith proviso only, with no mention of negligence. Typical of such bills is H.B. 744, Alaska Legislature (1976), which provides that:

A physician who in good faith and in accordance with the provisions of this chapter causes withdrawal of life-sustaining mechanisms is not guilty of a criminal offense or subject to civil liability for his action, and is

not in breach of a professional oath, affirmation, or standard of care.

The Alaska provision is also illustrative of those proposals which address themselves to the matter of professional responsibilities. Euthanasia legislation puts the cooperating physician in conflict with the Hippocratic Oath. The oath itself is somewhat contradictory; it requires the physician to pledge his efforts both to preserve his patient's life and to relieve his suffering.[136] Euthanasia will accomplish the latter goal, but in doing so, the physician will violate his pledge to preserve the life of his patient. It is questionable whether the Hippocratic Oath has much impact on physician conduct anyway, since many physicians admit to practicing nonstatutory euthanasia, and few, if any, are the subjects of action by the profession.[137] Once the decision is made to permit euthanasia, however, the participating physician must be protected from professional as well as civil and criminal liability.

Finally, the immunity provisions also should apply to persons who assist the physicians (e.g., nurses and medical technicians) as well as to hospitals, clinics, and other medical facilities which may be subject to liability. If, in the judgment of the legislature, participants in the euthanasia process should be immune from liability, then all such participants should be covered by their state's statute.[138]

I. Penalties for Abuse of the Statute

It was noted in Part III that only two of the proposed statutes make non-compliance with a patient's declaration a punishable offense. A number of bills, however, establish penalties for other methods of tampering with the statutory euthanasia process.

For example, S.B. 1177, Arizona Legislature (1976) provides as follows:

Any person who wilfully conceals, destroys except by direction of the maker, falsifies or forges a declaration or revocation of any other person made pursuant to this article is guilty of a felony.[139]

This provision is well-drafted because it recognizes that the statutory purpose may be abused not only by tampering with a declaration, but also by tampering with a revocation. A number of bills have failed to make this distinction.[140]

The severity of punishment varies among the proposals. Some declare tampering with a declaration or revocation to be a felony,[141] others a misdemeanor.[142] One bill specifies a punishment of life imprisonment,[143] while another declares that one who tampers with a declaration is "guilty of murder in the first degree."[144] Because the violative act is the mere *tampering* with the declaration, the criteria of the provision may be met even though euthanasia has not been performed and the patient is still alive. The impossibility of a murder without a death points up the desirability of making a violation of the provision a crime in and of itself, rather than finding the violator guilty of some other crime.

In S.B. 179, Oregon Legislature (1973), an additional distinction is made. Unlike the draftsmen in other states, the draftsmen of S.B. 179 not only recognized the need to protect against tampering with both declarations and revocations, but also drew a distinction between the two and punished the former more severely than the latter. S.B. 179 provides as follows:

1. It shall be an offense punishable, upon conviction, by a sentence of life imprisonment for any person wilfully to conceal, destroy, falsify or forge a declaration with intent to create the false impression that another person *desires* euthanasia.
2. It shall be an offense punishable, upon conviction, by a sentence up to 10 years imprisonment or a fine of up to $5,000, or both, for any person wilfully to conceal, destroy, falsify or forge a declaration with intent to create the false impression that another person *does not desire, or no longer desires,* euthanasia. [Emphasis added.]

If the purpose is to prevent abuse of the statutory machinery, such a distinction might be questioned; whereas if the purpose is to favor life over death and to prevent needless death, the distinction has merit.

J. Role of the Courts

As noted earlier, two of the American bills do not permit the execution of an advance declaration of intent, but instead require that a court be petitioned for permission to perform euthanasia.[145] Inasmuch as these bills deny to the individual the ability to make his own decision on euthanasia, they are in a sense contrary to the basic philosophy underlying the Model Act and almost all of the American proposals.

Only two of the "advance declaration" bills establish any specific role for the courts (other than as a depository for declarations, revocations, and certifications of qualifying condition).[146] These almost identical bills permit any person who is "adversely affected by an act or omission permitted or prohibited" by the proposal to bring a court action for injunctive relief in the county "in which such act or omission occurred." The bills also allow physicians to seek a declaratory judgment with regard to the validity of a declaration or revocation made by a person to whom he is administering medical treatment.

The "injunctive relief" provision if somewhat vague because it is unclear whether it can be used to attack the effectiveness of a declaration of revocation, or the acts or omissions which make up the euthanasia itself. If it is the former, it may add nothing to one's rights under general statutes permitting injunctions. If it is the latter, the use of the word "occurred" in the statute suggests that an action for injunctive relief could be brought only after euthanasia was accomplished, in which case injunctive action would obviously be moot.

The "declaratory judgment" provision, on the other hand, may well be a desirable provision, at least in those statutes which (unlike the Model Act) do not establish presumptions as to the validity of the patient's consent in the absence of knowledge by the physician to the contrary. Where a statute has established such a presumption of validity, in most cases the physician would have no need to petition a court to establish the validity or invalidity of the declaration. In special cases where the physician feels such need exists, there would seem to be no reason why he could not seek declaratory relief even in the absence of the specific provision.

Courts will, of course, serve their usual role in interpreting euthanasia statutes. However, there seems to be little reason to draft a statute which would involve a court every time a decision in favor of euthanasia is made.

K. Maintenance of Documents

Some of the proposed statutes provide for filing of declarations and revocations with the hospital in which the patient is being treated,[147] with the physician himself,[148] with the county clerk,[149] with the sheriff's office,[150] with the registrar of deeds,[151] or with some other person or office.

On the one hand, it is desirable that the Model Act specify some place which can serve as a central location of declarations and revocations. This would enable revocations to be matched with declarations so that the true intent of the patient is ascertainable. It also would enable those involved in the euthanasia process to know where to look for such documents.

On the other hand, in a mobile society, there will be many cases in which a declaration might be filed in one location and a revocation in another; or a patient might become hospitalized with a qualifying illness in a location far from the location of his declaration. In many cases, the euthanasia document simply would not be filed properly. Thus, to establish a statutory requirement for filing declarations and revocations in a specified place might well result in unwarranted assumptions that because the document is not there, there is no document. A mandatory filing provision simply undertakes too great a task. For this reason, it seems preferable to relegate to the declarant the responsibility for distributing copies of his declaration and revocation among his family, physicians, and friends, as well as seeing to it that they are included in his medical records and carried on his person at all times.

Oral revocations present a problem. Unless such oral statements are recorded mechanically, they are impossible to file. States permitting oral revocations may wish to follow the example set by S.B. 1177, Arizona Legislature (1976), and require, to the extent possible, persons having knowledge of an oral revocation to record it in writing and file it just as one would file any other euthanasia document.

L. Miscellaneous Provisions

The draftsmen in several states have included provisions which state that euthanasia shall not impair any insurance policy which has been in force for more than a prescribed length of time.[152] Such provisions, enacted independently of controlling insurance laws and of the policies themselves, may not be enforceable, and it therefore is suggested that draftsmen check the insurance laws and regulations of their respective states and ascertain the changes, if any, that would be necessary to give the insurance provisions in proposed euthanasia statutes their intended vitality.

Finally, any euthanasia statute must be squared with state laws dealing with suicides. In many states committing suicide or aiding another in committing suicide is still a crime.[153] Euthanasia, especially in its "passive" form, may not fit even conventional notions of suicide. However, the voluntary signing by the patient of a declaration authorizing euthanasia arguably brings even passive euthanasia within a broad definition of suicide. Therefore, it is advisable for the draftsmen to proceed on the assumption that laws against suicide implicitly include deaths involving euthanasia. A statutory provision should be included relieving from liability for suicide participants in the euthanasia process.[154] Prevailing laws regarding suicide should be examined to avoid all doubt and, if appropriate, rewritten to exclude death involving statutory euthanasia.

V. MODEL EUTHANASIA ACT WITH ANALYSIS

This Part sets forth and analyzes the author's model euthanasia statute. The Model Act is restricted to voluntary passive euthanasia for the reasons given in the Introduction. The overall intention of the Model Act is to provide a smooth-working voluntary passive euthanasia system which minimizes the problems heretofore considered and facilitates the resolution of those problems which are unavoidable.

The analysis of the Model Act overlaps to a certain extent with the discussion in Part IV and, to avoid repetition, will be considerably briefer than Part IV. In addition, nonproblematic portions of the Model Act are not analyzed.

The Model Act is presented section by section with an analysis immediately following each section. The analysis occasionally refers the reader to Parts I-IV of this Article.

A. Introduction and Definitions

MODEL ACT

BE IT ENACTED BY the Legislature of the State of _____ : (introductory statement of purpose may be inserted).

SECTION 1. As used in this Act, unless the context otherwise requires:

(1) "Physician" means any person licensed to practice medicine under (insert the appropriate state statutory provision).

(2) "Physician in charge" means the primary medical attendant of a person who has made (or has had made on his behalf pursuant to Section 6 of this Act) a declaration pursuant to Section 3 of this Act.

(3) "Qualified patient" means a person with respect to whom two physicians, including the physician in charge, have certified in writing that said person has an irremediable condition.

(4) "Irremediable condition" means either:

   (a) A condition of physical illness, physical injury, or other physical disability which is diagnosed as incurable and terminal; or

   (b) A condition of brain damage or deterioration such that a person's normal mental faculties are severely and irreparably impaired to such an extent that the person is deemed to have suffered brain death.

(5) "Declaration" means a declaration made pursuant to and complying with Section 3 of this Act.

(6) "Declarant" means a person on whose behalf a declaration is made.

(7) "Extraordinary medical treatment" means medical treatment which is designed solely to prolong the life of the person being given such treatment without improving the chances for a cure or reversal of his irremediable condition.

Analysis of Section I

The definitions are to apply "unless the context otherwise requires." The inclusion of such a clause carries with it the possibility for abuse, since an interested party may argue that his situation is contemplated by the phrase "otherwise requires." A specific definition should be abandoned only when it is absolutely clear that a particular case was intended to be excluded from coverage. Where it can be shown that a particular situation was not even considered by the draftsmen, the adjudicatory body can and should be less strict in adhering to the stated definitions.

For the reasons given in Part IV(B) of this Article, "euthanasia" is not defined in the Act. Instead, in Section 2 the Act refers to "withholding or terminating" treatment. This language has a two-fold advantage. It clarifies the fact that the Act permits only "passive" (as opposed to "active") euthanasia and it establishes in the simplest possible terms that the permissible passive euthanasia contemplated by the Act may include affirmative acts (e.g., pulling the plug on a respirator) as well as omissions.

The term "physician in charge" is one which rarely is used in the American proposals,[155] but which enables the statute to provide that the individual who performs or directs the performance of euthanasia will have knowledge of the patient's most recent expression of intent regarding euthanasia. Although most proposed statutes allow only the physician to perform euthanasia, many do not provide any statutory procedure to inform him that a declaration has been made or revoked.[156] Thus, as a practical matter, the patient's wishes may go unheeded. The Model Act attempts to solve this problem by defining a "physician in charge" and then tying this definition to Section 8 (requiring the physician in charge to honor the patient's declaration) and Sections 3(3), 5(4), and 9 (providing some assurance that the physician in charge will have the patient's most recent desire before him).

At the legislature's discretion, the definition of "qualified patient" may include a minimum age requirement. If it does, and if the statute also includes a vicarious consent provision (here, Section 6), the difference between the two provisions must be understood clearly. The vicarious consent provision simply circumvents the minor's common-law consent disability by allowing another to consent on his behalf. Once such vicarious consent is given, however, the minor's status as a qualified patient is not necessarily established. If the definition of "qualified patient" includes a minimum age requirement, the minor for whom vicarious consent has been given still cannot be given euthanasia until he has reached the minimum statutory age; conversely, one reaching the statutory age will not be given euthanasia automatically unless consent previously has been given. Unlike many American proposals, the Model Act omits a minimum age requirement, and thus permits the patient's condition rather than his age to be the sole determinant of whether or not he qualifies for euthanasia.

The remainder of the definition of "qualified patient" is straightforward and similar to the definition used in several of the recent legislative proposals. If there is no physician in charge for a particular patient, then one should be appointed by the hospital or board of health for purposes of this Act; failure to do so should not make the Act inapplicable, although it will negate the advantages described above with respect to the definition of a physician in charge. The two physicians who certify the existence of an irremediable condition are protected from liability by Section 7(3).

The definition of "irremediable condition" is related to that of a "qualified patient," since the latter is one who suffers from an irremediable condition. The definition chosen for the Model Act incorporates the two-fold concept of physical and mental death which was discussed in Part IV of this Article. However, it departs from the definitions used in many of the state proposals in several respects. Most notably, it eliminates completely the "incapable of leading a rational existence" standard which was employed in several of the bills.[157] Such a subjective standard only adds uncertainty to an otherwise reasonably objective definition. In addition, the Model Act definition omits the requirement, used in several bills,[158] that the condition be "expected to cause a person severe distress." This requirement is simply too vague. If "distress" means "pain," the term "pain" could easily be used. If it means something more general, it is too vague; presumably, the mere existence of a condition which is both incurable and terminal causes the patient "severe distress," so that these extra words add nothing to the definition. Admittedly, any definition short of a listing of specific illnesses and disabilities will be somewhat vague; but it is best not to add clauses which make the definition more subjective than is necessary.

The major innovation in defining "irremediable condition" is the use of the "brain death" standard in subparagraph (b). As noted earlier, the medical and forensic sciences have been attempting to define "brain death," but no single definition has emerged. Nevertheless, it is necessary to include the concept of "brain death" in subparagraph (b), because without it the defini-

tion would seem to include a large number of the mentally retarded, who are certainly not intended to be covered. Simply including the "brain death" concept in its most general terms rather than attempting to define it further has the advantage of bringing within the statute's coverage those persons whose conditions meet any of the most widely accepted definitions of "brain death." Where the state has enacted a statute defining "death" to include "brain death" that definition would apply.

Pain alone is not an irremediable condition within the definition of the Model Act. Its inclusion would undercut the Act's goal of freedom from the negative constructions of "mercy-killing" legislation.

The definition of "declaration" is elaborated in Sections 3 and 4. The form in Section 4, while not required to be used word for word by the declarant, is not merely a suggested form; the declaration must be in *substantially* that form, or it will fail. This requirement is intended to protect the declarant and to facilitate the application of the statute.

"Extraordinary medical treatment" is defined so as not to diminish any possibility there may be of saving the patient's life. Treatment designed to improve the patient's condition is "ordinary" and cannot be withheld. However, since, by definition, a qualified patient's condition cannot be improved by ordinary treatment, the patient will die after extraordinary treatment is discontinued, thus carrying out the statutory purpose. If the patient does not die within a given time after cessation of extraordinary treatment (as was the case with Karen Quinlan), his condition, by definition, has been misdiagnosed; in that event, extraordinary treatment should be resumed immediately.

B. The Basic Operative Provision of the Model Act

SECTION 2. Subject to the provisions of this Act, it shall be lawful for a physician (or a nurse or other medical personnel acting at a physician's direction), in accordance with the terms of the patient's declaration, to withhold or terminate extraordinary medical treatment in the case of a qualified patient who has made (or has had made on his behalf pursuant to Section 3 of this Act) a declaration that is lawfully in force at the time of

the withholding or termination of such extraordinary medical treatment.

Analysis of Section 2

This is the basic operative provision of the Model Act. Unlike some American bills,[159] it allows euthanasia to be performed only by a physician or by persons acting under the direction of a physician.

Euthanasia is lawful under Section 2 only where the declaration is lawful. To permit otherwise would make a mockery of the declaration requirement. On the other hand, the physician should not be required to assume the risk that the declaration was not made lawfully. This is especially true where, as in the Model Act, the physician is to honor the patient's request. To avoid a "damned if he does and damned if he doesn't" conflict, Section 7(2) of the Act gives the physician immunity in most cases even if the declaration does not comply with the Act. Therefore, the possibility exists that a defective declaration will be honored. In many cases, no harm will be done because the defect will be merely a technical one (e.g., failure to date the declaration). In other, more serious cases, however, the defect (e.g., a forged declaration) may result in euthanasia which is clearly involuntary. This risk is probably one which must be taken in order to achieve the larger social goals of assuring that legitimate requests will be honored and that physicians will not be motivated to seek ways of avoiding their duties under the Model Act. Hopefully, sanctions for tampering with declarations and revocations, such as those provided in Section 10 of the Model Act, will maintain at a tolerably low level the number of cases in which unauthorized euthanasia is performed.

C. Who May Execute the Advance Declaration

SECTION 3. (1) Any person of majority age or over for purposes of giving legal consent whether or not he has at that time an irremediable condition, may make a declaration directing that extraordinary medical treatment be withheld or terminated from use in his case if he should become a qualified patient. Such declaration shall be: (a) written, printed or typed, although not necessarily by the declarant; (b) signed by the declarant or, if the declarant is physically unable to sign it, by any person at the direction of the de-

clarant; (c) dated; (d) witnessed in writing by two persons, neither of whom is a person who has signed the declaration at the direction of the declarant; and (e) in substantially the form prescribed in Section 4 of this Act.

(2) A declaration signed by a person other than the declarant at the declarant's direction shall be deemed to be a declaration made by the declarant himself.

(3) It shall be the declarant's responsibility to communicate the execution of a declaration to the physician in charge of his case.

(4) A declaration shall remain in effect until revoked.

Analysis of Section 3

This section makes it clear that the Act is limited to voluntary euthanasia, since only the declarant may execute a declaration. There are two limited exceptions. One exception is the case in which a declarant physically is unable to sign the declaration; the execution of his declaration by another person is nevertheless within the scope of truly voluntary euthanasia because the declaration can be executed only at the direction of the declarant.

The other exception is the one raised in Part II of this Article and put into operative effect by Section 6 of the Act—the application of the Act to the incompetent and to the minor. While the Act therefore may not be truly voluntary, the author feels that the benefits of the Act should extend to all those who desire them, young as well as old, incompetent as well as competent, and that no other certain method exists by which to apply the Act to one who arguably cannot execute a lawful declaration. A legislature which is more concerned with maintaining a truly voluntary statute than with assuring universal coverage may opt to omit Section 6.

The requirements listed in (a) through (e) are procedural safeguards. Requirement (a) prohibits solely oral records of such declarations which easily could be ignored or abused. Requirement (b) is necessary lest a large group of potential declarants be denied the benefits of the Act. Requirement (c) is essential to the operation of Section 5(5). Other safeguards may be added at the option of the drafting legislature.

Section 3(2) is included so that the use of the word "declarant" in other sections of the Act (e.g., Section 5(1)) always will refer to the person on whose behalf a declaration is made, not necessarily to the person actually signing the declaration.

Subsection (3) recognizes the need for the physician in charge to be kept informed as to whether euthanasia is or is not authorized in a given case. Unfortunately, there is no way of assuring that this is done. A central depository for declarations (such as the county clerk) will be unable to keep track of the location of declarants and the identities of their physicians. Placing the burden on the physician himself to determine whether, for example, an unconscious patient has executed a declaration very well may result in many valid declarations going unheeded (since most bills contain no requirement that the physician honor a declaration he knows to exist, it is hardly likely that the physician will actively seek out the existence of a declaration). The fairest alternative is to place the burden on the one who will receive the benefit—the declarant. Much like a will, the declarant must, while he can do so, let it be known that he has executed a legal document. His efforts to that end are aided by a provision similar to Section 9 of the Act.

D. The Form of the Advance Declaration

SECTION 4. (1) The form for a declaration shall be substantially as follows:

DECLARATION made on this _____ day of _____ , 19 ___ , by _____ (name of declarant) of _____ (address, city, county, and state of declarant).

I DECLARE that I am of sound mind and, having considered the seriousness of this declaration, do hereby voluntarily consent to the following:

A. If at any time I should have a physical illness, injury or disability diagnosed by two physicians as incurable and terminal, I hereby direct voluntarily that medical treatment which prolongs my life without improving the chances for a cure or reversal of my condition be withheld or terminated.

B. If at any time I should have a condition of brain damage or deterioration such that my normal mental faculties are diagnosed by two physicians as severely and irreparably impaired to the extent that I may be deemed to have suffered brain death, I hereby direct voluntarily that medical treatment which prolongs my life without improving the chances for a cure or reversal of my condition be withheld or terminated.

C. This declaration shall remain in force until such time as I revoke it by a signed and dated written revocation of this declaration, which revocation also must be signed by two witnesses. I understand that I should communicate any revocation or subsequent declaration I may make to my physician, family, and friends, so that those responsible for my care will know my true wishes regarding the subject matter of this declaration.

SIGNED _____ (Declarant's signature)
DATED _____

I TESTIFY that the above-named declarant (signed) (was unable to write but directed that there be signed on his behalf by a person other than a witness) this declaration in my presence, that he appeared to do so voluntarily, and that he appeared to me to appreciate its full significance.

SIGNED _____ (Witness's signature)
DATED _____
SIGNED _____ (Witness's signature)
DATED _____

(2) Any person who makes a declaration in the form set forth above may strike to omit (if he is physically unable to do so, he may direct another to strike to omit) either paragraph A or B, provided that next to the omitted paragraph the declarant (or, if the declarant is unable, the person directed by him) shall sign his name, and provided, in any case, that the witnesses shall sign their names next to the omitted paragraph.

Analysis of Section 4

The primary purpose of the advance declaration is to avoid the problem of incompetent consent by enabling any person to consent to euthanasia at a point in time when he is competent to do so. Those persons who arguably are never competent are covered by Section 6.

There is no optimal language to be used in the declaration. The only requirement should be that the declaration paraphrase the statutory language as to the type of euthanasia allowed. The declaration used in the Act paraphrases the provisions dealing with "irremediable condition," withholding and terminating treatment, revocation, and communication to the physician. Not only does this assure that the patient's request will be within the permissible bounds of the Act, but it also informs the declarant of the procedure to which he is consenting.

Section 4(2) recognizes that, just as a person need not consent to euthanasia at all, he may limit his consent to euthanasia to some but not all circumstances.

The attestation by witnesses at the end of the declaration is a procedural safeguard. If the legislature wishes, it may provide for notarization in place of attestation, or may omit entirely such safeguards.

E. When, by Whom, and How an Advance Declaration May Be Revoked

SECTION 5. (1) A declaration made by the declarant may be revoked at any time only by the declarant. Said revocation shall be in the manner described in subsection (3) of this section.

(2) A declaration made on behalf of a declarant by a person other than the declarant, pursuant to Section 6 of this Act, may be revoked at any time only by the person who made the declaration or by the declarant if he subsequently should become capable of such revocation, and shall be in the manner described in subsection (3) of this section.

(3) The revocation of a declaration shall meet the same criteria enumerated in (a) through (d), inclusive, of Section 3(1) of this Act. In addition thereto, but not in lieu thereof, the declarant may destroy the declaration being revoked or may mark or alter it so as to indicate that it has been revoked.

(4) It shall be the declarant's responsibility to communicate the revocation of his declaration to the physician in charge of his case.

(5) In the event of conflicting declarations and/or revocations, the most recently dated document shall control.

Analysis of Section 5

The revocation provision focuses on the "when," "who," and "how" questions addressed in Part IV.

Under Section 5 of the Act, a declaration may be revoked at any time. As noted in Part IV of this Article, the common-law competency requirement should be implicit in this provision, so that the patient in effect may revoke such declaration "at any time that he is competent to do so."

Section 5 provides that a declaration, with one exception, may be revoked only by the person who made it. This preserves the integrity of the statute by assuring that the declarant's wishes will not be supplanted by another person. Section 5(1) covers the revocation of those declarations made by the declarant or at his direction. Section 5(2) covers the revocation of declarations made vicariously.

Only a single exception is provided under the Model Act to the rule that the person who made a declaration is the only one who can revoke it. Section 5(2) permits the patient himself to revoke a consent made vicariously on his behalf, should he become competent to do so. It is felt that the individual whose life is affected by the declaration should be permitted to change his mind regarding euthanasia in all cases where he is mentally competent to do so.

The Model Act answers the "how" question by requiring a revocation to be made in essentially the same manner as a declaration. For the reasons given in Part IV(F) of this Article, simply destroying or defacing the declaration is not acceptable by itself, but either method is permitted by the Act so that a defaced declaration may be questioned and the declarant consulted as to his true intentions prior to the performance of euthanasia. A legislature may wish to make revocation easier so as to disfavor euthanasia in cases where there is uncertainty as to whether a declaration has been revoked; but to the extent it does so, it also makes it easier for a person other than the declarant to thwart the declarant's wishes.

The explanation given in Section 3 as to the burden of notification being placed on the declarant applies to revocations as well as to declarations.

F. Vicarious Consent of Minors and Incompetent Adults

SECTION 6. (1) If any person is a minor for purposes of giving consent, or is an adult who lacks the capacity to execute a declaration and if

that person, to the best information and belief of the signer, never was capable of executing the same, a declaration may be executed, pursuant to the requirements of this Act, on his behalf:

    (a) If the person is a minor or unmarried incompetent adult, by both parents (or by one parent if the other has not expressed a contrary desire after a reasonable attempt has been made to ascertain that other parent's desire);

    (b) If the person is a married incompetent adult, by his or her spouse;

    (c) If the person is an incompetent widow, widower or divorceé, by the person's child of the age of consent or over; or if more than one such child, by a majority of such children; or if without children, by one or both parents pursuant to subsection (a) above;

    (d) (This list may be continued at the discretion of the legislature.)

(2) The foregoing list is to be followed in the stated order of priority when individuals in prior classes are unable or unwilling to make a decision regarding euthanasia. If the appropriate individual makes a decision not to consent to euthanasia on the declarant's behalf, no other individual shall have the right to consent on the declarant's behalf, but the declarant shall have such right if he subsequently becomes capable of executing a declaration.

Analysis of Section 6

A legislature that wishes to maintain a system of truly voluntary euthanasia may omit this vicarious consent provision. It should be included, however, where the legislature wishes its statute to apply to all qualified patients, their lack of age or mental capacity notwithstanding.

As discussed in Part IV(E) of this Article, the primary difficulty in drafting a vicarious consent provision is to avoid creating a loophole by which a person's affirmative decision *against* euthanasia could be overruled subsequent to his becoming a qualified patient. By limiting vicarious consent on behalf of an adult to those adults who never were competent to execute a declaration, the Model Act in effect establishes a conclusive presumption that one who has not executed a declaration desires not to have euthanasia performed. Just as Section 8 assures

that decisions in favor of euthanasia will be honored, this section assures that decisions against euthanasia similarly will be honored.

Section 6(2), unlike most of the American bills, expressly recognizes that it should not be the purpose of this section to enable one to run down the list of relatives until he comes to someone who will consent to euthanasia. Rather, if the first eligible vicarious consentor decides against euthanasia, that decision should be binding, just as if the patient himself affirmatively had decided against euthanasia. The language of Section 6(2) carries out this philosophy. It also reinforces the right of a person to execute a declaration "at any time" by permitting him to overrule a contrary decision made vicariously if subsequently he should become competent to do so.

G. Criminal, Civil, and Professional Sanctions

SECTION 7. (1) Any physician (including a nurse or other medical personnel acting at the direction of a physician), hospital or other medical institution that, in good faith, withholds or terminates extraordinary medical treatment pursuant to the provisions of this Act shall, in the absence of proof of negligence, be immune from civil or criminal liability that might otherwise be incurred and as a matter of law shall not be in violation of any professional oath or affirmation.

(2) In the absence of reason(s) to believe otherwise, a physician (including a nurse or other medical personnel acting at the direction of a physician), hospital, or other medical institution may presume that a declaration of which the person or institution has become aware is lawfully in force at the time of the withholding or termination of extraordinary medical treatment. If said declaration was in fact not lawfully in force, but the physician or other prescribed person had no reason to believe it was not lawfully in force, such person, if he otherwise complies with the provisions of this Act, shall have the same immunities described in subsection (1) of this section.

(3) A physician, hospital or other medical institution that certifies the existence of an irremediable condition shall be presumed to do so in good faith, and, in the absence of proof of negligence, said person or institution shall be immune from civil or criminal liability that might otherwise be incurred, and as a matter of law shall not be in violation of any professional oath or affirmation.

Analysis of Section 7

Section 7(1) is the operative provision with respect to immunity from liability for participating in euthanasia. Liabilities to which the immunity applies are stated expressly and include liability for breach of a professional oath. The immunities also apply to those persons assisting the physician. Hospitals and other medical institutions also are included, but it should be understood that physician immunity does not automatically preclude hospital liability; if the hospital's negligence can be proven, then liability will exist, regardless of the absence of negligence on the physician's part.

Section 7(3) is the equivalent of Section 7(1) with respect to the physician's role in certifying an irremediable condition.

The negligence standard is used in the Model Act both for the protection of the patient and because there is little unfairness in holding the physician to his common law standard of care. However, Section 7(2) establishes a presumption in favor of the physician with respect to at least one type of negligence. Section 7(2) raises, but does not resolve, the issue of whether a physician has a duty to make an *inquiry* concerning the validity of a declaration.

H. Mandatory Compliance

SECTION 8. It shall be unlawful for the physician in charge to fail to withhold or terminate extraordinary medical treatment in the case of a qualified patient whom he knows or has reason to know has executed a declaration pursuant to this Act. Any violation of this section shall be a [misdemeanor; felony].

Analysis of Section 8

This provision, missing from most of the American bills,[160] *requires* that the patient's declaration be honored. Only the physician in charge (rather than "any physician") is required to honor the declaration; otherwise, physicians only remotely involved with a patient's case (or not involved at all) would violate this section.

A number of bills employ the alternative of permitting a physician who does not wish to participate in euthanasia to "pass the buck," in effect, by transferring the patient to another physician.[161] The requirement of the Model Act is felt to be preferable because it avoids the possibility (however unlikely) that no physician could be found who would participate in euthanasia, and also permits the patient to remain under the care of his own physician with whom, presumably, he feels most secure.

I. Duty to Communicate Known Wishes of the Declarant

SECTION 9. All persons who have knowledge thereof shall be under a duty to report to the physician in charge within thirty-six hours of admission any wish, including the signing or revocation of a declaration, signified by a hospitalized person with regard to euthanasia, and the physician in charge shall ensure that any patient who to his knowledge wishes to make, revoke, amend, or alter a declaration is enabled to do so.

Analysis of Section 9

As previously noted with respect to Section 3, the declarant must assume the primary responsibility for making his wishes known to his physician. However, Section 9 may provide additional assurance that his wishes will be made known even if he fails or is unable to notify his physician.

This section is designed to promote the smooth functioning of the Model Act. However, the "duty" established is a duty without a statutory penalty for its breach, because in many (if not most) cases the person having knowledge of the declarant's wishes simply will not know soon enough that the declarant has been hospitalized or will not know the identity of declarant's physician.

J. Punishment for Willful Concealment, Destruction, Falsification, or Forgery of a Declaration or Revocation

SECTION 10. (1) It shall be an offense punishable, upon conviction, by a sentence of [insert appropriate sentence] for any person willfully to conceal, destroy, falsify, or forge a declaration or revocation with intent to create the false impression that another person desires the withholding or termination of extraordinary medical treatment.

(2) It shall be an offense punishable, upon conviction, by a sentence of [insert appropriate sentence] for any person willfully to conceal, destroy,

falsify, or forge a declaration or revocation with intent to create the false impression that another person does not desire, or no longer desires, the withholding or termination of extraordinary medical treatment.

(3) A person signing a declaration or revocation as a witness who willfully puts his signature to a statement he knows to be false shall be deemed to have committed an offense under [insert appropriate state statute dealing with perjury or witnesses' signatures].

Analysis of Section 10

This section is designed to assure that the true wishes of the declarant are carried out by dissuading those who might attempt to tamper with the system. Each legislature must formulate its own penalties. As noted in Part IV(I) of this Article, the legislature may determine that it is worse to commit fraud which may result in the undesired death of the patient than to commit fraud which may result in the continuance of the administration of extraordinary medical treatment contrary to his wishes, and to punish accordingly.

K. Immunity from Liability for Death Caused by the Administration of Drugs Required to Relieve the Patient of Pain

SECTION 11. Notwithstanding any contrary provision of this Act, a qualified patient may be given whatever quantity of drugs may be required to relieve him of pain. A physician (including a nurse or other medical personnel acting at the direction of a physician), hospital, or other medical institution administering drugs pursuant to this section shall have the same immunities prescribed in Section 7(1) of this Act.

Analysis of Section 11

As discussed in Part IV(B) of this Article, the purpose of this section is to clarify the fact that the administration of drugs is permitted, even though arguably it constitutes "active" euthanasia. If the drugs result in the patient's death, the physician administering them will be immune from liability. However, this is true only if the drugs were *required* to relieve the patient of pain. If a significantly greater dose than required is given, so as to cause the patient's death, there will be no immunity.

L. Enforceability of Life, Accident, and Health Insurance

SECTION 12. No policy of insurance that has been in force for [insert number] months prior to the insured's death shall be vitiated or impaired legally in any way by any act or omission authorized by this Act.

Analysis of Section 12

This provision is relatively simple and was discussed in Part IV(L) of this Article. Its inclusion may necessitate changes in the drafting state's insurance laws.

M. Immunity from Laws Prohibiting Suicide

SECTION 13. (1) No person signing a declaration in good faith pursuant to the provisions of this Act shall be found or be deemed to be in violation of [insert the section(s) of the state statute making it a criminal offense to commit suicide; if no such state statutes exist, this paragraph should be deleted].

(2) No person participating in good faith in any acts or omissions authorized by the provisions of this Act shall be found or be deemed to be in violation of [insert the section(s) of the state statutes making it a criminal offense to assist another in committing suicide or homicide; if no such state statutes exist, this paragraph should be deleted].

Analysis of Section 13

If the state has laws prohibiting suicide, this section will provide immunity both to the patient and to those who assist him under the terms of the Act. Of course, it is not clear that even active euthanasia, which the Act does not permit, is in fact considered to be suicide; *a fortiori,* it is unlikely that the passive euthanasia authorized by the Act would fall within the state's suicide prohibition, if any. Nevertheless, this section removes even the possibility of an argument that euthanasia constitutes suicide.

N. Severability of Provisions

SECTION 14. The provisions of this Act are hereby declared to be severable and if any provision of this Act or the application of such provision to any person or circumstance is declared

invalid for any reason, such declaration shall not affect the validity of remaining portions of this Act.

Analysis of Section 14

This section operates as a "safety valve" provision that prevents the invalidity of one section from destroying the entire statute. It is particularly important in preserving the immunities granted under the Act in the event that any portion of the Act is found invalid.

VI. CONCLUSION

The Model Act proposed by the author is to a degree a careful synthesis of recent euthanasia proposals. Legislative draftsmen must consider all proposals and build upon their strengths while, at the same time, avoiding their weaknesses. In many respects, earlier draftsmen have seen the kinds of problems that are likely to arise in the euthanasia process. However, for the most part they have delved too superficially into those problems. Furthermore, the statutory language they have chosen often has been inadequate to deal with such complex matters.

This Article has attempted to raise and confront a variety of issues concerning the drafting of effective euthanasia legislation. In such a new field, however, it is difficult to predict the results of any legislation, even the best conceived and most carefully drafted. It is hoped that this Article has made suggestions which will aid in the future drafting of euthanasia legislation which is unambiguous and effective.

NOTES

1. The word "euthanasia," which is derived from the Greek for "good death," is often used interchangeably with such terms as "mercy killing," "death with dignity," "right to die," and "painless inducement of death." However, there are some subtle—but nevertheless significant—distinctions between these terms, which are discussed in various places throughout the text. While recognizing its often negative connotations, the author has chosen to use the word "euthanasia" in this Article purely for the sake of convenience. The meaning intended, however, is as described in the text. The word "euthanasia" is *not* used in the Model Act.

2. For an overview of a variety of issues relating to euthanasia, *see generally* Survey, *Euthanasia: Crimi-*

nal, Tort, Constitutional and Legislative Considerations, 48 NOTRE DAME LAWYER 1202 (1973) [hereinafter cited as Survey].

3. 381 U.S. 479 (1965). *Griswold* recognized the existence of a "penumbra of rights," including a "right of privacy," guaranteed by the federal Constitution although not specifically enumerated therein. The exact parameters of the right of privacy are not clearly defined, although the right has been held applicable to such activities as abortion, *see* Roe v. Wade, 410 U.S. 113 (1972), and contraception, *see Griswold,* and Eisenstadt v. Baird, 405 U.S. 438 (1972). In the recent and much-publicized case of In the Matter of Karen Quinlan, 137 N.J. Super. 227, 348 A.2d 816 (1975), 70 N.J. 10, 355 A.2d 647 (1976), the lower court refused to extend the right of privacy to include the right to die; however, the New Jersey Supreme Court overruled the lower court's decision, in large part because it felt that "Presumably this right [of privacy] is broad enough to encompass a patient's decision to decline medical treatment under certain circumstances." The court did not use the term "right to die," although in practical effect the "right of privacy" becomes a "right to die" in the circumstances of that case. *See* In the Matter of Karen Quinlan, 70 N.J. 10, 355 A.2d 647 (1976).

4. *See generally* Forkosch, *Privacy, Human Dignity, Euthanasia—Are These Independent Constitutional Rights?,* 3 U.S.F.V. L. REV. 1 (1974).

5. A Life Magazine poll of 41,000 readers in 1972 showed that "91% believe a terminal patient should be permitted to refuse further treatment that will artificially prolong life." LIFE, Aug. 11, 1972, at 38–39.

6. The first proposals for euthanasia legislation in the United States were made in New York and Nebraska in 1938.

7. *See* Kutner, *Due Process of Euthanasia: The Living Will, A Proposal,* 44 IND. L.J. 539, 546 (1969) [hereinafter cited as Kutner]. In some modern European criminal codes, motive is among the elements used in determining the nature of the offense.

8. *See generally* Sanders, *Euthanasia: None Dare Call It Murder,* 60 J. Crim. L.C. & P.S. 351 (1969).

9. *See, e.g.,* In The Matter of Karen Quinlan, 137 N.J. Super. 277, 348 A.2d 816 (1975); 70 N.J. 10, 355 A.2d 647 (1976). In that case, the father of an incompetent adult asked the court to authorize expressly the discontinuance of all extraordinary means of keeping his daughter alive. The father asserted, *inter alia,* that his daughter had a "constitutional right to die." In ruling that "there is no constitutional right to die that can be asserted by a parent for his incompetent adult child," the lower court may have intended deliberately to bypass the question of whether there exists a constitutional right to die assertable by the individual on his own behalf. On appeal, the New Jersey Supreme Court held that the constitutional "right of privacy"

encompasses "a patient's decision to decline medical treatment under certain circumstances." By stating that ". . . the State's interest *contra* weakens and the individual's right to privacy grows as the degree of bodily invasion increases and the prognosis dims," the court seems to have limited the right to decline treatment only to those extreme situations (like Karen Quinlan's) in which death is a virtual certainty. Hence, the right enunciated by the court becomes a functional, though not a literal, equivalent of the right to die. 70 N.J. 10, 355 A.2d, 647 (1976).

10. Roe v. Wade, 410 U.S. 113 (1972).

11. The recent case of Dr. Kenneth Edelin, Commonwealth v. Edelin, Crim. No. 81823 (Super. Ct. Mass. Feb. _____ , 1975), is an example. Dr. Edelin performed an abortion within the guidelines set forth in Roe v. Wade, but was nevertheless found guilty of manslaughter, apparently on the grounds that the aborted fetus was viable at the time it was aborted.

12. *See generally* Kamisar, *Some Non-Religious Views Against Proposed "Mercy-Killing" Legislation,* 42 Minn. L. Rev. 969 (1958) [hereinafter cited as Kamisar]. Professor Kamisar, writing in 1958, concluded that "the only Anglo-American prosecution involving an alleged mercy-killing *physician* seems to be the case of Dr. Herman Sander" (emphasis added).

A second case involving an alleged mercy-killing physician recently resulted in the defendant's acquittal. Dr. Vincent A. Montemarano was acquitted by a jury on February 5, 1974 of murdering a terminally ill cancer patient with an intravenous injection of potassium chloride. Boston Globe, Feb. 6, 1974, at 2, col. 4.

13. Among the alternatives not discussed in the text are the "living will" and the "antidysthanasia contract."

First proposed in 1969, the so-called living will is a document quite similar to the advance declaration of the Model Act. Kutner, *supra* note 7. It is an expression of an individual's consent to euthanasia. By itself, however, it has no legal effect, and therefore has limited practical value without accompanying legislation. *See* Vodiga, *Euthanasia and the Right to Die—Moral, Ethical and Legal Perspectives,* 51 CHI-KENT L. REV. 1 (1974) [hereinafter cited as Vodiga].

The antidysthanasia contract is a contract between the patient and those who will be responsible for his care. In one sense it improves upon the living will because it legally is binding. It falls short of the Model Act, however, because it treats the individual's written declaration as merely an "offer" which must be "accepted" by a physician before it has any legally binding effect. Thus, the individual does not maintain the same degree of control over the euthanasia decision as he does under the Model Act. *See* Smyth, *Anti-Dysthanasia Contracts: A Proposal for Legalizing Death With Dignity,* 5 PACIFIC L.J. 738 (1974) [hereinafter cited as Smyth].

14. Vodiga, *supra* note 13, at 3.

15. Rep. Walter W. Sackett, Jr., M.D., sponsor of several bills in Florida, stated to the United States Senate Special Committee on Aging that his proposed statute ". . . has nothing to do with Euthanasia." Address by Rep. Walter W. Sackett, Jr., M.D., to U.S. Senate Special Committee on Aging, Aug. 7, 1972, at 1. Rep. Sackett prefers the term "Death With Dignity" because he feels it does not carry the same controversial and misunderstood connotation that "euthanasia" carries.

16. The following comment on two 1973 Oregon euthanasia bills is illustrative of the controversies stirred by the legislative proposals:

The public response to both pieces of legislation was highly emotional and many persons, particularly those in the senior citizen category, misunderstood the intent of the bill—that this decision would remain a personal and voluntary one and not become mandatory.

Letter from Cecil L. Edwards, Secretary of Oregon State Senate, to Ronald P. Kaplan, Jan. 29, 1974, on file in the offices of the AMERICAN JOURNAL OF LAW & MEDICINE.

17. One of the most complete legal studies of euthanasia has concluded that "American law has established few instances in which the taking of human life is permissible." Survey, *supra* note 1, at 1247.

18. *See, e.g.,* Smyth, *supra* note 13.

19. Louisell, *Euthanasia and Biathanasia: On Dying and Killing,* 22 CATHOLIC U.L. REV. 723 (1973) [hereinafter cited as Louisell].

20. The most frequent criticism of euthanasia (and especially of involuntary euthanasia) along ethical or sociological grounds has been based upon the so-called "wedge" theory, which refers to the possibility that any system of involuntary euthanasia, however limited, will open the door to the subsequent "benefit" extinction of the aged, the mentally ill, and other persons whose lives are, to some, not worth living or not worth saving. *See* Kamisar, *supra* note 12.

21. One such argument was suggested by the limited holding of the lower court in the *Quinlan* case, 137 N.J. Super. 227, 348 A.2d 816 (1975); 70 N.J. 10, 355 A.2d 647 (1976). That holding implicitly suggests that if there is a constitutional right to die, it is assertable only by the individual himself. If this is the case, then any statute permitting euthanasia where the individual has played no role in the decision (and perhaps even some in which he plays only a minor or indirect role) would be unconstitutional. On appeal of the Quinlan case, the New Jersey Supreme Court appeared to disagree, stating that:

Our affirmation of Karen's independent right of choice, however, would ordinarily be based upon her competency to assert it. The sad truth, however, is that she is grossly incompetent and we cannot discern her supposed choice based on the testimony of her previous conversations with friends, where such testimony is without probative weight. 137 N.J. Super. at 260. Nevertheless, we have concluded that Karen's right of privacy may be asserted on her behalf by her guardian under the peculiar circumstances here present.

22. Kamisar, *supra* note 12; Louisell, *supra* note 19.

23. *See generally* Comment, *Informed Consent and the Dying Patient,* 83 YALE L.J. 1632 (1974).

24. Louisell, *supra* note 19.

25. *See, e.g.,* H.B. 251 (1973), H.B. 30 (1975), Del. Legislature.

26. G. WILLIAMS, THE SANCTITY OF LIFE AND THE CRIMINAL LAW 331 (1957) [hereinafter cited as WILLIAMS].

27. *Id.* at 334.

28. Survey, *supra* note 1, at 1252.

29. Kamisar, *supra* note 12, at 986.

30. Survey, *supra* note 1, at 1253.

31. WILLIAMS, *supra* note 26, at 331.

32. Survey, *supra* note 1, at 1253.

33. N. ST. JOHN-STEVAS, THE RIGHT TO LIFE 55 (1963).

34. Survey, *supra* note 1, at 1253.

35. *See, e.g.,* H.B. 137, Mont. Legislature (1973) and S.B. 179, Ore. Legislature (1973), both of which permit euthanasia in certain situations of "brain death," a condition which may not meet the technical requirement of "terminal" illness. The problem of defining "death" is discussed in the text at page 64.

36. Survey, *supra* note 1, at 1253.

37. H. TROWELL, THE UNFINISHED DEBATE ON EUTHANASIA 17 (1973) [hereinafter cited as TROWELL].

38. Voluntary Euthanasia Act of 1969.

39. Kutner, *supra* note 7, at 544.

40. TROWELL, *supra* note 37, at 24.

41. *Id.* at 17.

42. The proposal would have amended Section 2 of Article I of the Florida Constitution to read:
Basic rights—All natural persons are equal before the law and have inalienable rights, among which are the right to enjoy and defend life and liberty, to pursue happiness, to be rewarded for industry, *to die with dignity, . . . etc.* [The amendment would have added the italicized portion.]

43. Sackett, *Death With Dignity,* 64 S. MED. J. 330, 331 (1971).

44. H.B. 3184, Fla. Legislature (1969).

45. Note, *Death With Dignity: A Recommendation for Statutory Change,* 22 U. FLA. L. REV 368 (1970). Rep. Sackett's proposal did not specify a form for the advance declaration, as many bills have done.

46. The figures in the text are based on responses of the various state legislatures to the author's request for proposed euthanasia legislation introduced in the legislatures and the status thereof.

47. H.B. 744, Alas. Legislature (1976); S.B. 1177, Ariz. Legislature (1976); A.B. 3060, Cal. Legislature (1976); H.B. 251 (1973), H.B. 30 (1975), Del. Legislature; H.B. 407 (1973), H.B. 239 (1975), H.B. 2463 (1976), Fla. Legislature; H.B. 1679 Ga. Legislature (1976); H.B. 342, Hawaii Legislature (1975); H.B. 143 (1969), H.B. 95 (1975), Idaho Legislature; H.B. 74 (1974), H.B. 11 (1975), H.B. 618 (1975), Ill. Legislature; S.B. 207, Iowa Legislature (1975); H.B. 265, Ky. Legislature (1976); S.B. 700 (1974), H.B. 764 (1975), S.B. 596 (1975), Md. Legislature; H.B. 3641 (1974), H.B. 2297 (1975), Mass. Legislature; H.B. 1082, Mo. Legislature (1975); H.B. 137 (1973), H.B. 256 (1975), Mont. Legislature; S.B. 179, H.B. 2997, Ore. Legislature (1973); H.B. 5196, R.I. Legislature (1975); H.B. 1384, Tenn. Legislature (1976); H.B. 620, Va. Legislature (1976); S.B. 2881, Wash. Legislature (1975); S.B. 358, W. Va. Legislature (1972); S.B. 670 (1971), S.B. 715 (1971), A.B. 1207 (1975), Wis. Legislature.

The above listing does not include a bill proposing euthanasia legislation which has just been introduced, but as this Article goes to press has not yet been printed, in the Ohio Legislature.

In addition to these bills, a number of states have dealt with euthanasia in other ways. For example, as noted in the text, several attempts have been made in Florida to amend the state constitution to include as a basic right the right "to die with dignity." *See, e.g.,* H.J.R. 3007 (1974), H.J.R. 2575 (1976), Fla. Legislature.

Article I, Section 10 of the Louisiana Constitution of 1974 provides, in part, that "No law shall subject any person to euthanasia, to torture, or to cruel, excessive, or unusual punishment." The categorization of euthanasia with torture and punishment is contrary to the whole notion of euthanasia as an avoidance of torture and punishment. Interestingly, Louisiana also has a statute (40 L.R.S. §1299.46, added in 1975) which implicitly declares a "right of a person eighteen years of age or over to refuse to consent to medical or surgical treatment as to his own person." In light of the above constitutional provision, §1299.46 would appear to be unconstitutional, although the issue has not yet come before the courts.

A.B. 4444, introduced in California in 1974, would have added to the enumeration of personal rights in the state's Civil Code a provision that "Every person has the right to die without prolongation of life by extraordinary medical means." The proposal, which died in committee, was not accompanied by any implementing legislation.

Colorado and Massachusetts have introduced resolutions calling for the study of possible euthanasia legislation. The Colorado resolution is still being considered. H.J.R. 1007, Colo. Legislature (1976). In 1974, Massachusetts adopted H.B. 5944, calling for a study of euthanasia legislation, only after a bill proposing actual euthanasia legislation was reported out of committee adversely. The following year, H.B. 6043, a measure almost identical to H.B. 5944, was defeated by a greater than 2–1 margin.

H.B. 2097 and S.B. 2005, Minn. Legislature (1976), provide that it is no defense to a wrongful death action or to certain felonies that after the tortious or criminal act was committed medical treatment was withdrawn from the victim. Query, whether the proposal would apply where the tortious or criminal act *is* the withdrawal of medical treatment.

The recently-enacted "Protection of the Abused or Neglected Elderly Act" in North Carolina provides, in part, that the state will provide services to prevent the abuse or neglect of the elderly. "Abuse" includes "the willful deprivation by a caretaker of services which are necessary to maintain mental and physical health." Whether this can be read to prohibit euthanasia is unclear. N.C.G.S. §108–91 *et seq.*

48. H.B. 407, Fla. Legislature (1973), is the only bill to have passed a vote of an entire branch of a state legislature. Under the sponsorship of Dr. Sackett, it passed the Florida House of Representatives by a vote of 56–50 in 1973, after having been defeated on its first consideration by that body only nine days earlier. However, it died on the Senate calendar in the same year. H.B. 137, Mont. Legislature (1973), was defeated in the House of that state by a vote of 76–15. Letter from Edwin A. Smith, Clerk of Montana House of Representatives to Ronald P. Kaplan, January 31, 1974 on file in the offices of the AMERICAN JOURNAL OF LAW & MEDICINE. The author's information as to the history and status of these bills is based largely upon responses from the various state legislatures to his request for such information.

49. H.B. 342, Hawaii Legislature (1975); H.B. 143, Idaho Legislature (1969); H.B. 137 (1973), H.B. 256 (1975), Mont. Legislature; H.B. 251 (1973), H.B. 30 (1975), Del. Legislature. Note, however, that Sections 8(5) and 9(2) of the Montana bill speak of giving a "death medication" to the patient.

50. H.B. 2997, Ore. Legislature (1973); S.B. 358, W. Va. Legislature (1972).

51. H.B. 1679, Ga. Legislature (1976); H.B. 265, Ky. Legislature (1976).

52. *See, e.g.,* Vaughn, *The Right to Die,* 10 CALIF. WESTERN L. REV. 613, 624 (1974).

53. Section 5 of H.B. 1082, Mo. Legislature (1975), provides:

Failure of any authorized physician to cease maintenance medical treatment upon presentment of the documents as provided in this act is guilty of a misdemeanor and, upon conviction, shall be punished as provided by law.

Section 3 of H.B. 618, Ill. Legislature (1975), provides:

It is unlawful for any physician or hospital to whom a written document authorized by Section 2 has been given, or who knows or should know of the existence of such document, to administer any medical treatment specifically indicated in that document solely to prolong human life. Any violation of this Section is a Class A misdemeanor.

54. *See, e.g.,* H.B. 744, Alas. Legislature (1976), which provides:

No physician or medical facility is under a duty to participate in withdrawal of life-sustaining mechanisms authorized by this chapter, but a physician or medical facility not honoring a patient's authorization has a duty to make arrangements to transfer the patient to another physician or medical facility that will give effect to an authorization made in accordance with this chapter.

55. *See, e.g.,* H.B. 1384, Tenn. Legislature (1976). Some bills specifically provide that a physician need not honor a patient's request for euthanasia. *See, e.g.,* S.B. 1177, Ariz. Legislature (1976).

56. H.B. 251 (1973), H.B. 30 (1975), Del. Legislature.

57. *See, e.g.,* A.B. 3060, Cal. Legislature (1976) ["The Legislature finds that adult persons have the fundamental right to control the decisions relating to the rendering of their own medical care . . . . ; H.B. 256, Mont. Legislature (1975) ["This legislation is written for the primary purpose of giving to every citizen the right to choose for himself how he wishes to die . . . ."]; S.B. 358, W. Va. Legislature (1972) ["Every person shall have the right to die with dignity . . . ."].

58. *See* discussion at footnote 3, *supra.*

59. One can think of several illustrations: cases permitting capital punishment [e.g., Furman v. Georgia, 408 U.S. 238 (1972)]; cases permitting refusal of life-sustaining treatment [e.g., Erickson v. Dilgard, 44 Misc. 2d 27. 252 N.Y.S.2d 705 (1962); *In Re* Estate of Brooks, 32 Ill.2d 361, 205 N.E.2d 435 (1965)]; and perhaps even the abortion cases [Roe v. Wade, 410 U.S. 113 (1972)].

60. *See, e.g.,* H.B. 342, Hawaii Legislature (1975).

61. S.B. 207, Iowa Legislature (1975).

62. H.B. 1384, Tenn. Legislature (1976).

63. H.B. 620, Va. Legislature (1976).

64. An example of a statute which does not reflect a recognition of the issue is H.B. 744 in Alaska, which provides only for the "withdrawal of life-sustaining mechanisms." Such language seems equivalent only to "termination" and not to "withholding." A more blatant example is H.B. 30, Del. Legislature (1975), which provides that in certain cases "death with dignity shall be granted," but does not give even a hint as to how this is to be carried out.

65. *See, e.g.*, H.B. 744, Alas. Legislature (1976), described in footnote 64, *supra*, which contains no clue as to what is a "life-sustaining mechanism."

66. *See, e.g.*, S.B. 358, W. Va. Legislature (1972) [". . . artificial, extraordinary, extreme or radical medical or surgical means or procedures calculated to prolong . . . life"].

67. *See, e.g.*, H.B. 1082, Mo. Legislature (1975). *See also* H.B. 265, Ky. Legislature (1976), which, in addition to the general language quoted in the text, is the only proposal to spell out specific types of treatment which may be refused. These include:

(a) Artificial respirators to promote breathing;
(b) Heart massage, pacemakers or other machines for stimulation of the heart muscle;
(c) Kidney machines;
(d) Transplantation of vital organs; and
(e) Prolonged intravenous feeding.

68. S.B. 207, Iowa Legislature (1975).

69. The "locality" standard is similar to that often used in malpractice cases in determining the standard of care owed by a physician. It may well be that, in a prosecution for wrongful termination of treatment under the Act, a "locality" standard would be imposed judicially even though not expressly written into the statute.

70. S.B. 1146, Ariz. Legislature (1976). *See also* H.B. 95, Idaho Legislature (1975), and H.B. 620, Va. Legislature (1976).

71. H.B. 618, Ill. Legislature (1975).

72. H.B. 342, Hawaii Legislature (1975). *See also* H.B. 143, Idaho Legislature (1969).

73. The statute should distinguish between illness and injury, which several had failed to do. *See, e.g.*, H.B. 2997, Ore. Legislature (1973), and H.B. 30, Del. Legislature (1975). *See also* H.B. 1082, Mo. Legislature (1975), which covers only "illness or accident."

74. *See, e.g.*, H.B. 744, Alas. Legislature (1976), which permits euthanasia only where a physician determines "that there is no expectation that the declarant will regain health and that but for the use of life-sustaining mechanisms the declarant would *immediately* die" (emphasis added). *See also* H.B. 239, Fla. Legislature (1975), which permits euthanasia where the patient is suffering from an "illness or injury that would result in natural expiration of life regardless of the use of discontinuance of medical treatment to sustain the life processes." A shorter form of this provision is found in H.B. 764, Md. Legislature (1975), which permits euthanasia "[w]hen there is no reasonable expectation of the person's recovery from a terminal illness, disease or condition." It should be noted, however, that the latter two proposals do not require an assessment that death *immediately* would follow the cessation of treatment.

75. H.B. 342, Hawaii Legislature (1975), which permits euthanasia where there is a "serious physical illness or impairment medically thought in the patient's case to be incurable and expected to cause him severe distress or render him incapable of rational existence."

76. *See, e.g.*, H.B. 137 (1973) and H.B. 256 (1975), Mont. Legislature, which permit euthanasia where the patient has either:

(a) a serious physical disability which is diagnosed as incurable and terminal, with no expectation of regaining health; or
(b) a condition of brain damage or deterioration such that a person's normal mental faculties are severely and irreparably impaired to the extent that he has been rendered incapable of leading a rational existence.

Note, however, that the Montana bills do not distinguish adequately between illness and injury. *See* footnote 73, *supra*. H.B. 143, Idaho Legislature (1969), which otherwise is similar to the Montana proposals, is superior in this respect; it separates paragraph (a) of the Montana bills into two separate paragraphs. *See* paragraphs (a) and (b) of H.B. 143, quoted in footnote 80, *infra*.

77. *See generally* Compton, *Telling the Time of Human Death by Statute: An Essential and Progressive Trend,* 31 WASH. AND LEE L. REV. 521 (1974); and Harvard Medical School Ad Hoc Committee to Examine the Definition of Brain Death, *Report: A Definition of Irreversible Coma,* 205 J.A.M.A. 337 (1968).

A substantial number of state legislatures have introduced (and several have passed) bills creating a statutory definition of death. Most of these bills permit a determination of death based on cessation of the functioning of the brain, even though the patient otherwise remains "alive." *See, e.g.*, CAL. HEALTH & SAFETY CODE 7180, which provides that:

A person shall be pronounced dead if it is determined by a physician that the person has suffered a total and irreversible cessation of brain function. There shall be independent confirmation of the death by another physician.

Nothing in this chapter shall prohibit a physician from using other usual and customary procedures for determining death as the exclusive basis for pronouncing a person dead.

78. *See, e.g.*, H.B. 137 (1973) and H.B. 256 (1975), Mont. Legislature, and H.B. 251, Del. Legislature (1973).

79. *See* the discussion of the so-called "wedge theory" at footnote 20, *supra*.

80. H.B. 143, Idaho Legislature (1969), permits euthanasia where the patient has either:

(a) a condition of physical illness thought in the patient's case to be incurable and terminal and expected to cause him severe distress; or

(b) a condition of grievous physical affliction occasioning the patient serious injury or disability thought to be permanent and expected to cause him severe distress; or

(c) a condition of physical brain damage or deterioration such that the patient's normal mental faculties are severely and irreparably impaired.

81. Some proposed bills do not require the patient to execute a declaration, but instead require him to petition the court for an order permitting euthanasia. *See* H.B. 1679, Ga. Legislature (1976), and H.B. 265, Ky. Legislature (1976).

82. *See, e.g.,* H.B. 342, Hawaii Legislature (1975).

83. *See, e.g.,* H.B. 239, Fla. Legislature (1975). *See also* H.B. 251, Del. Legislature (1973), which allows the declaration to be oral rather than written.

84. At least one state would permit a person, at his option, to consent to euthanasia in some but not all of the circumstances in which he qualifies for it, by allowing him to strike from his declaration those conditions under which he does not want euthanasia performed. Thus, for example, he could consent to euthanasia if he should suffer "brain death," but not if he should suffer a terminal illness. *See* H.B. 143, Idaho Legislature (1969).

85. *See, e.g.,* H.B. 744, Alas. Legislature (1976).

86. *See, e.g.,* H.B. 1082, Mo. Legislature (1975).

87. *See, e.g.,* H.B. 256, Mont. Legislature (1975).

88. *See, e.g.,* S.B. 207, Iowa Legislature (1975).

89. *See, e.g.,* H.B. 1384, Tenn. Legislature (1976).

90. Kamisar, *supra* note 12, at 986.

91. *See, e.g.,* S.B. 358, W. Va. Legislature (1972).

92. *See, e.g.,* H.B. 137, Mont. Legislature (1973), which provides that:

. . . a declaration may be made by any individual . . . that he voluntarily submits to euthanasia if he should become a qualified patient.

The final clause strongly suggests that the declarant need not be ill at the time he makes his declaration.

An even clearer example is H.B. 256, Mont. Legislature (1975), which states that:

. . . a declaration may be made by any individual, preferably years ahead of necessity. . . .

93. H.B. 143, Idaho Legislature (1969).

94. The other bill, H.B. 342, Hawaii Legislature (1975), is only slightly different than the Oregon proposal.

95. *See, e.g.,* S.B. 1146, Ariz. Legislature (1976).

96. Some bills permit a person who is unable to sign his own declaration to direct another to execute it on the declarant's behalf. *See, e.g.,* H.B. 95, Idaho Legislature (1975).

97. S.B. 670, Wis. Legislature (1971); S.B. 358, W. Va. Legislature (1972); H.B. 2997, Ore. Legislature (1973); H.B. 1679, Ga. Legislature (1976); H.B. 30, Del. Legislature (1975).

98. S.B. 670, Wis. Legislature (1971); S.B. 358, W. Va. Legislature (1972).

99. If the declaration is nonbinding, this might not always be the case.

100. H.B. 2997, Ore. Legislature (1973), limits vicarious consent to situations in which there is ". . . an absence of actual notice of contrary indications by the individual who is terminally ill. . . ."

101. *See, e.g.,* S.B. 670, Wis. Legislature (1971).

102. H.B. 30, Del. Legislature (1975).

103. H.B. 1679, Ga. Legislature (1976).

104. H.B. 30, Del. Legislature (1975).

105. *See, e.g.,* H.B. 2997, Ore. Legislature (1973).

106. *See, e.g.,* S.B. 358, W. Va. Legislature (1972).

107. *See, e.g.,* A.B. 3060, Cal. Legislature (1976) [72 hours]; H.B. 342, Hawaii Legislature (1975) [30 days].

108. H.B. 618, Ill. Legislature (1975), and S.B. 358, W. Va. Legislature (1972) are the only bills which contain no revocation provision.

109. *See, e.g.,* S.B. 1146, Ariz. Legislature (1976).

110. A.B. 3060, Cal. Legislature (1976), states that the declaration ". . . may be revoked at any time by the declarant, without regard to his mental state or competency. . . ."

111. *See, e.g.,* H.B. 342, Hawaii Legislature (1975).

112. S.B. 715, Wis. Legislature (1971), in providing that "Such document [advance declaration] may be revoked . . . in writing or orally," at least raises the possibility that one other than the declarant may revoke a declaration.

113. *See, e.g.,* A.B. 3060, Cal. Legislature (1976).

114. *See, e.g.,* H.B. 95, Idaho Legislature (1975).

115. *See, e.g.,* H.B. 342, Hawaii Legislature (1975).

116. The Euthanasia Education Council suggests that the declaration ("living will") be distributed to the declarant's doctor, clergyman, lawyer, and family members.

117. The successor of H.B. 137, H.B. 256, proposed in Montana in 1975, contains an unusual provision which restricts a declarant to one revocation. If subsequently he should execute a second declaration, it could not be revoked.

118. A.B. 3060, Cal. Legislature (1976), requires a revocation to be communicated to the attending physician before it becomes effective.

H.B. 620, Va. Legislature (1976), provides that:

It shall be the burden of such person [the declarant] to deliver the said revocation, if in writing, to the medical personnel administering medical treatment to such person, or it shall be the burden of such witnesses to communicate such oral revocation to the said medical personnel.

119. *See, e.g.*, H.B. 95, Idaho Legislature (1975).

120. One bill which does require a dated declaration is S.B. 1177, Ariz. Legislature (1976). However, that same bill does not require a revocation to be dated.

121. The extent to which the physician should control the euthanasia process is a topic of considerable disagreement among the commentators. *Compare* Kamisar, *supra* note 12, with WILLIAMS, *supra* note 26.

122. H.B. 1082, Mo. Legislature (1975).

123. Kutner, *supra,* note 7, at 551.

124. Even those bills which involve the courts in the euthanasia process require the participation of physicians in the decision-making process. *See, e.g.*, H.B. 1679, Ga. Legislature (1976).

125. Kamisar, *supra* note 12, at 998. Professor Kamisar feels that there is a significant danger of erroneous diagnoses. In addition, even where a diagnosis is correct, Kamisar is concerned that euthanasia may be performed on patients who could have benefited from new medical procedures which might be perfected during their lifetimes.

126. H.B. 744, Alas. Legislature (1976), provides that:

(a) Before withdrawing life-sustaining mechanisms from a patient, the physician in charge must be satisfied that the patient has authorized the action as provided in this chapter, the conditions of the authorization are met, and all steps proposed to be taken under it are in accord with the patient's last known wishes.

(b) Before withdrawing life-sustaining mechanisms from a mentally incompetent patient or one who is incapable of communication, the physician in charge shall ascertain that the patient authorized the action as provided in this chapter, and the conditions of the authorization are met.

See also A.B. 3060, Cal. Legislature (1976); H.B. 342, Hawaii Legislature (1975); H.B. 137 (1973) and H.B. 256 (1975), Mont. Legislature; and S.B. 179, Ore. Legislature (1973).

127. *See, e.g.*, S.B. 1177, Ariz. Legislature (1976), which provides that:

Medical personnel administering medical treatment . . . may presume that the person who executed such document was of sound mind when the document was executed unless such personnel has reliable information to the contrary in which event the document shall not be given force and effect unless and until a court of competent jurisdiction so orders.

See also H.B. 95, Idaho Legislature (1975); H.B. 3641 (1974) and H.B. 2297 (1975), Mass. Legislature; H.B.

2997, Ore. Legislature (1973); H.B. 5196, R.I. Legislature (1975); H.B. 1384, Tenn. Legislature (1976); and H.B. 620, Va. Legislature (1976).

128. *See, e.g.*, A.B. 3060, Cal. Legislature (1976).

130. H.B. 256, Mont. Legislature (1975).

130. *See, e.g.*, S.B. 1177, Ariz. Legislature (1976).

131. The possible exception is in California, where A.B. 3060 grants immunity only to physicians and health facilities, but seems to permit other persons to withhold or terminate treatment ["Nothing in this chapter shall impair or supersede any right which any person may have to effect the withholding or withdrawal of extraordinary life-sustaining procedures in any lawful manner."].

132. Only H.B. 251, Del. Legislature (1973), and H.B. 618, Ill. Legislature (1975), contain no immunity provision.

133. S.B. 358, W. Va. Legislature (1972).

134. *See, e.g.*, H.B. 143, Idaho Legislature (1973), and S.B. 179, Ore. Legislature (1973).

135. S.B. 1177, Ariz. Legislature (1976).

136. Note, *Death With Dignity: A Recommendation for Statutory Change, supra* note 45, at 371.

137. *See, e.g.*, Address by Rep. Walter W. Sackett, Jr., M.D., *supra* note 15, at 4.

138. *See, e.g.*, S.B. 1177, Ariz. Legislature (1976).

139. H.B. 95, Idaho Legislature (1975), and H.B. 620, Va. Legislature (1976), are virtually identical to the Arizona bill.

140. *See* H.B. 342, Hawaii Legislature (1973), and H.B. 143, Idaho Legislature (1969). *See also* A.B. 3060, Cal. Legislature (1976), which makes an unusual distinction by punishing one who conceals or withholds knowledge of an *oral*, but not a *written*, revocation.

141. *See, e.g.*, S.B. 1177, Ariz. Legislature (1976).

142. *See* A.B. 3060, Cal. Legislature (1976).

143. H.B. 137 (1973) and H.B. 256 (1975), Mont. Legislature.

144. H.B. 143, Idaho Legislature (1969).

145. H.B. 1679, Ga. Legislature (1976), and H.B. 265, Ky. Legislature (1976).

146. S.B. 1177, Ariz. Legislature (1976), and H.B. 95, Idaho Legislature (1975).

147. *See, e.g.*, S.B. 1177, Ariz. Legislature (1976).

148. *See, e.g.*, H.B. 143, Idaho Legislature (1969).

149. *See, e.g.*, S.B. 207, Iowa Legislature (1975).

150. *See, e.g.*, H.B. 256, Mont. Legislature (1976).

151. *See, e.g.*, S.B. 715, Wis. Legislature (1971).

152. *See, e.g.*, H.B. 256, Mont. Legislature (1975).

153. *See generally* Kutner, *supra* note 7, at 543, 544.

154. *See, e.g.*, H.B. 407, Fla. Legislature (1973).

155. *See, e.g.*, H.B. 143, Idaho Legislature (1969).

156. *See, e.g.,* H.B. 764, Md. Legislature (1975), which permits, but does not require, the filing of the declaration.

157. *See, e.g.,* S.B. 179, Ore. Legislature (1973).

158. *See, e.g.,* H.B. 143, Idaho Legislature (1969).

159. *See, e.g.,* H.B. 256, Mont. Legislature (1975).

160. The only exceptions are H.B. 1082, Mo. Legislature (1975), and H.B. 618, Ill. Legislature (1975).

161. *See, e.g.,* H.B. 744, Alas. Legislature (1976).

5.4 A Dilemma for the Legal and Medical Professions: Euthanasia and the Defective Newborn

RICHARD A. MUELLER and G. KEITH PHOENIX

Reprinted with permission from 22 *St. Louis University Law Journal* 501–518 (1978).

I. INTRODUCTION

In the spring of this year, twelve-year old Carl Huszar, a former March of Dimes poster child, committed suicide.[1] Carl had been born with a birth defect—his intestines were on the outside of his body. It was a condition that required numerous operations and left him with an unsteady gait and a hunchback posture. Although his physical and medical conditions were treated with remarkable skill, the defect apparently left its scar on Carl emotionally and eventually killed him.

The question of whether or not doctors should prescribe and perform extraordinary medical measures in treating defective newborns has perplexed the medical profession for years. Approximately 275 defective or malformed children are born in this country every day.[2] Only recently with the advent of the right-to-die statutes and the medical malpractice crisis has the question come to the attention of the legal community with any regularity. The issue now presented in a number of courts across the country is whether or not parents of defective newborn children have the right to refuse potentially lifesaving treatment.

This article will probe the peculiar problems attendant upon euthanasia in the case of a defective newborn child. It touches briefly upon the potential criminal liability which could befall both doctors and parents in this situation.[3] The article next discusses the more complicated and pragmatic problem of the potential civil liability which could arise from the actions of doctors and parents who permit the death of defective newborns. Finally, recommendations are proposed for the doctors and parents involved in these tragic situations and for the lawyers who may be called to represent them.

A. Major Infant Defects

There are several major birth defects in which the survival of affected infants is problematic without substantial medical intervention. One major birth defect involving the brain is hydrocephaly, which is characterized by a large accumulation of free fluid in the cranial cavity resulting in a marked enlargement of the head.[4] Another defect, which occurs in approximately one out of 700 live births, is Downs Syndrome,[5] more commonly referred to as mongolism which is related to a chromosomal disorder. In the infant stage, Downs Syndrome victims tend to be placid, rarely cry, and as they grow older, it becomes obvious that their physical and mental development is retarded.

Another defect sometimes seen in the newborn is spina bifida.[6] This defect, which has a dim prognosis, normally involves the posterior aspects of the vertebral column. The effects of this disease result from a defective closure of the vertebral column. It is commonly seen in the lower back and normally extends over an area covering three to six vertebral segments. The presence of this defect increases the risk of meningeal infections which may lead to death or brain damage and, when the spinal cord or lumbosacral nerve roots are involved, which is common, there may be degrees of paralysis of the lower extremities.[7]

Depending on the severity of the case, treatment of spina bifida may require the services of a number of specialists from a multitude of disciplines, including neurosurgical, urological, orthopedic, pediatric, and various other services. The decision whether or not to treat should be made before any neurosurgery is performed, as the closure of the vertebral column where the defect occurs assures at least temporary survival.[8]

Thus, with these major defects and others, extraordinary surgical and medical intervention may be required merely to preserve life. Not many years ago, before recent medical and technological advancements, these infants would have died soon after birth. Today, a large percentage of them can continue to "live" for extended periods of time even though most of them will be severely handicapped and unable to lead a normal life.

B. Beyond Quinlan

The question of whether to treat or withhold treatment, in cases where this decision may mean the difference between life and death, has been raised in courts with increasing frequency. The issue was most dramatically illustrated in the case of In re Quinlan,[9] a case in which the New Jersey supreme court confronted the question of whether life-prolonging medical techniques should be applied to forestall the natural death of one who is in an irreversible unconscious state. The court found, in allowing the patient's guardian to assert her constitutional right to privacy, that the patient had a right to die based on the right to privacy.[10] The legal questions presented in this case prompted much debate[11] although the potential civil and criminal liability for euthanasia involving adults has been an issue probed in legal literature for years.[12] The Quinlan case, however, has provoked additional discussion by legal scholars,[13] actions by state legislatures[14] and resolutions of the American Bar Association.[15] The discussion of the euthanasia problem for the most part, however, has centered around the constitutionally based right to die and proposed state legislation.

A distinction commonly drawn in the literature on euthanasia is between (1) voluntary and involuntary euthanasia.[16] Voluntary euthanasia occurs when the death of the individual results at the instigation and with the actual consent of the decedent. Involuntary euthanasia occurs, as in the Quinlan case, when the individual involved does not have the capacity to express his desire regarding medical treatment.[17] In the case of a defective newborn, all euthanasia cases therefore would be deemed involuntary because the defective newborn lacks the capacity to express a desire regarding that treatment.

Another distinction usually drawn is between extraordinary and ordinary medical care,[18] a distinction that is not always clear. Some authorities refer to extraordinary medical care as that which involves a substantial interference with the bodily privacy of the patient.[19] Others refer to extraordinary medical care as that which is not designed to cure the disease or illness but rather is only designed to preserve, prolong, or sustain life.[20] Much of the right-to-die legislation, and particularly those statutes modeled after the pioneering California legislation,[21] refers only to "life-sustaining procedures" which are defined as procedures which "would only serve to artificially prolong the moment of death and where . . . death is imminent."[22] Both definitions present obvious problems in application which will be discussed below. To the extent that "extraordinary medical care" refers only to life-sustaining procedures, the treatment outlined above is clearly "ordinary medical care." To the extent that the term takes on any meaning only with reference to the degree of bodily interference, however, many of the procedures outlined above constitute "extraordinary medical care." The definition utilized to determine whether or not the treatment is ordinary or extraordinary may well determine whether or not the medical care may be lawfully withheld.

II. CRIMINAL LIABILITY

Although the number of criminal prosecutions in cases involving defective newborns is extremely small,[23] there is the possibility of criminal liability for parents and physicians for euthanasia involving defective newborns. The notion that euthanasia may be regarded as a crime has had a substantial impact on the patient's legal ability to consent to it.[24] Additionally, whether or not the withholding of treatment is a crime is important because civil liability may be premised upon the commission of a criminal act.[25] This section analyzes the legal theories upon which a prosecution for murder, manslaughter, or child abuse can be based and considers the defenses available to prospective defendants in infant euthanasia cases.[26]

A. Physicians' Liability

Most euthanasia cases, though not all,[27] involve a death as a result of the doctor's failure to render some type of essential treatment. Thus, unless it is a case involving the withdrawal of life-supporting techniques, most euthanasia cases do not involve any affirmative acts by the physician resulting in death. The traditional rule has been, however, that one may be held criminally responsible for a death resulting from one's failure to act where there is a duty to take an action that would have avoided death.[28] It is also true that neither the fact that a patient is already dying nor the good intentions and moral beliefs of one who shortens the life of another will be a shield against criminal liability.[29] Consequently, the same standards of intent that apply to murder, in which the prosecution need prove only malice aforethought,[30] also have similar application to euthanasia. The California Supreme Court in *People v. Conley*[31] stated this position clearly: "One who commits euthanasia bears no ill will towards his victim and believes his act is morally justified, but he nonetheless acts with malice if he is able to comprehend that society prohibits his act regardless of his personal belief."[32]

The question, therefore, becomes one of the scope and duty of the physician to act in these circumstances. Doctors do not have a legal responsibility to care for any person who is in need of medical care.[33] Once a doctor has assumed responsibility for a patient, however, he is under a duty to render all medical care and treatment as the patient needs.[34] Thus, a doctor is civilly liable for injuries caused the patient after a doctor has abandoned that patient.[35] The duty of the doctor to the patient may be discharged by the patient at any time or by the doctor, provided he gives the patient sufficient notice so that he may obtain the services of another physician.[36] Assuming that the patient has not discharged his

physician and that the doctor has not given reasonable notice to the patient, the question of the scope of the physician's duty remains.[37] In this context, the distinction between the doctor's responsibility to render ordinary medical care as opposed to extraordinary medical care becomes pertinent.[38] Ordinary medical care has been defined to mean "all medicines, treatments, and operations, which offer a reasonable hope of benefit and which can be obtained and used without excessive expense, pain, or other inconvenience."[39] Extraordinary medical care has been defined to mean "all medicines, treatments, and operations, which cannot be obtained or used without excessive expense, pain or other inconvenience, or which, if used, would not offer a reasonable hope of benefit."[40] This distinction between ordinary and extraordinary medical care, however, has not been expressly recognized by most legal authorities.[41]

Courts have imposed different standards of duty to act on physicians based on whether the required treatment is ordinary or extraordinary. Generally, a physician may be required to render ordinary care such as would sustain life but will not be bound to embark upon extraordinary interventions which offer small hope for success and high risk to the patient. Thus, in the latter circumstance, it is far less likely that a court would impose liability on a physician for failure to intervene to prevent death. This matter will be explored more fully later in the context of the constitutional right to die.[42]

In the "normal" euthanasia case involving a terminally ill adult, these distinctions may be applied without great difficulty. By definition, in these cases the patient is terminally ill and the medical treatment given is "life sustaining" and is not designed to cure the patient's condition. In the words of the above definition, there is no "reasonable hope of benefit."

In the case of the defective newborn, though, it is more difficult to determine whether the care is ordinary or extraordinary. Frequently, the medical care will involve excessive pain, expense and inconvenience but, on the other hand, the medical care will preserve life in the sense that it will avert the immediate threat of death. If given proper medical treatment, a defective newborn may live a significant period of time.

The fact that the child normally will be faced with significant mental and physical handicaps is a factor that is and must be rejected as determinative in the decision of whether the doctor may withhold medical treatment. The argument that the doctor may withhold medical treatment based upon his conclusion as to the quality of life that will be experienced by the patient after treatment has little support in the law.[43] Under well-established common law principles, life is regarded as sacred without regard to its quality.[44]

It seems apparent that where the procedure or treatment will substantially prolong the life of a defective newborn, it must be considered ordinary medical care. If the doctor fails to render care in these circumstances, then the breach of his duty to the patient will have caused his death, thus exposing the doctor to criminal liability for murder or manslaughter.

B. Parents' Liability

As in the case of the physician, the criminal liability of the parents is premised upon their failure to act when they are under a duty to do so. It is a well-established principle that the parents of a minor child have a duty to provide necessary medical assistance.[45] This duty, which was recognized at common law, has been incorporated in the child abuse statutes of most states.[46] These statutes establish that parents of minor children are criminally liable for the failure to provide necessary medical assistance regardless of their ignorance, economic status[47] or religious beliefs.[48]

Whether the parent's refusal to provide these medical services constitutes child abuse depends upon the risks accompanying the medical procedure and whether the procedures are necessary to sustain life.[49] Where the medical care at issue involves a substantial risk of harm and is not necessary to sustain life, the parents are permitted a degree of discretion with regard to their decision to withhold medical treatment.[50] On the other hand, where the risk of harm is insignificant and the benefits from the procedure are substantial, a refusal to provide those services may constitute child abuse.[51]

C. Defenses to Criminal Prosecution

1. Common Law Defenses

As already noted, neither the good intentions of the defendant, whether a physician or a par-

ent, their religious beliefs nor their intent to benefit the child will constitute a defense in a criminal prosecution.[52] Inasmuch as the criminal liability of the physician and parent is premised upon their failure to act when they are under duty to do so, it is always open to these defendants to assert that they did not have such a duty. In other words, the physician may try to show that the medical care required was "extraordinary" and, therefore, that he was not obliged to provide it.[53] Similarly, the parents may try to show that the medical care was not "necessary" and, thus, that failure to provide it could not constitute neglect.[54]

In the absence of these defenses, the only other defense apparently available is proof that the failure to act was not the cause of the death.[55] Proof of lack of causation may not be premised upon the argument that the child would have died whether or not the treatment was given because, as noted above, prosecution for murder is allowed even though the killing merely accelerated an already certain or imminent death.[56]

Both the parents and the physician may contend that the withheld medical care only would have extended the child's life for a short period of time and, as a consequence, that they were not under a duty to provide such care. The difficulty with this argument, however, given the advanced state of medical art, is that it would not be medically accurate[57] in most of the conditions discussed previously. Nor is it likely that the parents or physician will be able to look to each other as intervening causes.[58] Logic suggests that in causation defense would seem to be available, although some decisions in this area have adopted a very relaxed view of causation which may provide a basis, in some circumstances, for a defense.[59]

2. Defense Based on a Constitutional Right To Die

The notion of a patient's constitutional right to die has been frequently raised in the literature[60] and was recently accepted by two state courts.[61] Obviously, where the patient has a constitutional right to die, there can be no criminal or civil prosecution against one who does not attempt to prohibit the patient from exercising his constitutionally protected choice.[62] The main difficulty facing doctors and parents in the case of a defective newborn in this circumstance is whether there has been a "lawful" exercise of this constitutional right and who may legally exercise it.[63]

The constitutional right to die is based upon the constitutional right to privacy including the right to privacy against unwarranted infringement of one's bodily integrity.[64] The position that this right to privacy prohibits a state from forcing unwanted medical care upon the patient was adopted in *In re Quinlan*[65] by the New Jersey supreme court. There the court stated that the right of privacy "is broad enough to encompass a patient's decision to decline medical treatment under certain circumstances, in much the same way as it is broad enough to encompass a woman's decision to terminate pregnancy under certain conditions."[66]

The question, of course, is in what circumstances does this right exist. The right to privacy is not inviolate. If the state can show a sufficient interest in preserving the life of the individual in question, then medical treatment may be ordered by a court.[67] Generally, the state has claimed an interest in requiring medical treatment because: (1) it has an interest in the preservation of human life; (2) it has a responsibility to protect the interest of innocent third parties (in the usual euthanasia case these are the children of the parents facing death); (3) it has an interest in preventing suicide; and (4) it has an interest in maintaining the ethical integrity of the medical profession.[68] In the case of defective newborns, there will be no "innocent third persons"[69] and the factor of ethical integrity has been rejected because the current practice of many physicians is to permit defective newborn individuals to die.[70] Also, the action or inaction of the patient *wishing* euthanasia has not been viewed as constituting suicide,[71] which leaves only the state's interest in preserving the value of human life. The strength this factor has in relation to the patient's possible constitutionally protected choice to select euthanasia is uncertain. Clearly, where the treatment is only life-prolonging and involves a large degree of interference with the bodily privacy of the patient, the patient's choice prevails.[72] For example, in *Superintendent of Belchertown State School v. Saikewicz*,[73] a sixty-seven year old patient, who had been a resident of state institutions since 1923 and who had a mental age of approximately two years and eight months, contracted leukemia and the state

institution desired to withhold medical treatment. The Massachusetts Supreme Court held that the state institution could withhold chemotherapy treatment because it would not permanently cure the patient's condition and would involve many painful side effects. In so holding, the court stated:

> It is clear that the most significant of the asserted State interests is that of the preservation of human life. Recognition of such an interest, however, does not necessarily resolve the problem where the affliction or disease clearly indicates that life will soon, and inevitably be extinguished. The interest of the state in prolonging a life must be reconciled with the interest of the individual to reject the traumatic cost of that prolongation. There is a substantial distinction in the state's insistence that the human life be saved where the affliction is curable, as opposed to the state interest where, as here, the issue is not whether but when, for how long, and at what cost to the individual that life may be briefly extended.[74]

Similarly, in *In re Quinlan,* the recommended life-prolonging treatment involved a large degree of bodily interference and was not designed to permanently cure the patient's condition. In relation to the state's interest in preserving the sanctity of human life, the court stated:

> The claimed interests of the State in this case are essentially the preservation and sanctity of human life and defense of the right of the physician to administer medical treatment according to his best judgment. ** ** ** We think that the State's interest *contra* weakens and the individual's right of privacy grows as the degree of bodily invasion increases and the prognosis dims. Ultimately, there comes a point at which the individual's rights overcome the State interest. (emphasis original)[75]

Thus, where the interference with the bodily privacy of the patient is large and the prognosis is poor, the individual's choice overcomes the state interest in protecting the value and sanctity of human life. Conversely, if the interference with the bodily privacy of the patient is minimal and the prognosis is good, then the state's interest should prevail. Cases involving defective newborns, however, do not easily fall into either of these two extremes. Usually the bodily interference required to preserve the life of a defective newborn is extensive but the prognosis is good, for in most cases a child will be "cured" by the treatment in the sense that his life expectancy will be relatively normal. Frequently, though, the resulting children will experience severe mental and physical handicaps. There is authority to the effect, however, that the severity of impairment may not be an appropriate consideration. In *Belchertown,* for example, although the Massachusetts supreme court did not address itself to impaired children, the court specifically rejected any "quality of life" analysis, stating:

> The sixth factor identified by the judge as weighing against chemotherapy was "the quality of life possible for [the patient] even if the treatment does bring about remission". To the extent this formulation equates the value of life with any measure of the quality of life, we firmly reject it.[76]

On the other hand, some courts have approved physically "harmful" medical procedures for minors and incompetents and have justified their actions based upon the psychological benefits to these individuals.[77] To the extent that such psychological factors can be equated with quality of life considerations, these cases are contrary to the position taken by the court in *Belchertown.*

Finally, it is of paramount importance that the exercise of this constitutional right be "lawful." In the case of the defective newborn, this requires a determination of what procedures are required in order to obtain a lawful consent to withhold medical treatment, which will be examined in the next section in the context of potential civil liability for euthanasia in the case of defective newborns.

III. POTENTIAL CIVIL LIABILITY

Civil liability for euthanasia involving a defective newborn, as in the case of criminal liability, is based upon the duty of the physicians and parents to act for the benefit of the newborn child. The potential civil liability, as opposed to

the potential criminal liability, of the participants in a euthanasia case has been given much less consideration by legal scholars.[78] In fact, research has failed to locate any case in which such a civil action has been filed. Theoretically, this action would arise from the wrongful death of the deceased.[79] Equally theoretical would be a civil action premised upon a violation of the constitutional rights of the patient under 42 U.S.C. §1983.[80]

The main difference between the potential criminal and civil liability is that normally the consent of the injured party is a defense in a civil action but not in a criminal action.[81] Obviously, though, in the case of a defective newborn, it will be impossible to obtain the actual consent of the patient. The current practice in a significant portion of the medical profession assumes that the consent[82] of the child's parents is sufficient to authorize the physician to withhold medical treatment.[83]

Therefore, the focus of this section will be on the potential civil liability for physicians and parents who withhold treatment from a defective newborn under the assumption that the consent of the parent is a defense.

A. Physicians' Liability

The civil liability of the physician who withholds medical care from a defective newborn, as in the criminal case, is based upon his duty to act for the benefit of his patient. This liability could be based either upon his negligent failure to provide medical treatment or upon the theory of abandonment. The duty to act for the benefit of the child could arise by virtue of the doctor/patient relationship with the parents,[84] the assumption of care for the child at birth,[85] or his responsibility to report child neglect under most child abuse statutes.[86]

The physician may be forced to walk a tightwire between the potential liability for failing to withhold medical treatment in violation of the newborn's constitutional right to die and the potential liability for failing to render medical assistance resulting in the child's wrongful death without due process of law.[87] For example, in *Holmes v. Silver Cross Hospital,* the representatives of the deceased patient at the defendant hospital brought an action under 42 U.S.C. §1983 for the defendant's violation of the deceased's constitutional rights. The decedent was a twenty-year-old minor who refused blood transfusions on religious grounds. When the decedent's condition became critical, the doctors and hospital representatives, without notice to the patient or his family, petitioned the probate court to declare the decedent a neglected minor and to appoint a guardian for the specific purpose of consenting to the blood transfusion. The probate court appointed the guardian and the representatives of the decedent brought a §1983 action against the doctors, the hospital and the guardian alleging a conspiracy to violate the decedent's constitutional rights under the first amendment. The court granted the guardian's motion to dismiss, based upon his judicial immunity, but otherwise held that the complaint stated a cause of action.[88] To the extent that the first amendment's protection of freedom of religion is analogous to the constitutional right to die, this case suggests the proposition that the doctor and the hospital may be sued by a minor's legal representatives for rendering medical assistance without the consent of a minor.

Similarly, in *Winters v. Miller*,[89] the plaintiff, a fifty-nine-year-old Christian Scientist, became involved in a dispute with her landlord and was taken to Bellevue Hospital where she was involuntarily committed for a sixty-day examination period. During her stay at Bellevue Hospital, Miss Winters informed the medical officials of her religious beliefs, but, nonetheless, over her continued objections, was given forced medication. Upon being released from the hospital, Miss Winters brought suit against numerous defendants and the trial court granted the defendants' motion for summary judgment. On appeal, the Second Circuit reversed the trial court's decision on the grounds that forced medication violated the plaintiff's first amendment rights.

As these two cases demonstrate, not only may the doctor be sued for failing to render medical care, but he may also be sued for failing to withhold medical care. Furthermore, if the doctor proceeds to render medical care without the consent of the parents, he may be sued for battery.[90]

The main difficulty with this state of the law is that the circumstances in which medical care may be withheld, or must be given, are not clearly defined. Under well-accepted constitutional principles, the right to die is subject to a balancing test in which the interests of the patient must be weighed against the interests of the state.[91] Such a test is not subject to a quick and easy application. The common law solution to this problem is equally complicated. As previously discussed, a doctor is under a duty to render ordinary medical care but need not render extraordinary medical care. The dilemma is compounded in that the terms "extraordinary" and "ordinary" medical care are not subject to exact definition. Furthermore, where there is a substantial risk of harm to the child from the medical treatment, the parents are permitted a degree of discretion whereby, without being guilty of neglect, they may require the doctor to withhold medical treatment.[92] In this situation, the doctor presumably will be relieved from legal responsibility. The law provides no clear guideposts, however, to aid in the weighing of the risk of harm against the potential benefits from medical treatment.

Under situations of this type, the only legally sensible solution for the physician is to petition the court for the appointment of a guardian. In most states, this proceeding requires a finding by the court that the child is dependent or neglected.[93] This requirement usually can be satisfied if the parents intend to withhold their consent to necessary medical treatment.[94] On the other hand, it is possible that a juvenile or probate court may have inherent authority to appoint a guardian in these circumstances, even in the absence of a finding of neglect or dependency. In light of the state of the law, a physician may shield himself from potential civil liability by petitioning the court for a guardian.

B. Parents' Liability

As in the case of criminal liability, the potential civil liability of parents of defective newborns is premised upon their common law duty to provide necessary medical services. In addition, this responsibility is imposed upon the parents by statute in most states.[95] Parents who refuse to provide these medical services may be found guilty of neglect. For example, in *State v. Perricone*,[96] the parents brought their child to the hospital with a heart malfunction, stated that they were Jehovah's Witnesses and that, consequently, no blood transfusions would be permitted. After the child's condition became critical, the hospital petitioned the court for the appointment of a guardian in order to obtain consent to the blood transfusion. The parents contested the jurisdiction of the juvenile court on the grounds that their refusal to consent to the transfusion did not constitute abuse or neglect within the terms of the state statute. The court held that the probate court had jurisdiction to appoint a guardian under these circumstances. In *Hoener v. Bertinato,*[97] a case relied upon by the court in *Perricone,* the parents refused to consent to a blood transfusion for their suspected RH negative child. The court stated:

> There is no doubt of the defendants' good faith as to their religious principles; nor is there any doubt as to their being good and devoted parents, except in their refusal to consent to the transfusions.
> Nevertheless, I have no difficulty in finding that, by their refusal to consent to the blood transfusions, defendants are neglecting to provide the child to be born with proper protection within the meaning of N.J.S.A. 9:2–9.
>
> ** ** **
>
> Since the blood transfusions are required in order for the child to live, the defendants' refusal to consent thereto constitutes "neglect to provide the child with proper protection" under the statute. Failure or refusal to take necessary steps to protect a child's life is obviously neglect of the child even if the parents have not failed in their duty to the child in other respects and even if such failure or refusal is grounded on genuine religious beliefs. The parents constitutional freedom of religion, although accorded the greatest possible respect, must bend to the paramount interest of the state to act in order to protect the welfare of a child in its right to survive.[98]

Thus, both at common law and by statute, parents may have a duty to provide medical care necessary to sustain the life of the child. The parents' breach of this duty will expose them to liability.[99] In addition, the parents' refusal to consent to necessary medical care will constitute neglect, thus triggering the reporting requirements of most child abuse statutes.[100]

IV. CONCLUSION

It should be evident from the foregoing that no clear rule exists as to when a physician or parent may withhold necessary medical treatment from a defective newborn without potentially exposing themselves to criminal or civil liability. Perhaps the only "safe" course of action may be to petition the court for the appointment of a guardian. This leaves unanswered the further question of whether a court-appointed guardian or the courts themselves will be competent to cope with the web of medical and ethical considerations attendant upon these decisions.[101]

Courts seemingly have not shied away from making decisions to order treatment necessary to sustain life,[102] an area that was once the sole province of the physician. It is unlikely, however, especially in light of the superior medical technology and skills that physicians may now marshal, that the courts soon will articulate a clear standard governing decisions bearing on the euthanasia of defective newborns.

NOTES

1. St. Louis Globe-Democrat, April 17, 1978.

2. Compiled from the United States Census, 1975, and Perinatal Medicine Diseases of the Fetus and Infant 79 (R. Behrman, M.D., ed. 1975) [hereinafter cited as Behrman].

3. For an excellent discussion of the potential criminal liability of parents and physicians as a result of their decision to withhold medical services from a defective newborn, *see* Robertson, *Involuntary Euthanasia of Defective Newborns: A Legal Analysis,* 27 Stan. L. Rev. 213 (1975) [hereinafter cited as Robertson]. For a discussion of potential criminal liability in any euthanasia case, *see* Note, *Euthanasia: Criminal, Tort, Constitutional and Legislative Considerations,* 48 Notre Dame L.J. 1202, 1203–16 (1973) [hereinafter cited as Survey].

4. *See* Behrman *supra* note 2, at 811. The appearance of the bones in the skull resembles the appearance of beaten metal, as these bones sometimes become very thin. One of the possible treatments is surgery and the insertion of a shunt into the skull, which is only occasionally removed. A hydrocephalic child cannot hold his head up and walking and talking are delayed. The legs are spastic and convulsions are not uncommon. As a rule, a hydrocephalic child is dull and lethargic. Blindness also occurs occasionally, and with the shunt in place, the risk of infection is also increased. *Id.* at 817.

5. Pathology of Infancy and Childhood 8 (2d ed., J. Kissane ed. 1975). Few individuals with Downs Syndrome attain an IQ of fifty. Downs Syndrome victims have an increased susceptibility to acute leukemia and congenital heart defects, which often account for a decreased life span, are found in about thirty-five per-

cent of its victims. *Id.* at 134–135. In the absence of such defects and with good medical care, however, their lifespan can be expected to approach normal. *See generally* NELSON TEXTBOOK OF PEDIATRICS, 10th ed., V. Vaughn III, M.D. & R. McKay, (M.D., eds. 1975) [hereinafter cited as NELSON].

6. *See* NELSON, *supra* note 5, at 1412.

7. *Id.*

8. *Id.* Ones who do survive are severely restricted by motor disability and fifty percent of them are mentally retarded. *Id.* at 1413.

9. 355 A.2d 647 (N.J. 1976).

10. *Id.* at 662–63.

11. *See, e.g.,* Note 8 RUT.-CAM. L.J. 37 (1976).

12. *See, e.g.,* Note, *Euthanasia—The Individual's Right to Freedom of Choice,* 5 SUF. L. REV. 190 (1970); Note, *The Right to Die,* 7 HOUS. L. REV. 654 (1970).

13. *See, e.g.,* Collester, *Death, Dying and the Law: A Prosecutorial View of the Quinlan Case,* 30 RUTGERS L. REV. 304 (1977); Note, *A Hypothetical: Quinlan Under Ohio Law,* 10 AKRON L. REV. 145 (1976); Note, *Euthanasia: The Physician's Liability,* 10 J. MAR. L. REV. 148 (1976); Note, *In Re Quinlan: Defining the Basis for Terminating Life Support Under Right of Privacy,* 12 TULSA L.J. 150 (1976); Vodiga, *Euthanasia and the Right to Die—Moral, Ethical, and Legal Perspectives,* 51 CHI.-KENT L. REV. 1 (1974).

14. *See, e.g.,* IDAHO CODE §§39–4501 - 39–4509 (Supp. 1977); ARK. STAT. ANN. §82.3801 (Supp. 1976); TEX. CODE ANN. 4590h (Supp. 1978).

15. *See* Recommendation of A.B.A. Section of Insurance, Negligence and Compensation Law (1977) (unpublished).

16. *See, e.g.,* Robertson, *supra* note 3, at 214 n.16.

17. *Id.*

18. *See, e.g.,* McKenney, *Death and Dying in Tennessee,* 7 MEMPHIS STATE U.L. REV. 503, 538 (1977); Foreman, *The Physician's Criminal Liability for the Practice of Euthanasia,* 27 BAYLOR L. REV. 68 (1975).

19. Robertson, *supra* note 3, at 223–224.

20. *See, e.g.,* Robertson, *supra* note 3, at 235–37; SURVEY, *supra* note 3, at 1209.

21. CAL. HEALTH & SAFETY CODE §§7185–95 (West Supp. 1977).

22. *See supra* note 14.

23. Research has not revealed any criminal prosecutions for the cause of death of a defective newborn. Parents have been prosecuted for negligent failure to provide care, Stehr v. State, 139 N.W. 676, *aff'd on rehearing,* 142 N.W. 670 (Neb. 1913); for refusing medical treatment on religious grounds, Bradley v. State, 84 So. 677 (Fla. 1920); and for neglect, Eaglen v. State, 231 N.E.2d 147 (Ind. 1967); Mathews v. State,

126 So.2d 245 (Miss. 1961); State v. Perricone, 181 A.2d 751 (N.J. 1962). Similarly, doctors have been prosecuted for affirmative acts of euthanasia resulting in death. *See* SURVEY, *supra* note 3, at 1213.

24. Whether or not the patient's act of consenting to euthanasia constitutes suicide has had an effect on the utilization of that consent as a defense in a civil action. *See, e.g.,* Superintendent of Belchertown State School v. Saikewicz, 370 N.E.2d 417, 426 n.11 (Mass. 1977); John F. Kennedy Memorial Hosp. v. Heston, 279 A.2d 670, 673 (N.J. 1971); Erickson v. Dilgard, 252 N.Y.S.2d 705 (1962).

25. *See, e.g.,* W. PROSSER, LAW OF TORTS §2 (4th ed. 1971) [hereinafter cited as PROSSER].

26. Much of this section is based on Professor Robertson's article on the potential criminal liability of physicians and parents. *See* Robertson, *supra* note 3.

27. *See supra* note 23.

28. *See, e.g.,* Robertson, *supra* note 3, at 217; SURVEY, *supra* note 3, at 1207–10.

29. *See, e.g.,* People v. Conley, 411 P.2d 911, 918 (Cal. 1966); SURVEY, *supra* note 3, at 1204.

30. LAFAVE & SCOTT, HANDBOOK OF CRIMINAL LAW §§68, 69 (1st ed. 1972).

31. 411 P.2d 911 (Cal. 1966).

32. *Id.* at 918.

33. *See, e.g.,* Robertson, *supra* note 3, at 255 n.81; SURVEY, *supra* note 6, at 1207.

34. *Id.*

35. *See generally,* Annot., 57 A.L.R.2d 432 (1958).

36. *Id.*

37. Theoretically, the patient may discharge the physician. In such a circumstance, however, the doctor may become responsible for aiding and abetting a suicide or as a member of a conspiracy to commit a suicide. Furthermore, the action of the patient in discharging the physician under these circumstances would be analogous to consenting to murder, which is not a defense. Therefore, it is arguable that the action of a patient discharging a physician under circumstances where the doctor is aware of the impending death is not a defense. Finally, in the case of a defective newborn, it is clear that the newborn child would not have the awareness to discharge his physician.

Similarly, the action of a doctor in giving notice of intent to terminate services where the doctor is aware of the patient's intent not to seek other medical assistance might make the physician guilty of aiding and abetting a suicide. Moreover, in the case of a defective newborn it is apparent that no notice to the child would be sufficient. Whether or not notice to the parents under circumstances where the physician is aware of the parent's intent not to seek further medical assistance will excuse the physician from liability is a question which will be discussed later. *See* notes 81–83, *infra,* and accompanying text.

38. *See, e.g.,* Superintendent of Belchertown State School v. Saikewicz, 370 N.E.2d 417, 423–24 (Mass. 1977); Robertson, *supra* note 3, at 235; SURVEY, *supra* note 3, at 1209; Elkinton, *The Dying Patient, the Doctor, and the Law,* 13 VILL. L. REV. 740, 743 (1968); Rabkin, Gillerman & Rice, *Orders Not to Resuscitate,* 293 NAT'L. A.J. MED. 364 (1976); Lewis, *Machine Medicine and its Relation to the Fatally Ill,* 206 J. AM. MED. ASS'N. 387 (1968); Collins, *Limits of Medical Responsibility in Prolonging Life,* 206 J. AM. MED. ASS'N 389 (1968); Williamson, *Life or Death—Whose Decision?,* 197 J. AM. MED. ASS'N. 793 (1966).

39. Robertson, *supra* note 3, at 236.

40. Kelly, *The Duty to Preserve Life,* 12 THEOL. STUD., 550 (1951); N. ST. JOHN-STEVAS, LIFE DEATH AND THE LAW, 275–76 (1961); 48 NOTRE DAME LAW 1203, 1209 (1973); Robertson, *supra* note 3, at 236.

41. Robertson, *supra* note 3, at 236.

42. *See* notes 60–77 and accompanying text, *infra.*

43. Superintendent at Belchertown State School v. Saikewicz, 370 N.E.2d 417, 432 (Mass. 1977); Gleitman v. Cosgrove, 227 A.2d 689 (N.J. 1967).

44. *See generally* WILLIAMS, THE SANCTITY OF HUMAN LIFE AND THE CRIMINAL LAW (1957).

45. *See, e.g.,* State v. Perricone, 181 A.2d 751 (N.J. 1962); Hoener v. Bertinato, 171 A.2d 140 (N.J. Super. 1961); People v. Labrenz, 104 N.E.2d 769 (Ill. 1952); Robertson, *supra* note 3, at 218.

46. *See, e.g.,* 5 ARIZ. REV. STAT. ANN. §13–801(1) (1956); COLO. REV. STAT. 19-10-103 (Supp. 1973); 10 CONN. GEN. STAT. §17–38 (1975); KAN. STAT. §38–802(g) (Supp. 1977).

47. Stehr v. State 139 N.W. 676 (Neb. 1913).

48. In Bradley v. State, 84 So. 677 (Fla. 1920), the court found that a father's refusal to provide medical service based on his religious beliefs constituted culpable negligence but held that the father's action did not "cause" the death. *Cf.* Craig v. State, 155 A.2d 684 (Md. 1959); State v. Barnes, 212 S.W. 100 (Tenn. 1919); State v. Chenoweth, 71 N.E. 197 (Ind. 1904).

49. For example, some treatments for spinal bifida involve a substantial risk of death but are not necessary to sustain life.

50. *See, e.g.,* Robertson, *supra* note 3, at n.67–70; People v. Labrenz, 104 N.E.2d 769 (Ill. 1952).

51. *Id.*

52. *See supra* notes 46, 47.

53. *See* Robertson, *supra* note 3.

54. *See supra* note 52.

55. *See supra* note 48.

56. *See, e.g.,* State v. Mally, 366 P.2d 868 (Mont. 1961); People v. Ah Fat, 48 Cal. 61 (1874); LaFave & Scott, *supra* note 30, at 250 n.28.

57. *See* text accompanying notes 4–8, *supra.*

58. *See* Robertson, *supra* note 3, at 238–39.

59. *See, e.g.,* Bradley v. State, 84 So. 677 (Fla. 1920), in which the father of a minor epileptic daughter refused to obtain medical care for burns suffered during a seizure. The court held the burns to be the cause of death instead of the father's failure to obtain medical care. *But see* State v. Pickles, 218 A.2d 609 (N.J. 1965); State v. Staples, 148 N.W. 283 (Minn. 1974).

60. *See, e.g.,* Note, *The Legal Aspects of the Right to Die: Before and After the Quinlan Decision,* 65 KY. L.J. 823 (1976); Note, *In Re Quinlan, Defining the Basis for Terminating Life Support Under Right of Privacy,* 12 TULSA L.J. 150 (1976); Brown & Truitt, *Euthanasia and the Right to Die,* 3 OHIO N.U.L. REV. 615 (1976); Steele & Hill, *A Plea for a Legal Right to Die,* 29 OKLA. L. REV. 328 (1976); Vodiga, *Euthanasia and the Right to Die—Moral, Ethical and Legal Perspectives,* 51 CHI.-KENT L. REV. 1 (1974); Delgado, *Euthanasia Reconsidered—The Choice of Death as an Aspect of the Right of Privacy,* 17 ARIZ. L. REV. 474 (1975).

61. *See* Superintendent of Belchertown State School v. Saikewicz, 370 N.E.2d 417 (Mass. 1977); In re Quinlan, 355 A.2d 647 (N.J. 1976).

62. In re Quinlan, 355 A.2d at 669–70.

63. *Cf.* Holmes v. Silver Cross Hosp., 340 F. Supp. 125 (N.D. Ill. 1972), wherein the representatives of a deceased patient brought an action under 42 U.S.C. §1983 alleging a conspiracy to violate decedent's freedom of speech in that, contrary to the decedent's religious belief prohibiting blood transfusions, the defendant doctors and hospital, without notice and hearing to the decedent, had the 20-year-old decedent declared an incompetent and obtained a court order permitting the transfusion. The court held that the petition stated a cause of action. *See also* Winters v. Muller, 446 F.2d 65 (2nd Cir. 1971).

64. Roe v. Wade, 93 S. Ct. 705 (1973); Griswold v. Connecticut, 85 S. Ct. 1678 (1965).

65. 355 A.2d 647 (N.J. 1976).

66. *Id.* at 663.

67. *Id.* at 663–64; Superintendent of Belchertown State School v. Saikewicz, 370 N.E.2d 417, 424 (Mass. 1977).

68. In re Quinlan, 355 A.2d at 663; Superintendent of Belchertown State School v. Saikewicz, 370 N.E.2d at 425.

69. The notion that the state has an interest in protecting innocent third parties developed in cases in which a parent of a minor, who was a Jehovah's Witness, refused a blood transfusion for the child on religious grounds. In this circumstance, the courts frequently have ordered the transfusion. *See* Application of President and Directors of Georgetown College, Inc., 331 F.2d 1000 (D.C. Cir. 1964); United States v. George, 239 F.Supp. 752 (D. Conn. 1965); Raleigh Fitkin-Paul Morgan Mem. Hosp. v. Anderson, 201

A.2d 537 (N.J. 1964). In cases involving an adult, however, the individual's right to refuse medical treatment generally has been honored. *See* In Re Richardson, 284 So.2d 185 (La. App. 1976); In Re Osborne, 294 A.2d 372 (D.C. App. 1972); In Re Estate of Brooks, 205 N.E.2d 435 (Ill. 1965). *See also* Annot., 35 A.L.R.3rd 692 (1971).

70. Superintendent of Belchertown State School v. Saikewicz, 370 N.E.2d 417, 426–427 (Mass. 1977); In re Quinlan, 355 A.2d 647, 664–669 (N.J. 1976).

71. In Superintendent of Belchertown State School v. Saikewicz, 370 N.E.2d at 426–427, the Massachusetts Supreme Court responded to the state's argument that the proposed action would constitute suicide by stating:

> The interest in protecting against suicide seems to require little if any discussion. In the case of the competent adults refusing medical treatment such an act does not necessarily constitute suicide since (1) in refusing treatment the patient may not have the specific intent to die, and (2) even if he did, to the extent that the cause of death was from natural causes, the patient did not set the death producing agent in motion with the intent of causing his own death. [citations omitted]. Furthermore, the underlying state interest in this area lies in the prevention of irrational self-destruction. What we consider here is a competent, rational decision to refuse treatment where death is inevitable and the treatment offers no hope of cure or preservation of life. There is no connection between the conduct here at issue and any state concern to prevent suicide.

72. These were the circumstances in Superintendent of Belchertown State School v. Saikewicz, 370 N.E.2d 417 (Mass. 1977), and In re Quinlan, 355 A.2d 647 (N.J. 1976).

73. 370 N.E.2d 417 (Mass. 1977).

74. *Id.* at 425–426.

75. In re Quinlan, 355 A.2d at 663–64.

76. Superintendent of Belchertown State School v. Saikewicz, 370 N.E.2d at 432.

77. In several cases, courts have been faced with the question of whether or not they should authorize the transplant of an internal organ from a minor or incompetent to a sibling of that minor or incompetent. *See, e.g.*, In Re Guardianship of Pescinski, 226 S.W.2d 180, 182 (Wis. 1975); Hart v. Brown, 289 A.2d 386, 389 (Conn. App. 1972); Strunk v. Strunk, 445 S.W.2d 145, 146 (Ky. App. 1969). The courts that allowed this "detrimental" procedure did so based upon the fact that the minor or incompetent would be benefited psychologically by the continued existence of the sibling. The *Pescinski* case may be reconciled with the other two decisions based upon the fact that Pescinski was a catatonic schizophrenic and therefore it was highly unlikely that he would psychologically benefit by the

continued existence of his sister. In fact, there was no medical testimony offered, as in the other cases, to demonstrate any psychological benefit.

78. The physician's potential civil liability has received some consideration. *See, e.g.*, Note, *Euthanasia: The Physician's Liability*, 10 J. MAR. L. REV. 148, 163–169 (1976); Note, *Death With Dignity, The Physician's Civil Liability*, 27 BAYLOR L. REV. 86 (1975); SURVEY, *supra* note 3, at 1216–1227. These articles do not consider the problem of euthanasia involving a defective newborn. To the extent that these articles discuss the problem of obtaining the consent of the minor, they concluded that neither the minor nor any third party could consent to euthanasia.

79. *See* SURVEY, *supra* note 3, at 1217 n.121. This article takes the position that liability for euthanasia would exist even though the physician was acting with the consent of the deceased. *Id.* at 1218 n.123. The citation to W. PROSSER, LAW OF TORTS 107 (4th ed. 1971) is presumably intended to state that consent in such a situation is never a defense. As discussed in this section of this article this position is erroneous. *The Physician's Civil Liability*, 27 BAYLOR L. REV. 86, 97 (1975) (minor cannot consent); SURVEY, *supra* note 3, at 1221 (parents probably cannot consent). Aside from this brief discussion, the potential liability of parents in this situation was not addressed by these articles.

80. *See* SURVEY, *supra* note 3, at 1217 n.121. This article takes the position that liability for euthanasia would exist even though the physician was acting with consent of the deceased. To the extent that the authors of the SURVEY concluded that consent in this circumstance may never be a defense, the instant authors disagree.

81. *See* text accompanying notes 60–77. *See generally* Holmes v. Silver Cross Hosp., 340 F. Supp. 125 (N.D. Ill. 1972); Winters v. Miller, 446 F.2d 65 (2nd Cir. 1971); United States v. George, 239 F. Supp. 752 (D. Conn. 1965). A §1983 action theoretically could be premised upon the wrongful failure to withhold medical services as well as the wrongful failure to render medical services resulting in the patient's death without the due process of law.

82. *See* PROSSER, *supra* note 25, §18 at 101. Note, however, if the doctor provides medical assistance against the wishes and without the consent of the parent his actions will constitute battery. *See, e.g.*, Bonner v. Moran, 126 F.2d 121 (D.C. Cir. 1941); *accord*, Winters v. Miller, 446 F.2d 65, 68 (2nd Cir. 1971). In these circumstances, the child's consent does not constitute a defense. *Id.* If the physician feels that the medical assistance should be rendered he will have to have the child declared "neglected" under the local child abuse statute and he will have to obtain a court order permitting the medical procedure. *See, e.g.*, State v. Perricone, 181 A.2d 751 (N.J. 1962); Hoener v. Bertinato, 171 A.2d 140 (N.J. Super. 1961); People v. Labrenz, 104 N.E.2d 769 (Ill. 1952).

83. The term consent as utilized in this discussion refers to consent as a defense under traditional tort principles as well as the exercise of the patient's constitutional right to die.

84. This article does not attempt to discuss the question of the sufficiency of the information given to the individual consenting to the medical treatment. For an excellent discussion of the doctrine of informed consent as it relates to euthanasia, *see* Note, *Informed Consent and Dying Patient,* 83 Yale L.J. 1632 (1974).

85. This theory is based upon the assumption that the physician's duty to the mother includes an implied promise of care for the child upon birth. This responsibility presumably cannot be retracted by the parents after birth because the child is a third party beneficiary of that contract. *See* Robertson, *supra* note 3, at 226.

86. This theory of liability is based upon the assumption that immediately after birth the doctor normally will assume the responsibility for the care of the child before withholding medical treatment. It is a well-established principle of law that one who is not normally under a duty to care for another is under that duty to care if he has assumed that responsibility. In other words, once a doctor assumes responsibility to care for the child, a doctor-patient relationship is established. *See* Robertson, *supra* note 3, at 227–229.

87. Civil liability may be premised upon the breach of a duty imposed by statute. Under most state child abuse statutes, the physician is under a duty to report instances of child abuse. A patient's refusal to consent to the rendering of further medical treatment probably constitutes child abuse and, therefore, the doctor would be under a duty to report this to the juvenile authorities. The doctor's failure to report this to the juvenile authorities and failure to render required medical services likely would be considered the cause of the child's death. *See* Robertson, *supra* note 3, at 233–34.

88. *See supra* note 82; *Cf.* Annot., 22 A.L.R.3rd 1441 (1968).

89. 340 F. Supp. 125 (N.D. Ill. 1972). The court by implication suggested that the patient's constitutional right to die should be given the same constitutional priority as the patient's freedom of religion. *Id.* at 129–30.

The court also held that the "state action" requirement under §1983, with regard to the hospital, was satisfied by the pervasive regulatory system governing the hospital. The state action requirement with regard to the doctors was satisfied by virtue of the alleged conspiracy between the hospital and the doctors, thus making the doctors the agents of the hospital. *Id.* at 132–36.

90. 446 F.2d 65 (2nd Cir. 1971).

91. *See, e.g.,* Bonner v. Moran, 126 F.2d 121 (D.C. Cir. 1941).

It is not entirely clear whether or not the parents may exercise the right-to-die choice. It is clear that the parents have no such right by themselves, with regard to the continued life of their child. In re Quinlan, 355 A.2d at 664. The only cases which have discussed this constitutional right to die have involved proceedings wherein a separate guardian was appointed to represent the child. *See, e.g.,* Superintendent of Belchertown State School v. Saikewicz, 370 N.E.2d 417 (Mass. 1977). Courts, as in *Quinlan,* often have applied the doctrine of "substituted judgment" in order to determine the desires of the minor or incompetent. *See, e.g.,* Custody of a Minor, No. 78–6816 (Mass. Sup. Ct., April 18, 1978); Hart v. Brown, 289 A.2d 386 (Conn. App. 1972); Strunk v. Strunk, 445 S.W.2d 145 (Ky. App. 1969); *contra,* In Re Guardianship of Pescinski, 226 N.W.2d 180 (Wis. 1975).

92. *See* text accompanying notes 60–77, *supra.*

93. *See, e.g.,* State v. Perricone, 181 A.2d 751 (N.J. 1962); Hoener v. Bertinato, 171 A.2d 140 (N.J. Super. 1961); People v. Labrenz, 104 N.E.2d 769 (Ill. 1952). *See generally,* Annot., 30 A.L.R.2d 1138 (1953).

94. *Id. See also* the statutes cited *supra* note 14.

95. *Id.*

96. *See supra* note 46.

97. 181 A.2d 751 (N.J. 1962).

98. 171 A.2d 140 (N.J. Super. 1961).

99. *Id.* at 142–143. Similarly, in People v. Labrenz, 104 N.E.2d 769 (Ill. 1952), the court stated:

The question here is whether a child whose parents refuse to permit a blood transfusion, when lack of a transfusion means a child will almost certainly die or at best will be mentally impaired for life, is a neglected child. In answering that question it is of no consequence that the parents have not failed in their duty in other respects. We entertain no doubt that this child, whose parents were deliberately depriving it of life or subjecting it to permanent mental impairment, was a neglected child within the meaning of the statute. The circuit court did not lack jurisdiction. *Id.* at 773.

100. One difficulty here is the intrafamily immunity doctrine. The trend, however, is towards the abolition of this doctrine. *Cf.* Annot., 41 A.L.R.3d 904 (1972).

101. Under most of these statutes, the doctor is under a duty to report instances of child neglect. *See supra* note 86.

102. Recently, a Massachusetts court in Custody of a Minor, No. 78–6816 (Mass. Sup. Ct., April 18, 1978), substituted its judgment for that of the parents in a case involving a two-year-old child with acute lymphocytic leukemia. The parents had withdrawn the child from chemotherapy prescribed by a physician and instituted treatment of special nutrition and

prayer. One of the court's findings of fact was that with continued chemotherapy, the child had a better than fifty percent chance of survival and that dietary manipulation offered no prophylactic or curative benefits. After weighing the arguments for and against treatment, and after balancing the interest of the state preserving life with the individual's right to privacy (assuming competency to assert that right), the court invoked the "substituted judgment" doctrine in favor of chemotherapy.

ISSUES FOR CONSIDERATION AND SUGGESTIONS FOR FURTHER READING

The issue of who should decide whether life-saving therapy is appropriate for those unable to decide for themselves is resolved in two different ways in *Quinlan* (patient's guardian, family, attending physicians, and hospital's ethics committee) and *Saikewicz* (judge). Which approach is correct? What role does the *Saikewicz* decision see for the judge?

In a note on the *Saikewicz* case in 298 *New Eng. J. of Med.* 499 (Mar. 2, 1978), Professor Curran criticizes the *Saikewicz* "court procedure" approach on the grounds that it "is clearly too slow and cumbersome to fit most of the decisions made in intensive-care units." Do you agree?

How should questions of euthanasia be handled? By physicians? By families? By ethics panels? By anyone?

For additional materials on *Quinlan* and *Saikewicz,* see Baron, "Assuring 'Detached But Passionate Investigation and Decision': The Role of Guardians Ad Litem in *Saikewicz*-type Cases," 4 *Am. J. of Law & Medicine* 111 (1978);

Relman, "The *Saikewicz* Decision: A Medical Viewpoint," 4 *Am. J. of Law & Medicine* 233 (1978); Baron, "Medical Paternalism and the Rule of Law: A Reply to Dr. Relman," 4 *Am. J. of Law & Medicine* 337 (1979); Annas, "Reconciling *Quinlan* and *Saikewicz:* Decision Making for the Terminally Ill Incompetent," 4 *Am. J. of Law & Medicine* 367 (1979); and Coburn, "In re Quinlan: A Practical Overview," 31 *Ark. L. Rev.* 59 (1977) (written by the court-appointed guardian for Karen Ann Quinlan).

How much technology should society devote to those at the end stage of their life?

What legal problems are suggested by the hospice movement? You may wish to consult K. Cohen, *Hospice: Prescription for Terminal Care* (1979), and the works cited in its extensive bibliography, or R. Weir, ed., *Ethical Issues in Death and Dying* (1977), a collection of articles.

Finally, you may wish to consider whether other topics dealt with in this work (for example, alcohol abuse, Chapter 4) can be effectively approached through legislation.

CHAPTER 6

THE REGULATION OF PUBLIC HEALTH RESEARCH BY INSTITUTIONS AND GOVERNMENT

OVERVIEW

The articles in this chapter explore diverse approaches to the regulation of biomedical and behavioral research and examine a variety of legal issues in the regulation of scientific research with particular application to public health.

The article by Hogue examines the origins and functions of the institutional review process for research involving human subjects mandated by federal law and argues that its procedural safeguards should not be overextended to interfere in projects that do not pose the sorts of risks that Congress and the Department of Health, Education, and Welfare (HEW) considered in enacting the regulations. The article proposes a restrained interpretation of the regulations that Institutional Review Boards (IRBs) charged by law with carrying out the regulations may wish to follow in applying the rules to research at their own institutions.

Chalker and Catz consider the regulation of controversial DNA recombinant research (i.e., moving genes between organisms that ordinarily

would have no genetic contact) by means of the National Environmental Policy Act of 1969 (NEPA) and the technique of the environmental impact statement (EIS). The authors contend that the EIS prepared by the National Institutes of Health (NIH), an agency within HEW, was inadequate and did not consider the possibility of precluding recombinant research altogether. The authors urge more public input into the decision whether such research should be permitted and, if so, what restraints should be imposed on it.

Shapiro's article on new drug research examines the incentives in the drug industry to compile accurate data for submission to the Food and Drug Administration (FDA) to support that agency's determination as to whether a new drug is safe and beneficial for humans. The author suggests expanded involvement in the testing and data-gathering process for both the FDA and independent parties.

Finally, Tancredi's article explores the ethical dimensions of the clinical trial on human subjects and suggests a methodology of disclosure to patient/subjects and compensation for misadventures.

6.1 Institutional Review Boards and Public Health Research: An Analysis*

L. LYNN HOGUE

Reprinted with permission from 1 *UALR Law Journal* 428–454 (1978). Copyright © 1978 by the Board of Trustees of the University of Arkansas. All rights reserved.

A flexible policy is essential. Research, development, and the reduction to practice of new ideas are not carried out in a practical, ethical, or legal vacuum. The public interest obviously would not be served by an inflexible approach to what can or should be done. Ultimately, the decisions required . . . must depend upon the common sense and sound professional judgment of reasonable men.[1]

D.T. Chalkley, Ph.D.

INTRODUCTION

Experimental medical procedures have been subjected to litigation,[2] numerous studies,[3] and congressional hearings investigating abuses,[4] as has human experimentation in educational[5] and psychological[6] research. This article explores another area of nonmedical, experimental research on human subjects—public health research[7]—and suggests a proper analytic framework for those concerned with the protection of human subjects of such research. It is assumed that institutional review by boards designed to prevent abuses in experimental, therapeutic[8] medical research can and does unduly restrict public health researchers whose projects do not involve the dangers to subjects that institutional review was designed to mitigate or avoid.[9]

The current requirements for institutional review[10] are imposed by the United States Department of Health, Education, and Welfare (DHEW) on institutions administering studies involving biomedical or behavioral research on human subjects under authority of a provision of title II of the National Research Act of 1974.[11] The necessity for some regulation in this area is apparent from hearings conducted by the Subcommittee on Health of the Senate Committee on Labor and Public Welfare. The concerns reflected in testimony before the Subcommittee shaped both the statutory requirement for institutional review boards (IRBs) and the content of subsequent regulatory guidelines.[12]

The Subcommittee heard accounts of the unapproved use of drugs approved by the Food and Drug Administration (FDA) for other uses, other types of nonpharmaceutical medical experiments, and medical experiments and treatment without informed consent. In each of these instances, patients or subjects were not fully informed about the nature of the experiments in

---

*The author would like to acknowledge the helpful suggestions of Professor Robert H. Marquis of the UALR School of Law, who read an early draft of this article.

At this writing the National Commission was in the process of debating successive drafts of IRB Recommendations. To the extent possible under publishing deadlines, this article will consider the latest position taken by the Commission with respect to the implementation of DHEW regulations on the protection of human subjects.

which they were involved or, in some instances, were not told that they were involved in a medical experiment at all. Specific instances presented in subcommittee testimony included the following: (1) the use of Depo-Provera, a drug approved by the FDA for the treatment of endometrial cancer and endometriosis, as a three-month injectable contraceptive given to more than 1500 women under the Tennessee Maternal Health Family Planning Program without FDA approval and without informing the women involved;[13] (2) use of diethylstilbestrol (DES) as a post-coital contraceptive at several universities, although DES was not approved for this use;[14] (3) psychosurgery on patients in mental hospitals;[15] (4) use of a "supercoil" experimental intrauterine device developed by a nonphysician and implanted in several out-of-state women by a physician;[16] (5) the Tuskegee Syphilis Study;[17] (6) biomedical research in prisons and research on the effects of the biomedical research testing program on the rest of the prison social structure;[18] (7) the sterilization of minor welfare recipients without their parents' informed consent.[19] The Subcommittee also learned that, in some instances, research was not scrutinized by the researcher's scientific or professional peers and that some physician researchers simply conducted biomedical research as an adjunct to their medical practices.

Several bills were introduced in Congress to correct these abuses.[20] One approach was to establish a permanent national commission for the protection of human subjects that would have power to investigate and report on human subjects research; the commission would establish guidelines for IRBs and publish and distribute the decisions made by IRBs. Congress did not fully adopt this approach in the legislation finally enacted. It was also proposed, but rejected, that IRBs would be required to have a two-part structure: (1) a subcommittee that would review the scientific merits of research protocols submitted to it; and (2) a subcommittee that would "focus primarily on ensuring that the individual subjects of biomedical and behavioral research . . . are as well informed about the nature of the research as possible and that their rights are protected to the maximum extent."[21]

What emerged out of this legislative concern over abuses in experimental biomedical and behavioral research was a law establishing a temporary National Commission for the Protection

of Human Subjects of Biomedical and Behavioral Research (National Commission), and a requirement that DHEW mandate institutional review by IRBs and issue guidelines to govern them.[22] The guidelines on "Protection of Human Subjects," published in final form in the *Federal Register* in 1975, reflect many of the concerns already discussed that were before Congress.[23] For example, an elaborate definition of "informed consent" was set out to eliminate the abuses resulting from widely differing interpretations of that term as it was used by researchers.[24]

1. INSTITUTIONAL REVIEW BOARD REGULATIONS AND THE REVIEW PROCESS

a. Scope

The regulations on the protection of human subjects are applicable to all DHEW grants and contracts supporting research, development, and related activities in which human subjects are involved. This includes nonmedical, educational,[25] and other research. Special protection is extended to pregnant women and fetuses under other parts of the regulations,[26] which are beyond the scope of this article.

b. Policy

The regulations are designed to safeguard the rights and welfare of subjects "at risk" in activities supported by DHEW contracts and grants.

c. Procedure

IRBs are to review research proposals and determine whether subjects will be placed "at risk." If they will be, the IRB is then further to determine (1) whether "[t]he risks to the subject are so outweighed by the sum of the benefit to the subject and the importance of the knowledge to be gained as to warrant a decision to allow the subject to accept these risks"; (2) whether "[t]he rights and welfare of such subjects will be adequately protected"; and (3) whether "[l]egally effective informed consent[27] will be obtained by adequate and appropriate methods in accordance with the provisions of the regulations."[28]

The regulations also provide for the periodic review of projects involving subjects "at risk."[29] There is also a requirement that projects not initially involving human subjects must be brought under review by the IRB if such subjects are later involved.[30]

d. Sanctions

The responsibility for enforcing these safeguards to subjects belongs to the institution that receives the funding or is accountable to DHEW for it.[31] Institutions must assure DHEW that review will be instituted.[32] Unapproved studies are not eligible for DHEW funding.[33] Negative determinations by an IRB are the primary sanction against an investigator, and a negative IRB determination can only be reversed by the IRB. IRB approval does not obligate an institution to a particular research project if institutional administrators disapprove, but the findings of the IRB cannot be rescinded administratively if they are negative.[34]

Since DHEW research is funded by the government and presumably serves a public interest, it could be argued that the government should assume responsibility for the programs it funds and scrutinize programs for the protection of human subjects. The bureaucratization this approach would entail has precluded adoption or even serious consideration of it.[35]

The government could also protect human subjects by focusing on bad results and providing compensation for them.[36] This could be done through an insurance pool built up by the profits of new research, thereby letting the technical benefits of research bear the burdens of their discovery, or a no-fault system like workers' compensation for human subjects injured through research. As a less comprehensive remedy, the Federal Tort Claims Act[37] could be extended to cover subjects injured through negligence or wrongful conduct in government-funded research programs, including projects conducted by others under a contract or grant. Compensation mechanisms would have the advantage of assuming the cost of misadventures in such research as a public cost of advancing knowledge while at the same time fostering research.

e. Membership and Organization

The membership and organization of the IRBs are controlled by federal regulation.[38] A minimum of five persons is required, and a quorum for the IRB is a majority of its members. The regulations require that not all members of the board come from within the institution itself[39] or from any single professional group.[40] A board member is prohibited from participating in a review of his own project or one in which he is involved, except to the extent of providing information to the board.[41] Documentation of the training and experience of board members is required.[42]

An underlying assumption of the regulations is that IRB members must be competent to determine when a human subject is placed "at risk" and, when "subjects at risk" are identified, to be able to weigh intelligently the risk to the subject against the benefits to him and to society through the knowledge to be gained by the research. IRB members must also be knowledgeable enough to know whether the welfare of the subject will be protected and whether legally effective informed consent will be obtained. One proposal considered by Congress but rejected, as was noted earlier, was to provide for a two-part IRB: one subpart of the board to weigh the scientific merits of the proposed research protocols and the other to provide for the protection of the human subjects "at risk."[43] Although Congress did not include this two-part IRB in the final language of the National Research Act of 1974, elements of both functions are to be found in the present system. They are not clearly delineated, however. Implicit in weighing the risks and benefits of a given project is determining whether the research is worth doing from a scientific point of view and also whether a particular project is a good way in which to gain the information sought.[44]

The congressional choice to compel institutions to provide protection, rather than assuming that responsibility within DHEW, has forced researchers' peers in an IRB to undertake a fairly complex evaluative task without much legal guidance. Once an IRB determines that a subject is "at risk" it must consider (1) whether "[t]he risks to the subject are so outweighed by the sum of the benefit to the subject and the importance of the knowledge to be gained as to warrant a decision to allow the subject to accept these risks''; (2) whether "[t]he rights and welfare of any such subjects will be adequately protected''; and (3) whether "[l]egally effective informed consent will be obtained by adequate and appropriate methods. . . .''[45]

The procedural steps in arriving at the issue of risk are well illustrated by *Crane v. Mathews*,[46] wherein the State of Georgia secured permission from DHEW to impose co-payment requirements on its Medicaid recipients[47] in an effort to reduce steadily rising Medicaid costs.[48] The project was approved as an experiment on "Recipient Cost Participation in Medicaid Reform" designed to test whether co-payment "would curtail overutilization in Georgia of 'marginally needed' health care."[49]

An action brought by plaintiff Medicaid recipients in federal district court sought, among other things, a preliminary injunction against the imposition of co-payment requirements. The preliminary injunction was denied,[50] as was a motion by the Secretary of DHEW for summary judgment.[51] Following a trial, the court found that the co-payment project was covered by the regulations for the protection of human subjects[52] and required submission of the project to the state's IRB[53] for review:

> The question . . . before the Court is: Are human subjects involved in the Georgia co-payment project in such a way as to trigger the provisions of 45 C.F.R. §46? The Court need not determine whether the subjects are at risk; this is a determination to be made by the IRB, only after a determination is made that human subjects are involved.[54]

Although the cutbacks in benefits were ostensibly justified as "experiments," they were in fact merely reductions which could be permitted under applicable Medicaid law only when characterized as "experimental."[55] The *Crane* court held that IRB review was required, but it did not address the definitions applicable in that review.[56] The court then denied a motion by the defendant to dismiss and granted plaintiff's motion for a permanent injunction to take effect only if certain conditions, one of which was submission of the project for IRB approval, were not met. According to plaintiff's attorney in *Crane,* the Georgia IRB "determined [on remand] that the 'human subjects' [identified by

the court in the *Crane* case] were 'subjects at risk' and that potential benefits of the experiment were so outweighed by the risks that the project should be discontinued."[57] The experiment was accordingly ended July 30, 1976.[58] It should be noted that the result reached by the Georgia State IRB in *Crane* may have been compelled in part by the virtual impossibility of applying the protective safeguards required by the regulations, such as legally effective informed consent,[59] after subjects were found to be at risk. Since the co-payment requirement was imposed statewide,[60] securing informed consent would be difficult or impossible because few welfare recipients would voluntarily choose to make co-payments. An even more important factor in *Crane* was the use of the human subjects research regulations as a legal strategy to stave off a statewide reduction in Medicaid benefits. While the reduction was styled as an "experiment" by the State of Georgia and the cooperation of DHEW secured on that basis, the Medicaid reduction "experiment" was probably not the sort contemplated by the National Research Act of 1974,[61] if the hearings preceding it are any guide.

2. DEFINING AND DETERMINING RISK

The determination of whether a human subject of a research project is "at risk" is the IRB's principal function, and it is central to research project approval. It is in this step that an IRB, particularly one in an institution doing public health research, has the greatest opportunity to avoid hampering its institution's research effort. Public health-related IRBs should weigh carefully how they understand and apply these guidelines.

The function of any IRB in determining subject risk can most appropriately be viewed as a two-step process. The initial inquiry is whether human subjects are involved in the research.[62] If they are not, then review under these regulations proceeds no further. If they are, the next step is a determination of whether a subject of the research will be placed "at risk." This determination is crucial. If no human subjects are placed "at risk," the further requirements of the regulations are obviated.[63] "This review shall determine whether these subjects will be placed at risk, and if risk is involved,"[64] then the IRB must consider risk versus benefit, protection of the subject's rights, and the matter of consent, as previously mentioned. The form certifying that review has taken place[65] echoes this procedural view, for IRBs must certify for each project:

- Human Subjects: Reviewed, Not at Risk.
- Human Subjects: Reviewed, At Risk, Approved.

The words "at risk" have a special definition, supplied by the regulations themselves.[66]

a. Defining Risk to Subjects

Under the DHEW regulations, a "subject at risk" is any individual who may be exposed to the possibility of injury, including physical, psychological, or social injury, as a consequence of participation as a subject in any research, development, or related activity *which departs from the application of those established and accepted methods necessary to meet his needs, or which increases the ordinary risks of daily life, including the recognized risks inherent in a chosen occupation or field of service.*[6]

The definition clearly does not treat all risks as placing a subject "at risk." The inclusive category of "any individual . . . who may be exposed to the possibility of injury . . . as a subject in any research" is carefully limited by the two clauses beginning with "which" that follow it. Although it is possible to interpret the definition in a more expansive fashion (more restrictive to researchers), a construction stressing the language concerning "the possibility of injury" and viewing any subject as "at risk" who is so exposed should be rejected for public health research.

This is true because an IRB finding that a subject is "at risk" in turn mandates the use of DHEW-required procedural protections such as fully documented,[68] legally effective[69] informed consent[70] which includes (1) a fair explanation of the procedures to be followed and their purposes, including identification of any procedures which are experimental; (2) a description of any attendant discomforts and risks reasonably to be expected; (3) a description of any benefits rea-

sonably to be expected; (4) a disclosure of any appropriate alternative procedures that might be advantageous for the subject; (5) an offer to answer any inquiries concerning the procedures; and (6) an instruction that the person is free to withdraw his consent and to discontinue participation in the project or activity at any time without prejudice to the subject. One option open to IRBs is to assume that all research on humans places them at risk. If the additional procedural requirements are imposed on all human research, then at least two positive results follow: (1) Subjects are extended maximum protection even against remote, highly contingent, or speculative risks. Pushed to an extreme, research might protect human subjects by reducing even ordinary dangers through an excess of caution exercised in the experimental environment. (2) Any possibility of error or liability for error by the IRB in the assessment of "risk," such as errors in applying the definition to the research protocol,[71] is reduced to nil. This safe path also affects research by limiting it, by making it more costly, and, in some instances, by adversely affecting research protocols.

If all subjects are given the maximum procedural protection available under DHEW guidelines, then these subjects of any research would be extended the same protection as subjects of experimental, therapeutic, medical research. Put another way, a person asked simply to answer a questionnaire[72] would be given the same protection as someone undergoing experimental cancer chemotherapy.

Under such constraints, some types of public health research are made more difficult, if not impossible, by procedures that require fully documented, legally effective informed consent of a type appropriate by and large only for medical research. An experiment, for example, may be spoiled if those in either the experimental or the control group are told that they are involved in an experiment in which their attitudes or preferences are being observed and evaluated. The fact that the subjects are aware of the experiment, its purposes, and the alternative paths of behavior may hopelessly prejudice the outcome of the experiment.

Another problem is that simple experiments, such as telephone surveys, may become pointless when subjected to rigid formal requirements of informed consent. Telephone surveys minimize the cost and effort required by personal contact; but if a rigid application of the "at risk" notion requires prior, documented, legally effective informed consent for a simple telephone interview, then the researcher might as well rely on the traditional interviewer who can take a consent form along or he may forego gathering the information altogether because of such a restrictive research climate.[73]

At some point it becomes valid to inquire how important it is to evaluate both innovations and long accepted notions about health and health care delivery involving human subjects. If any differentiation for experimental purposes is presumed to entail "risk," then society faces the unhappy prospect of permitting innovations without being able to evaluate them because disclosure to the control and acquisition of his consent will destroy the effectiveness of having a control. If research involving human subjects is desirable and even necessary, then the IRB can be seen as exercising a crucial role in the future of research because it can either facilitate or hamper research by its interpretation of the rules it applies. Some research, even though it involves humans, does not involve the risks inherent in novel biological or psychological manipulation or medical research of a therapeutic nature. In short, elaborate safeguards should not be required if research does not involve "risk."

b. Determining When Human Subjects Are Placed at Risk

If not every research project involving human subjects places them at risk, then it is necessary to distinguish between that research which does and that which does not involve risks. The Georgia IRB's finding that human subjects were "at risk" used a broader interpretation of "subject at risk" than one suggested by the situations before Congress when it imposed IRB review; Congress legislated in response to projects which departed from established treatment regimens, such as the use of FDA-approved drugs for unapproved purposes, psychosurgery, and other techniques of behavior manipulation.

It should be noted that the areas of concern addressed by the legislative hearings on the National Research Act of 1974 were the source of the examples of "risk" cited by DHEW Secretary David Mathews in a notice published in the *Federal Register*, "Secretary's Interpretation of 'Subject at Risk,'"[74] issued in the midst of the *Crane* litigation. The Secretary's interpretation pointed out several examples of DHEW-funded, welfare-related research in which subjects were not considered by DHEW to be "at risk." It was not surprising that the instances cited in the Secretary's interpretation included projects designed to test methods for reducing welfare benefits and their attendant burden on the public fisc in some states.[75]

The examples cited by the Secretary of how DHEW interprets the definition of "subject at risk" in the context of the Medicaid cutback program are, as will be seen, consistent with a careful reading of the regulations. They also offer public health researchers an opportunity to avoid problems resulting from unnecessary or inappropriate procedural requirements and to achieve greater flexibility in designing study protocols and appropriate protection for human subjects of public health research. The Medicaid experiments were as follows: (1) Some welfare recipients were to report their incomes more frequently than others for purposes of determining their eligibility for, or the level of, their welfare benefits. (2) Some, but not all, able-bodied welfare recipients were required to work as a condition of eligibility. (3) The level of welfare benefits (within prescribed boundaries) payable to some, but not all, similarly situated welfare beneficiaries was diminished. (4) Some, but not all, welfare recipients were required to make a co-payment toward the cost of governmentally-financed medical care (as in *Crane*).[76]

In his interpretation, the Secretary urged that these four experiments

[did] not constitute burdens or effects of the nature that the regulations [for the protection of human subjects] are intended to encompass and, therefore, would not place the individuals subject to these burdens or effects "at risk" within the meaning of the regulation. In the context of the regulations, there would be no departure from the range of "established and accepted methods necessary to meet [the] needs [of the individual]" in these types of circumstances.[77]

The standard used by the Secretary to measure a "departure" from the norm was "the average American in his daily life."[78] Since the average able-bodied American must work, it is no departure from the norm to require able-bodied welfare recipients to work, even though the norm for welfare recipients is not working. Similarly, income reporting, lowered incomes, and some payment for medical care[79] are not departures from normal experience. The Secretary contended that

the regulations for the protection of human subjects are not intended to protect individuals from the "ordinary risks of daily life." There are certain risks which may reasonably be encountered by anyone, for example, the risks inherent in having to make a decision as to how to allocate funds, or in deciding whether to meet certain conditions, such as performing work, which are required in order to obtain funds. The exposure to the risks which emanate from these choices does not constitute the type of situation against which the Department's regulations are designed to guard.[80]

The Secretary's interpretation of the definition of "subject at risk," probably an interpretative rule,[81] is entitled to considerable weight,[82] particularly by members of IRBs, researchers, and those who may practice before such boards. Board members can in good faith[83] rely on the interpretation in determining how to apply the definition.

IRBs are not bound by expansive interpretations of risk by other boards such as that in Georgia,[84] and that is particularly true where those interpretations are in conflict with interpretations promulgated by the Secretary of DHEW, the agency that is responsible for the regulations. Boards are free to interpret "risk" more narrowly, so long as they do not evade the minimal protective purpose of the DHEW regulations already discussed.

Whether boards adopt a narrow or restrictive definition of "subject at risk," such as the Secretary of DHEW urged in his interpretation, or a broader definition, such as that applied by the Georgia State IRB, can have a substantial impact on public health research. In terms of permissible methodologies of experimental research, the definition of risk can operate constrictively since, under the regulations, a determination that a subject is placed "at risk" triggers procedural safeguards which do not apply to other research. Put another way, under the

regulations research in which subjects are not placed "at risk" is under no greater constraint than is research not involving human subjects at all (except that it must be passed on initially by the IRB).[85] It should be noted, of course, that professional ethics may impose constraints on research on human subjects that would not apply to research with mice or dice, but ethical considerations are not a part of the DHEW regulations and are not considered further here.[86]

Subject "risk," as has been noted, is defined as "the possibility of injury, including physical, psychological, or social injury."[87] Consistent with the intent of the National Research Act of 1974, the regulations on institutional review leave considerable discretion[88] to the IRB members to define when risk exists for the human subjects of specific research projects. The use of the term "including" in connection with the catalog of potential areas of harm suggests that the scope of harm is not limited to those set out in the regulations.

Physical risk is perhaps the easiest example to understand, in large measure because medical and other researchers and even clinicians are familiar with physical consequences, iatrogenic (arising from therapeutic misadventures) and otherwise, which can and do occur, as well as their potential liability for intentionally and negligently caused physical harm. Risk of psychological harm is more difficult because of its emergent nature and nascent legal contours.[89] Although the concept of risk is not limited to what is defined in law to be a physical, psychological, or social risk, such an independent reference point in law may serve to guide an IRB in its determinations. Risks of harm which are not redressable at law may also be de minimis for research purposes as well and should be disregarded by IRBs along with conjectural and hypothetical views of harm.

Social harm includes such things as the risk of embarrassment, humiliation, stigma, and social or economic reprisal. It implicates, but probably differs from, the right to privacy.[90] Legal harm is an important adjunct to social risk and probably a distinct category of subject risk. Legal risks to subjects can arise from research into the use and effects of narcotics or alcohol when information supplied by the subject could serve as the basis for his criminal prosecution or for a civil action against him. Legal harm as a risk is suggested but not explored in the DHEW *Institutional*

Guide to the regulations on human subjects' protection.[91] Congress has specifically provided for eliminating subject risk with respect to drug and alcohol studies.[92] Of course, the failure of an investigator to avail himself of this provision or the approval of such a project by an IRB without requiring the investigator to secure authorization to protect the subjects' privacy pursuant to the statute would expose the subject to risk, thus evidencing negligence on the part of the investigator and possibly a lack of good faith by members of the IRB.

Despite the provision for special protection of information and subject identities obtained in connection with drug and alcohol studies, other areas of research have no such safeguards. For instance, substantial probability of legal risk to subjects follows venereal disease research, which could give rise to information useful in a civil action for tortious infection,[93] or research into the battered child syndrome,[94] which could result in both civil[95] or criminal[96] liability.

3. INSTITUTIONAL REVIEW BOARDS AND ADMINISTRATIVE LAW

Two problems with IRBs are readily apparent, only one of which can be addressed at the local level without revision of the DHEW Guidelines. The first problem concerns the excess discretion vested in IRBs and the need for a clear and coherent definition of subject "risk." A second and more fundamental problem is the allocation by DHEW of primary responsibility for protecting human subjects to the IRB rather than to a human subjects' advocate or ombudsman.

IRBs are creatures both of the federal regulations that require them of research institutions and of the institutions themselves. IRBs are bound to apply in good faith[97] the federal rules promulgated by DHEW. They may also, consistent with state law and institutional limitations, if any, promulgate their own rules—procedural and substantive.[98] Without attempting to set forth a complete model of such rules, it is sufficient to suggest here the need for a substantive definition of "risk" so that investigators will know what protocols and activities will result in a higher level of scrutiny and will trigger protective safeguards. An absence of a definition can lead to overzealous application of human sub-

jects' protection by IRBs to the detriment of research to which the protection has little application.

Hershey and Miller, in their work on the function of the IRB in a predominantly medical setting, depict the review process as informal, with the investigator and the IRB members apparently collaborating in the design of an inoffensive protocol. They state that "[i]nstitutional review should be an interactional process between the [IRB] and the investigator, striving to find a way that the proposed study can be performed in a manner consistent with public policy and the rights and welfare of the subjects, without destroying the worth of the study."[99]

Ordinarily, interactional processes are unobjectionable, even salutary, in the academy, but interaction with an IRB guided by loosely defined and largely subjective concepts of risks to subjects is likely to lead to a one-sided contest with a detrimental effect to innovative research. Under federal regulations, investigators are dependent upon IRB approval for funding and for authority to conduct even unfunded studies. Review is pervasive. Investigators must expect repeated encounters with IRBs if their research routinely involves human subjects, and it is not likely that they will risk arguing over details at the expense of an ongoing relationship which every investigator must hope will be marked by good will.

Proposed recommendations have suggested continuity and stability in IRBs. These measures would foster competence and familiarity in dealing with problems but will likewise place active investigators further at the mercy of IRBs.[100] Since negative decisions by an IRB are not appealable,[101] there are substantial opportunities for abuse of discretion by a board.

Concerning such abuses, Professor Kenneth Davis, who has written extensively about the problem of delegation,[102] has proposed the following reformulation of the nondelegation doctrine to protect "against unnecessary and uncontrolled discretionary power":

The focus should no longer be exclusively on standards; it should be on the totality of protections against arbitrariness, including both safeguards and standards. The key should no longer be statutory words; it should be the protections the administrators in fact provide, irrespective of what statutes say or fail to say.[103]

An effective prophylactic against abuse of IRB procedure would be a proper allocation of functions according to traditional administrative law models. For example, an IRB should consider limiting the scope of its inquiry into risk by a definition of "risk" as it is recognized in the department, school, or institution of which the IRB is a part. Such a definition should be arrived at after soliciting information and proposals from affected parties.[104] Such a definition would circumscribe the work of the IRB and prevent the abuse of its discretion in the interaction between investigators and the board.[105]

As a second step, the review process should be tailored along the lines of an adjudicatory hearing with minimal due process required.[106] Since the investigator will have had an opportunity in most instances to explain his protocol, it is worth emphasizing that due process would require notice of an adverse decision, its basis, and an opportunity to respond orally and/or in writing to the reasons given. Oral argument is particularly desirable in view of the absence of any appeals process. It is interesting to note that a recommendation for more protection than is currently required by due process was incorporated in the proposals of the National Commission.[107]

In some instances it may be desirable to achieve greater procedural protection for investigators by bringing the IRBs at state-owned institutions under the state's administrative procedure act.[108] The Model State Administrative Procedure Act[109] provides a useful example amply solicitous of investigators' interests. Any inclusion of IRBs within a state administrative procedure act would, however, have to be approved by the Secretary of DHEW[110] as a part of an institution's general assurances of compliance.

It is important to note that merely because an IRB responds to the supposed interests of human subjects does not mean either that such subjects are properly represented or even that their interests are adequately articulated. Nor does the presence of a nonprofessional on the IRB, a "consumer" or community member, alleviate the problem. The purpose of the community member is to enhance the collective expertise of the board and alleviate the possibility of professional bias in the ethical perspective of the board. So the addition needed in the IRB review

process is an independent spokesman for the interests of potential human subjects, a human subjects' advocate or ombudsman[111] charged with identifying and articulating the interests of subjects and representing their position before the board. It is submitted that this proposal would require a change in the DHEW regulations since present regulations impose primary responsibility for subject protection on the IRB. Inherent in this proposal is a partial transfer of that responsibility from the IRB, which would become more neutral in its stance and better able to weigh independently the information presented to it by the investigator and the human subjects' rights advocate. At the same time, primary responsibility for advocating subjects' interests would rest with the ombudsman. Institutions could, however, experiment with this proposal without shifting responsibility, assuming they file a revised general assurance with DHEW and secure the Secretary's approval.

Many of the problems explored in this article, such as IRB abuses in expansively construing the concept of risk, can be traced directly to the structure of the IRB and its procedure as prescribed by DHEW regulations. Under present rules, the board is to function both as an advocate for the human subjects of the experiment and as an impartial decision-maker passing on a project's acceptability. The fusion of these functions naturally leads to a blurring of responsibility that should be kept distinct. The IRB has the power to approve or disapprove a proposal; it is the expert decision-making body. The investigator presents his view of the proposal to the board, including his perspective on potential harm to subjects. What is lacking is an independent assessment by an individual charged with presenting the subjects' interests. The present regulations require both the investigator and the IRB to consider subjects' interests, but obviously an investigator's other responsibilities affect his ability to discharge that duty. In fact, the IRB requirement arose out of an obvious inability to entrust investigators with sole responsibility for subjects. It is not surprising that IRBs saddled with a dual task—protecting subjects and approving (or disapproving) projects—tend to give considerable attention to interests of the unrepresented. Lawyers who have witnessed a court's solicitude for a pro se litigant matched against qualified legal counsel will recognize the problem.

CONCLUSION

The requirement of ethical peer review in the form of IRBs to protect human subjects of biomedical and behavioral research was a much-needed response to some obvious abuses, particularly in medical research. The protection provided by IRBs should be for real and substantial harms defined in advance by a process of rule-making reflective of scientific consensus in a given department, school, or institution. This is particularly appropriate for public health and other types of nontherapeutic research. At the same time, some consideration should be given to protecting investigators from an abuse of discretion by IRBs by adopting standards and incorporating practices based on minimal notions of due process.

NOTES

1. U.S. Dep't of Health, Educ., and Welfare, The Institutional Guide to DHEW Policy on Protection of Human Subjects, iii (1971) [hereinafter cited as Institutional Guide].

2. *E.g.*, Hyman v. Jewish Chronic Disease Hosp., 21 App. Div. 2d 495, 251 N.Y.S.2d 818 (1964), *rev'd*, 15 N.Y.2d 317, 206 N.E.2d 338, 258 N.Y.S.2d 397 (1965) (hypodermic injection of cancer cells into 22 human patients).

3. *E.g.*, H. Beecher, Research and the Individual (1970); Biomedical Ethics and the Law (J. Huber & R. Almeder eds. 1976) [hereinafter cited as Biomedical Ethics]; Experimentation with Human Subjects (P. Freund ed. 1970); C. Fred, Medical Experimentation: Personal Integrity and Social Policy (1974); N. Hershey & R. Miller, Human Experimentation and the Law (1976) [hereinafter cited as Hershey & Miller]; J. Katz, Experimentation with Human Beings (1972); Houlgate, *Rights, Health, and Mental Disease*, 22 Wayne L. Rev. 87 (1975); Ladimer, *Ethical and Legal Aspects of Medical Research on Human Beings*, 3 J. Pub. L. 467 (1954); Mullen, *Human Experimentation Regulations of HEW Bar Georgia Medicaid Cutbacks*, 10 Clearinghouse Rev. 259 (1976); *Viewpoints on Behavioral Issues in Closed Institutions*, 17 Ariz. L. Rev. 1 (1975); Note, *Medical Experiment Insurance*, 70 Colum. L. Rev. 965 (1970); Note, *Experimentation on Human Beings*, 20 Stan. L. Rev. 99 (1967); Comment, *Non-therapeutic Medical Research Involving Human Subjects*, 24 Syracuse L. Rev. 1067 (1973).

4. *E.g.*, *Hearings on Quality of Health Care— Human Experimentation before the Senate Comm. on Labor and Public Welfare*, S. Rep. No. 381, 93d Cong., 2d Sess., *reprinted in* [1974] U.S. Code Cong. & Ad. News 3634, 3638 [hereinafter cited as *Hearings*].

5. *E.g.*, DuVal, *Educational Research and the Protection of Human Subjects*, 1977 Am. B. Foundation Research J. 477, 519:

Historically the emphasis in the regulation of research for the protection of subjects has been in the biomedical context. The nature of harm that students and teachers may sustain as a consequence of their participation in educational research differs markedly from, and on the whole is less dramatic than, that which may arise from biomedical research. Educational research does not present the risk of physical injury that is often inherent in biomedical research. Educational research may result in psychological stress and may invade the privacy interests of teachers and students. But while both the intentional infliction of psychological harm and the invasion of privacy are actionable, the likelihood that substantial damages will be imposed is less than in biomedical research.

6. Ad Hoc Comm. on Ethical Standards in Psychological Research, Ethical Principles in the Conduct of Research with Human Participants (1973); London, *Experiments on Humans: Where To Draw the Line*, Psychology Today, Nov. 1977, at 20. *E.g.*, Ethical and Legal Issues of Social Experimentation (A. Rivlin & P. Timpane eds. 1975); Social Research in Conflict with Law and Ethics (P. Negelski ed. 1976).

7. A fundamental characteristic differentiating "public health" from other health and medical disciplines is its corporate focus or emphasis on more than just individuals. This concept has been described as follows:

In scientific public health, we no longer treat the individual—the segment of the community—but the total body politic—mental, physical, social, and economic. We no longer treat individuals with communicable diseases, but we prevent, control, or eradicate the disease in the body politic. The total patient is our responsibility [*i.e.*, the community], and not the individuals who are a part of it.

McGavran, *What is Public Health?* 44 Canadian J. Pub. Health 441, 444 (1953). "*Public Health is the scientific diagnosis and treatment of the body politic or community.*" *Id.* at 447 (emphasis in original).

As will be seen, this corporate or community focus has significant legal implication since the "risk" to which study populations may be exposed in studies involving community measurements, demographic characteristics, etc., is substantially attenuated when compared with that inherent in medical research. The traditional assumption, however, is that all research is therapeutic and aimed at treatment of individuals: "Most biomedical investigators are . . . interested in taking care of patients and making them well." Barber,

The Ethics of Experimentation With Human Subjects, Scientific Am., Feb. 1976, at 25, 30. No more articulate expression of the erroneous assumption that all research is necessarily therapeutic could be found. It is to assist in righting this notion and urging a proper understanding of institutional review for nontherapeutic research that this article was written.

8. *Therapeutic research, nontherapeutic research.* The Commission recognizes problems with employing the terms "therapeutic" and "nontherapeutic" research, notwithstanding their common usage, because they may convey a misleading impression. Research refers to a class of activities designed to develop generalizable new knowledge. Such activities are often engaged in to learn something about practices designed for the therapy of the individual. Such research is often called "therapeutic" research; however, the research is not solely for the therapy of the individual. In order to do research, additional interventions over and above those necessary for therapy may need to be done, *e.g.,* randomization, blood drawing, catheterization; these interventions may not be "therapeutic" for the individual. Some of these interventions may themselves present risk to the individual—risk unrelated to therapy of the subject.

Nat'l Comm'n for the Protection of Human Subjects of Biomedical and Behavioral Research, Research Involving Prisoners (1976) [hereinafter cited as National Commission].

The special considerations applicable to therapeutic research are further apparent in the following caveat—part of Nat'l Comm'n for the Protection of Human Subjects of Biomedical and Behavioral Research, IRB Recommendations, Recommendation (3)(D), Comment (D) at 16 (Draft March 3, 1978) [hereinafter cited as Commission Draft]: "The involvement of a physician or therapist as an investigator may have significant advantages for patients and make available to them new forms of therapy. However, research interests may compromise the therapist's sound judgments regarding therapeutic goals."

9. "In recent years . . . widespread societal concern for privacy and confidentiality, often manifest in confusing or ambiguous regulations, has made many types of epidemiologic and other medical investigation increasingly difficult to conduct and, in fact, now threatens to make many such studies virtually impossible." Gordis, Gold, & Seltser, *Privacy Protection in Epidemiologic and Medical Research: A Challenge and a Responsibility,* 105 Am. J. of Epidemiology 163, 163 (1977).

10. The development of institutional review is surveyed in Ratnoff, *Who Shall Decide When Doctors Disagree? A Review of the Legal Development of Informed Consent and the Implications of Proposed Lay Review of Human Experimentation,* 25 Case W. Res. L. Rev. 472 (1975).

11. 42 U.S.C. §2891–3(a) (Supp. V 1975).

12. 45 C.F.R. §§46.101–.301 (1976); *Hearings, supra* note 4, at 3638.

13. *Hearings, supra* note 4, at 3638.

14. *Id.* at 3639.

15. *Id.* at 3640.

16. *Id.* at 3642.

17. *Id.*

18. *Id.*

19. *Id.* at 3645.

20. *See* Ratnoff, *supra* note 10, at 517 n.280 for list.

21. *Hearings, supra* note 4, at 3656.

22. 42 U.S.C. §2891–3(a) (Supp. V 1975).

23. 40 Fed. Reg. 11, 854 (1975), 45 C.F.R. §§46.101–.301 (1976).

24. The range of practice in securing "informed consent" is reflected in the following episodes excerpted from the hearings of the Senate Committee on Labor and Public Welfare preceding the legislation and regulations on human subjects research:

DepoProvera research (use of FDA-approved drug for an unapproved purpose): "Anna Burgess, one of the women who received [DepoProvera as an injectable contraceptive] testified that she was never informed of the potential side effects, never signed a consent form, and experienced a significant degree of discomfort after taking the drug. Dr. Kase and Ms. Greenberger reported on the results of a field investigation in which six women in Cumberland County, Tennessee[,] including Miss Burgess, were interviewed about the use of DepoProvera. Dr. Kase concluded that informed consent was not obtained in any of the six cases, no attempt was made to achieve patient awareness, and the potential short and long term hazards of the drug were not discussed."

Hearings, supra note 4, at 3638–39.
The following position of the American Medical Association is analogous: Dr. Barclay, testifying on behalf of the American Medical Association, said that the final responsibility for the treatment of patients rests with the individual physician, and that it was proper for him to have the right to use an unapproved drug or to perform experimental surgery if that was, in his, the physician's opinion in the best interest of the patient.

Id. at 3643.
On "informed consent" to medical treatment, as the term is used in its more conventional sense, *see* Schneyer, *Informed Consent and the Danger of Bias in the Formation of Medical Disclosure Practices,* 1976 Wis. L. Rev. 124; Waltz & Scheuneman, *Informed Consent to Therapy,* 64 Nw. U.L. Rev. 628 (1970).

25. *See* DuVal, *supra* note 5.

26. 45 C.F.R. §§46.102(c), .201–.211 (1976). IRBs' additional responsibilities are found in 45 C.F.R. §46.205 (1976).

27. "As originally proposed the regulation did not contain the words 'legally effective.' . . . The insertion of the phrase was suggested in comments on the proposed rule. . . . No explanation of the significance of the addition was given." DuVal, *supra* note 5, at 509 n.121.

28. 45 C.F.R. §46.102 (1976).

29. *Id*. §46.102(d).

30. *Id*. §46.114.

31. *Id*. §46.102(a).

32. *Id*. §46.104.

33. Failure to conform to the agreement between an institution and DHEW, as set out in the institution's assurance to DHEW, could lead to a loss of research funding by DHEW. With respect to sanctions, the Commission Draft, *supra* note 8, at 9, has proposed the following:

> *Recommendation (2)*(A) Federal law should be enacted or amended to authorize the secretary of Health, Education, and Welfare to carry out the following duties:
>
> . . . .
>
> (ii) Compliance activities, including site visits and audits of institutional review board records, to examine the performance of the boards and their fulfillment of institutional assurances and regulatory requirements. . . .
>
> . . . .
>
> *Comment:* . . .
>
> . . . .
>
> Site visits, audits of IRB records, and other compliance activities should be conducted routinely to assure continuing quality control of the performance of IRBs. The compliance effort should be aimed at educating, improving performance of IRBs and providing needed advice. Where necessary, however, failure by investigators, institutions or IRBs to meet their responsibilities should be subject to sanctions ranging from warnings to loss of IRB accreditation and consequent ineligibility to receive federal funds for research involving human subjects or refusal by a regulatory agency to accept data.

34. 45 C.F.R. §46.118 (1976).

35. For instance, even the essentially aggrandizing recommendations of the National Commission eschew national review in favor of local IRB screening as follows:

> The Commission believes that the rights of the subjects should be protected by local review committees operating pursuant to federal regulation and located in institutions or other entities where research involving human subjects is conducted. Compared to the possible alternatives of a regional or national review process, local committees have the advantage of greater familiarity with the actual conditions surrounding the conduct of research . . . [and] can work in cooperation with local investigators to assure that [subjects are protected] and . . . that [policies are fairly applied to investigators] . . . .

Commission Draft, *supra* note 8, at 1–2.

36. For discussion of an analogous program designed to absorb catastrophic costs of medical care, see Havighurst, Blumstein & Bovbjerg, *Strategies in Underwriting the Costs of Catastrophic Disease*, 40 L. & Contemp. Prob. 122, 127–34 (1976).

37. 28 U.S.C. §§1346, 1402, 1504, 2110, 2401, 2402, 2411, 2412, 2671–2680 (1970). *See* W. Prosser, Law of Torts §131, at 972 (4th ed. 1971).

38. 45 C.F.R. §46.106(b) (1976). *See also* Hershey & Miller, *supra* note 3, at 79–85.

39. 45 C.F.R. §46.106(b)(4) (1976). Commission Draft, *supra* note 8, at 14, suggests that an institution provide remuneration to nonemployees serving on an IRB.

40. 45 C.F.R. §46.106(b)(5) (1976).

41. *Id*. §46.106(b)(3).

42. *Id*. §46.106(b)(2).

43. *Hearings, supra* note 4, at 3656.

44. Proposals to define further the role of the IRB in exercising scientific oversight have been advanced. *E.g.*, Commission Draft, *supra* note 8, at 17 states as follows:

> *Recommendation (4)* The Secretary of Health, Education and Welfare should require by regulation that all research involving human subjects that is subject to federal regulation shall be reviewed by an institutional review board and that the approval of such research shall be based upon affirmative determinations by the board that:
>
> (a) The research methods are appropriate to the objectives of the research and the field of study.

The effect of this recommendation would be to compel a double peer review of the scientific protocols of many projects. *See* 42 U.S.C. §2891–4 (Supp. V 1975). Peer review has come under attack recently as unduly limiting research by channeling it in directions already sanctioned by scientific consensus. One possible effect of this limitation is to foreclose new ideas and new technologies by denying them funding and thereby perpetutating the commonplace. *See* Rosenbaum, *Cancer Research: Ordeal By Peers*, New Times, Feb. 20, 1978, at 10 (denial of continued funding to Dr. Raymond Damadian of the Biophysical Laboratory, S.U.N.Y. Brooklyn for continued research on the use of nuclear magnetic resonance (NMR) for the detection of malignant tissue); Damadian, Minkoff, Golfsmith, Stanford, & Koutcher, *Field Focusing Nuclear Magnetic Resonance (FONAR): Visualization of a Tumor in a Live Animal*, 194 Science 1430 (1976).

45. 45 C.F.R. §46.102(b)(1)-(3) (1976). The adequacy and appropriateness of methods used to secure informed consent are described in detail at *id.* §§46.103(c).110.

46. 417 F. Supp. 532 (N.D. Ga. 1976). *See also* Clay v. Martin, 509 F.2d 109, 111–13 (2d Cir. 1975) (prisoner's pro se complaint was based on an experimental drug program in 1970 in which plaintiff suffered a serious heart attack after injection with Naltrexone; consent was based on physician's assurance that the dosage involved would be too small to cause harm).

47. Under the Medicaid portion of the Social Security Act, states instituting a Medicaid plan must do so in conformity with the Act and with the approval of the Secretary of DHEW. 42 U.S.C. §1396 (1970). Assistance is required for individuals receiving grants under the Act's cash assistance program, the "categorically needy." *Id.* §1396a(a)(1)(A). The Georgia program included only the categorically needy.

The Medicaid program includes both mandatory and optional services. *Id.* §1396d(a)(1)-17 (1970 & Supp. V 1975). Categorically needy recipients cannot be required to contribute to the costs of mandatory services, and any charges for optional services must be nominal in accordance with standards approved by the Secretary of DHEW and included as a part of the state's plan. *See* Crane v. Mathews, 417 F. Supp. 532, 536 (N.D. Ga. 1976).

48. It is clear that the Medicaid program has important cost considerations.

The incurring of excess costs with respect to one phase of the Medicaid program may very well mean a reduction of the program in another area. The public purse, both that of the state and even of the United States, is not absolutely unlimited. Accordingly, public officials must make some effort to provide the greatest good possible at the least possible costs.

Crane v. Mathews, 417 F. Supp. 532, 540 (N.D. Ga. 1976).

49. The Social Security Act, 42 U.S.C. §301 (1970), provided for "experimental, pilot, or demonstration project[s] which, in the judgment of the Secretary [of DHEW are] likely to assist in promoting the objectives of [the public assistance program]." *Id.* §1315. Such projects require a waiver by the Secretary. Crane v. Mathews, 417 F. Supp. 532, 536–37 (N.D. Ga. 1976); 42 U.S.C. §1315(a) (1970). The *Crane* court held that projects approved under a §1315 waiver were subject also to the regulations of the protection of human subjects, 45 C.F.R. §§46.101–.301 (1976). Crane v. Mathews, 417 F. Supp. 532, 545 (N.D. Ga. 1976).

50. Crane v. Mathews, 417 F. Supp. 532, 540 (N.D. Ga. 1976). The denial was predicated on plaintiff's failure to meet the tests of Canal Auth. of Fla. v. Callaway, 489 F.2d 567 (5th Cir. 1974).

51. Crane v. Mathews, 417 F. Supp. 532, 540 (N.D. Ga. 1976).

52. *Id.* at 545; 42 U.S.C. §1315(b) (1970); 45 C.F.R. §§46.101–.301 (1976).

53. *See* Crane v. Mathews, 417 F. Supp. 532, 543 n.2 (N.D. Ga. 1976) (on the Georgia State IRB).

54. *Id.* at 544.

55. *Id.* at 536–37; 42 U.S.C. §§1315(a), 1396 (1970 & Supp. IV 1974); 45 C.F.R. §§46.101–.301 (1976).

56. The *Crane* court, which did not reach the issue of "risk," was solely concerned with the lack of definitions for "grants and contracts supporting research, development, and related activities" in 45 C.F.R. §46.101(a) (1976), which it had to construe in *pari materia* with the scope of the §1315 waiver and with "human subjects" in 45 C.F.R. §46.101(a) (1976). Crane v. Mathews, 417 F. Supp. 532, 544 (N.D. Ga. 1976). Since "risk" was not before the court, its definition was worth only a passing footnote. *Id.* n.3, which does not clearly establish the definition of "risk."

57. Quoted in Mullen, *supra* note 3, at 260.

58. *Id.*

59. 45 C.F.R. §46.102(b)(3) (1976); *see also* Mullen, *supra* note 3, at 260 n.7.

60. A blanket reduction in welfare benefits would entail some but not all of the procedural safeguards of Goldberg v. Kelly, 397 U.S. 254 (1970). *See* Burr v. New Rochelle Mun. Housing Auth., 479 F.2d 1165, 1169 (2d Cir. 1973), in which the court held "that due process does not require an adversary hearing before a general rent increase or service charge can be imposed." *See generally* Friendly, *"Some Kind of Hearing,"* 123 U. Pa. L. Rev. 1267 (1975).

61. 42 U.S.C. §§218, 241–2a, 282, 286a, 286b, 287b, 287d, 288a, 289c–1, 289g, 289k, 289*l*–1 to –3, 295f–2 to –3(b), 295f–3(q), 300a–7 (Supp. IV 1974). *Cf.* Dodson v. Parham, 427 F. Supp. 97 (N.D. Ga. 1977) (proposed restriction of list of drugs for Medicaid recipients for which reimbursement of pharmacists would be available).

62. "The regulations only apply if a determination is made that the project in question involves human subjects." Crane v. Mathews, 417 F. Supp. 532, 543, 547 (N.D. Ga. 1976).

63. 45 C.F.R. §46.102(b) (1976). It is apparently the intent of Commission Draft, *supra* note 8, at 2–4, to extend review into the conduct of research involving human subjects who are not "at risk." Any such expansion of IRB authority should be viewed with caution by institutions that are seriously interested in innovative research.

64. 45 C.F.R. §46.102(b) (1976).

65. *Id.* §46.111(a).

66. *Id.* §46.103(b).

67. *Id.*

68. *Id.* §46.110. *See also* Hershey & Miller, *supra* note 3, at 29.

69. *See* DuVal, *supra* note 5.

70. 45 C.F.R. §46.103(c) (1976). *Cf.* Berger & Stallones, *Legal Liability and Epidemiological Research,* 106 J. of Epidemiology 177, 178 (1977) ("Determination of informed consent in epidemiologic studies is particularly difficult").

71. 45 C.F.R. §46.102(b)(3). *See also* Mullen, *supra* note 3, at 260 n.7.

72. *Cf.* Hershey & Miller, *supra* note 3, at 29:

Questionnaires raising issues that might be emotionally disturbing or might elicit potentially embarrassing information also place a subject at risk. Thus, an investigator should be seeking neutral information through methods that add no risk of physical or psychological injury before he requests a determination that subjects are not at risk.

The extreme or categorical position taken by Hershey & Miller apparently disregards the potential "risks" in the normal assaults of daily social intercourse. Consider these questions: "Haven't you had three martinis already?" "Didn't your first pregnancy end in a miscarriage?" "Have you ever had (an abortion, a vasectomy, venereal disease, tuberculosis, an ingrown toenail, a disturbing sexual experience, etc.)?" The potential for harm from blunt, nosey questions is always present but is taken in stride by most as part of the "ordinary risks of daily life." While the calculated effort on the part of an investigator to ask a blunt or socially embarrassing question might distinguish it from the chance inquiry at a social gathering, in fact the reply/response (if any) in an experimental context is less exposed to the chance of disclosure, embarrassment, or coercion than if the question is put at a social occasion.

73. Commission Draft, *supra* note 3, at 25–26, leaves some latitude for the conduct of simple surveys without consent formalities, but the force of these in freeing investigators will largely depend on the definition of "risk" adopted by the IRB.

74. 41 Fed. Reg. 26,572–73 (1976).

75. Crane v. Mathews, 417 F. Supp. 532, 540 (N.D. Ga. 1976); 41 Fed. Reg. 26,572–73 (1976).

76. Crane v. Mathews, 417 F. Supp. 532 (N.D. Ga. 1976).

77. 41 Fed. Reg. 26,573 (1976).

78. *Id.*

79. *Cf.* Crane v. Mathews, 417 F. Supp. 532, 546 (N.D. Ga. 1976):

Certainly the imposition of co-payments, which financially burden recipients defined as the categorically needy in the Georgia Medicaid Program, may inhibit such individuals from seeking necessary medical services. The Georgia co-

payment project has the effect of diminishing the amount of money that a family might have available for basic living needs and forces the family to make a determination whether to apply that money to basic living needs or to apply it to purchase medical care. Such an activity . . . [is one] which "deliberately and personally imposes" upon these human beings.

The court's language in dealing with the issue of whether the project implicated "human subjects" seems to comment almost poignantly, albeit indirectly, on the circumstances of those subjects as related to the issue of risk reserved by law to the IRB. The degree to which this influenced the subsequent deliberations cannot be known.

80. 41 Fed. Reg. 26,573 (1976).

81. 5 U.S.C. §553(b)(A) (1970). *See* 1 K. Davis, Administrative Law Treatise §5.03 (1958).

82. *See* 1 K. Davis, *supra* note 81, §5.05.

83. On the importance of "good faith" as a necessary predicate for avoiding possible liability as an IRB member, *see* note 97 *infra.*

84. The Georgia State IRB's expansive view of "risk" following *Crane* illustrates an important problem with Commission Draft, *supra* note 8, at 9–10, as follows:

Recommendation (2)(A) Federal law should be enacted or amended to authorize the Secretary [of DHEW] to carry out the following duties:

. . . .

(iii) Educational Activities to assist members of institutional review boards in recognizing and considering the ethical issues that are presented by research involving human subjects.

In its comment on this recommendation, the Commission explains that "DHEW should develop . . . mechanisms for reporting key IRB decisions to promote uniform treatment of similar protocols. Caution should be exercised, however, to avoid usurping the IRB's decision-making authority." *Id.* at 11.

It would be regrettable if the Georgia decision following *Crane* were to achieve the status of a "key decision." But compare the following:

In general ethical peer review is hampered by the fact that each committee operates in isolation and must consider every new issue on its own and without benefit of precedent. A case-reporting system, such as operates in the law, would make that unnecessary and would promote both equity among institutions and high standards.

Barber, *The Ethics of Experimentation with Human Subjects,* 234 Scientific Am., Feb. 1976, at 25, 29–30 (1976).

85. 45 C.F.R. §46.102(b) (1976). *See also* Crane v. Mathews, 417 F. Supp. 532, 544–46 (N.D. Ga. 1976); 45 C.F.R. §46.111(a) (1976).

86. *Cf.* Hershey & Miller, *supra* note 3, at 29: "Even though there might be no legal requirement to obtain consent when there are no risks, *investigators should seriously consider obtaining consent out of respect for human dignity*" (emphasis added).

On the ethical considerations of human experimentation, *see, e.g.*, Barber, *The Ethics of Experimentation with Human Subjects,* Scientific Am., Feb. 1976, at 25; Beecher, *Ethics and Clinical Research,* 274 New Eng. J. Med. 1354 (1966), *reprinted in* Biomedical Ethics, *supra* note 3, at 193; Dyck & Richardson, *The Moral Justification for Research Using Human Subjects, Use of Human Subjects in Safety Evaluation of Food Chemicals—Proceedings of a Conference* 229 Nat'l Acad. Sci. & Nat'l Research Council Pub. No. 1491 (1967), *reprinted in* Biomedical Ethics, *supra* note 3, at 243; Fletcher, *Human Experimentation: Ethics in the Consent Situation,* 32 L. & Contemp. Prob. 620 (1967); Fletcher, *Realities of Patient Consent to Medical Research,* 1 Hastings Center Studies 39 (1973), *reprinted in* Biomedical Ethics, *supra* note 3, at 261; Jonas, *Philosophical Reflections on Experimenting with Human Subjects,* 98 Daedalus 219 (1969), *revised in* H. Jonas, *Philosophical Essays: From Ancient Creed to Technological Man* (1974), *reprinted in* Biomedical Ethics, *supra* note 3, at 217; Shimkin, *Scientific Investigations on Man: A Medical Research Worker's Viewpoint, Use of Human Subjects in Safety Evaluation of Food Chemicals—Proceedings of a Conference* 217 Nat'l Acad. Sci. & Nat'l Research Council Pub. No. 1491 (1967), *reprinted in* Biomedical Ethics, *supra* note 3, at 207. "It is to be understood that no [statement of ethical] principles [that will assist the institution in discharging its responsibilities for protecting the rights and welfare of subjects] supersede[s] DHEW policy or applicable law." Institutional Guide, *supra* note 1, at 5.

87. 45 C.F.R. §46.103(b) (1976).

88. For a discussion of various aspects of IRB discretion, *see* pp. 449–50 *infra* and authorities cited notes 101–105 *infra.*

89. Leong v. Takasaki, 55 Haw. 398, 520 P.2d 758 (1974) (recovery for any resulting physical injury or objective manifestations of emotional distress). *See also* Billings v. Atkinson, 489 S.W.2d 858 (Tex. 1973); Comment, *Negligently Inflicted Mental Distress: The Case for an Independent Tort,* 59 Geo. L.J. 1237 (1971).

90. *See* W. Prosser, *supra* note 37, §117.

91.

There are . . . medical and biomedical projects concerned solely with organs, tissues, body fluids, and other materials obtained in the course of the routine performance of medical services such as diagnosis, treatment and care, or at autopsy. The use of these materials obviously involves no element of physical risk to the subject.

However, their use for many research, training, and service purposes may present psychological, sociological, or legal risks to the subject or his authorized representatives.

Institutional Guide, *supra* note 1, at 3. *Cf.* Hershey & Miller, *supra* note 3, at 26, 52. *See also* Commission Draft, *supra* note 8, at 25, which states as follows:

In some studies, subjects would be placed at risk by the creation of documents linking them with an illegal or stigmatizing characteristic or behavior under study. The most secure method of protecting confidentiality of subjects in such studies is to create no written record of their identity, since such records are generally vulnerable to subpoena. Confidentiality assurances are available from the Department of Justice and the Department of Health, Education, and Welfare that may effectively protect such documents from subpoena in certain studies of illegal behavior or drug abuse. When such protection is not available in studies in which a breach of confidentiality may be harmful to subjects, and subjects might prefer that there be no documentation linking them with the research, the IRB may waive the requirement for documentation of consent in the interest of protecting the subject.

92.

The Secretary [of DHEW] may authorize persons engaged in research on mental health, including research on the use and effect of alcohol and other psychoactive drugs, to protect the privacy of individuals who are the subject of such research by withholding from all persons not connected with the conduct of such research the names or other identifying characteristics of such individuals. Persons so authorized to protect the privacy of such individuals may not be compelled in any Federal, State, or local civil, criminal, administrative, legislative, or other proceeding to identify such individuals.

42 U.S.C. §242a(a) (1970 & Supp. IV 1974). The statute was upheld in People v. Still, 80 Misc. 2d 831, 364 N.Y.S.2d 125 (1975) (quashed subpoena duces tecum issued to employees of the methadone maintenance clinic), *modified,* 48 App. Div. 2d 366, 369 N.Y.S.2d 759 (1975); People v. Newman, 32 N.Y.2d 379, 298 N.E.2d 651, 345 N.Y.S.2d 502 (1973) (disclosure of pictures of patients taken in connection with a methadone program barred).

93. *E.g.,* Crowell v. Crowell, 180 N.C. 516, 105 S.E. 206 (1920), *rehearing denied,* 181 N.C. 66, 106 S.E. 149 (1921). *See* W. Prosser, *supra* note 37, §18 at 105 & n.73.

94. *See* The Battered Child (2d ed. R. Helfer & C. Kempe eds. 1974). *See also* Hogue, Book Review, 65 Am. J. Pub. Health 414 (1975).

95. *See* W. Prosser, *supra* note 37, §122 at 864–69.

96. Ark. Stat. Ann. §42–807 (Repl. 1977). An example of a statute providing immunity to those reporting child abuse in good faith is Ark. Stat. Ann. §42–814 (Repl. 1977). The following observations of Berger & Stallones, *supra* note 70, at 181, appear somewhat wide of the mark:

A final example of areas where confidentiality of research data conflicts with police powers concerns studies of causes and possible prevention of child abuse. Substantially standardized reporting laws in most states guarantee immunity from civil or criminal liability to anyone *who reports* suspected child abuse; indeed, legal pressure is oriented toward ensuring that suspected cases *are reported* to the appropriate state agency (usually the Welfare Department). Such legal provisions are strengthened by stipulations that fines, imprisonment or both may be levied against those who knowingly fail to report even suspected cases of child abuse or neglect. Implementation of this requirement is facilitated by provision for anonymous reporting.

(Emphasis added.)

The liability of subjects of research (*e.g.*, abusing parents or guardians), not investigators, is what the regulations for the protection of human subjects are concerned with. There is thus a real danger that, for example, research into accidents, accidents involving children (or their parents), or, more narrowly yet, child abuse, could expose subjects of such research to prosecution.

97. "Good faith" is necessary to avoid the imposition of liability and is a necessary predicate to indemnification in Arkansas. Ark. Stat. Ann. §12-3401 (Repl. 1968 & Cum. Supp. 1977) provides indemnification for

damages adjudged . . . or . . . a compromise settlement . . . against officers or employees of the State of Arkansas . . . based on an act or omission by the officer or employee while acting without malice and in good faith within the course and scope of his employment and in the performance of his official duties.

See also Wood v. Strickland, 420 U.S. 308, *rehearing denied,* 421 U.S. 921 (1975); Hogue, *Board Member and Administrator Liability Since Wood v. Strickland,* 7 (U.N.C.) Sch. L. Bull. 1 (Oct. 1976).

98. *See* 45 C.F.R. §46.106 (1976).

99. Hershey & Miller, *supra* note 3, at 14, 71–74.

100.

IRB members should be appointed for a fixed term of at least a year and should not be removed during this term except for good cause. An IRB's membership should be relatively stable from year to year in order to enhance the experience of the IRB and to introduce stability into standards applied by the IRB.

Commission Draft, *supra* note 8, at 14.

101. "Board approvals, favorable actions and recommendations are subject to review and to disapproval or further restriction by the institutional officials. Board disapprovals, restrictions, or conditions cannot be rescinded or removed except by action of a Board described in the assurance approved by DHEW." 45 C.F.R. §46.118 (1976).

In its proposed comment to *Recommendation (5),* the National Commission has addressed this review problem as follows:

The Commission has not recommended a mechanism for appeal from IRB determinations, since it believes that an IRB should have the final word at its institution regarding the ethical acceptability of proposed research involving human subjects. . . . Should an institution wish to establish an appeals process, the Commission suggests that it be restricted to investigation of prejudice or unfairness and that the appeals board not be given authority to conduct a secondary review of the protocol or to reverse the IRB decision.

Commission Draft, *supra* note 8, at 32.

102. *E.g.,* K. Davis, Discretionary Justice—A Preliminary Inquiry (1969).

103. Davis, *A New Approach to Delegation,* 36 U. Chi. L. Rev. 713 (1969). *See also* Environmental Defense Fund, Inc. v. Ruckelshaus, 439 F.2d 584, 598 (D.C. Cir. 1971) (Bazelon, C.J.):

Judicial review must operate to ensure that the administrative process itself will confine and control the exercise of discretion. Courts should require administrative officers to articulate the standards and principles that govern their discretionary decisions in as much detail as possible. Rules and regulations should be freely formulated by administrators, and revised when necessary. Discretionary decisions should more often be supported with findings of fact and reasoned opinions.

(Citing K. Davis, Discretionary Justice—A Preliminary Inquiry (1969)) (footnotes omitted). *Cf.* Sax, *The (Unhappy) Truth About NEPA,* 26 Okla. L. Rev. 239 (1973) ("I know of no solid evidence to support the belief that requiring articulation, detailed findings or reasoned opinions enhances the integrity or propriety of the administrative decisions. I think the emphasis on the redemptive quality of procedural reform is about nine parts myth and one part coconut oil").

104. For discussion of rule-making hearings based on legislative facts, *see* 1 K. Davis, Administrative Law Treatise, §7.04 (1958); Davis, *An Approach to Problems of Evidence in the Administrative Process,* 55 Harv. L. Rev. 364, 402–16 (1942); Friendly, *"Some Kind of Hearing"* 123 U. Pa. L. Rev. 1267 (1975).

105. *E.g.,* Yick Wo v. Hopkins, 118 U.S. 356, 366 (1886) ("The power given . . . is not confided to their discretion in the legal sense of that term, but is granted

to their mere will. It is purely arbitrary and acknowledges neither guidance nor restraint"). For a discussion of the constitutional dimension of this problem, see Hogue, *Eastlake and Arlington Heights: New Hurdles in Regulating Urban Land Use?* 28 Case Wes. Res. L. Rev. 41, 70 n.174 (1977).

106. Londoner v. Denver, 210 U.S. 373 (1908). *Cf.* Bi-Metallic Inv. Co. v. State Bd. of Equalization, 239 U.S. 441 (1915).

107. Commission Draft, *supra* note 8, at 28 states as follows: *"Recommendation (5)* . . . The Secretary should require, further, that an institutional review board inform investigators of the basis of decisions to disapprove or require the modification of proposed research and give investigators an opportunity to respond in person or in writing."

108. *E.g.,* Ark. Stat. Ann. §§5-701 to -715 (Repl. 1976); N.C. Gen. Stat. §150A-1 (Repl. 1974 & Cum. Supp. 1977).

Independent bodies such as IRBs are apparently not subject to the federal Administrative Procedure Act (APA), 5 U.S.C. §§500–706 (1970). *See* Washington Research Project, Inc. v. Department of HEW, 366 F. Supp. 929 (D.D.C. 1973), *modified,* 504 F.2d 238 (D.C. Cir. 1974), *cert. denied,* 421 U.S. 963 (1975) (initial review groups (IRGs) of outside consultants required for project approval not subject to APA's freedom of information provisions).

Some states expressly exclude educational institutions and their constituent bodies from state administrative procedure acts. For example, the North Carolina exclusion is as follows:

> Article 4 of this Chapter, governing judicial review of final agency decisions, shall apply to the University of North Carolina and its constituent or affiliated boards, agencies, and institutions, but the University of North Carolina and its constituent or affiliated boards, agencies, and institutions are specifically exempted from the remaining provisions of this Chapter.

N.C. Gen. Stat. §150A-1(a) (Cum. Supp. 1977).

See generally Daye, *North Carolina's New Administrative Procedure Act: An Interpretive Analysis,* 53 N.C.L. Rev. 833, 842 n.44 (1975).

Final negative determinations by an IRB under 45 C.F.R. §46.118 (1976) at a branch of the state university would appear to be reviewable in superior court under N.C. Gen. Stat. §150A-43 to -52 (Repl. 1974 & Cum. Supp. 1977). The scope of review is limited, but where the record of the proceeding is inadequate and at the discretion of the trial judge, review may be de novo. N.C. Gen. Stat. §§150A-50 to -51 (Repl. 1974 & Cum. Supp. 1977).

109. 13 U.L.A. 347 (Supp. 1978), enacted with variations as follows: Ark. Stat. Ann. §§5-701 to -715 (Repl. 1976); Conn. Gen. Stat. Ann. §§4-166 to -189 (West Supp. 1978); D.C. Code §§1-1501 to -1510 (Supp. II

1975); Ga. Code Ann. §§3A-101 to -124 (Rev. 1975); Haw. Rev. Stat. §§91-1 to -18 (Repl. 1976); Idaho Code §§67-5201 to -5218 (1973 & Cum. Supp. 1977); Ill. Ann. Stat. ch. 127, §§1001-1021 (Smith-Hurd Cum. Supp. 1978); Iowa Code Ann. §§17A.1-.23 (West 1978); La. Rev. Stat. Ann. §§49:951-:967 (West Cum. Supp. 1978); Md. Code Ann. §§41-244 to -256A (Repl. 1971); Mich. Comp. Laws Ann. §§24.201-.315 (Cum. Supp. 1978); Mo. Ann. Stat. §§536.010-.150 (Vernon 1953 & Cum. Supp. 1978); Mont. Rev. Codes Ann. §§82-4201 to -4225 (Cum. Supp. 1977); Neb. Rev. Stat. §§84-901 to -919 (Supp. 1973); Nev. Rev. Stat. §§233B.010-.160 (1975); N.H. Rev. Stat. Ann. §§541-A:1 to -A:9 (Repl. 1974); N.Y. State Admin. Proc. Act (McKinney Special Pamphlet 1977); N.C. Gen. Stat. §§150A-1 to -64 (Repl. 1974 & Cum. Supp. 1977); Okla. Stat. Ann. tit. 75, §§301-327 (West 1976 & Cum. Supp. 1978); R.I. Gen. Laws §§42-35-1 to -35-18 (Reen. 1977); S.D. Compiled Laws Ann. §§1-26-1 to -26-40 (Rev. 1974); Tenn. Code Ann. §§4-502 to -527 (Repl. 1971 & Cum. Supp. 1977); Vt. Stat. Ann. tit. 3, §§801-820 (1975 Cum. Supp.); Wash. Rev. Code Ann. §§34.04.010-.940 (1965 & Supp. 1976); W. Va. Code §§29A-1-1 to -7-4 (Repl. 1976 & Cum. Supp. 1977); Wis. Stat. Ann. §§227.01-.26 (West 1957); Wyo. Stat. §§9-276.19 to -276.33 (Cum. Supp. 1975).

110. *See* 45 C.F.R. §46.106 (1976). The Commission Draft, *supra* note 8, at 32, recognizes the possibility of IRBs being subject to state as well as federal law. Thus, the Commission "supports the principle of open meetings. The public generally should have access to IRB meetings, limited only by local law or a decision by the IRB to close a meeting in order to discuss personal or proprietary information." The impact of state open meetings or sunshine laws should probably be noted in the general assurance to DHEW. Laws will, of course, differ in their applicability to IRBs; some will be required to comply while others will not. *But see* Student Bar Ass'n Bd. of Governors v. Byrd, 293 N.C. 594, 239 S.E.2d 415 (1977) (North Carolina's open meetings statute, N.C. Gen. Stat. §143-318.1 to -318.6 (Repl. 1974 & Cum. Supp. 1977) held inapplicable to meetings of the faculty of the law school; the law faculty held not a part of a governmental body acting as body politic). *Accord,* Fain v. Faculty of the College of Law, 552 S.W.2d 752 (Tenn. 1977); McLarty v. Board of Regents, 231 Ga. 22, 200 S.E.2d 117 (1973) (faculty-student committee to recommend allocation of revenues from student fees), *cited with approval in* Arkansas Gazette Co. v. Pickens, 258 Ark. 69, 79, 522 S.W.2d 350, 356 (1975) (Fogleman, J., concurring). *Contra,* Cathcart v. Andersen, 85 Wash. 2d 102, 530 P.2d 313 (1975) (law faculty).

Open meetings in Arkansas are governed by the Freedom of Information Act (FOIA) Ark. Stat. Ann. §12-2805 (Repl. 1968), which requires public meetings of "all boards, bureaus, commissions, or organizations" of the state "supported wholly or in part by public funds, or expending public funds" to be open. Exceptions are limited to sessions "considering employment, appointment, promotion, demotion, disciplining or resignation of any public officer or employee." The sanction for noncompliance is to void any public business not within the exception that is conducted in executive session and not reenacted in a public session. *Id.* §12-2805(b). Injunctions are available to excluded parties. *Id.* §12-2806. Arkansas' FOIA incorporates two standards. Its application to units of local government is limited by §12-2805 to "governing bodies" and is possibly subject to the narrow construction followed in other states in the *Student Bar Ass'n* and *Fain* cases discussed above. The broad scope of §12-2805, however, would preclude a narrower application of the statute when units of state government are involved. Arkansas Gazette Co. v. Pickens, 258 Ark. 69, 522 S.W.2d 350 (1975) (committees of the university's board of trustees). The Commission proposal that "IRBs should make provision to consider requests by investigators to close meetings or portions of meetings at which their research proposals will be discussed," Commission Draft, *supra* note 8, at 32, is not within the authorized exceptions to Arkansas' FOIA. *See also* Nat'l Comm'n for the Protection of Human Subjects of Biomedical and Behavioral Research, Disclosure of Research Information under the Freedom of Information Act (1977).

111. The term "ombudsman" is not intended in a limited, technical sense. *See* Verkuil, *The Ombudsman and the Limits of the Adversary System,* 75 Col. L. Rev. 845, 847 & n.10 (rejecting the narrower concept espoused in *The Ombudsman: Citizen's Defender,* xii (D. Rowat ed. 1968)). The human subjects' rights advocate is analogous to the public counsellor incorporated into the administrative procedure of some state and federal agencies. *E.g.,* 45 U.S.C. §§715(a),(d)(2) (Supp. 1976) (Rail Service Planning Office within the Interstate Commerce Commission); Cal. Pub. Res. Code §§25217(b), 25222 (West Cum. Supp. 1975) (advisor to California Energy Resources Conservation and Development Commission); 14 C.F.R. §§302.9, 384.7 (1975) (consumer advocate participating in deliberations of the Civil Aeronautics Board). *See also* Bloch & Stein, *The Public Counsel Concept in Practice: The Regional Rail Reorganization Act of 1973,* 16 Wm. & Mary L. Rev. 215 (1974); Comment, *The Office of Public Counsel: Institutionalizing Public Interest Representation in State Government,* 64 Geo. L.J. 895 (1976).

The literature on the ombudsman is extensive. *E.g.,* W. Gellhorn, When Americans Complain: Governmental Grievance Procedures (1966); Cramton, *A Federal Ombudsman,* 1972 Duke L.J. 1; Davis, *Ombudsman In America: Officers to Criticize Administrative Action,* 109 U. Pa. L. Rev. 1057 (1961); Frank, *The Nebraska Public Counsel—The Ombudsman,* 5 Cum.—Sam. L. Rev. 30 (1974); Comment, *A State Statute to Create the Office of Ombudsman,* 2 Harv. J. Legis. 213 (1965).

The role of ombudsman or public counsel is allocated by law in some instances to the state's attorney general. *E.g.,* Ark. Stat. Ann. §§70-901 to -929 (Cum. Supp. 1977) (Consumer Protection Division within the office of the Attorney General).

6.2 A Case Analysis of NEPA Implementation: NIH and DNA Recombinant Research*

SUSAN M. CHALKER and ROBERT S. CATZ

Reprinted with permission of Susan M. Chalker, Robert S. Catz, and the *Duke Law Journal*, from 1978 *Duke Law Journal* 57–67, 92–112. Copyright © 1978 by the *Duke Law Journal*. All rights reserved.

Can the human mind master what the human mind has made?
Paul A. Valery
French Poet and Philosopher
(1871–1945)

I. INTRODUCTION

A biological revolution is underway which promises and threatens radical changes in plant and animal life as it now exists. Since 1950, biologists have been quietly at work, largely unnoticed, unravelling the mysteries of life. The new scientific knowledge that has emerged—the knowledge of the molecular basis of heredity—gives scientists the potential power to manipulate the genetic code that determines the physical development of all living organisms. For the first time there exists the technology to cross large evolutionary boundaries and to move genes between organisms that would not, under natural processes, have any genetic contact. This process of gene transference between unrelated organisms is called "recombinant DNA technology."[1] While the pace of scientific achievement has accelerated, government's ability to keep up with it has not.

The most prominent characteristic of recombinant DNA research is its potential for enormous benefit or catastrophic harm. The precise nature of the long- and short-range risks, whether the expected benefits outweigh the anticipated social, philosophical, moral or ecological risks, and whether this research should be undertaken at all, are subjects of current unresolved debate.[2] Anticipated beneficial impacts include developing cures for cancer and a variety of hereditary diseases such as sickle cell anemia, diabetes, Tay-Sachs disease and phenylketonuria,[3] producing inexpensive and abundant quantities of oral vitamins and hormones, and providing childless couples with a method of producing offspring. On the negative side, it may be stated that probably no scientific breakthrough since the discovery of nuclear power has such an enormous potential for creating large-scale and irreversible damage to life forms, to future generations and to the biosphere on which we all depend. In addition to the possible accidental creation and dispersion of new destructive bacteria,[4] the misuse of biological technology portends implications for biological warfare. Moreover, serious moral, ethical and philosophical questions arise when natural human and animal evolutionary processes become the subject of deliberate manipulation which could potentially disrupt the complex and delicate balance among living things in the name of producing "desirable" improvements in humankind.[5]

---

*The views expressed herein are those of the authors and do not necessarily represent the views of any agency of the United States.

367

At this point both proponents and opponents of continued and accelerated DNA research concede the speculative nature of both the potential benefits and detriments. This realm of uncertainty regarding consequences, however, is unlikely to persist much longer. The pace of advances in the field have occurred so rapidly that the complex, basic knowledge—the breaking of the genetic code—is available to scientists throughout the world. The capacity to apply this new knowledge will follow in relatively short order[6] unless the pace of the research and experimentation is abated or circumscribed in some manner by outside forces.

A second significant characteristic of recombinant DNA research in the United States is that although some research is sponsored by private industry and by private educational institutions, the vast majority of it has been funded by the federal government.[7] The federal commitment has been, and continues to be, the mainstay of molecular biological research in this country.[8] The largest single federal agency sponsoring genetic research is the National Institutes of Health (NIH), an agency of the U.S. Department of Health, Education and Welfare (HEW).[9] The system employed by NIH for allocating its limited financial resources among competing researchers, although theoretically providing for input from lay persons, is in practice effectively controlled by the scientific establishment.[10] Moreover, the NIH regulations and criteria used to review applicants for federally funded research projects are quite broad.[11] This systematic exclusion of the public from the institutional decision-making processes concerning if, when and how to proceed with DNA research is an additional characteristic of the research effort in the field.[12] The exclusion is even more pervasive in the DNA research efforts undertaken by private educational institutions and by private industry.

Recognition of the hazards associated with recombinant DNA research is not a recent phenomenon. In July 1973, at the Gordon Research Conference on Nucleic Acids, the potential hazards of this research and technology were discussed; those in attendance voted to send an open letter to the Residents of the National Academy of Sciences and the Institute of Medicine suggesting that the Academy "establish a study committee to consider this problem and to recommend specific action or guidelines, should that seem appropriate."[13]

The following year, a committee of the National Academy of Scientists chaired by Paul Berg called for a voluntary moratorium on all recombinant activities. The committee also proposed an international meeting of scientists to more thoroughly assess the risks and to devise appropriate guidelines for the safe conduct of DNA research.[14] An international meeting was held at the Asilomar Conference Center in February 1975 to discuss recombinant DNA research.[15] Participants at the conference, after reviewing progress in the research and the potential biohazards of the work, concluded that experiments on construction of recombinant DNA molecules should proceed, provided that appropriate containment is utilized. The conference made recommendations for matching levels of containment with levels of possible hazard for various types of experiments. Certain experiments were judged to pose such serious potential dangers that the conferees recommended against their being continued at that present time.[16]

Immediately after the conference, NIH adopted the recommendations of the conference as guidelines for research until an advisory committee[17] had an opportunity to draft more specific guidelines. After meeting three more times, in December 1975 the advisory committee submitted its own proposed guidelines to the Director of NIH,[18] and in February 1976 the Director called a special meeting of the advisory committee to review the proposed guidelines. The public was invited to comment and participate in the meeting. After revisions were made in response to the comments at the meeting, the final Guidelines were released and published in the Federal Register;[19] the voluntary moratorium on recombinant DNA research ended. On August 23, 1976, NIH, in an effort to comply with the provisions of the National Environmental Policy Act of 1969 (NEPA).[20] issued a Draft Environmental Impact Statement (EIS) on the DNA Research Guidelines and published the Draft EIS in the Federal Register on September 9, 1976.[21]

This Article contends that, substantively and procedurally, the Draft EIS belatedly issued by NIH is in violation of the letter and spirit of NEPA and that the defects are so fundamental as to render it invalid. The purposes of NEPA have been thwarted, and any improvements that may be made in the final EIS will be of no avail in influencing the reality of continued and accelerated research in the field. This will be so because the major philosophical and ethical issues have never been effectively aired in a public forum, a fact that is unacceptable in an area where the well-being of the public is at stake.[22] Dramatic legislative intervention, national in scope, is needed; unfortunately, it is too late in the day for NEPA to fulfill its promise.

II. THE NATIONAL ENVIRONMENTAL POLICY ACT AND DNA RECOMBINANT RESEARCH

In 1969, in an effort to protect and preserve the quality of the human environment, Congress enacted NEPA.[23] The ensuing seven years have spawned a proliferation of increasingly lengthy and complex EIS's[24] as federal agencies have attempted to comply with the numerous court decisions interpreting the Act and, more specifically, with the mandate of the impact statement requirement contained in the Act. While controversy exists as to whether judicial decisions have expanded the scope of the Act beyond legislative intent or whether the courts have done too little to give teeth to the Act in light of the broad evils which the Act was intended to remedy,[25] there is little question that the environmental consciousness of federal agencies has been raised as they have been forced, at least in form, to take environmental factors into consideration when formulating policies and programs[26] and when appropriating funds.[27] However, a review of the voluminous EIS's filed over the last seven years indicates that such statements almost invariably concerned themselves with assessing the impact on the physical environment of easily quantifiable factors, such as the number of persons who would be displaced by the construction of an interstate highway,[28] or the sewage, heat and water displacement problems engendered by the construction of an office building.

Prior to August 1976, no EIS had been issued by NIH on recombinant DNA research.[29] Indeed, no evidence exists that the applicability of NEPA to such endeavors had even been considered by the appropriate NIH officials.[30] In August 1976, however, when the NIH issued and circulated a Draft EIS on recombinant DNA research, it embraced for the first time the principle that NEPA's coverage extends to areas of basic research and development. Despite the laudable advance in conceptualization the issuance of the EIS represents, an examination of the purposes and requirements of NEPA indicates that the Draft EIS has dismally failed to meet the high standards required by the Act and has failed to serve its statutory functions as either an aid to internal agency decision-making or as an informational vehicle for the public.[31]

The National Environmental Policy Act of 1969 is an effort to halt the destruction of the environment and to preserve its quality.[32] It shows that Congress recognizes that human activities, including the actions and nonactions of federal agencies, have had adverse effects on our natural environment, and is committed to the principle that "each person should enjoy a healthful environment."[33] NEPA sets forth three basic purposes:

1. to declare a national policy which will encourage productive harmony between man and his environment,
2. to promote efforts which will prevent or eliminate damage to the environment and biosphere and stimulate the health and welfare of man,
3. to enrich the understanding of the ecological systems and natural resources important to the nation.[34]

"New and expanding technological advances" are explicitly recognized as one factor having a profound influence on the natural environment,[35] and the legislative history cites many instances where the failure to take environmental and health concerns into account prior to implementation of innovative technologies resulted in disastrous environmental consequences.[36] The Act establishes as a national policy the commitment "to use all practicable means . . . to create and maintain conditions under which man and nature can exist in productive harmony."[37] To effectuate this policy it is the responsibility of the federal government to "improve and coordinate Federal plans, functions, programs and resources to the end that the Nation may . . . attain the widest range of beneficial uses of the environment without degradation, risk to health or safety, or other undesirable and unintended consequences."[38]

Section 101[39] articulates a policy of enlightened substantive values and recognizes the need for improved environmental planning by requiring all agencies to consider values of environmental planning preservation in their spheres of activity. The section's broad goal is a major first step in the congressional scheme to eliminate shortsightedness in the conduct of human affairs having environmental consequences. It is only the first step, however. Congress went on in section 102 to prescribe a methodology for implementing these substantive concepts to ensure that the stated values are in fact fully respected.[40] Unlike the substantive policy provisions of the Act, which are flexible and leave room for a responsible exercise of discretion, the "procedural" provisions of section 102 impose non-discretionary obligations and require a strict standard of compliance. They form the very essence of the Act.[41]

The section 102 procedures must be complied with "to the fullest extent possible"[42] in making decisions having environmental impact. Among the most important are the requirements that every federal agency "utilize a systematic, inter-disciplinary approach";[43] make efforts to quantify presently unquantified environmental values and give them appropriate consideration along with economic and technical considerations;[44] "recognize the worldwide and long-range character of environmental problems and . . . lend . . . support to initiative . . . and programs designed to maximize international cooperation in environmental improvement";[45] and "study, develop and describe . . . alternatives to recommended courses of action" involving "unresolved conflicts concerning alternative uses of available resources."[46]

In many ways the most important procedural requirement is that every federal agency proposing "legislation and other major Federal actions significantly affecting the quality of the human environment" must issue a "detailed statement" accounting for all of the impacts of the action.[47] The statement must evaluate any alternatives to the proposed action,[48] take into account the action's long range consequences,[49] and delineate the unavoidable adverse consequences of the action.[50] This justification document, the EIS, is the most concrete of the mandatory procedures of section 102 and is the action-triggering keystone of the NEPA edifice.

Although theoretically all the procedural requisites outlined in section 102 must be complied with regardless of whether an agency issues an EIS,[51] and although the statutory language throughout the Act is sweeping and obscure, judicial assistance for the most part has been sought only with regard to enforcement of the EIS requirement. Even more rarely has judicial intervention been sought to enforce the substantive provisions of section 101.

When an EIS is filed, a procedure must be established to circulate copies to the public, Congress and other federal, state and local agencies, secure the comments of those with special expertise in the subject matter of the statement, solicit the views of the public, file the statement with the Council on Environmental Quality (CEQ)[52] and ensure that the statement accompany the proposed legislation or action through agency review processes.[53] It is at this stage, prior to implementation of a policy or program, that deliberations should be most open to the public and decisions about the action subject to public participation and intervention.

The overall purpose of NEPA is to compel federal agencies to consider the environmental consequences of their actions. The purpose of the requirement of a written justification is to provide a practical vehicle for implementing that purpose. The statement informs the public of environmental consequences of and alternatives to proposed actions and enables evaluation, comment and intervention from interested parties outside the agency process who presumably will not be biased with the same self-interest in the particular project as those within the promoting agency who are responsible for its development and stand to gain the most from its adoption. It ensures that environmental considerations are placed before the ultimate decision-maker—the public—before federal agencies undertake environmentally damaging actions. It opens up technology-dominated decisions to public inspection.[54] The expectation is that if the public has timely access to all the relevant information it can operate politically, and if need be judicially, to attain environmentally sound policies.[55]

Requiring the statement to be "detailed," to include specifically for each case project an assessment of the environmental costs weighed against the expected benefits—economic, technical, environmental—and to consider the outlined alternatives that would affect the cost-benefit balance[56] affords some assurance that the agency's own decision-makers will receive and use the information and will incorporate environmental values into their policy-making internal balancing processes at a time *before* projects are hardened and resources irrevocably committed.[57] It provides some assurance that all possible approaches to a particular problem will be taken into account and that the most beneficial decision will be made.[58] Additionally, such a statement constitutes some evidence that the correct decision-making process has taken place and provides a judicially reviewable record against charges of noncompliance with NEPA. Whether the public and agency informational role of the EIS serves or can potentially serve to fulfill its implicit statutory promise to protect the national environmental well-being in the case of DNA recombinant technology will be discussed further.

* * *

C. The Substance

Recombinant DNA research and technology initiates a new era of synthetic biology. Techniques for gene transplantation are not simply novel research tools, but instruments for the manufacture of new organisms. Few doubt that these techniques have the potential for deliberate misuse to produce pathogenic organisms capable of disrupting the ecosystem or initiating deadly forms of disease.[168] Considering the incomplete understanding of the biological implications of novel combinations of genes, it is also possible that comparably disastrous effects might result from "peaceful" research and development. As in the case of other hazardous activities, the guiding principle for policy formation ought to be the well-being and security of human life. It is by this principle that NIH's actions must be analyzed.

The Draft EIS contains some expression of the primacy of public safety. The objective of the Guidelines is stated to be "the protection of laboratory workers, the general public, and the environment from infection by possibly hazardous agents that may result from recombinant DNA research."[169] The conclusion drawn by the Draft EIS is that by promulgating the Guidelines, NIH has fully satisfied that objective. According to the statement, if the Guidelines are followed, the probability that a

pathogenic organism will be created is extremely low.[170] Even if created, the probability of escape from its restrictive environment is equally low.[171] Statements such as "any potential release of high-risk materials to the environment should be prevented by adherence to the NIH Guidelines"[172] suggests that the Guidelines have adequately taken into account all possible ways in which any potential biological hazard arising from recombinant DNA research could enter the environment, that there is little further need to improve them or to explore alternative courses of action and that the public can afford to rest easy in the well-supported blanket of protection provided by responsible science.

Yet there is nothing within the impact statement that provides a rational basis for such sanguine conclusions. On the other hand, both what is stated and omitted casts significant doubt on the validity of the impact statement. Indeed, the statement is, on the whole, in substantive noncompliance with NEPA. While the procedural directives of section 102 have received most of the judicial attention in NEPA litigation,[173] it is clear that these procedures are not ends in themselves but are intended to trigger and ensure the implementation of the less precise substantive policies of environmental protection enunciated in section 101 of the Act.[174] The courts have recognized that each agency has an obligation to carry out the substantive as well as the procedural requirements of NEPA and that purely mechanical compliance with section 102 is not sufficient to satisfy the provision of the Act. Furthermore, the courts will not hesitate to review substantive agency decisions on the merits.[175] NEPA was intended to effect substantive results and to be more than an environmental full disclosure law.

In reviewing agency decisions on the merits, the court will examine whether the agency engaged in a full and good faith consideration and balancing of all relevant environmental factors[176] and whether, in the light of the standards set forth in sections 101(b)[177] and 102(1)[178] of the Act, "the actual balance of costs and benefits that was struck was arbitrary or clearly gave insufficient weight to environmental values."[179] The standard of review thus articulated is a narrow one in the sense that it is not within the court's power to substitute its judgment for that of the agency.[180] NIH's Draft EIS fails to pass such a test.

The impact statement is not the "detailed statement," in either quantity or quality of environmental information, required by NEPA in order to fulfill its purpose of providing a basis for informed decision-making on the key question of whether recombinant DNA technology should proceed.[181] The agency's conclusion that it is currently environmentally sound to proceed with recombinant DNA research and experimentation, performed as specified in the NIH Guidelines, is based on incomplete, inadequate and untested data, and is not the result of a full and good faith effort to set forth all the competing environmental considerations.

In order for the impact statement to provide rational assurance to the public that the most environmentally sound decision has been made, four general categories of information should be provided: first, a description of the proposed action, its probable environmental effects and all reasonably available alternatives; second, estimates of the likelihood and magnitude of the environmental effects of the action and of the alternatives; third, where possible to calculate, the monetary cost of such effects; and fourth, an analysis of the resultant cost-benefit balance. The complete impact study must be more than just a catalogue of the above categories of data. The agency must also "explicate fully its course of inquiry, its analysis and its reasoning."[182] The analysis must be objective.

The most significant failures of NIH's Draft EIS as a detailed, intelligent description and quantification of the probable environmental effects of recombinant DNA research, and its failures in meeting the "good, full faith consideration" test are its lack of objectivity, its unsatisfactory discussion of alternatives and its inadequate and inaccurate description and quantification of the hazards of recombinant DNA research. These individual failures contribute to the document's unfounded and highly misleading claims regarding the efficacy of the containment measures outlined in the Guidelines to ensure public safety.

1. Lack of Objectivity

NIH's Draft impact statement can be characterized as an exercise in justification. Its dominant tone is adversarial, radiating an urgent sense of "let's get on with it," and its content never adequately addresses the central policy questions regarding genetic manipulation and development. As an exercise in justification, it is violative of NEPA's mandate to federal agencies to undertake major actions affecting the quality of the human environment only after a full and good faith consideration and balancing of all economic and environmental concerns. Without such a requirement, the impact statement provision of section 102(2)(C) would serve only a disclosure function and assurances that the substantive policies of section 101 would be respected would be lessened considerably. Judicial enforcement of NEPA standards requires a determination of whether the agency has reconstructed its decision-making apparatus in a way that ensures review of environmental considerations disclosed in impact statements and whether the agency has actually considered the information and analysis adduced in the statement in making its decision.

> If the decision [the major action significantly affecting the quality of the human environment] was reached procedurally without individualized consideration and balancing of environmental factors—conducted fully and in good faith—it is the responsibility of the courts to reverse.[183]

Even the mere probability that an impact statement will, because of self-interest of the authors in the proposed project, be based on "self-serving assumptions"[184] is enough to render the procedure in noncompliance with NEPA.

No decision or decision-making procedure can meet the standard of "full, good faith consideration" if the agency is committed in advance to a particular course of action. If the ultimate decision-maker were so committed, there obviously could be no "good faith" consideration of alternatives to the preselected course of action. Thus, the environmental costs of proceeding with the chosen course of action could not be said to have been actually "considered," but merely to have been recognized. Substantial evidence exists which indicates that NIH determined to continue the funding of recombinant DNA research prior to development of the Draft EIS and that this determination affected the objectivity of the agency's consideration of the matter.[185] For example, by misdefining its "major . . . action" to be the promulgation of the safety measures contained in its Guidelines rather than its financial support of recombinant DNA research, NIH established a framework for the EIS discussion that effectively ignored the key question that the statement ought to address—whether, on balance, it is environmentally wise to proceed with widespread recombinant DNA technology. The whole impact statement discussion proceeds from the implicit assumption that it is environmentally wise and that NIH will continue funding such research.[186] The timing of the Draft EIS, years after grants had been awarded by NIH for recombinant DNA research and when the research was fast approaching the applied technology state, as well as after the promulgation of the Guidelines themselves, is a procedural violation of NEPA and constitutes further evidence that the impact statement is nothing more than "post-hoc environmental rationalizations of decisions already fully and finally made."[187]

Scientific controversy and debate have raged around the issue of recombinant DNA research and technology. The potential dangers have been likened in magnitude by many scientists to those of applied nuclear technology. The scientific community was sufficiently concerned in 1974 to impose an unprecedented moratorium on such activities.[188] Responsible scientific literature on the subject is extensive.[189] Yet nowhere in NIH's discussion of the biological aspects of recombinant DNA technology or of the containment measure to safeguard experiments is reference made to the large body of scientific opinion that is in disagreement with NIH's positions.[190] Indeed, very few of the claims advanced are backed up by reference to any authoritative source material. For the most part assertions are advanced in a conclusory fashion; the reader, left uncertain of their basis, is asked to accept NIH's controversial statements on little more than blind faith. An impact statement based substantially on unsupported conclusions and without reference to responsible opposing views is contrary to the objective process required by NEPA;[191] "actions" based on such a statement are arbitrary.

2. The Hazards and the Safeguards

The Draft EIS offers explicit assurance that the Guidelines adequately safeguard human and environmental health, thereby implying that all potentially dangerous possibilities arising from gene transferences can be, and have been, accurately assessed and that adherence to the Guidelines will be universal. Both propositions are doubtful.

When the moratorium on DNA recombinant experimentation was called in June 1974, it was proposed to last until the potential hazards of such recombinant DNA molecules have been better evaluated or until adequate methods are developed for preventing their spread.[192] Although neither of these conditions have been met, NIH has approved proliferation of the technology. Present scientific knowledge of much of the genetic function in existing organisms remains very slim; there is an even greater absence of hard facts about the risks of the infinite variety of genetic combinations that might result from recombinant gene transference. Admissions of this knowledge gap and uncertainty are found in various parts of the impact statement, as well as the Guidelines. An implicit acknowledgement can be found in the Introduction to the Draft EIS, which states: "In issuing the Guidelines, the NIH Director pointed out that they will be subject to continuous review and modification in the light of changing circumstances."[193] More explicit admissions exist in the impact statement:

> Current knowledge does not permit accurate assessment of whether such changes [in the properties of the host cell or virus from the stable insertion of DNA derived from a different species] will be advantageous, detrimental or neutral, and to what degree, when considering a particular recombinant DNA experiment. At present it is only possible to speculate on ways in which the presence of recombinant DNA in a cell or virus could bring about these effects.[194]

The Draft impact statement is laced with optimistic predictions based on these admittedly uncertain data and untested theories. A few of the more significant statements are illustrative.

A central assumption of the EIS is that if the physical and biological containment measures of the Guidelines are strictly observed in DNA experiments, hazardous organisms will not be created (biological containment), or that if they are created, they will not escape from laboratories (physical containment), and that an acceptable degree of safety has thereby been provided. There is, however, no realistic assurance that the system devised is scientifically sound. The system for classifying experiments as outlined in the Guidelines is elaborate.[195] A given experiment is assigned to a category according to the type of recombinant DNA involved. It is then assigned to one of four physical containment levels and one of three biological containment levels.[196] Extremely hazardous experiments are prohibited outright.[197] The physical containment measures describe laboratory conditions ranging from "P1" to "P4," with P4 being the most restrictive and also the most expensive to construct and operate.[198] It is assumed and considered to be within the range of acceptable risk that a certain amount of accidental release will occur in P1 and P2 facilities.[199] NIH assumes that because only organisms which have been rated low or moderate risks are handled in P1 or P2 laboratories, such exposure will not harm laboratory workers or others.[200] The biological containment provisions are based on the theory that certain organisms carry a greater potential for toxic spread and contamination than others and therefore require a more secure laboratory.[201]

Although the complexity of the containment system is impressive, the repeated admissions by NIH that it does not know enough about the hazards of recombinant DNA and the effects of any particular genetic recombination make highly doubtful the accuracy of the risk evaluations on which the 13-tiered classification of containment levels is premised. There is no scientific evidence for the assumption that organisms which are rated low-risk by NIH's classification system will prove harmless. For example, the central assumption underlying the biological classification system and the biological containment measures is that most cells with foreign DNA from higher organisms are more hazardous than those from lower organisms. Therefore, more containment is required for experiments that take DNA from primates than for those that take DNA from birds or plants.[202] But there is no scientific basis for assuming that philogenic order or any other single factor can accurately predict risk[203] when the Draft EIS itself lists thirteen factors that determine the likelihood that a particular organism will cause harm.[204] Whatever single factor is selected to rank hazards, it will always be possible to make a credible argument that some experiments which are rated as low risks are in fact more risky than some of those that were rated as high risks.

The larger question of whether there can ever be any biological containment is never addressed by the EIS. Even if a disabled strain—one that could not survive outside the laboratory—were developed, we could never be sure of its safety because, by definition, a recombinant experiment would add new traits to the disabled strain that might cancel out its disability.[205] The EIS itself presents a good example of just this phenomenon. It describes an experiment in which an histidine deficient E. coli (a disarmed host) lost its disability when recombined with yeast DNA.[206] Since after recombination a new organism is developed, the premise of biological containment is possibly an invalid one.[207]

Because the likelihood of harm cannot be calculated with precision, the Guidelines essentially provide for the ranking of experiments on the basis of untested theories which may be inaccurate or not comprehensive enough to be used as the basis for predicting risk. Since recombinant DNA molecules are placed in living host cells, which have the potential of surviving and multiplying in the environment, even one experiment that is mistakenly considered harmless could cause widespread and irreversible damage. Given the magnitude of possible adverse impacts and the imprecision of present estimates of risks of different experiments, all organisms should be presumed hazardous to the environment if they should escape. Although some recognition of this presumption and incorporation of cautionary measures can be found in the impact statement, the overall effect of NIH's action is to promote the proliferation of the number of facilities engaged in gene transplantation and to create a false sense of security by using sweeping, unsupported generalizations that consistently downgrade the estimates of the potential risks. Such a statement as "[T]here is no known instance in which a hazardous agent has been created by recombinant DNA technology"[208] is typical. Given the fact that a moratorium has been in effect since 1974, and that this area of scientific inquiry is not even seven years old, this statement is less elucidating on the point of safety than it might appear.[209] The same statement would have applied to uranium enrichment prior to the summer of 1945 when the first nuclear bomb was actually tested.

A policy formulation premised on the presumption that, given the absence of hard data, all organisms with DNA must be considered hazardous would confine all research to one or a few heavily secured facilities until the dangers could be more accurately assessed.[210] The research efforts should be directed to the determination of the nature and level of the risks inherent in gene transplantation, the development of a host organism that is not a resident of the normal human environment and does not exchange DNA with organisms in that environment, and the determination of the effectiveness of biological containment with this new host organism.[211]

Human safety cannot be compromised. The implicit framework of the impact statement discussion appears to revolve around the question of whether the Guidelines balance scientific responsibility to the public with scientific freedom to pursue new knowledge. Presentation of the issue as one of "balancing" suggests the propriety of a compromise between the two—a misleading and dangerous position. With a process that has such a high level of possible risks, the only concern that cannot be compromised is public safety. If that means a longer wait for benefits while procedures for better identifying potential risks and for preventing their occurrence and spread are developed, it is a small price to pay.

Furthermore, NIH's implicit expectation that its Guidelines will command universal adherence is unrealistic. The Guidelines expressly regulate only NIH grantees, calling for voluntary compliance on the part of other researchers.[212] Thus far the call for voluntary compliance from private institutions and industry has been less than resounding; there is little realistic expectation that this will change.[213] Only the National Science Foundation (NSF) has given its formal commitment; the pharmaceutical industry has, in principle, agreed to abide by the safety measures, but it has been unwilling to give teeth to its commitment by disclosing all of its activities[214] to the public (or competitors), citing a claimed need to protect marketing and patent information.[215]

An unsettling paradox becomes apparent here. DNA research conducted under the auspices of NIH and NSF is more likely to be motivated by scientifically pure reasons than that of private industry where the desire for profit and the competition for lucrative patents might tempt scientists to dispense with the extra time, effort and care necessary to conduct experiments according to the Guidelines.

Because the "strict" adherence[216] upon which NIH's predictions are implicitly premised is unlikely to materialize, the optimistic "environmental impact" statement is misleading. The EIS would be improved by a discussion of the environmental impact of DNA research conducted without the biological and physical restrictions described in the Guidelines. To state, as does the Draft EIS, that an analysis of such unknown quantities is "speculative and therefore not quantifiable"[217] is somewhat disingenuous in light of the fact that any discussion of potential risks and benefits in this field is equally uncertain. Yet this did not deter NIH from concluding that its Guidelines sufficiently protect our environmental well-being.

There is an additional reason to doubt that the Guidelines will provide sufficient protection. For the Guidelines to be as effective as NIH assures us they are, it must be assumed that the restrictive measures contained therein can be, and will generally be, implemented without consequential human and technological error—a questionable premise. Moreover, the Draft EIS does not discuss the "impact" of such potentialities. The need to do so is particularly striking when one considers the admitted lack of scientific certainty surrounding the concept of biological containment in general and the soundness of the biological and physical containment measures of the Guidelines in particular,[218] and the potentially grave consequences of even one error. The fact that potentially hazardous biological materials or infectious agents are insidious makes the need even more urgent. The presence of such agents can be detected only when they are properly labelled and one has a thorough knowledge of what has taken place in the laboratory. They cannot be detected by the five senses.[219] Despite this, no mention is made in the EIS of specific training or protection of the personnel handling these agents, which would be required to ensure the safe operation of the facility.

The Draft EIS assures us that "[a]ny potential release of high-risk materials to the environment should be prevented by adherence to the NIH Guidelines."[220] In support of this claim, brief reference is made to the supposed success of similar containment measures at Fort Detrick, the U.S. Army's biological warfare facility.[221] Nonetheless, there is substantial support for the view that NIH's interpretation of the Fort Detrick experience is not accurate and that the more favorable experience of recent years at the Fort Detrick installation is the consequence principally of the development of means of vaccinating the personnel against the agents under study, rather than, as NIH contends, the development of more effective containment facilities.[222] Moreover, the impact statement adds that those infections that did occur at Fort Detrick occurred as a result of the "absence of genuine efforts to control contaminated air, liquid wastes, refuse and laundry."[223] If "genuine efforts" can be lacking in a national biological warfare facility dealing with known pathogens, it is unrealistic to expect that such efforts be made in hundreds of gene transplantation laboratories across the country when the risks are unknown to those engaged in the research.

The element of human error can never be eliminated. Mistakes are made under even the most ideal of conditions; nature is more complex and we are more fallible than we realize. The participants in the Asilomar Conference acknowledged this:

> Stringent physical containment and rigorous laboratory procedures can reduce but not eliminate the possibility of spreading potentially hazardous agents. Therefore, each investigator bears a responsibility for determining whether, in his particular case, special circumstances warrant a higher level of containment.[224]

There is no guarantee therefore, even if the Guidelines are in effect, that a recombinant molecule will not escape the laboratory. Reported laboratory infections among scientists who work in containment facilities reveal that only a limited protection is provided to scientific workers.[225] Neither the NIH Guidelines nor the Draft EIS satisfactorily acknowledge the element of human error or incorporate it into their risk equations.[226]

A particularly critical factor in determining the possible harm to the public, not considered in the impact statement, is the number of facilities engaged in gene transplantations. To allow, or actually promote, the proliferation of DNA research centers, as the Guidelines do, is to create a push for new discoveries, causing greater numbers of laboratory personnel to become involved in research and increasing the likelihood of laboratory accidents resulting from human and mechanical failures. Such proliferation negates the effectiveness of the proposed physical containment procedures. Even if the Guidelines were ideal, it is unrealistic to hope that the ideal will be universally attained in hundreds of institutions across the country. Because of these factors, research should presently be confined to one national facility. Public safety is incompatible with the present policy of proliferation, which appears to protect the research to a much greater extent than it protects the human environment.

Additionally, the mechanisms for enforcing the Guidelines are insufficient to ensure the high level of compliance and error-free performance on which the safety predictions of the Guidelines are implicitly based. Obviously, the enforcement provisions are directly applicable only to NIH grantees. Others comply with the Guidelines voluntarily. Under the Guidelines, grantees are essentially allowed to police themselves. The chief responsibility for enforcement rests with the principal investigator, the individual or the institution under the grant, and on the "biohazards committee," which is required to be established by the principal investigator. The principal investigator is specifically responsible for evaluating the biohazards of the experiments, training staff and ensuring compliance with safety procedures. The biohazards committee of the institution must certify to the NIH staff that the experiment and facility comply with the Guidelines.[227]

The role and responsibilities of the NIH staff are so extensive that it is unrealistic to expect that they will have both the time and resources sufficient to adequately ensure universal compliance with the Guidelines.[228] Given the increasing number of NIH grantees currently conducting DNA research, the time demands on the staff will prevent the effective monitoring of the hundreds of facilities, as well as the safety of laboratory workers for "leaks" of recombinant DNA particles.[229] Because of the number of complex factual determinations the staff is required to make,[230] virtually all of its time is likely to be spent reviewing applications. The task of monitoring is made even more difficult because the Guidelines do not limit the number of facilities where recombinant DNA research can be conducted. The only sanction for non-compliance is revocation of denial of a grant; there is no force of law behind the Guidelines, no penalties are assessed even if they are deliberately flouted.

Grantees cannot be expected to police themselves effectively. There will always be a strong competitive interest in pushing research ahead and when the progress of research conflicts with adherence to the Guidelines, safety procedures may be bent. The competitive pressures on NIH grantees will be particularly great because non-NIH researchers are not subject to any mandatory safety restraints. Thus, the conclusions of the EIS regarding the nature and extent of the potential hazards of DNA research and technology and the degree of protection afforded by the promulgation of the Guidelines are not sufficiently supported by reason or authority either to be convincing or to meet the rigorous procedural and substantive standards of NEPA.

3. Inadequate Analysis of Alternatives

The Draft EIS issued by NIH is seriously deficient in its analysis of the many important alternatives to recombinant DNA technology. To suggest that the statement fulfills its function of providing a comparative basis upon which significant policy planning decisions can be made is to strain credulity to the breaking point. The cursory treatment given the "alternatives" raises grave question as to whether any options besides the Guidelines were ever actually weighed by NIH. Section 102(2)(E) of NEPA requires that the agency "study, develop, and describe appropriate alternatives to recommended courses of action in any proposal which involves unresolved conflicts concerning alternative uses of available resources."[231] This provision follows and adds to the requirement that alternatives to the proposed action be included in the environmental impact statement, which is found in section 102(2)(C).[232] Since it has been seen to be the "essence and thrust of NEPA that the pertinent statement serve to gather in one place a discussion of the relative environmental impact of alternatives,"[233] it would seem that the more extensive treatment of alternatives required by section 102(2)(D) should be incorporated in the EIS.

The requirements that the impact statement be "detailed," that it include an assessment of the

environmental costs weighed against the expected benefits and that it outline all alternatives that would affect the cost-benefit balance are intended to ensure that agency decision-makers incorporate environmental values into their ultimate decisions and that the public has a basis for evaluating the decision. The legislative history indicates the importance of alternatives as a source of environmental input into the process:

> [T]he agency shall develop information and provide descriptions of the alternatives in adequate detail for subsequent reviewers and decision makers, both within the executive branch and the Congress, to consider the alternatives along with the principal recommendations.[234]

In addition, the Guidelines issued by the Council on Environmental Quality indicate the importance of adequately analyzing alternatives:

> A rigorous exploration and objective evaluation of alternative actions that might avoid some or all of the adverse environmental effects is essential. Sufficient analysis of such alternatives and their costs and impact on the environment should accompany the proposed action through the agency review process in order not to foreclose prematurely options which might have less detrimental effects.[235]

To fulfill the mandates of NEPA, the impact statement study should not just list the alternatives but should also include the result of the agency's own investigation and evaluation of alternatives so that the reasons for the choice of a course of action are clear. The complete impact study must contain more than a mere catalogue of environmental facts. The agency must also "explicate fully its course of inquiry, its analysis and its reasoning."[236]

NIH's discussion of alternatives fails to comply with NEPA by failing to mention many of the important alternatives to DNA research and technology and discussing others only superficially.[237] The alternative options, discussed in less than ten pages of double-spaced standard sized paper, include: no action, NIH prohibition of funding of all experiments with recombinant DNA, development of different Guidelines, no Guidelines but NIH consideration of each project on an individual basis before funding, and general federal regulation of all such research. Each is hardly noted; the average length of the comments on each option is one page.

General federal regulation is mentioned, for example. An incomplete list of agencies with potential authority to regulate DNA technology is provided,[238] but there is no real discussion of the form such regulation might take, nor are comparisons made between the statutory powers of these agencies, where it is noted, for example, that the Occupational Safety and Health Administration (OSHA) has authority to proscribe laboratory conditions, it is not noted that OSHA is powerless to regulate transportation of recombinant materials.[239] The no action alternative, defined by NIH as continuation of NIH-funded experiments without any restrictions or controls, should more properly address itself to terminating federal governmental financial support for all recombinant DNA research. The Draft impact statement should apply not only to NIH's funding of genetic research but to all federal agency activities in this area; NIH is merely acting as the lead agency for purposes of NEPA. Recombinant research supported by other federal agencies should therefore also be discussed and evaluated in the Draft impact statement. Additionally, the no action alternative does not discuss the impact that cessation of NIH funding of genetic technology would have on the environment; it only describes the impact it would have on American research in the field.

The alternatives of issuing national safety standards regulating the conduct of all DNA research is not adequately discussed, despite the fact that HEW has the authority to issue such standards.[240] The alternative of developing regional containment facilities designed to keep the experimentation away from areas of high population density was included, but the increase in safety that such a policy would offer was not discussed.[241] The possibility of confining all federally funded research to one central, highly secure facility while potential hazards and the means to control them are more carefully assessed is not considered, nor is the possibility of a temporary moratorium covering federal, state and private research discussed. Also absent from the EIS are the options of maintaining a federal monopoly over recombinant DNA activities, such as exists in the case of nuclear weapons research and manufacture, and estab-

lishing international control over DNA research utilizing multilaterally supervised sites, as was done in recent initiatives toward supernational uranium fuel enrichment and reprocessing facilities.[242]

The Draft EIS makes no attempt to do a cost-benefit analysis as required by NEPA.[243] Not one of the alternatives is weighed in a serious manner. Each course of action will have its own environmental risks and benefits and its own monetary costs. For example, because of their significant expense, it is imperative that an analysis be done on the costs of having multiple P3 and P4 containment laboratories throughout the country. This cost would probably weigh heavily toward establishing regional centers. Other factors will favor different alternatives, but they should at least be the subjects of thorough analyses. In addition to analysis of the environmental considerations of funding DNA recombinant technology, the impact statement should consider the key question of how NIH may best advance its goals of preventing and curing disease. These are the principal benefits which may possibly be achieved through DNA research. But alternative methods of accomplishing these objectives may be less expensive—monetarily and environmentally. If so, the dispersion of grants should reflect these factors. The information provided on alternatives is not minimally sufficient to permit a reasoned choice of options so far as environmental aspects are concerned. NIH has not taken the "hard look" at the environmental consequences of this significant new technology it is helping to create.

IV. CONCLUSION

The DNA recombinant research controversy is a classic illustration of the law's inability to keep up with the pace of scientific inquiry. NIH's draft environmental impact statement, assessing its research Guidelines for the conduct of experiments relating to a technology already in the applied state of development, is a legal formality offered only to justify a *fait accompli*. A more far-reaching and fundamental flaw is NIH's failure to consider in its EIS the question of whether it is appropriate to fund DNA research at all. Given the potential for catastrophic harm to humankind inherent in this technology, this question should have been addressed at the outset. Since NIH has proven ineffective in regulating the pace and scope of the genetic research which it funds, separate legislation will be needed to protect the public interest. Several bills are now pending in Congress,[244] but, because of the powerful scientific lobby, the likelihood of any forceable action is doubtful.[245] Since this is a highly technical field, and as has been noted, most legislators are "technically illiterate,"[246] it will not be an easy task to develop appropriate legislative safeguards in an area in which the scientific community is divided. In the meantime, strict adherence to NIH's research guidelines is mandatory. In addition, while Congress debates the appropriate mode of regulating genetic engineering, it should at the very least codify the guidelines so that they will apply with equal force to the private and commercial sector not receiving federal research monies. The quality of life, in the final analysis, is more important than the unfettered sanctity of scientific inquiry.

NOTES

1. Recombinant DNA technology or "genetic engineering" involves combining a strip of genes from a cell of a higher organism with the genes in a lower organism, such as a bacteria, so that the foreign genes can be studied in a simpler environment. Genes, which are the units that control heredity, consist of deoxyribonucleic acid, DNA. This process technically creates new kinds of living cells. *See* J. KATZ, EXPERIMENTATION WITH HUMAN BEINGS 492 (1972). *See generally* Green, *Genetic Technology: Law and Policy for the Brave New World,* 48 IND. L.J. 559 (1973).

2. Fields, *Debate Over Genetic Research Spreads Across the Country,* Chronicle of Higher Education, Jan. 31, 1977, at 1, cols. 1–3; *see* Smith, *Manipulating the Genetic Code: Jurisprudential Conundrums,* 64 GEO. L.J. 697 (1976).

3. Phenylketonuria is a congenital deficiency of phenylalanine hydroxylase, which if untreated will produce brain damage and mental retardation. STEADMAN'S MEDICAL DICTIONARY 1072–73 (Williams & Wilkins Co., ed., 23d ed. 1976).

4. Grobstein, *A New Genie Is Out of the Bottle,* L.A. Times, Aug. 29, 1976, pt. IV, at 5, cols. 1–4.

5. *See The Law and the Biological Revolution,* 10 COLUM. J.L. & SOC. PROB. 47 (1973) (Gaylin, moderator; Callahan, Edgar & Michels, commentators); Davis, *Ethical and Technical Aspects of Genetic Intervention,* 285 NEW ENG. J. MED. 1799 (1971); Friedman, *The Federal Fetal Experimentation Regula-*

tions: An Establishment Clause Analysis, 61 MINN. L. REV. 961 (1977); Gorney, *The New Biology and the Future of Man,* 15 U.C.L.A. L. REV. 273 (1968); Robinson, *Genetics and Society,* 1971 UTAH L. REV. 487; Vukowich, *The Dawning of the Brave New World—Legal, Ethical, and Social Issues of Eugenics,* 1971 U. ILL. L.F. 189; Waltz & Thigpen, *Genetic Screening and Counseling: The Legal and Ethical Issues,* 68 NW. U.L. REV. 696 (1973).

6. Dr. Joseph E. Grady, head of infectious disease research, Upjohn Company, testifying before a Senate science subcommittee, indicated that Upjohn expects marketable by-products of genetic engineering in less than five years. Cohn, *"Products" of Genetic Engineering Seen Less Than Five Years Away,* Washington Post, Nov. 11, 1977, at A-2, cols. 4–6.

In a recent landmark patent case, *In re* Bergy, 563 F.2d 1031 (C.C.P.A. 1977), the U.S. Court of Customs and Patent Appeals ruled that Upjohn Company can patent certain forms of life developed in its laboratories. The court's 3-2 decision (Kashiwa, J., concurred in the reasoning and result of the two judge "majority") opened the door for a broad spectrum of food and drug manufacturers to patent processes creating new forms of life. *See also In re* Chakrabarty, 571 F. 2d 40 (C.C.P.A. 1978).

7. S. REP. No. 381, 93d Cong., 1st Sess. 4–11 (1973).

8. *Id.*

9. *Id.* 19. Biomedical research under the aegis of NIH is of two types: inhouse and grantee. *See id.* 5–7. The Institute employs over 1000 scientists to engage in full-time research; in addition, millions of dollars are awarded by way of grants to successful applicants.

10. *See* Parenteau & Catz, *Public Assessment of Biological Technologies: Can NEPA Answer the Challenge?,* 64 GEO. L.J. 679, 687 (1976). For an excellent analysis of the DNA recombinant controversy, see Note, *Recombinant DNA and Technology Assessment,* 11 GA. L. REV. 785, 845–60 (1977).

11. 42 C.F.R. §52.13(a) (1976).

12. *See* Bazelon, *Technology and the Legal Process,* 62 CORNELL L. REV. 817, 824–25 (1977) (urging greater public participation).

13. HOUSE COMM. ON SCIENCE & TECH., 93D CONG., 2D SESS., GENETIC ENGINEERING—EVOLUTION OF A TECHNOLOGICAL ISSUE, SUPP. REPORT I 8–10, 73 (Comm. Print 1974).

14. The members of the committee published the following resolutions:

First, and most important, that until the potential hazards of such recombinant DNA molecules have been better evaluated or until adequate methods are developed for preventing their spread, scientists throughout the world join with the members of this committee in voluntarily deferring . . . [certain] experiments. . . .

Second, plans to link fragments of animal DNAs to bacterial plasmid DNA or bacteriophage DNA should be carefully weighed. . . .

Third, the Director of National Institutes of Health is requested to give immediate consideration to establishing an advisory committee charged with (i) overseeing an experimental program to evaluate the potential biological and ecological hazards of the above types of recombinant DNA molecules, (ii) developing procedures which will minimize the spread of such molecules within human and other populations, and (iii) devising guidelines to be followed by investigators working with potentially hazardous recombinant DNA molecules.

Fourth, an international meeting of involved scientists from all over the world should be convened early in the coming year to review scientific progress in this area and to further discuss appropriate ways to deal with the potential biohazards of recombinant DNA molecules.

Id. 8–9.

15. One hundred and fifty-five participants attended, including fifty-five foreign scientists from fifteen countries, four attorneys and representatives of the press. HOUSE COMM. ON SCIENCE & TECH., 94 CONG., 2D SESS., GENETIC ENGINEERING, HUMAN GENETICS, AND CELL-BIOLOGY—EVOLUTION OF TECHNOLOGICAL ISSUES 20, 91–95 (Comm. Print 1976).

16. Berg, Baltimore, Brenner, Roblin & Singer, *Summary Statement of the Asilomar Conference on Recombinant DNA Molecules,* 72 NAT'L ACADEMY SCIENCES PROC. 1981, 1983 (1975).

17. The Director of NIH established the Recombinant DNA Molecule Advisory Committee to investigate the potential dangers of recombinant DNA research and to recommend guidelines for future projects. 39 Fed. Reg. 39306 (1974).

18. The result was the "Proposed Guidelines for Research Involving Recombinant DNA Molecules," which was referred to the Director of NIH for a final decision in Dec. 1975. HOUSE COMM. ON SCIENCE & TECH., *supra* note 15, at 21–22.

19. 41 Fed. Reg. 27902 (1976).

20. NEPA §102(2)(C), 42 U.S.C. §4332(2)(C) (1970). The issuance of an EIS by NIH was the first time that the agency ever considered its research activities subject to NEPA. *See* Parenteau & Catz, *supra* note 10, at 692.

21. 41 Fed. Reg. 38426 (1976).

22. *See generally* Asimow, *Public Participation in the Adoption of Interpretive Rules and Policy Statements,* 75 MICH. L. REV. 521 (1977); DiMento, *Citizen Environmental Litigation and the Administrative Process: Empirical Findings, Remaining Issues and a Direction for Future Research,* 1977 DUKE L.J. 409; Green, *Public Participation in Nuclear Power Plant*

Licensing: The Great Delusion, 15 WM. & MARY L. REV. 503 (1974).

23. Pub. L. 91–190, 83 Stat. 852 (current version at 42 U.S.C. §§4321–4347 (1970 & Supp. V 1975)).

24. NEPA §102(2)(C), 42 U.S.C. §4332(2)(C) (1970). The EIS must contain the following elements:

(i) the environmental impact of the proposed action,

(ii) any adverse environmental effects which cannot be avoided should the proposal be implemented,

(iii) alternatives to the proposed action,

(iv) the relationship between local short-term uses of man's environment and the maintenance of enhancement of long-term productivity, and

(v) any irreversible and irretrievable commitments of resources which would be involved in the proposed action should it be implemented.

25. *See* McGarity, *The Courts, the Agencies, and NEPA Threshold Issues,* 55 TEX. L. REV. 801 (1977).

26. *See* Note, *Program Environmental Impact Statements: Review and Remedies,* 75 MICH. L. REV. 107 (1976).

27. *See* Note, *The Application of Federal Environmental Standards to the General Revenue Sharing Program: NEPA and Unrestricted Federal Grants,* 60 VA. L. REV. 114 (1974).

28. *See, e.g.,* Sierra Club v. Volpe, 351 F. Supp. 1002 (N.D. Cal. 1972).

29. HOUSE COMM. ON SCIENCE & TECH., *supra* note 15, at 32.

30. Parenteau & Catz, *supra* note 10, at 692. Between 1970 and 1977, NIH issued several EIS's. Almost all of these involved simple construction activities, even though the major activity undertaken by the agency is biomedical research. One statement did touch upon a more sophisticated environmental problem—a proposal to construct an incinerator for the disposal of hazardous laboratory wastes at the Bethesda, Md. campus of NIH. Interestingly, the decision to build was postponed after the EIS turned up significant problems with the proposed facility.

31. *See generally* Hanks & Hanks, *An Environmental Bill of Rights: The Citizen Suit and the National Environmental Policy Act of 1969,* 24 RUTGERS L. REV. 230 (1970).

32. Other congressional acts evidencing a similar commitment to enhance the quality of the environment, although less extensive in scope, are the Environmental Education Amendments of 1974, 20 U.S.C. §§1531–1532 (Supp. V 1975); Water Quality Improvement Act of 1970, 33 U.S.C. §§1151, 1155–1156, 1158, 1160–1172, 1174 (1970); Air Quality Act of 1967, 42 U.S.C. §§1857–1857*l* (1970); Environmental Quality Improvement Act of 1970, *id.* §§4371–4374.

33. NEPA §101(c), 42 U.S.C. §4331(c) (1970). This section derives from a provision of the Senate bill, S. 1075, 91st Cong., 1st Sess., 115 CONG. REC. 19008 (1969), which stated that Congress "recognizes that each person has a fundamental and inalienable right to a healthful environment." *Id.* §101(b), 115 CONG. REC. 19008 (1969). The Conference Report states: "The compromise language was adopted because of doubt on the part of the House conferees with respect to the legal scope of the original Senate provision." H.R. REP. NO. 765, 91st Cong., 1st Sess. 8, *reprinted in* [1969] U.S. Code Cong. & Ad. News 2767, 2768–69.

34. NEPA §2, 42 U.S.C. §4321 (1970).

35. NEPA §101(a), *id.* §4331(a). Other aspects of human activity specifically recognized as having an impact include population growth, high density urbanization, industrial expansion and resource exploitation.

36. *See generally* 115 CONG. REC. 40 (1969).

37. NEPA §101(a), 42 U.S.C. §4331(a) (1970).

38. NEPA §101(b), *id.* §4331(b).

39. NEPA §101, *id.* §4331.

40. NEPA §102, 42 U.S.C. §4331 (1970 & Supp. V. 1975), prescribes a methodology. It does not tell the decision-maker what values to prefer. This provision was not in S. 1075 as it was originally introduced by Sen. Henry Jackson (D-Wash.). As introduced, S. 1075 was intended primarily to authorize the Secretary of the Interior to conduct ecological investigations, and to establish a Council on Environmental Quality. Section 102 was generated in large part by the experience with the Miami jetport, an ongoing controversy during the same period that S. 1075 was under consideration in the Senate. A lesson thought to be learned from that controversy was that the process of coordinating is not a reliable means by which to provide for environmental protection, or indeed to identify the environmental issues, in connection with major public works projects. Instead it seemed necessary to require articulation along the lines provided by section 102. *See* Brennan, *Jetport: Stimulus for Solving New Problems in Environmental Control,* 23 U. FLA. L. REV. 376 (1971); Kessler & Teply, *Jetport: Planning and Politics in the Big Cypress Swamp,* 25 U. MIAMI L. REV. 713 (1971).

41. Perhaps because of the vagueness of the statutory language, the mandatory nature of the procedural duties, and the courts' view that their reviewing authority is limited, there are few judicial interpretations of the broad substantive provisions of section 101. Most judicial attention has focused on section 102's impact statement requirement.

42. NEPA §102, 42 U.S.C. §4332 (1970). This strong language in the procedural section should be contrasted with the weaker standard in substantive section 101(b), which requires agencies to "use all practicable means consistent with other essential considerations."

Id. §4331(b). The difference in approach, apparent from a surface language comparison, is made express in the words of the Senate and House conferees who explained the "fullest extent possible" language as follows:

The purpose of the new language is to make it clear that each agency of the Federal Government shall comply with the directives set out in . . . [section 102(2)] *unless the existing law applicable* to such agency's operations *expressly prohibits or makes full compliance with one of the directives impossible.* . . . Thus, it is the intent of the conferees that the provision "to the fullest extent possible" shall not be used by any Federal agency as a means of avoiding compliance with the directives set out in section 102.

H.R. REP. NO. 765, *supra* note 33, at 9–10, *reprinted in* [1969] U.S. CODE CONG. & AD. NEWS 2767, 2770 (emphasis added). The Senators' views are contained in "Major Changes in S. 1075 as Passed by the Senate," 115 CONG. REC. 40417–18 (1969). The Representatives' views are contained in a separate statement filed with the Conference Report, 115 CONG. REC. 40427 (1969).

43. NEPA §102(2)(A), 42 U.S.C. §4332(2)(A) (1970).

44. NEPA §102(2)(B), *id.* §4332(2)(B). "The legislative history indicates that one of the strong motivating forces behind NEPA, and section 102 in particular, was to make exploration and consideration of environmental factors an integral part of the administrative decision-making process." City of N.Y. v. United States, 337 F. Supp. 150, 160 (E.D.N.Y. 1972). "Perhaps the greatest importance of NEPA is to require . . . agencies to *consider* environmental issues just as they consider other matters within their mandates." Calvert Cliffs' Coordinating Committee, Inc. v. United States Atomic Energy Commission, 449 F.2d 1109, 1112 (D.C. Cir. 1971). *See also* S. Rep. No. 296, 91st Cong., 1st Sess. (1969); 115 CONG. REC. 40416 (1969) (remarks of Sen. Jackson).

45. NEPA §102(2)(F), 42 U.S.C. §4332(2)(F) (Supp. V 1975).

46. NEPA §102(2)(E), 42 U.S.C. §4332(2)(E) (Supp. V 1975).

47. NEPA §102(2)(C), 42 U.S.C. §4332(2)(C) (1970).

48. NEPA §102(2)(C)(iii), *id.* 4332(2)(C)(iii).

49. NEPA §102(2)(C)(iv), *id.* §4332(2)(C)(iv).

50. NEPA §102(2)(C)(ii), *id.* §4332(2)(C)(ii).

51. Hanly v. Mitchell, 460 F.2d 640, 644 (2d Cir.), *cert. denied,* 409 U.S. 990 (1972); National Resources Defense Council v. Morton, 458 F.2d 827, 834 (D.C. Cir. 1972).

52. CEQ Guidelines, 40 C.F.R. §1500 (1977).

53. NEPA §102(2)(C), 42 U.S.C. §4332(2)(C) (1970).

54. "It is important that we take people into our confidence before the fact rather than after the fact, in

order to provide the opportunity for discussion of the many approaches which can bring a catalyst into being." 115 CONG. REC. 40425 (1969) (remarks of Sen. Randolph). There are also examples of instances where well-focused public input has influenced the agency decision-making process. *See* Andrews, *NEPA in Practice: Environmental Policy or Administrative Reform?*, in WORKSHOP ON THE NEPA 21, 29–30 (1976) (Report Prepared Pursuant to the Request of the Subcomm. on Fisheries and Wildlife Conservation and the Environment of the House Comm. on Merchant Marine and Fisheries by the Environment and Natural Resources Policy Division, Congressional Research Service, Library of Congress). Robert Cahn cites the example of a toll bridge in San Francisco that was scrapped because of public pressure resulting in the rejection of the EIS prepared for the project. Cahn, *Impact of NEPA on Public Perception of Environmental Issues,* in WORKSHOP ON THE NEPA, *supra,* at 62, 65. *See also* 1 CEQ ANN. REP., ENVIRONMENTAL QUALITY 211–12 (1970).

55. There are various avenues open to members of the public to secure environmental redress. They can petition agencies. If that is unsuccessful, they can petition Congress. An impact statement can be the basis for a court attack on agency action under the Administrative Procedure Act (APA), §10(e), 5 U.S.C. §706(2) (A) (1970). *See* Andrews, *supra* note 54, at 28.

56. This does not imply that only environmental factors need be considered but that they should be given weight along with other legitimate factors such as cost and time.

57. *See, e.g.,* Brooks v. Volpe, 350 F. Supp. 269 (W.D. Wash. 1972), *aff'd per curiam,* 487 F.2d 1344 (9th Cir. 1973); Environmental Defense Fund v. TVA, 339 F. Supp. 806 (E.D. Tenn.), *aff'd,* 468 F.2d 1164 (6th Cir. 1972). *See also* 115 CONG. REC. 40416 (1960) (remarks of Sen. Jackson). "The requirement to prepare as EIS has had the salutary effect of continually reminding the decisionmaker that environmental factors must be given adequate attention in all phases of planning." *National Environmental Policy Act Oversight: Hearings Before the Subcomm. on Fisheries and Wildlife Conservation and the Environment of the House Comm. on Merchant Marine and Fisheries,* 94th Cong., 1st Sess. 5 (1975) (statement of Kenneth McIntyre).

58. The lower courts have almost uniformly recognized NEPA's public informational purpose. *See, e.g.,* Scenic Hudson Preservation Conference v. FPC, 407 U.S. 926, 933 (1972) (Douglas, J., dissenting from denial of certiorari); Maryland Nat'l Capital Park & Planning Comm'n v. United States Postal Serv., 487 F.2d 1029 (D.C. Cir. 1973); Iowa Citizens for Environmental Quality, Inc. v. Volpe, 487 F.2d 849 (8th Cir. 1973); National Helium Corp. v. Morton, 486 F.2d 995 (10th Cir. 1973), *cert. denied,* 416 U.S. 993 (1974);

International Harvester Co. v. Ruckelshaus, 478 F.2d 615, 650 n.130 (D.C. Cir. 1973).

* * *

168. Federation of American Scientists, Public Interest Report: Recombinant DNA 1 (Apr. 1976) (Position Paper, Document 9).

169. 41 Fed. Reg. 38427 (1976). The Introduction continues: "The Guidelines are meant to ensure that experiments are carried out under conditions and safeguards that minimize the possibility of harmful exposure of any human being or other component of the environment to these possibly hazardous agents." *Id.*

170. *Id.*

[I]t is believed that the containment measures specified in the Guidelines make the escape of potentially harmful recombinant organisms into the environment highly improbable. . . . [I]t is also believed that, even if an experiment performed in accordance with the Guidelines does result in accidental release of recombinant organisms, adverse effects will either not occur or not be serious.

171. *Id.*

172. *Id.*

173. Most particularly courts have tended to focus on the sufficiency of the impact statement requirement and of the bureaucratic procedures followed in considering that statement. Presumably the reason for this focus is that these are the most concrete incidents of agency environmental considerations and hence most easily subjected to judicial evaluation. Furthermore, challenges to agency action under NEPA tend to focus on the sufficiency of the impact statement and agency procedures for its consideration. Although a NEPA complaint will generally allege violations of each section of the Act, complainants tend to focus on the more concrete sections of the Act when filing affidavits or making formal offerings of proof of agency noncompliance with NEPA standards.

174. S. REP. NO. 296, *supra* note 44, at 19.

175. Environmental Defense Fund v. Corps of Engineers, 470 F.2d 289, 298–99 (D.C. Cir. 1972). "NEPA is silent as to judicial review, and no special reasons appear for not reviewing the decision of the agency. To the contrary, the prospect of substantive review should improve the quality of agency decisions and should make it more likely that the broad purposes of NEPA will be realized." *See also* Conservation Council of N.C. v. Froehlke, 473 F.2d 664 (4th Cir. 1973); Natural Resources Council, Inc. v. Morton, 458 F.2d 827 (D.C. Cir. 1972); National Helium Corp. v. Morton, 455 F.2d 650 (10th Cir. 1971); Scenic Hudson Preservation Conference v. FPC, 453 F.2d 463 (2d Cir. 1971), *cert. denied,* 407 U.S. 926 (1972) (Douglas, J., dissenting); Ely v. Velde, 451 F.2d 1130 (4th Cir. 1971); Calvert Cliffs' Coordinating Comm. v. AEC,

449 F.2d 1109 (D.C. Cir. 1971). See also the third annual report of the CEQ which concludes that "after an agency has considered environmental effects, its decision to act is subject to . . . limited judicial review." 3 CEQ ANN. REP., ENVIRONMENTAL QUALITY 254 (1972).

176. Calvert Cliffs' Coordinating Comm. v. AEC, 449 F.2d 1109, 1115 (D.C. Cir. 1971).

177. Agencies have an obligation "to use all practical means, consistent with other essential considerations of national policy, to improve and coordinate Federal plans, functions, programs and resources" to preserve and enhance the environment. NEPA §101(b), 42 U.S.C. §4331(b) (1970). To this end, section 101 sets out specific environmental goals to serve as a set of policies to guide agency action affecting the environment.

178. NEPA §102(1), *id.* §4332(1), directs that the policies, regulations and public laws of the U.S. be interpreted in accordance with these policies to the "fullest extent possible."

179. Calvert Cliffs' Coordinating Comm. v. AEC, 449 F.2d 1109, 1115 (D.C. Cir. 1971). This standard of review in its totality focuses on two main aspects of the bureaucratic process. First, a court will review agency decisions for failure to take into account all relevant factors or values or for misuse of authority in basing decisions on irrelevant factors or values. Secondly, a court will review to see that no single factor or value has been given too much or too little weight in the decision. This is in addition to the court's review of the sufficiency of bureaucratic procedures for ensuring the consideration of environmental factors. NEPA mandates a "particular sort of careful and informed decisionmaking." *Id.*

180. Citizens to Preserve Overton Park v. Volpe, 401 U.S. 402, 416 (1971). Some judges have argued for a stricter standard of review. *See, e.g.,* Scenic Hudson Preservation Conference v. FPC, 453 F.2d 463, 482 (2d Cir. 1971), *cert. denied,* 407 U.S. 926 (1971) (Oakes, J., dissenting), as well as the dissent of Mr. Justice Douglas from the order denying certiorari, in which it was argued that a standard of review stricter than the arbitrary or capricious test should have been used, 407 U.S. at 930–31. Similarly, a three-judge court in City of New York v. United States, 344 F. Supp. 929, 939–40 (E.D.N.Y. 1972), made a limited review on the merits of an agency decision. The question as to whether or not a stricter standard of review should be used was left open.

181. The Guidelines themselves, although comparatively more detailed and objective in tone than the brief conclusory Draft EIS, are nevertheless deficient in providing a rationally convincing basis for its assurances that the public is now well protected from the potential hazards of DNA recombinant technology.

182. Ely v. Velde, 451 F.2d 1130, 1139 (4th Cir. 1971).

183. Calvert Cliffs' Coordinating Comm. v. AEC, 449 F.2d 1109, 1115 (D.C. Cir. 1971). This case, which involved the licensing of a nuclear power plant, indicated that NEPA requires actual and active consideration of environmental factors in agency planning, and also requires internal organization and procedures to ensure such consideration. The AEC rule in dispute in the case forbade the AEC hearing board to consider nonradiological environmental factors in reviewing applications for nuclear power plants unless such factors were "affirmatively raised" by intervenors or AEC regulatory staff. This ad hoc reliance on interested third parties to raise environmental issues was held to be insufficient to meet NEPA's requirements.

184. Greene County Planning Bd. v. FPC, 455 F.2d 412, 420 (2d Cir. 1972). FPC regulations, 18 C.F.R. §2.80–.82 (1972), allowed power plant applicants to prepare their own impact statements which the FPC staff would then circulate to other federal agencies for comment. The FPC, however, would file its own impact statement only after its final decision to license the plant. Such a procedure was deemed by the court to be inadequate because it did not evidence independent FPC research and analysis nor did it provide an FPC statement for comment and debate prior to the agency's final decision.

185. This is not to suggest that the standard required by NEPA is that of subjective impartiality. "NEPA assumes as inevitable an institutional bias within an agency proposing a project and erects the procedural requirements of §102 to insure that 'there is no way [the decision-maker] can fail to note the facts and understand the very serious arguments advanced by the plaintiffs if he carefully reviews the entire environmental impact statement.'" Environmental Defense Fund v. Corps of Engineers, 470 F.2d 289, 295 (8th Cir. 1972). Thus NEPA requires that prior to embarking on an action an agency must objectively evaluate the environmental costs and benefits and that the evaluations process be reflected in an impact statement.

186. See notes 111–19 *supra* and accompanying text. [*Text and notes omitted.*]

187. Jones v. District of Columbia Redevelopment Land Agency, 499 F.2d 502, 511 (D.C. Cir. 1974), *cert. denied,* 423 U.S. 937 (1975). See notes 120–67 *supra* and accompanying text. [*Text and notes omitted.*]

188. See notes 13–16 *supra* and accompanying text.

189. *See* materials cited in notes 1–5 *supra*.

190. An example of this failure is NIH's discussion of the organism E. coli. The biological containment safeguards of the Guidelines depend upon the safety of the use of E. coli (strain K12) as the bacterial host. In sanctioning the use of E. coli as a recipient for recombinant DNA molecules, it is stated that "[T]his organism has been studied extensively and is well suited to recombinant research." 41 Fed. Reg. 38435. The statement goes on to admit that "[I]t has been argued

. . . that E. coli should not be used at the present time. This is because many E. coli strains are intimately associated with humans and other living things, and because they readily exchange DNA [genes] with certain other bacteria in nature." *Id.* No reference is given to the many scientific publications which assert in essence that there is probably a no more inappropriate organism to use than E. coli for such work. *E.g.,* Anderson, *Viability of, and Transfer of a Plasmid from, E. coli K-12 in the Human Intestine,* 255 NATURE 502 (1975). *See also* Chargaff & Simring, *On the Dangers of Genetic Meddling,* 192 SCIENCE 938 (1976) (letter to the editor); Dyson, *Costs and Benefits of Recombinant DNA Research,* 193 SCIENCE 6 (1976); Hubbard, *Recombinant DNA: Unknown Risks,* 193 SCIENCE 834 (1976); Simring, *Recombinant DNA Risks and Benefits,* 192 SCIENCE 940 (1976). No relevant information on the K12 strain is given such as its rates of genetic exchange with other wild type E. coli, or the mechanisms by which K12 could be made pathogenic through recombinant research both intentionally and unintentionally. There is no discussion of the fact that many pathogenic E. coli strains exist. For example, two out of 1000 patients that enter Boston hospitals die from E. Coli infections. 294 NEW ENG. J. MED. 61 (1976). The statement made by NIH that the organism has been "extensively studied" has also been refuted. "As of October 1976, only a few experiments to test the innocuousness of K12 have been performed, and these under only the most normal conditions. The conditions under which accidents occur are notable for their non-normality." Lappé, *Regulating Recombinant DNA Research: Pulling Back from the Apocalypse,* II MAN AND MEDICINE, Summer 1976, at 103, 106. Scientists have also urged that research efforts should first be directed to the development of a host organism that is not a resident of the normal human environment and does not exchange DNA organisms in that environment. These are not referred to. In general, the hazard of using a bacteria whose niche is the mammalian gut and the possible repercussions of this are in no way discussed in an adequate, informed manner.

191. A function of the court is

to assure that the statement sets forth the opposing scientific views, and does not take the arbitrary and impermissible approach of completely omitting from the statement, and hence from the focus that the statement was intended to provide for the deciding officials, any reference whatever to the existence of responsible scientific opinions concerning possible adverse environmental effects.

Committee for Nuclear Responsibility, Inc. v. Seaborg, 463 F.2d 783, 787 (D.C. Cir.), *application for injunction in aid of jurisdiction denied,* 404 U.S. 917 (1971). In that case, the court agreed with plaintiff's claim that omission of all reference to existing respon-

sible scientific opinion as to possible adverse consequences is contrary to the process described in NEPA. *Cf.* Environment Defense Fund v. TVA, 339 F. Supp. 806, 809 (E.D. Tenn.), *aff'd,* 468 F.2d 1164 (6th Cir. 1972) (draft impact statement on the Tellico dam project insufficient because its cost-benefit analysis consisted almost entirely of unsupported conclusions and requiring that a final statement be filed).

192. *See* Berg, Baltimore, Brenner, Roblin & Singer, *supra* note 16, at 1984.

193. 41 Fed. Reg. 38427 (1976).

194. *Id.* 38429. Other admissions are: "In the absence of an adequate base of data derived from either experiments or experience, it must be recognized that future events may not conform to these judgments [the Guidelines containment levels]." *Id.* 38427. "Different assessments of the hazards could have been made and consequently more stringent precautions could have been taken." *Id.* "[T]he use of these physical containment] measures reduces but does not prevent the potential for laboratory-acquired infections." *Id.* 38436. "Lack of knowledge about the real risks of such molecules makes it impossible to determine either the nature of the hazards or the extent to which laboratory personnel are endangered by exposures to the materials." *Id.*

195. The system is only superficially noted in the Draft EIS itself. *Id.* 38432–34.

196. *Id.* 38456–57.

197. *Id.* 38454.

198. *Id.* 38452–54.

199. In describing the protection provided by P1 and P2 facilities, the Draft EIS states: "These measures do not provide absolute protection from exposures, and the required primary barriers can be compromised by lack of attention to technique, poor placement of equipment, and human error." *Id.* 38436.

200. *Id.*

201. *Id.* 38452, 38454.

202. *Id.* 38454–58.

203. It is possible to imagine an experiment with primate DNA which is less hazardous than one with prokaryote DNA. For example, an experiment that puts primate DNA into E. coli might produce an organism with such a low probability of survival and such a low probability that the primate DNA would be fully expressed and create a primate protein, that it poses virtually no risk to humans. Another experiment in which DNA from a prokaryote is inserted in E. coli might improve the survival ability of E. coli, be transmitted to a pathogenic strain of E. coli and make it more virulent, thereby substantially increasing the risk of disease in humans. Some of the assumptions underlying the classification system are contradictory. In some situations higher containment levels are required because almost nothing is known about the hazards; in

other situations, stricter containment is required because concrete information about the hazards exists. For example, one of the reasons for requiring a high level of containment for experiments with primate DNA is that we know so little about such recombinations. On the other hand, the reason for prohibiting experiments which would transfer antibiotic resistance to nonresistant species is that we know such transfers will certainly impair the ability to cure human disease. Similarly, special provision is made in the Guidelines for experiments using E. coli host-vector systems because we know that E. coli colonizes in the human intestine. But other prokaryotic host-vectors, which do not colonize in humans, may prove equally harmful to the environment in ways we cannot now foresee.

204. The EIS walks the reader through a complex series of hypothetical events which would have to happen simultaneously to create a biohazard. The genetically engineered organism which possesses a potentially harmful gene must first escape from the experimental situation (risk: 1 in 100); it must survive after escape (risk: 1 in 10,000); it must grow and reproduce in its new environment (risk: 1 in a million). Successful epidemic conditions would then require that the first infected organisms contact other hosts, that the bacteria leave the first host in infectious form, and grow and multiply once again. The aggregate risk (which the authors consider conservative) is given as 1 in a trillion (1×10^{12}). 41 Fed. Reg. 38438 (1976).

205. The very brief discussion on the ideal use of a strain of bacteria that could not survive outside of the laboratory does not in any sense serve as a real discussion on the important area of biological containment. *Id*. 38432–38435.

206. *Id*. 38430.

207. Other problems with biological containment which should have been discussed in the EIS include the possibility that the biologically enfeebled host organisms could spontaneously revert to a wild type organism, or could survive and propagate by otherwise circumventing the disabling characteristics forced upon it. Another possibility that was never addressed in the Draft EIS is that since the crippled organism will grow more slowly due to its disability a contaminant might fall into the culture and grow at a faster rate than the disabled organism. Thus, the researcher will unknowingly end up with a culture not of the disabled host, but of a wholly different viable organism. Another potentially hazardous situation would occur if a non-pathogenic culture became contaminated with a virulent species. The researcher could continue to treat it as harmless, subjecting it to the stricter containment care it should receive. No periodic check for culture purity is recommended in the impact statement or the Guidelines. The Guidelines should require a continual checking of host organisms to ensure that they always contain the full complement of disabling characteristics. *See* Comments of Hon. Louis J. Lef-kowitz, Atty. Gen. of N.Y., on the Guidelines and Draft EIS for Recombinant DNA Research, Submitted to the Director of NIH, at 11–12 (Oct. 19, 1976).

All of the above mentioned problems and limitations of biological containment should have been thoroughly discussed. An extensive review of microbiological strategies whereby host organisms could lose their disabling characteristics, plus a risk analysis of the likelihood of this happening, is an essential requirement for an adequate impact statement.

208. 41 Fed. Reg. 38429 (1976).

209. The possibility of the totally unexpected is emphasized in the impact statement's discussion of "Benefits," but is not addressed adequately in the discussion of "Hazards." In discussing potential benefits, it is stated: "It is important to stress that the most significant results of this work, as with any truly innovative endeavor, are likely to arise in unexpected ways and will almost certainly not follow a predictable path." *Id*. 38431. Similar statements could be made about the hazards. For example, an organism containing chimeric DNA could possess properties exhibited by neither the host nor the organism providing the source of the recombinant DNA.

210. The experience with atomic energy provides an example of how unreliable future risk predictions can be. When the decision was made in 1941 to proceed with the technology, very little was known about the biological effects of radiation, particularly low level effects. DNA had just been discovered; the mechanism of mutation was unknown. The designers of the Bomb knew that $E=MC^2$, but did not anticipate radioactive fallout from the atmosphere as more than a trivial problem. "Allowable" exposures to radiation were many times higher than the current 5 rem/year, itself under much attack for being too high. No one imagined, or cared, that plutonium would turn out to be a potent carcinogen. In short, all the hazards, the undesirable effects and "environmental impacts" of the governmental action to develop atomic energy have been much worse than anyone imagined in 1941. The benefits (if this term can be legitimately used), including nuclear power, were fairly well anticipated in 1941. *Hearing Before the Subcomm. on Health and Scientific Research of the Senate Comm. on Human Resources*, 95th Cong., 1st Sess. 259–60 (1977) (comments of Burke K. Zimmerman, Ph.D., Staff Scientist, Environmental Defense Fund, on the Draft Environmental Impact Statement for the NIH Guidelines for Research Involving Recombinant DNA molecules submitted to the Director of NIH (Oct. 18, 1976)). Thus the history of nuclear energy undermines the Draft impact statement which implies that we know enough about the potential hazards so that "strict adherence" to the Guidelines should render "harmful effects from research with high risk recombinant DNA molecules . . . extremely unlikely." 41 Fed. Reg. 38437 (1976). Such a statement cannot be justified in the context of DNA research.

211. The experience with the use of radioactive materials in the laboratory, an area under strict government regulation, reveals that a number of abuses occur for a variety of reasons. The situation is somewhat different with DNA recombinant research because radioactivity, if released, is diluted in the environment, while an organism capable of survival and reproduction could multiply and spread. *See Hearings Before the Subcomm. on Health and Scientific Research of the Senate Comm. on Human Resources, supra* note 210, at 268–69 (comments of Burke K. Zimmerman, Ph.D.)

212. The impact statement points out that it is currently impossible to assign specific probabilities to events related to risk assessment and that NIH is supporting research designed to improve this deficiency. 41 Fed. Reg. 38436 (1976).

213. As discussed earlier at notes 118–19 *supra [text and notes omitted]*, NIH made a decision not to regulate non-NIH supported techniques even though the Secretary of HEW has the authority under Section 361 of the Public Health Services Act, 42 U.S.C. §264 (1970), to regulate all such activities.

214. Experiments conducted in violation of the Guidelines will pose the same hazards as experiments which are not covered by the Guidelines. The Draft EIS should, but does not, evaluate the likelihood that the Guidelines will be followed by non-NIH grantees and the risk to the public from noncomplying experiments.

215. The presumed requirement of secrecy is in conflict with the spirit and letter of the Guidelines under which all projects require, at the very least, an impartial peer review as well as scrutiny by an institutional biohazards committee. Moreover, the implications of this industrial attitude are antithetical to the notion that any form of research and technology with a potential for impairing the health of the environment should proceed only with the informed consent of the public. Grobstein & Clifford, *Recombinant DNA Research: Beyond the NIH Guidelines*, 194 SCIENCE 1133, 1133–35 (1976).

216. 41 Fed. Reg. 38437 (1976).

217. *Id.* 38446.

218. See notes 195–201 *supra* and accompanying text.

219. *See Oversight Hearing on Implementation of NIH Guidelines Governing Recombinant DNA Research: Joint Hearings Before the Subcomm. on Health of the Senate Comm. on Labor & Public Welfare and the Subcomm. on Administrative Practice and Procedure of the Senate Comm. on the Judiciary,* 94th Cong., 2d Sess. 115 (1976) (comments of Burke K. Zimmerman, Ph.D., Staff Scientist, Environmental Defense Fund).

220. 41 Fed. Reg. 38437 (1976). The statement continues:

All high-risk materials are required to be isolated in physically contained, absolute primary bar-

riers. All effluents from these barriers are sterilized. The barriers themselves are located in maximum-security facilities, which are provided with additional barriers to prevent any accidental release. Air locks, negative air pressure, clothes-change rooms, filtration and incineration of all air exhausted from the facility, and the secondary sterilization of all liquid and solid wastes, provide additional protection to the environment. *Id.*

221. *Id.* "An analysis of 36 reported laboratory-acquired micro-epidemics in the period 1925–1975 involving over 1,000 infections . . . demonstrated no infections among persons who were never in the laboratory building or who were not associated in some way with the laboratory." The citation given by NIH is Wedum, A.G., The Detrick Experience as a Guide to the Probable Efficacy of P4 Microbiological Containment Facilities for Studies on Microbial Recombinant DNA Facilities (1976) (Unpublished Report to the National Cancer Institute).

222. *See, e.g., Oversight Hearing on Implementation of NIH Guidelines Governing Recombinant DNA Research, supra* note 219, at 76–88 (comments of Dr. Robert L. Sinsheimer).

223. 41 Fed. Reg. 38437 (1976).

224. Berg, Baltimore, Brenner, Roblin & Singer, *supra* note 16, at 1982.

225. *See* CONFERENCE ON BIOHAZARD IN BIOLOGICAL RESEARCH 59,331 (A. Hellman, M. Oxman & R. Pollack eds. 1973).

226. Instead, conclusions are drawn on the basis of qualified statements expressing the ideal—that under standardized procedures research personnel will be well-trained and proficient. 41 Fed. Reg. 38437 (1976). To assume this level of perfection in all cases is unrealistic.

227. The EIS's discussion of Enforcement appears at 41 Fed. Reg. 38458–60 (1976).

228. The staff is also required to make a number of factual determinations: assigning containment levels, approving applications for lower containment levels, approving host-vector systems for biological containment and approving large scale experiments. *Id.* 38459.

229. No truly reliable means seem to exist for detecting or giving warning of accidental release to the environment of potentially hazardous materials. Nor is there sufficient discussion on environmental-spill contingency plans. See discussion of risks, HOUSE COMM. ON SCIENCE & TECH., *supra* note 15, at 36–39. *See also Oversight Hearing on Implementation of NIH Guidelines Governing Recombinant DNA Research, supra* note 219, at 115 (comments of Burke K. Zimmerman, Ph.D., Staff Scientist, Environmental Defense Fund). This is true when the "hazard or potential hazard cannot be seen, heard or smelled." *Id.* 123.

230. *See* 41 Fed. Reg. 38459 (1976). For the number of NIH grantees conducting DNA-related research, see note 90 *supra*. [Text and note omitted.]

231. NEPA §102(2)(E), 42 U.S.C. §4332(2)(E) (Supp. V 1975); *see* Comment, *NEPA—The Purpose and Scope of the Duty to Discuss Alternatives*, 7 URB. L. ANN. 390 (1974).

232. NEPA §102(2)(C), 42 U.S.C. §4332(2)(C) (1970).

233. Natural Resources Defense Council v. Morton, 458 F.2d 827, 834 (D.C. Cir. 1972). In that case the court affirmed the district court's action in enjoining the sale of oil leases in excess of $500 million, based upon an alleged failure of the government to discuss certain alternatives in its Final EIS.

234. S. REP. NO. 296, *supra* note 44, at 21.

235. 36 Fed. Reg. 7724–25 (1971).

236. Ely v. Velde, 451 F.2d 1130, 1139 (4th Cir. 1971) (agency in question was the Law Enforcement Assistance Administration).

237.
We reject the implication of one of the Government's submissions which began by stating that while the Act requires a detailed statement of alternatives, it "does not require a discussion of the environmental consequences of the suggested alternative." A sound construction of NEPA . . . requires a presentation of the environmental risks incident to reasonable alternative courses of action.
Natural Resources Defense Council v. Morton, 458 F.2d 827, 834 (D.C. Cir. 1972) (citation omitted).

238. The agencies include the Center for Disease Control and the Occupational Health and Safety Administration. 41 Fed. Reg. 38436 (1976).

239. *Id.*

240. Section 361 of the Public Health Services Act, 42 U.S.C. §264 (1970), gives the Secretary of HEW the authority to promulgate regulations to protect the public from communicable diseases. The draft EIS repeatedly recognizes that DNA activities may create or increase the virulence of infectious agents, making regulation under section 361 appropriate.

241. 41 Fed. Reg. 38435 (1976).

242. These latter choices appear certain to grow in public favor. The widespread publicity which followed the mysterious outbreak of "Legion fever" in Pennsylvania, the first instance of disease which implicates recombinant organisms, will probably result in the rapid imposition of general federal regulation. The next serious outbreak may well precipitate federal monopoly, and the next, internationalization. Detailed planning for the possible implementation of these likely steps should begin now, lest proliferation of techniques, apparatus materials and know-how make their later achievement extremely difficult. Early institution of arrangements congruent with the assumption of high hazard will avoid the possibilities of calamitous health damage, political overreaction and resultant expensive modification or scrapping of facilities adjudged no longer acceptable. *See, e.g.,* Atomic Energy Act of 1954, 42 U.S.C. §§2131–2140 (1970) (as amended) (licensing the use of atomic energy). Legislation to regulate recombinant research, covering the private sector, was proposed in the 95th Congress. See note 244 *infra*.

243. *See* Comment, *Cost-Benefit Analysis in the Courts: Judicial Review Under NEPA*, 9 GA. L. REV. 417 (1975).

244. S. 1217, 95th Cong., 1st Sess., 123 CONG. REC. S 5335–37 (daily ed. April 1, 1977) (Kennedy D-Mass.) ("The Recombinant DNA Regulation Act"); H.R. 4232, 95th Cong., 1st Sess. (1977) (Solarz D-N.Y.) ("Commission on Genetic Research and Engineering Act of 1977"); H.R. 7897, 95th Cong., 1st Sess. (1977) (Rogers D-Fla.) ("A Bill to Amend the Public Health Services Act").

245. *See* Cohn, *Scientist Lobby Successful—DNA Research Control Dims,* Washington Post, Sept. 28, 1977, at A-1, cols. 1–2. *See also* Fields, *Opposed by Scientists—Kennedy Withdraws Bill to Regulate DNA Research,* Chronicle of Higher Educ., Oct. 3, 1977, at 10, cols. 1–5. *See generally* Morgenthau, *Modern Science and Political Power,* 64 COLUM L. REV. 1386 (1964).

246. *See* Ethyl Corp. v. EPA, 541 F.2d 1, 67 (D.C. Cir.) (*en banc*) (concurring opinion, Bazelon, C.J.), *cert. denied,* 426 U.S. 941 (1976) (referring to judges).

6.3 Divorcing Profit Motivation from New Drug Research: A Consideration of Proposals to Provide the FDA with Reliable Test Data*

SIDNEY A. SHAPIRO

Reprinted with permission of Sidney A. Shapiro and the *Duke Law Journal*, from 1978 *Duke Law Journal* 155–168, 172, 181–183. Copyright © 1978 by *Duke Law Journal*. All rights reserved.

I. INTRODUCTION

Under present federal regulation, a pharmaceutical company that is attempting to gain Food and Drug Administration (FDA) approval for marketing a new drug is responsible for conducting the necessary drug experimentation.[1] It has been forcefully argued that because the company has a financial interest in successful test results, the present drug testing system contains an inherent bias[2] that adversely affects the accuracy and acceptability of drug research.[3] Concern about these effects has led to proposals that pharmaceutical research be conducted by independent parties with no financial interest in the outcome of the research.[4] To evaluate whether such regulatory changes are necessary, this Article will examine the relationship between the profit-oriented testing of drugs and the need for both ethical human experimentation and accurate experimental data. Consideration will be given to what improvements, if any, might be made in the present system.

II. THE DRUG TESTING PROCESS

Before new drugs[5] can be marketed, they must be proven safe and effective to the satisfaction of the FDA.[6] The necessary proof includes a three phase test[7] of the drug on human beings[8] and at least two well-controlled clinical studies.[9] However, even before the research on humans can be initiated, the sponsor of the drug must submit to the FDA a Notice of Claimed Investigation Exemption for a New Drug (IND)[10] containing information—including results of *in vitro*[11] and animal studies[12] on the pharmacologic and toxic effects of the drug—from which the FDA can determine whether the drug appears to be reasonably safe and effective for human use.[13]

If human tests are permitted,[14] the sponsor may, upon completion of the necessary tests, file a New Drug Application (NDA), seeking FDA approval for marketing the drug.[15] The FDA then has 180 days in which to approve or disapprove an NDA, although this review period often may be extended.[16] In evaluating an NDA, the FDA reviews the sponsor's summary of the raw data derived from all the studies that were conducted.[17] In addition, most FDA reviewers

*This Article is based on a report prepared for the Review Panel on New Drug Regulation of the Department of Health, Education and Welfare. However, the views expressed herein reflect the personal opinion of the author, and thus are not necessarily the views of either the Review Panel or of HEW.

The author would like to express his appreciation to the members of the Review Panel—Dr. Allen Astin, Professor Marsha Cohen, Dr. Charles Cornelius, Professor Norman Dorsen, Professor Robert Hamilton, Dr. David Rall and Dr. Norman Weiner—who evaluated the report on which this Article was based. The author also is appreciative of the assistance of Ms. Kathleen Buto and Mr. Jeffrey Miller, members of the Review Panel staff, who provided criticism of the same report.

randomly audit certain sections of the several hundred volumes of raw data. They find it impossible, however, to review every page of the submitted information.[18] If the NDA is not approved, the FDA must give the sponsor "notice of an opportunity for a hearing . . . on the question whether such application is approvable,"[19] after which the FDA issues a final order either approving or refusing to approve the NDA.[20]

Throughout this drug testing process, all human testing is commercially sponsored. Accordingly, it is essential that certain safeguards be built into the testing system. The public must be assured that the testing of unapproved drugs in humans is conducted in an ethical manner.[21] Further, the FDA must be confident that the data submitted to it by the sponsor are complete and accurate before it determines if a drug is safe and effective for its intended use.[22]

III. ETHICAL CONSIDERATIONS IN HUMAN TESTING

The testing of new drugs on human beings involves subjecting selected portions of the population to a certain amount of risk for possible but unestablished benefits to the general public.[23] The risks may be minimized and the benefits approximated by preliminary experimentation with animals,[24] by thoughtful chemical analysis and through a review of past experience with similar drugs.[25] Nevertheless, until a drug is tested in humans, the extent of its safety and effectiveness cannot be fully assessed.[26]

Human testing involves a number of ethical considerations. Among the most serious and widely discussed of these is the selection of subjects for tests.[27] Subjects should be accepted only after they have given their informed consent, indicating they are fully aware of the nature and purpose of the tests and the possible risks involved.[28] Thus, special problems arise in seeking the consent of persons such as prisoners, children and the mentally retarded who have questionable ability to make such meaningful decisions.

Consideration also must be paid to safeguarding the public and test subjects from needless exposure to risks that result from poorly designed tests or inaccurate or biased evaluation of test data.[29] The number of test subjects exposed to experimental drugs must be large enough to establish significant levels of safety and efficacy, but not so large as to expose subjects unnecessarily to an experimental drug.[30] Additionally, tests should be sufficiently well-designed to avoid repetition.[31] Moreover, unless the FDA is given accurate information, a drug may be marketed under inaccurate claims of effectiveness or with inadequate warnings about its safe use. This not only results in risks to those for whom the drug is prescribed, but it also results in unnecessary exposure to test risks for the test subjects since the results of the test in which they participated will not be reflected in accurate labeling of the drug.[32]

In light of these ethical considerations, human drug testing can be viewed as a "public trust."[33] The concept of public trust has long been used by the legal system to denote a special or higher standard of care on the part of those who serve the public or who otherwise are charged with the maintenance of public assets.[34] Under this concept, while the responsibility for ethical drug investigation is shared by all of the participating entities,[35] the government, as the initiator of the research, would be the ultimate trustee charged with protecting the individuals involved.[36] To that end, the government should consider any changes in the existing system that would better protect the individuals involved in clinical testing. It is important to examine the present drug testing system to determine if the public interest is best served by industry sponsorship of drug research. In particular, it is essential to review whether industry's desire to gain maximum profits from drugs creates problems in either the ethical acceptability or the reliability of the present testing system.

IV. THE RELATIONSHIP OF THE PROFIT MOTIVE TO RELIABLE DRUG TESTING

The hallmark of the present system of drug development is the sponsorship of human drug testing by private concerns whose major motivation is the hope of realizing a profit from the eventual sale of the drug.[37] Consideration must be given to how their profit motivation might affect the objectivity and efficiency of the drug testing system.

A. The Role of the Sponsor in Drug Research

Conventional economic thought holds that a private corporation's estimate of the anticipated profit from a new product takes into account possible social or external damage caused by the product to the extent that the public's ill will might decrease sales[38] or that its profits may be diminished by tort actions against the company for injuries caused by the product.[39] Decisions within the pharmaceutical industry concerning the research and development of new drugs appear to fit this pattern. The sponsor's future financial planning with regard to a new drug depends on an accurate appraisal of the drug's therapeutic value,[40] including any dangers which might lead to tort liability.[41] Additionally, the anticipated cost of developing a drug includes the expense of further testing that may be required if the FDA finds test data to be inaccurate or inadequate.[42] For these reasons, there is a substantial corporate interest in obtaining accurate information. Moreover, there is a strong ethically motivated desire among drug sponsors to turn out effective products,[43] and this is only possible when production is preceded by thorough and valid research.

Nevertheless, because of the potential for profit from a successful drug, it is claimed that a pharmaceutical firm's view of information about its drugs may be colored by its natural desire to turn out commercially successful compounds,[44] and this bias may result in the firm interpreting data more favorably than would independent observers.[45] Dr. Louis Lasagna reports that he has observed such instances in scientific meetings, in personal discussions and in the sometimes acrimonious exchanges which follow evaluation of a firm's product by outside bodies such as the American Medical Association's Council on Drugs or the Medical Letter on Drugs and Therapeutics.[46]

Thus, the sponsor's motivation to obtain accurate information should not be considered sufficient to ensure the objectivity or reliability of test results. In fact, as presently constituted, the relationship between the sponsor and its researchers may have the effect of subtly biasing the results of studies in favor of drugs being tested, thereby undermining the accuracy of data submitted to the FDA.

B. The Relationship between Sponsors and Researchers

Most pharmaceutical companies contract out their clinical research on humans to university-affiliated hospitals.[47] Although some companies also contract out their preclinical animal tests,[48] this research usually can be done by private pharmaceutical firms. The contractual relationship between the sponsor and the physician doing clinical research varies, but it usually includes reimbursement for expenses incurred,[49] and it sometimes includes payment for services rendered.[50]

The fact that the testing physician or clinical laboratory receives financial support from the drug's sponsor has been viewed as creating a conflict of interest.[51] Some observers believe that a clinical researcher who is beholden to a sponsor for financial support cannot make a detached observation concerning the cause and significance of physical effects of the experimental drug,[52] and that in making subjective judgments, a researcher will be at least unconsciously influenced by the fact that a drug company is paying for the research and hoping for favorable results.[53]

The problem of objectivity that is inherent in the relationship between the sponsor and the investigator has been recognized for many years. In 1961, it was observed that the company's influence over researchers came not as much from financial payment as from personal contact.

Having spent some 6 years in the business of influencing clinical investigators, I can assure you that objectivity can be destroyed more frequently and more effectively by the soft sell than by the bribe. . . . A paternalistic attitude toward the detail man who is a "nice fellow" and who requests the "study"; the positive response to the medical director "who traveled all the way from New York" to "consult" the "investigator"; the wish to be an "investigator" and perhaps to be invited to give a paper at a "symposium"; the fantasy of prestige and of the respect of the medical community; the certain knowledge that no one ever won a Nobel Prize by publishing a negative paper about an obscure drug; the fantasy of the "pioneer" who blazes the trail to the discovery of a new drug—these are only a few examples of the really potent influences which determine objectivity in drug studies.[54]

There are other ways in which the objectivity of data may be compromised. When a sponsor is unable to obtain its first choice of an investigator, it is possible that the clinician who finally accepts the job may do so because he favored the drug in the first place.[55] In addition, the reliability of data from either animal or human testing may be affected if investigators find they are operating under rigid deadlines. If the sponsor desires to obtain results at the earliest possible moment to recover expeditiously its investment, it may communicate a sense of urgency to the researcher. Such time pressures may cause researchers to make errors in their analyses of data.[56]

While acknowledging the potential for misleading results under the present system, scientists assert that the professionalism of those involved provides a substantial guarantee of reliability.[57] One physician described the influence of professionalism on the drug testing process as follows:

> [T]here are going to be some people who will be found in any community who might bow to temptation, but . . . the vast majority of the drug testing being done now is being done in academic centers and with high standards regardless of who sponsors the testing. . . . Testing is being done by people who have their academic reputations on the line, not simply support for their future studies. The results they obtain will eventually be published in a reputable journal—the careers of the investigators are at stake. Thus there are check systems within the system which will guarantee you that good testing can be done.[58]

Undoubtedly, professionalism is an important factor in promoting accurate information, but recent events indicate that its effects must not be overestimated. Caution is necessary because fraud in research exists and apparently is rising.[59] Moreover, scientists have begun to examine critically the adverse impact that the sponsorship of research might have on the integrity of the resulting data.[60]

The criminal penalties for submission of fraudulent data to the FDA[61] reflect society's belief that government oversight is necessary. The FDA's policy of checking test results submitted by sponsors similarly reflects this concern.[62] The important questions are whether such checking is, or can be, sufficient to verify the submitted data and whether the criminal penalties are, or can be, sufficient incentive to sponsors to furnish reliable data. To answer these questions, it is important to assess the extent to which problems have arisen with regard to the reliability of data.

C. Misleading or Fraudulent Industry-Generated Research

The FDA has found that several animal and clinical test results have been fabricated or otherwise made misleading by sponsors or by toxicology laboratories working for sponsors.[63] Recent incidents have been sufficiently serious for FDA officials to call for a re-examination of the general reliability of industry animal test submissions.[64]

In early 1976, the FDA raised questions regarding the integrity of animal data submitted to it by G.D. Searle Company in support of the drugs Flagyl and Aldactone.[65] To determine the seriousness of the discrepancies in Searle's data, the FDA formed a task force which studied the data in question as well as data submitted in support of other Searle drug applications. On-site investigations were conducted of Searle laboratories.[66] Based on this investigation, the FDA reported to a Senate committee that

> Searle made a number of deliberate decisions which seemingly were calculated to minimize the chances of discovering toxicity and/or to allay FDA concern. . . .
>
> In addition, Searle made other decisions which may have been inadvertent or unintentional which produced similar results.[67]

On this record, the FDA recommended to the Department of Justice that grand jury proceedings be instituted to determine if Searle had violated the Federal Food, Drug and Cosmetic Act (FDCA).[68]

Additional investigations indicated that at least one other major pharmaceutical manufacturer had the same sort of serious deficiencies in its animal testing procedures,[69] that three other companies withheld adverse animal data from the agency,[70] and that several contract animal testing laboratories had problems similar to those at Searle.[71] Responding to a statement that the situation uncovered by the FDA is "serious and grave," the FDA Commissioner Alexander Schmidt replied:

> I would agree with that characterization. . . .
> It is certainly more widespread than I would have guessed. I think it represents an area in which we have never been active in regulating, and now clearly we must be.[72]

Similar problems were discovered in the early 1960s with respect to clinical testing. In 1963, two clinical researchers reported that they were approached by a pharmaceutical sponsor whose offer to finance research was predicated upon a return promise that the test results would be favorable.[73] In 1964, a clinical researcher pleaded *nolo contendere* to an indictment charging that he willfully submitted fictitious reports of clinical studies in support of five separate new drug applications.[74] Similarly, from 1963 to 1965 three pharmaceutical companies and several of their employees were convicted of, or pleaded *nolo contendere* to, charges that they had fraudulently withheld from the FDA information adverse to their drug applications.[75] All three of the drugs that were involved, MER-29 by Richardson Merrell, Inc., Dornwell by Wallace and Tiernan, and Flexin by McNeil Laboratories, were approved by the FDA in ignorance of the withheld information, and subsequently were prescribed for large numbers of patients.[76]

These clinical incidents predate the 1962 Amendments to the FDCA, which included provisions that require the registration of drug manufacturers, allow for the inspection of drug plants, and impose more rigid controls over the manufacture and approval of drugs.[77] Although comparable incidents have not been discovered since, the FDA apparently believes that problems still exist in the field of clinical research:

> We have looked more at clinical research, and . . . have not found the kinds of very serious errors . . . in clinical research

which we found in some of the animal toxicology research. . . . [Nevertheless] faults in protocol design can be found in both clinical and animal research. Inadequate training of research workers is to be found in both, and sometimes improper data handling is to be found in both clinical research and animal toxicology research.[78]

The FDA believes that potentially the problems are more serious in experiments involving animals than in those conducted on humans. Clinical research often is conducted in universities and the results may be published in the medical literature. Animal testing is conducted by the sponsor or a contract laboratory and is not as susceptible to peer scrutiny.[79] The FDA also requires the submission of raw data for clinical research, but not for animal studies.[80]

For both animal and clinical research, the FDA thinks that the problems which it finds result primarily from poor and sloppy procedures, rather than from deliberate distortions of data.[81] However, the effects of the two sources of error are the same; both prevent the FDA from obtaining accurate information upon which to base its decisions.[82]

* * *

Under the FDCA if the agency receives inaccurate or misleading data, it may use any of the following sanctions: an information letter advising a firm or person of violations of law and regulations;[111] a regulatory letter which cites specific violations, sets a deadline for a response regarding corrective actions and advises that administrative or legal action will be taken if corrective action is not undertaken;[112] disqualification of clinical investigators from eligibility to receive investigational new drugs if they repeatedly or deliberately violate the FDCA or its regulations;[113] termination of a sponsor's IND;[114] disapproval of an NDA;[115] or withdrawal of a marketed drug.[116] The following legal actions can be initiated through the Department of Justice: prosecuting an individual for use of the mails to submit fraudulent data to the government;[117] enjoining individuals or firms from violation of the FDCA or regulations;[118] seizing any drug which is adulterated or misbranded when introduced into, or while it is in, interstate commerce.[119]

* * *

VI. CONCLUSIONS AND RECOMMENDATIONS

Under the present drug testing system, there are few mechanisms to ensure that the FDA receives reliable data in its consideration of the safety and effectiveness of a new drug. Without accurate data, the agency may lack an adequate basis upon which to evaluate the risks and benefits associated with a drug's use. Serious questions can also be raised about the morality of human testing when data from such testing are not accurately presented to the FDA.

Despite the sponsor's financial interest in deriving precise information from clinical tests and the professionalism of researchers involved in testing, the possibility remains that data submitted to the agency will be at least unconsciously biased and, at worst, fraudulent. Likewise, criminal penalties for submission of fraudulent information and the FDA's monitoring of laboratory practices provide incentive for the submission of accurate information. However, these factors have not always prevented submission of fraudulent data and they are not useful mechanisms for deterring subtle bias in data analysis. Accordingly, five further steps should be taken to minimize problems of inaccurate and misleading test information.

First, the FDA already has proposed regulations concerning Good Laboratory Practice for Nonclinical Laboratories. The agency hopes to inspect each nonclinical laboratory every two years to determine if the laboratories are in compliance with the regulations. In addition to this inspection program, the FDA should use its authority for limited third-party testing to verify animal test information submitted to it. If such authority is limited to spot checks where sponsors have submitted misleading or inaccurate information in the past, limited third-party testing should serve as an additional incentive for the submission of reliable information. Spot checking would not slow the development process since it could be conducted simultaneously with the ongoing testing.

This form of limited third-party testing is thought to be preferable to complete third-party testing for animal experimentation. While completely removing animal testing from sponsors to an independent third party is a more direct method by which to eliminate some of the possibility of bias or distortion, it may also create a

research disincentive since the animal testing process is closely tied to sponsor innovation. Moreover, complete third-party testing could not be implemented as rapidly as the partial testing approach because presently animal testing expertise independent of the pharmaceutical industry is limited.

A second step would be for the FDA to finalize its guidelines for clinical research to ensure that sponsors are fully aware of the agency's requirements for such research. The inaccuracy and sloppiness of industry-generated data apparently results in part from lack of guidance from the FDA regarding the research requirements. Thus such guidelines could reduce inefficiency in the testing process, thereby minimizing the possibility that test subjects would be exposed to risks unnecessarily. Clinical guidelines also would provide the FDA with a further basis for evaluating the industry submissions of information.

In addition, if, in conjunction with the release of guidelines, the FDA were to increase its supervisory role during the clinical investigational period for new drugs, the quality of data submitted as a result of clinical studies would be enhanced. For example, the FDA might institute conferences with the sponsor at critical times during the drug development process, such as prior to initiation of large-scale clinical trials.

As a fourth innovation, the FDA should utilize its present authority to impose administrative sanctions against anyone found to have submitted inaccurate or misleading material information or, where appropriate, recommend criminal prosecutions. The FDA has assigned too low a priority to enforcement of the provisions of the FDCA and those of its regulations that are intended to ensure the accuracy of data. Although the FDA must take care to avoid a relationship with the industry that is so adversarial as to be counter-productive, its behavior must also convince researchers and drug sponsors that sanctions will be imposed on those who submit inaccurate or misleading information.

Finally, a pilot program should be implemented whereby HEW would contract with independent parties for the clinical testing of a class of drugs which the FDA would choose based on its assessment of which class of drugs could benefit most from the program. Additional assurance of the accuracy of clinical research could be best implemented through such a program of government contracting. The other possible alternatives appear to be less advantageous than the contracting approach. Limited third-party testing to verify existing clinical research information would pose ethical problems and would be difficult, costly and time-consuming. Complete testing by the government would necessitate a sizable government bureaucracy which might not be as efficient or innovative as the private sector. By comparison, government contracting would be a lesser regulatory intrusion. But since it would be a substantial change from the present system, it is difficult to foresee all of the possible complications which might arise if government contracting is adopted. For that reason, a pilot program would be a reasonable method to approach the implementation of this proposal.

NOTES

The following citations will be used in this article:

Examination of the Pharmaceutical Industry, 1973–74: Hearings Before the Subcomm. on Health of the Senate Comm. on Labor and Public Welfare, 93d Cong., 1st & 2d Sess., Part 5 (1974) [hereinafter cited as *Examination of the Pharmaceutical Industry (Part 5)*];

Hearings on Competitive Problems in the Drug Industry Before the Subcomm. on Monopoly of the Senate Select Comm. on Small Business, 90th Cong., 2d Sess., Part 7 (1968) [hereinafter cited as *Competitive Problems in the Drug Industry (Part 7)*];

Hearings on Competitive Problems in the Drug Industry Before the Subcomm. on Monopoly of the Senate Select Comm. on Small Business, 91st Cong., 1st Sess., Part 10 (1969) [hereinafter cited as *Competitive Problems in the Drug Industry (Part 10)*];

Hearings on Interagency Coordination in Drug Research and Regulation Before the Subcomm. on Reorganization and Internat'l Organizations of the Senate Comm. on Government Operations, 88th Cong., 1st Sess. (1963) [hereinafter cited as *Interagency Coordination in Drug Research and Regulation*];

Preclinical and Clinical Testing by the Pharmaceutical Industry, 1975, Joint Hearings Before the Subcomm. on Health of the Senate Comm. on Labor & Public Welfare and the Subcomm. on Administrative Practice and Procedure of the Senate Comm. on the Judiciary, 94th Cong., 1st Sess., Part 1 (1975) ([hereinafter cited as *Preclinical and Clinical Testing (Part 1)*];

Preclinical and Clinical Testing by the Pharmaceutical Industry, 1976, Joint Hearings Before the Subcomm. on Health of the Senate Comm. on Labor & Public Welfare and the Subcomm. on Administrative Practice and Procedure of the Senate Comm. on the Judiciary, 94th Cong., 2d Sess., Part 2 (1976) [hereinafter cited as *Preclinical and Clinical Testing (Part 2)*];

GENERAL ACCOUNTING OFFICE, FEDERAL CONTROL OF NEW DRUG TESTING IS NOT ADEQUATELY PROTECTING HUMAN TEST SUBJECTS AND THE PUBLIC, REPORT TO THE CONGRESS (1976) [hereinafter cited as FEDERAL CONTROL OF NEW DRUG TESTING];

NATIONAL ACADEMY OF SCIENCES, EXPERIMENTS AND RESEARCH WITH HUMANS: VALUES IN CONFLICT (1975) [hereinafter cited as VALUES IN CONFLICT];

NATIONAL ACADEMY OF SCIENCES, HOW SAFE IS SAFE? THE DESIGN OF POLICY ON DRUGS AND FOOD ADDITIVES (1974) [hereinafter cited as HOW SAFE IS SAFE?].

1. See text accompanying notes 5–22 *infra.*

2. "Bias" as used in this Article refers to a partiality toward a certain outcome. It is not intended to indicate that the partiality is necessarily malicious.

3. See text accompanying notes 37–82 *infra.* [*Text and notes 59–82 omitted.*]

4. See text accompanying notes 135–78 *infra.* [*Text and notes 135–167 omitted.*]

5. Section 201(p) of the Federal Food, Drug and Cosmetic Act, 21 U.S.C. §321(p) (1970), defines "new drug" as:

(1) Any drug . . . the composition of which is such that such drug is not generally recognized, among experts qualified by scientific training and experience to evaluate the safety and effectiveness of drugs, as safe and effective for use under the conditions prescribed, recommended, or suggested in the labeling thereof. . . .

(2) Any drug . . . the composition of which is such that such drug, as a result of investigations to determine its safety and effectiveness for use under such conditions, has become so recognized, but which has not, otherwise than in such investigations, been used to a material extent or for a material time under such conditions.

For a discussion of the difficulty faced in interpreting this section, see J. MASHAW & R. MERRILL, INTRODUCTION TO THE AMERICAN PUBLIC LAW SYSTEM 463–66 (1975).

6. 21 U.S.C. §355 (1970); *see* Weinberger v. Bentex Pharmaceuticals, 412 U.S. 645, 652–54 (1973).

7. Phase I of the human testing is directed at determining the drug's chemical effects on a small number

of healthy volunteers. *Primer on New Drug Development*, FDA CONSUMER 12, 12–13 (Feb. 1974). Phase II studies involve administering the drug to a limited number of patients who are affected with the specific disease the drug is intended to treat. During this phase, the investigators can begin to evaluate the effectiveness of the drug while additional safety testing on humans or animals continues. *Id.* 13. In Phase III, a large number of patients are treated in order to assess the drug's safety, effectiveness and most desirable dosage. *Id.* 13–14. For a detailed description of these phases, see J. GIBSON, MEDICATION, LAW AND BEHAVIOR 125–45 (1976).

8. *Primer on New Drug Development, supra* note 7, at 12, 13. The conditions under which such human experimentation may occur are prescribed by the Secretary of Health, Education and Welfare, acting pursuant to the Federal Food, Drug and Cosmetic Act. 21 U.S.C. §355(i) (1970).

9. As used in this Article, "clinical" refers to studies on human subjects.

10. 21 U.S.C. §355(a) (1970); 21 C.F.R. §312.1(a)(2) (1977). Human experimentation is necessary for several important reasons, such as that a drug may affect humans differently than animals. *See* HOW SAFE IS SAFE? 109 (remarks of Oliver H. Lowry, M.D.); *id.* 218 (remarks of Samuel S. Epstein, M.D.). Other reasons for human experimentation are discussed in *Preclinical and Clinical Testing (Part 1)*, at 4.

11. *In vitro* refers to studies performed outside of living organisms.

12. 21 C.F.R. §321.1(a)(2) (1977). Other information submitted includes the chemical composition of the new drug, a detailed protocol intended to be used in initial clinical studies, the qualifications of the clinical investigators who will carry out the studies, an agreement by the sponsor to notify FDA and all participating investigators of any adverse effects which arise during animal or human testing, an agreement by the sponsor that it will obtain the consent of the person on whom the drug is to be tested, and agreement to submit annual progress reports. *Primer on New Drug Development, supra* note 7, at 12.

13. 21 C.F.R. §312.1(a)(2) (1977); *Primer on New Drug Development, supra* note 7, at 12.

14. The sponsor may initiate the clinical studies unless the FDA prohibits it from doing so within 30 days of receiving the IND. 21 C.F.R. §312.1(a)(2) (1977).

15. 21 U.S.C. §355(c)-(d) (1970). The statute, which rejects use of uncontrolled studies, anecdotal reports and clinical testimonials to gain new drug approval, adopted the scientific viewpoint that in light of the unpredictable course of many diseases and the biases and expectations of both patients and physicians, quantification of therapeutic benefit was not possible in the absence of formal experimental controls. Weinberger v. Hyson, Westcott & Dunning, 412 U.S. 609,

617–20 (1973); Upjohn Co. v. Finch, 422 F.2d 944, 951–54 (6th Cir. 1970). *See also* Lasagna, *The Pharmaceutical Revolution: Its Impact on Science and Society*, 166 SCIENCE 1227, 1231 (1969).

16. 21 U.S.C. §355(c) (1970); Review Panel on New Drug Regulation, Department of Health, Education and Welfare, Interim Report: FDA's Review of Initial IND Submissions: A Study of the Process for Resolving Internal Differences and an Evaluation of Scientific Judgments (Feb. 28, 1977).

17. Review Panel on New Drug Regulations, *supra* note 16, at 40.

18. *Id.* 9, 41.

19. 21 U.S.C. §355(c) (1970).

20. *Id.* §355(d). Unfavorable decisions are appealable to the appropriate United States Court of Appeals. *Id.* §355(h).

21. See text accompanying notes 23–36 *infra*.

22. See text accompanying notes 37–82 *infra*.

23. HOW SAFE IS SAFE? 113 (statement of Oliver H. Lowry, M.D.); VALUES IN CONFLICT 153 (remarks of J. Katz, M.D.); Dyck & Richardson, *The Moral Justification for Research Using Human Subjects*, in BIOMEDICAL ETHICS AND THE LAW 243, 243–44 (J. Humber & R. Almeder eds. 1976); Lasagna, *supra* note 15, at 1227.

24. VALUES IN CONFLICT 196 (remarks of Richard Merrill and Oliver H. Lowry, M.D.); *id.* 218 (remarks of Samuel S. Epstein, M.D.); New York Acad. of Medicine, Comm. on Public Health, *The Importance of Clinical Testing in Determining the Efficacy and Safety of New Drugs*, 2 J. OF NEW DRUGS 135, 138 (1962).

25. VALUES IN CONFLICT 29 (remarks of Francis D. Moore, M.D.); Trout, *Problems in Drug Research and Development*, in INTERSECTIONS OF LAW AND MEDICINE 59–63 (G. Morris & M. Norton eds. 1972).

26. B. BARBER, DRUGS AND SOCIETY 83, 84 (1967); HOW SAFE IS SAFE? 30 (remarks of W. Clarke Wescoe, M.D.); *id.* 114 (remarks of Oliver H. Lowry); Dyck & Richardson, *supra* note 23, at 243.

27. *Preclinical and Clinical Testing (Part 1)*, at 350 (statement of the Pharmaceutical Manufacturers Association); VALUES IN CONFLICT 212 (remarks of Ivan Bennett, M.D.). *See generally Preclinical and Clinical Testing (Part 1);* B. BARBER, *supra* note 26; VALUES IN CONFLICT.

28. *Preclinical and Clinical Testing (Part 1)*, at 350–54 (statement of the Pharmaceutical Manufacturers Association); VALUES IN CONFLICT 4, 59–60; Dyck & Richardson, *supra* note 23, at 251–55; Shimkin, *Scientific Investigations on Man: A Medical Research Worker's Viewpoint*, in BIOMEDICAL ETHICS AND THE LAW 207, 212 (J. Humber & R. Almeder eds. 1976). The term "informed" has been viewed as a contradiction in itself. If an experiment is being done, it

REV. 858, 882–83 (1973). *Contra,* HOW SAFE IS SAFE? 135 (remarks of W. Clarke Wescoe, M.D.).

56. New York Acad. of Medicine, *supra* note 24, at 143; *Interagency Coordination in Drug Research and Regulation,* Part 4, at 1601.

57. HOW SAFE IS SAFE? 136, 200 (remarks of W. Clarke Wescoe, M.D.); *cf.* GENERAL ACCOUNTING OFFICE, FEDERAL CONTROL OF NEW DRUG TESTING IS NOT ADEQUATELY PROTECTING HUMAN TEST SUBJECTS AND THE PUBLIC 28 (1976).

58. *Examination of the Pharmaceutical Industry (Part 5),* at 2301–02 (testimony of Kenneth Melmon, M.D.).

59. Rensberger, *Fraud in Research is a Rising Problem in Science,* N.Y. Times, Jan. 23, 1977, at 1, cols. 1–3, at 44, cols. 3–6; Vonder Haar & Miller, *Warning: Your Prescription May be Dangerous to Health,* NEW YORK, May 16, 1977, at 54; *Violating Nature,* TIME, Mar. 14, 1977, at 54.

60. Horowitz, *Science, Sin and Sponsorship,* ATLANTIC, Mar. 1977, at 99, 101; Trippett, *Science: No Longer a Sacred Cow,* TIME, Mar. 7, 1977, at 72–73.

61. 18 U.S.C. §1001 (1970).

62. HOW SAFE IS SAFE? 172–74 (remarks of Phillip Handler, M.D.); see note 18 *supra* and accompanying text.

63. See text accompanying notes 65–76 *infra.*

64. *Preclinical and Clinical Testing (Part 2),* at 6–7.

65. *Id.* 5–6. *See generally* Vonder Haar & Miller, *supra* note 59, at 46–52.

66. Vonder Haar & Miller, *supra* note 59, at 57–58.

67. *Hearings on Preclinical and Clinical Testing by the Pharmaceutical Industry, supra* note 48, at 25, 27. In addition, animal studies done by a Searle contractor, Hazelton Laboratories, were also found to have serious flaws in research design and performance. *Id.* 27, 724.

68. *Id.* 724.

69. *Id.* 725.

70. *Preclinical and Clinical Testing (Part 1),* at 43–44.

71. *Hearings on Preclinical and Clinical Testing by the Pharmaceutical Industry, supra* note 48, Part 3, at 725.

72. *Id.*

73. *Interagency Coordination in Drug Research and Regulation* Part 3, at 1018.

74. *Interagency Coordination in Drug Research and Regulation,* Part 6, at 3197–98. *See generally* M. MINTZ, *supra* note 50, at 328–36.

75. *See generally* M. MINTZ, *supra* note 50, at 17–32, 36q, 230–47; Greenberg, *How Safe Are Your Drugs,* SCIENCE DIGEST, June 1975, at 54.

76. Flexin was used by 3 million people, Dornwell by 160,000 and MER-29 by 418,000. M. MINTZ, *supra* note 50, at 20, 27, 246.

77. 21 U.S.C. §§301–392 (1970), *as amended by* Act of Oct. 10, 1962, Pub. L. No. 87–781, 76 Stat. 780. *See* S. REP. NO. 1744, 87th Cong., 2d Sess. 8 (1962).

78. *Preclinical and Clinical Testing (Part 2),* at 46–47 (testimony of Alexander M. Schmidt, M.D.).

79. *Id.* 46.

80. *Id.*

81. *Preclinical and Clinical Testing (Part 1),* at 12 (testimony of Alexander M. Schmidt, M.D.).

82. *Preclinical and Clinical Testing (Part 2),* at 83 (statement of Alexander M. Schmidt, M.D.). *See also* Ladimer, *Quackery and the Consumer—Responsibility of the Medical Profession,* 18 FOOD DRUG COSM. L.J. 436, 448 (1963).

* * *

111. FEDERAL CONTROL OF NEW DRUG TESTING 21.

112. *Preclinical and Clinical Testing (Part 2),* at 369.

113. 21 C.F.R. §312.1(c)(1)-(2) (1977).

114. *Id.* §312.1(d).

115. 21 U.S.C. §355(d) (1970); 21 C.F.R. §314.111 (1977).

116. 21 U.S.C. §355(e) (Supp. V 1975); 21 C.F.R. §314.115 (1977).

117. 18 U.S.C. §1001 (1970).

118. *Id.* §332(a).

119. 21 U.S.C.A. §334 (West Supp. 1977). *See generally* CIBA Corp. v. Weinberger, 412 U.S. 640, 644 (1973).

* * *

6.4 The Ethics Quagmire and Random Clinical Trials

LAURENCE R. TANCREDI

Reprinted with permission of the Blue Cross Association, from *Inquiry*, Vol. XII, No. 3 (September 1975), pp. 171–179. Copyright © 1975 by the Blue Cross Association. All rights reserved.

Ethical appropriateness has become a common subject in discussing medical research plans, and in many cases has been the critical issue in determining whether a scientifically important study is to be conducted. Current interest in this dimension of medical research reflects the conceded abuses that have occurred where patients have unknowingly been made subjects of studies with high attendant risks for personal injury. Tuskegee (the long-term syphilis study) and similar incidents have contributed, and justifiably, to the current sensitivity to issues surrounding patient consent with the administration of new and experimental treatment, and highlight the patient's right to medical disclosure and the physician's duty to provide even unsolicited information on the nature, relevance and potential adverse effects of medical procedures.[1]

But ethical reasons have been evoked under certain conditions to curtail apparent abuses while in effect serving to unnecessarily restrict research that is essential if major strides are to be achieved in medical care. One of the primary targets is the random clinical trial, a method that allows for comparability between two groups by dividing the patients on the basis of a simple numerical device, such as the use of random numbers, and thereby avoiding the possibilities that the characteristics of the patients will influence the outcome. The scientific importance of such trials cannot be overestimated. As A.L. Cochrane beautifully shows in his book, *Effectiveness and Efficiency—Random Reflections on Health Services,* the random clinical trial is the major technique available for determining if a certain diagnostic or therapeutic procedure effectively serves the ends for which it was developed and, thereby, actually significantly alters for the better the natural history of a disease.[2] At the same time, the need for appropriate protection for patients involved in such trials cannot be ignored. The issue, however, is not whether random clinical trials should be allowed, nor whether protection should be afforded to patients, but rather what mechanisms could be constructed to both allow random trials and still provide protection to patients. Current proposals that would eliminate certain types of random clinical trials or establish more complicated bureaucracies through "protection committees" and "ethics review boards"[3] pose the danger of precluding valuable research that has at best minimal ethical conflicts—conflicts that might be resolved by the provision of effective disclosure mechanisms.

In general, epidemiological or population-based experiments refer to situations where the investigator has deliberately influenced a course of events for specific population groups, while other comparable groups receive an alternative program or no program, as in a controlled experiment.[4] Such experiments fall within two very broad categories: they are either interventional studies using primarily the random clinical trial, or non-interventional ones. The non-interventional type studies, either prospective or retrospective, attempt to determine causal factors for outcomes, such as disease or death; and outside of issues associated with confidentiality of information, they do not present any unique questions regarding the protection of patients' rights that are of present day concern. The interventional studies, on the other hand, because they involve alterations in diagnosis and treatment of diseases, do create important ethical and legal difficulties.

INTERVENTIONAL STUDIES

Interventional studies are either controlled clinical trials, with participants selected through random distribution, that are designed to compare specific medical treatment with no treatment; or controlled clinical trials, with random distribution, that are constructed to differentiate between usual care methods and special or intensive-care treatment programs. Ethical conflicts emerging from these experiments differ to some extent in kind, and certainly in degree. The controlled clinical trial characterized by random distribution of patients for a program of treatment or no treatment is often perceived as unethical from nearly all stand-points.[5] In spite of obtaining informed consent, such trials are considered unethical principally because one class of patients is denied any treatment at all which might be essential for the resolution of their diseased condition. It is further argued that even though society would benefit from knowing that existing or experimental treatments are effective, the nature of the benefit-risk ratio as between treatment and no treatment, when seen in terms of the individual subjects of the experiment, would be skewed to such a degree as to conceivably militate against the creation of a control group. Consistent with this, on balancing the benefit-risk equation, it seems apparent that those individuals placed in the control group receiving no treatment, or a yet untried experimental treatment, would be significantly at risk with little or no benefits to be gained by the society at large.

Without considering devices that could protect the patient even in the setting of such controlled trials, the position that random distribution of patients for a program of treatment or no treatment is universally ethically undesirable ignores the fact that there are many conditions for which an existing treatment is totally ineffective. Take, for example, the treatment for the com-

mon cold. Outside of various supportive measures that relieve some of the symptoms of that condition, there is no known treatment that will essentially accelerate the curative process. Some argue further that palliation of the symptoms may have no relationship at all to the ultimate resolution of the disease state.

Now assume that there is reason to believe, as has been proposed, that vitamin C taken in large doses will considerably ameliorate the symptoms of the common cold and in fact hasten the development and improve the effectiveness of the body's own defenses against the condition. In the face of such a proclamation, medical science could hardly ignore the potential benefits from vitamin C therapy for the common cold. On the other hand, it would not be serving society to its best interests if an attempt were not made to develop a body of data or establish proof that this treatment is effective.

In a case such as this, where there is no known treatment that has been shown in any way to alter the course of the disease and an experimental treatment is presented that could possibly serve this function, why would it be unethical to conduct a controlled trial between a population receiving therapy and one receiving no therapy as far as this disease is concerned? One could hardly say that an individual in the controlled, no-therapy group would be denied the opportunity to receive treatment that could possibly mitigate this discomfort. To a great extent, this same situation existed in proving the effectiveness of the polio vaccine. One could have hardly argued strongly at that time that conducting a randomized clinical trial with persons who were receiving the polio vaccine and those who were not would be denying those in the second category the right to well-proven preventive measures. The statement that random distribution between those receiving therapy and those not receiving therapy is under all conditions unethical does not deal appropriately with the realities of medical science; that is, that many diseases afflict mankind for which there is no known effective cure. On the other hand, there are circumstances in which the argument is justified that a random clinical trial between treatment and nontreatment is ethically unsound. In his now classic article, "Ethics and Clinical Research," Dr. Henry Beecher presented an example of a study that physicians would uniformly agree was ethically inappropriate.[6] This was a study to determine the effectiveness of treatment of streptococcal respiratory infections in preventing the secondary sequelae of this condition, rheumatic fever and acute glomerulonephritis. At the time the study was conducted, it was recognized that rheumatic fever could usually be prevented by adequate treatment of streptococcal respiratory infections through parenteral administration of penicillin. Beecher goes on to describe how treatment was withheld and placebos were given to a group of 109 men in the military service who were suffering from these respiratory infections. An equal number of men were treated with benzathine penicillin G. The decision as to who should receive the placebo therapy and who should receive the already recognized appropriate treatment of such respiratory conditions was determined automatically by the military serial number of the men who were involved in the study. The results of the study could have been predicted well before it was conducted. In the group of patients studied, two developed acute rheumatic fever and one developed acute glomerulonephritis. All of these cases were among those receiving placebos in the controlled population, whereas those men who were treated with benzathine penicillin G did not develop any of these more serious complications.

There could be little repugnance against vehement outcries concerning the unethical nature of this or similar experiments. A known treatment did exist that was considered to be effective for the prevention of the very serious conditions of rheumatic fever and acute glomerulonephritis. But perhaps more important than the recognition of the unethical nature of this experiment is the fact that, from the scientific perspective, such an experiment would not necessarily be considered good medical science. No doubt, it is very important to know that unequivocally penicillin G is effective in preventing the development of rheumatic fever. But much of this information had already been obtained through retrospective evaluations that established the efficacy of penicillin G. Denying this antibiotic to a patient population with the prior knowledge that a significant proportion of these patients will develop the very serious and often permanently damaging complications of rheumatic fever and acute glomerulonephritis can be considered not only gross negligence but inferior clinical research.

There are, however, therapies considered to be well established that have not been subjected to effectiveness tests. A most conspicuous example of such a therapy is the use of coronary care units in the treatment of acute ischemic heart disease. Until recently, care in such units was considered to be the most appropriate and beneficial way to treat an acute heart attack, particularly when the patient suffered from continuing arrhythmias, or when a large portion of the heart had been injured in the episode. No one questioned the efficacy of coronary care units because it seemed like common sense that by placing a patient in an environment where he could be constantly monitored by sophisticated electronic equipment, intervention, if needed, could be instituted immediately to offset the development of an exacerbation of the disease. Mather and his associates, however, conducted an interesting study in England using the randomized clinical trial to determine if, in fact, hospital treatment, including some time in a coronary care unit, resulted in significant medical advantages over drug treatment at home.[7] The results of his research study showed, to everyone's surprise, that there is essentially no medical gain in admission to a hospital with a coronary care unit as compared to being treated at home under the care of a physician.

But there is an important distinction between this study of the effectiveness of a well-established treatment and that which was conducted using benzathine penicillin G. The most important distinction is that in the penicillin experiment, the control group received no treatment, although it was well recognized that streptococcal respiratory infections could lead, if untreated, to rheumatic fever and possibly acute glomerulonephritis. In the experiment involving the care of acute ischemic heart disease, there had not been any proof of the association between the use of coronary care units and the prevention of disability or death. Furthermore, the alternative to the coronary care unit was not *no* treatment, but rather treatment in a different context, the home.

Responsibility to Participants

Random clinical trials can also be used to contrast well-established care programs with special services that are delivered to comparable populations. Such trials create a different set of ethical problems. Initially, this might be viewed as an ethically sound study in that usual care would be the method of treatment for everyone in the absence of a study, and no one would be denied what he would otherwise receive were he to enter into the hospital or into a medical care program. However, certain questions of an ethical nature can arise, particularly if viewed from the standpoint of the institution's responsibility to assure that the patient or the community, in the case of a broad study, understands the expected adverse results of such investigations. A host of questions emerge: At what point in the conduct of an experiment is there a special relationship between the investigator or health care institution and the populations that are used as subjects of the investigation? Is the duty of the investigator limited to disclosure of information; or is there also a duty to allow those who have not been selected for the project, or who have been selected to receive usual care to enter into a track that would allow them to benefit from a special care program? A case in point might be if an institution would like to test the advantages of a specialized and intensive maternal and child health program over its existing program, which may be characterized by somewhat infrequent visits, a minimum of physical examinations and laboratory studies, and only the required preventive measures for the child such as smallpox and diphtheria vaccines.[8]

As with the one-to-one physician-patient relationship, it is arguable that the issue is ultimately that of determining the nature of the informed consent that should be required in such a study if a level of comprehension is to be achieved whereby individuals are aware of the implications of entering the usual care instead of the specialized care track. After providing adequate disclosure, the issue might then be whether individuals who do not wish to participate in the experiment should be allowed to simply drop out of the research study, or if some mechanism should be available to allow those who might otherwise be in the usual care group to gain admission to the specialized program. To some extent, such a mechanism could in effect remove the ethical obligation of the investigator to the usual care group. On the other hand, the statistical validity of the study might be severely impaired. One could conceive of a situation where a large number of those who would otherwise be in the usual care track of maternal and child health would demand inclusion in the controlled, specialized care group, in which case a scientifically adequate comparison between the two groups, which is the objective of the study, would be virtually impossible.

Compatible with these ethical concerns in determining who should receive usual care versus a more thorough specialized service is the additional problem of how to handle those patients considered high risks—for example, a pregnant mother with diabetes—for certain untoward outcomes; and who would, therefore, receive special services even though they entered the existing usual health care program in the hospital. What could be the expected impact of not providing special care in these circumstances? Could one know with reasonable certainty that in not providing such services to certain high risk groups there would be an increase in the incidence and prevalence of untoward complications?

In some cases the purpose of the research project is to determine if there is a difference in the incidence and prevalence of certain outcomes as between traditional treatment regimens and more sophisticated programs. Certainly a comparison of usual maternal and child health with a more intensive program would be directed at determining if more circumspect attention would avert some of the serious problems that afflict pregnant mothers and infants. By the same token, if there is very good reason to believe that the experiment will come out disclosing that serious complications affect certain patient populations that fit within well-known risk categories, then the ethical features in channeling such patients into usual care methods to meet the requirements of an experiment become especially troublesome. Such an experiment would not be that much different from the one comparing patients with streptococcal respiratory infections who were treated with penicillin with those who were left untreated.

Protection of Participants

It is apparent from this discussion that random clinical trials are an essential feature of medical research because they provide a means of evaluating the effectiveness of diagnostic and treatment measures. It is equally apparent, however, that patients who become subjects of such experiments can be exposed to significant risks and must be protected against strong-arm tactics that would not allow them a major role in influencing what is done to their body for the sake of medical science. Some protective mechanism must be devised to achieve an ethically acceptable power balance between the physician or experimenter and his subjects, a device whereby the subject of an experiment is made adequately aware of the consequences of participating in specific research and allowed the option to withdraw if he so desires. No one would be likely to dispute this latter statement, although there might be much debate over the sufficiency of any protective measure where random clinical trials are used that distinguish treatment from non-treatment. However, the issue has been not whether or not patients should be protected in medical experiments but rather how this protection should be effected.

The trend at the present time seems to be distinctly in the direction of creating various review committees in institutions, on a regional basis, and at the national level that will screen out potentially unethical studies before they even become an issue for patient choice. A recent issue of the *Federal Register* included a lengthy statement by a National Institutes of Health Committee on the Protection of Human Subjects that advocated the establishment of protection committees in various institutions receiving HEW support to further shield particularly vulnerable groups like the mentally ill, children, and prisoners from coercive behavior by medical researchers.[3] In addition to ethical protection committees, other committees such as ethical review boards and the existing organizational review committees are advocated to assure that unethical conduct is avoided in the experimental setting.

Such committees may result in eliminating grossly unethical studies from being conducted in various settings. But in addition, they may tend to impede, in a major way, important scientific research or even prevent it from being completed, even though the ethical conflicts may be quite minor. Also, the scientific committees that approve and review research in their institutions seem to already screen out the grossly unethical studies. Of course, it may be questioned whether any committee will really have a major impact on preventing research that is undesirable from an ethical standpoint. Regulation committees, as has been shown in other settings, often serve the

objectives of those that are regulated despite the composition of the committee.[9] But perhaps even more important, the administrative effects of compounding bureaucracy on bureaucracy may lead to such inefficiency that the advantages of such committees become increasingly less impressive; and when compared with other possible checking mechanisms, such as legislatively defined informed consent requirements and equitable compensation for injuries incurred in research, they actually become a disadvantage. More effective in the long run than additional committees would be requirements for disclosure of information to participants in research and the implementation of systems for compensation for injuries.

INFORMATION DISCLOSURE AND INJURY COMPENSATION

Informed consent has been considered for a long time to be an important protective instrument for the patient in the physician-patient relationship.[10] In clinical situations where the patient can establish that he was not informed of specific medical procedures, nor gave his consent to the physician that they be performed on him, the physician has been held liable for a malfeasance.[11] For the most part, the lack of informed consent has been conspicuous in these cases. The difficulty arises in instances where some information has been given, but perhaps not enough to justify a position that the patient was indeed informed fully of a procedure; or where consent has been given but not sufficiently to support the physician's decision to use a certain treatment of the patient. It has been particularly troublesome in some cases to determine which risks in the procedure the patient had knowledge of before he consented to the treatment program.[12]

Because of these difficulties, the HEW guidelines on experimental research recommended that the following ingredients should be present if informed consent is to be a viable instrument of protection for the patient. Informed consent must designate physician responsibility for disclosure of information and determine the level, extent and nature of that information. Consistent with this, it must also take into account the patient's capacity to comprehend the information that is to be disclosed.[13] Therefore, the ultimate that should be achieved through informed consent is that a true understanding of the proposed medical procedure be conveyed, which would involve the patient's awareness of the nature of that procedure, the organs of the body that would be involved, the diseases or incapacities that are to be cured, and the possible results, both adverse or feasible, in that procedure.[14]

Even given these requirements, informed consent as a major protective instrument for the patient has often proved to be rather insubstantial. The difficulties with defining the appropriate level of information, the actors in the experimental drama, and the capacity of the patient to comprehend various levels of information can prevent informed consent from being as effective as it should be for equalizing the balance of power between the patient and the physician.[12] On the other hand, despite its weaknesses, informed consent is the most valuable tool yet devised for protecting patients. And, it appears to be serving as a major theoretical underpinning for legal liability.[11] Refinement of the concept of informed consent by establishing a hierarchy of physician obligations to the patient might possibly result in a delicately tuned legal instrument for the patient in the physician-patient relationship.

Population-Based Experiments

Different mechanisms from those employed in the individual physician-patient relationship would have to be used if informed consent is to be applied to population-based experiments that involve random clinical trials. The recipients of important medical information are of such large numbers that informed consent could not be realistically achieved on a person-to-person basis. Therefore, other methods for obtaining consent would have to be developed whereby information would be conveyed in readily understandable language and in a manner reasonably designed to reach all members of the experimental population. Equally important, the disclosure of information and obtaining of consent should be accomplished in such a manner as not to affect the validity of the experiment. To achieve this, the experimental population would likely have to be asked to consent to participate in the experiment without being informed of whether specific individuals will be included in the control or treatment groups.

Three mechanisms could be used for assuring that large populations are made aware of the nature of specific epidemiological experiments so that they can respond appropriately. First, members from the community could be identified to represent the community when population-based studies are being considered. These representatives, for the most part individuals in positions of responsibility and power in the community, could be delegated the responsibility of safeguarding the health of that community. The investigator would thereby have to obtain the informed consent of this representative body before implementing a research design in the community.

Second, health care institutions or investigators could be required to file public notification containing the details of the experiment that is being considered, the benefits to be gained, the adverse effects on the community population, and the means by which individuals selected for the control group could withdraw at any time from the study. This last requirement has been included as one of the important provisions in the HEW guidelines on informed consent in human experimentation.[13]

Third, the representatives of the community could form a health overseeing body, similar in design to the comprehensive health planning agencies,[15] which would make and publish its own analysis of the pros and cons of certain experiments. It could also be empowered to provide a forum, such as hearings, for community response when epidemiological experiments are about to be conducted, thereby assuring participation of the community as well as health care institutions in major decisions regarding such studies. This last mechanism would function only to disclose information to the community, not to serve as a screening device like the protection committees to prevent experiments from ever being conducted.

Compensation

In addition to informed consent, compensation to patients injured while participating in experiments would be an ethically important feature in an overall protection system. An automatic system of compensation could be constructed along the lines of a no-fault system; patients who were injured in the course of an experiment would be compensated to the extent of payment for additional medical services and for loss of wages during the period of disability.[16] Such a no-fault system is not only theoretically feasible but, with some modifications, has actually been put into practice at the University of Washington where research projects are covered by insurance for untoward outcomes that might afflict subjects during the course of an experiment.[17]

It is possible to further classify experimental procedures into those that are non-therapeutic and those that are therapeutic. Such a distinction may provide another basis for determining if compensation should occur and to what extent. In the case of the non-therapeutic experiment—that is, experiments where subjects would not benefit from the procedure—compensation might be more reasonably required for all untoward outcomes. The justification for this would be that the experiment benefits the researcher and society by advancing medical knowledge and is of little or no benefit to the subject. It could be argued that it would be unfair to have the subject who volunteers himself for medical science bear the expenses of medical care and loss of wages in the event of morbidity from the procedure.

A therapeutic experiment, on the other hand, may be of benefit to the patient and therefore poses a more complicated problem. Patients who receive experimental treatment because it is felt that the existing treatment is ineffective should possibly be handled differently than patients who receive experimental treatment in spite of the fact that the existing treatment is satisfactory.[18] For illustration, the existing treatment for the terminal stages of cancer of the colon is at the very best palliative. At a certain stage in the disease process, there is little if anything that medical science can do to prevent severe disability and death. However, let us assume that a new experimental drug has reached the level of safety for testing in a clinic population; and there would be an expectation that this drug could be highly effective in the treatment of end-stage cancer of the colon. It could then be argued strongly that patients who would receive this experimental treatment would likely be in a better position in terms of averting the inevitable consequences of terminal cancer than if they were maintained on the existing highly ineffec-

tive therapy. Under such conditions, it could also be argued that the untoward outcomes from the experimental treatment should not be compensable, for the risks to the patient overall would be significantly less than were he to continue on the known treatment program.

The distinction between therapeutic and non-therapeutic experimentation draws a sharp line for determining who qualifies for compensation in the event that an injury occurs. It is conceivable that some who derive therapeutic benefits from research might deserve ethically to receive some compensation for untoward outcomes. A patient with a disease that is not likely to lead to severe disability or death even were he to be treated through traditional measures would not benefit so significantly from a therapeutic trial to outweigh the risks of greater damage from an untoward event. Therefore, the important point of this argument is not that a distinction should necessarily be made, but that compensation along with informed consent provides major protection to patients or subjects of large-scale randomly distributed clinical trials. The protection provided by these two mechanisms, augmented by the screening that is conducted in scientific reviews of research projects, should provide maximum protection for subjects and still allow for very important clinical research.

CONCLUSION

The ethical issues of random clinical trials are concerned with the power prerogatives between the investigator and the subjects of the experiment, which might be a large population or community. In the traditional medical experiments involving individual physicians and patients, informed consent has been the major instrument for protecting the patient. The application of this tool to large-scale epidemiological experiments requires some modification of the concept, even though the questions that would be examined are very similar. The most important concern is developing a way for mapping in the consent of patients and perhaps their preferences regarding their involvement in the epidemiological experiment, and along with this assuring that the experiment will produce valid results.

In addition to the major role that disclosure has in protecting patients, a system for compensating those injured in experiments should also be implemented. Such a system could take into account the fact that in the majority of experiments, patients volunteer without any prospects of immediately benefiting from the research. There are a certain select group of cases where the prospects for severe disability and death are very high and the patients would likely receive more benefit from experimental treatment than existing therapies. But this group is small and possibly should be treated differently in a compensation system. Above all, however, the important consideration behind recommending the use of disclosure mechanisms and compensation for injuries is that the random clinical trial has been shown to be an extremely important instrument for determining the effectiveness of medical diagnosis and treatments. Every effort should be made to arrive at a system that is ethical from the standpoint of patient requirements and yet allows trials to be conducted in all facets of medical care.

REFERENCES

1. Myers, M.J. "Informed Consent in Medical Malpractice," *California Law Review* 55:1396 (1967).

2. Cochrane, A.L. *Effectiveness and Efficiency—Random Reflections on Health Services* (London: The Nuffield Provincial Hospitals Trust, 1972).

3. National Institutes of Health. "Protection of Human Subjects, Policies and Procedures," *Federal Register* 38:31738 (November 16, 1973). See also: Mulford, R. "Human Experimentation," *Stanford Law Review* 20:99 (November 1967).

4. Hutchison, G.W. "Evaluation of Preventive Measures," in: Clark, D.W. and MacMahon, B. (eds.) *Preventive Medicine* (Boston: Little, Brown and Co., 1967).

5. Plat, R. "The Ethical Basis of Medical Science," *Scientific Basis of Medicine: Annual Review* 1–15 (1966).

6. Beecher, H.K. "Ethics and Clinical Research," *New England Journal of Medicine* 274:1354 (June 16, 1966).

7. Mather, H.G.; Pearson, W.G.; Read, K.L.Q., *et al.* "Acute Myocardial Infarction: Home and Hospital Treatment," *British Medical Journal* 334 (August 7, 1971).

8. See: Kessner, D.M. *Infant Death: An Analysis by Maternal Risk and Health Care,* Vol. 1 (Washington, D.C.: National Academy of Sciences, 1973).

9. Noll, R.G. *Reforming Regulation,* An Evaluation of the Ash Council Proposal (Washington, D.C.: The Brookings Institution, 1971).

10. See: Holder, R. "Informed Consent. (I. Evolution)," *Journal of the American Medical Association* 214:1181 (1970); and Beecher, H.K. "Experimentation in Man," *Journal of the American Medical Association* 169:420 (1959).

11. Secretary's Commission on Medical Malpractice. *Report of the Secretary's Commission on Medical Malpractice,* Department of Health, Education and Welfare (Washington, D.C.: GPO, 1973) pp. 29–30.

12. Epstein, L.C. and Lasagna, L. "Obtaining Informed Consent—Form or Substance," *Archives of Internal Medicine* 123:682 (1969).

13. "Protection of Human Subjects, Proposed Policy," *Federal Register* 38:27882 (October 9, 1973).

14. Ratnoff, O.D. and Ratnoff, M.F. "Ethical Responsibilities in Clinical Investigations," *Perspectives in Biology and Medicine* 82 (Autumn 1967).

15. Curran, W. "National Survey and Analysis of Certificate of Need Laws: Health Planning and Regulation in the State Legislatures," in: Havighurst, C.C. (ed.) *Regulating Health Facilities Construction,* Proceedings of a Conference on Health Planning, Certificate of Need and Market Entry (Washington, D.C.: American Enterprise Institute for Public Policy Research, forthcoming).

16. Havighurst, C.C. and Tancredi, L.R. "Medical Adversity Insurance—A No-Fault Approach to Medical Malpractice and Quality Assurance," *Milbank Memorial Fund Quarterly: Health and Society* 51:125 (Spring 1973).

17. Insurance policy provided by Olympic Insurance Company.

18. "Medical Experiment Insurance," *Columbia Law Review* 70:970 (May 1970).

ISSUES FOR CONSIDERATION AND SUGGESTIONS FOR FURTHER READING

To what extent should the federal government be involved in the regulation of scientific research affecting health? Are the regulatory mechanisms explored in this chapter designed with sufficient flexibility to permit evolution that parallels research developments and innovations without inhibiting them? Should all research be government sponsored? Funded? Insured?

What is the proper role of law in the experimental environment? Are boards, expert or lay, helpful? Are impact statements helpful? How? How not? How would you balance the need to protect subjects of experiments and the public from irresponsible research or researchers?

You may wish to compare an exchange on the question of whether health care providers can be "subjects at risk" within the meaning of the human subjects regulations [45 C.F.R. §46.103(b)]. Compare Hogue, "Institutional Review Boards and Consumer Surveys," 60 *American Journal of Public Health* 649 (July 1979), with Levine, "Deceiving Dentists: Health Care Providers as 'Subjects at Risk,'" 1 *IRB: A Review of Human Subjects Research* 7 (August/September 1979). An earlier guide to IRBs is N. Hershey and R. Miller, *Human Experimentation and the Law* (1976).

You may also wish to consider Blank, "The Delaney Clause: Technical Naiveté and Scientific Advocacy in the Formulation of Public Health Policies," 62 *California L. Rev.* 1084 (1974) (regulation of carcinogens).

TABLE OF CASES

INDEX

ABOUT THE EDITOR

Dr. L. Lynn Hogue is on the faculty of the School of Law at the University of Arkansas at Little Rock. He received his J.D. degree from Duke Law School in 1974 and is a member of the bars of Arkansas and North Carolina. He is the author of numerous articles and a chapter entitled "A Comparative Survey of Abortion Legislation: International Perspective," in *Liberalization of Abortion Laws: Implications*, Abdel R. Omran, Editor (1976).

Professor Hogue serves as a reviewer for the *American Journal of Public Health* and is a member of the American Public Health Association and active in its Health Law Forum.